Cardiovascular Medicine Board Review and Self-Assessment

A Companion to Cardiovascular Medicine & Surgery

Cardiovascular Medicine Board Review and Self-Assessment

A Companion to Cardiovascular Medicine & Surgery

Editors

Debabrata Mukherjee, MD, MS, FACC, FAHA, MSCAI

Professor and Chair
Department of Internal Medicine
Paul L. Foster School of Medicine
Texas Tech University Health
  Sciences Center El Paso
El Paso, Texas

Sulagna Mookherjee, MD, MS, FACC

Program Director, Cardiovascular
  Disease Fellowship Program
Associate Professor of Medicine
Division of Cardiology
Department of Medicine
Albany Medical College
Albany Med Health System
Albany, New York

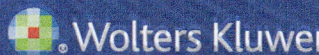

Philadelphia · Baltimore · New York · London
Buenos Aires · Hong Kong · Sydney · Tokyo

Acquisitions Editor: James Sherman
Senior Development Editor: Ashley Fischer
Editorial Coordinator: Priyanka Alagar
Marketing Manager: Kirsten Watrud
Senior Production Project Manager: Alicia Jackson
Manager, Graphic Arts & Design: Stephen Druding
Manufacturing Coordinator: Lisa Bowling
Prepress Vendor: S4Carlisle Publishing Services

Copyright © 2025 Wolters Kluwer.

All rights reserved. This book is protected by copyright. No part of this book may be reproduced or transmitted in any form or by any means, including as photocopies or scanned-in or other electronic copies, or utilized by any information storage and retrieval system without written permission from the copyright owner, except for brief quotations embodied in critical articles and reviews. Materials appearing in this book prepared by individuals as part of their official duties as U.S. government employees are not covered by the above-mentioned copyright. To request permission, please contact Wolters Kluwer at Two Commerce Square, 2001 Market Street, Philadelphia, PA 19103, via email at permissions@lww.com, or via our website at shop.lww.com (products and services).

9 8 7 6 5 4 3 2 1

Printed in the United States of America

Library of Congress Cataloging-in-Publication Data

ISBN-13: 978-1-975214-29-6

Library of Congress Control Number: 2024916364

This work is provided "as is," and the publisher disclaims any and all warranties, express or implied, including any warranties as to accuracy, comprehensiveness, or currency of the content of this work.

This work is no substitute for individual patient assessment based upon healthcare professionals' examination of each patient and consideration of, among other things, age, weight, gender, current or prior medical conditions, medication history, laboratory data and other factors unique to the patient. The publisher does not provide medical advice or guidance and this work is merely a reference tool. Healthcare professionals, and not the publisher, are solely responsible for the use of this work including all medical judgments and for any resulting diagnosis and treatments.

Given continuous, rapid advances in medical science and health information, independent professional verification of medical diagnoses, indications, appropriate pharmaceutical selections and dosages, and treatment options should be made and healthcare professionals should consult a variety of sources. When prescribing medication, healthcare professionals are advised to consult the product information sheet (the manufacturer's package insert) accompanying each drug to verify, among other things, conditions of use, warnings and side effects and identify any changes in dosage schedule or contraindications, particularly if the medication to be administered is new, infrequently used or has a narrow therapeutic range. To the maximum extent permitted under applicable law, no responsibility is assumed by the publisher for any injury and/or damage to persons or property, as a matter of products liability, negligence law or otherwise, or from any reference to or use by any person of this work.

shop.lww.com

For our families.
To the amazing cardiology fellows I have had the opportunity to work with; to my parents for their infinite patience, love, and understanding; to my nephew Rohin; to Asit Kumar Bhattacharya (Baba) for his incredible kindness; and to Suchandra, for her love and support.

—Debabrata Mukherjee

To my father, Dr Sakti Mookherjee, the first (and best) cardiologist I've ever known and in whose footsteps I've always tried to follow. You are the biggest inspiration in my life.
To my mentors and partners, thank you for everything through the years and for contributing your time and energy to this publication.
To my fellows: past, present, and future. Thank you for all the hard work in writing these questions. You are the future of cardiology and the best part of my career!
To Ria, Elise, Nina, Avinash, and Veera, my loves. To Mommy, Drs Disha, and Swagatam Mookherjee . . . my rocks.
To my husband, Dr Robert Millar. Thank you for all your support, unconditional love, and continued patience always.

—Sulagna Mookherjee

PREFACE

The field of cardiovascular medicine continues to rapidly evolve in both diagnostic and therapeutic arenas. Over the past decade, substantial advances have been made on many fronts including cardiovascular imaging, electrophysiology mapping and ablation techniques, heart failure diagnosis and management, percutaneous hemodynamic support, drug-eluting stents, drug-coated balloons, and structural heart endovascular techniques. Concurrent with advances in percutaneous techniques, cardiovascular surgery has also evolved with minimally invasive and robotic techniques. The evolution of newer drugs, devices, and improvements in both percutaneous and surgical techniques challenges providers to stay abreast of cutting-edge pharmacologic, endovascular, and surgical strategies for optimal patient care. The *Cardiovascular Medicine Board Review and Self-Assessment: A Companion to Cardiovascular Medicine & Surgery* aims to provide clinicians with key concepts on the topics of clinical cardiology, cardiovascular imaging, cardiac catheterization and intervention, electrophysiology, heart failure, vascular medicine, cardiovascular surgery, and importantly the field of preventive cardiology. The text derives its questions from the comprehensive *Cardiovascular Medicine and Surgery* textbook.

Of foremost importance, the topic areas covered are relevant to the daily practice of cardiovascular medicine and are considered essential knowledge for Cardiovascular Medicine Board Certification Examination. The content of this textbook reflects the rapidly changing field of cardiovascular medicine and surgery.

Essential to the quality and appropriateness of the text is the expertise of the chapter authors. We are fortunate to have assembled a stellar roster of cardiovascular medicine fellows and are greatly indebted to them. The practice of cardiovascular medicine is exciting, rewarding, and a privilege each of us enjoys. Likewise, it has been our personal honor to work with these superb contributors, our colleagues in cardiovascular medicine, as well as the editorial team at Wolters Kluwer. It is our hope that you will enjoy this book and that it will be a valuable resource to you in providing the highest quality of care to your patients.

Debabrata Mukherjee, MD, MS
Sulagna Mookherjee, MD, MS, FACC

CONTENTS

Preface vi

SECTION 1: CLINICAL CARDIOLOGY

1. Clinical Cardiology 1
John Tremblay, Mikhail Torosoff, and Sulagna Mookherjee

2. General Cardiovascular Examination 9
John Tremblay, Mikhail Torosoff, and Steven A. Fein

3. Clinical Pharmacology 17
Niranjan Ojha, Anojan Pathmanathan, and Robert L. Carhart

4. Stable Ischemic Heart Disease 21
Samuel Kim, Radmila Lyubarova, Neil Yager, and Mandeep S. Sidhu

5. Unstable Angina, Non–ST-Elevation Myocardial Infarction-Acute Coronary Syndrome 28
Natasha Babar, Ravi Kiran Vuthoori, and Anthony Gerald Nappi

6. ST-Elevation Myocardial Infarction 34
Natasha Babar, Ravi Kiran Vuthoori, and Anthony Gerald Nappi

7. Acute Myocardial Infarction Complications 41
Natasha Babar, Ravi Kiran Vuthoori, and Anthony Gerald Nappi

8. Refractory Angina 47
Natasha Babar, Ravi Kiran Vuthoori, and Anthony Gerald Nappi

9. Rheumatic Heart Disease 51
Natasha Babar, Radmila Lyubarova, Sulagna Mookherjee, and Robert D. Millar

10. Mitral Valve Disease 56
Matthew Derakhshesh and William Bachman

11. Aortic Valve Disease 62
Matthew Derakhshesh and William Bachman

12. Adult-Acquired Tricuspid and Pulmonary Valve Disease 68
Matthew Derakhshesh and Mohamed Khalid Munshi

13. Prosthetic Valve Dysfunction 71
Matthew Derakhshesh and Mohamed Khalid Munshi

| 14 | **Infective Endocarditis** . . . . 77 |

Matthew Derakhshesh and Mohamed Khalid Munshi

| 15 | **Pericardial Disease** . . . . 83 |

Ciril Khorolsky, Radmila Lyubarova, and Marisa A. Orgera

| 16 | **Pulmonary Hypertension** . . . . 90 |

Ciril Khorolsky and Mohammad El-Hajjar

| 17 | **Adult Congenital Heart Disease** . . . . 100 |

Harneet Bhatti and Robert L. Carhart

| 18 | **Pregnancy and Heart Disease** . . . . 103 |

Wen Qian (Jenny) Zheng, Joshua Schulman-Marcus, Radmila Lyubarova, and Sulagna Mookherjee

| 19 | **Women and Heart Disease** . . . . 111 |

Wen Qian (Jenny) Zheng, Kim A. Poli, Sulagna Mookherjee, and Radmila Lyubarova

| 20 | **Older Adults and Heart Disease** . . . . 116 |

Wen Qian (Jenny) Zheng, Sulagna Mookherjee, and Radmila Lyubarova

| 21 | **Cardiac Manifestation of Systemic Diseases** . . . . 121 |

Wen Qian (Jenny) Zheng, Joshua Schulman-Marcus, and Sulagna Mookherjee

| 22 | **Substance Abuse and the Heart** . . . . 127 |

Wen Qian (Jenny) Zheng, Joshua Schulman-Marcus, and Sulagna Mookherjee

| 23 | **Cardiac Trauma** . . . . 132 |

Nathan Centybear and Mohamed Khalid Munshi

| 24 | **Cardiac Tumors** . . . . 136 |

Ciril Khorolsky and Robert D. Millar

| 25 | **Cardiac Evaluation for Noncardiac Surgery** . . . . 143 |

Teni Olatunde and Robert L. Carhart

| 26 | **Cardio-Oncology** . . . . 151 |

Robert L. Carhart and Anojan Pathmanathan

| 27 | **Cardiac Disease in Human Immunodeficiency Virus Infection** . . . . 156 |

Anshu Shridhar

| 28 | **Dysautonomia** . . . . 162 |

Atika Azhar and Robert L. Carhart

29 **Environmental Exposures and Cardiovascular Disease** 167
Nathan Centybear and Mohamed Khalid Munshi

30 **Amyloid Cardiomyopathy.** 172
Ciril Khorolsky and Edward F. Philbin III

31 **Cardiovascular Imaging.** 182
Robert L. Carhart, Ashwini K. Ashwath, Sanchari Banerjee, and Hiba Zafar

SECTION 2: CARDIOVASCULAR IMAGING

32 **Chest Radiography** 189
Vishal Phogat and Robert L. Carhart

33 **Electrocardiographic Exercise Testing.** 196
Meet Patel

34 **Echocardiography** 204
Robert L. Carhart, Atika Azhar, and Subash Nepal

35 **Nuclear Cardiology and Molecular Imaging** 218
Bilal Talha and Alisha Khan

36 **Cardiac Computed Tomography.** 225
Alisha Khan and Vishal Phogat

37 **Cardiac Magnetic Resonance Imaging** 234
Rohan Desai, Bhavi Trivedi, Rakhee Makhija, and Debabrata Mukherjee

38 **Hybrid and Multimodality Imaging Correlation** 245
Karan Sarode and Debabrata Mukherjee

39 **Periprocedural Imaging** 253
Shweta Paulraj

SECTION 3: CARDIAC CATHETERIZATION

40 **Cardiac Catheterization and Hemodynamic Assessment** 257
Joseph Cade Owens and Mohamed Khalid Munshi

41 **Diagnostic Coronary and Pulmonary Angiography and Left Ventriculography** 263
Joseph Cade Owens and Mohamed Khalid Munshi

42 **Intracoronary Imaging** 270
Neil Yager and Joseph Cade Owens

43 Percutaneous Coronary Intervention 276
Joseph Cade Owens and Mohammad El-Hajjar

44 Percutaneous Valvular Intervention 283
Joseph Cade Owens and Mohammad El-Hajjar

45 Catheter Interventions in Congenital Heart Disease 288
Robert L. Carhart

46 Percutaneous Closure of Patent Foramen
Ovale and Atrial Septal Defect 293
Jacqueline Kenitz and Neil Yager

47 Ethanol Septal Ablation 297
Ciril Khorolsky and Mohammad El-Hajjar

48 Left Atrial Appendage Closure 304
Ravi Kiran Vuthoori and Mohammad El-Hajjar

49 Electrocardiogram 309
Robert L. Carhart, Shweta Paulraj, and Sean Byrnes

SECTION 4: ELECTROPHYSIOLOGY

50 Mechanisms of Cardiac Arrhythmias 315
Casey White and Amole Ojo

51 Genetics of Arrhythmias 320
Casey White and Amole Ojo

52 Ambulatory Rhythm Monitoring 325
Casey White and Amole Ojo

53 Electrophysiology Testing 331
Casey White and Amole Ojo

54 Bradycardias: Sinus Node Dysfunction and
Atrioventricular Conduction Disturbances 336
Casey White and Amole Ojo

55 Supraventricular Tachycardias. 340
Jeanwoo Yoo, Evan C. Adelstein, and Alfred M. Loka

56 Atrial Fibrillation and Atrial Flutter 348
Jeanwoo Yoo, Evan C. Adelstein, and Alfred M. Loka

| 57 | **Ventricular Tachycardia** 354
Jeanwoo Yoo, Evan C. Adelstein, and Alfred M. Loka

| 58 | **Antiarrhythmic Drugs** 363
Jeanwoo Yoo, Alfred M. Loka, and Evan C. Adelstein

| 59 | **Catheter Ablation Therapy** 371
Jeanwoo Yoo, Alfred M. Loka, and Evan C. Adelstein

| 60 | **Implantable Cardioverter-Defibrillators** 376
Amole Ojo and Casey White

| 61 | **Syncope** 381
Meet Patel

| 62 | **Sudden Cardiac Arrest** 387
Samuel Kim and Mohammad El-Hajjar

| 63 | **Permanent Pacemaker** 394
Amole Ojo and Casey White

| 64 | **Lead Extraction** 400
Nathan Centybear and Evan C. Adelstein

SECTION 5: HEART FAILURE

| 65 | **Heart Failure: Epidemiology, Characteristics, and Prognosis** 405
Robert L. Carhart and Anojan Pathmanathan

| 66 | **Pathophysiology of Heart Failure** 410
Phillip Olsen and Dmitri Belov

| 67 | **Genetics of Cardiomyopathy** 416
Nathan Centybear, Edward F. Philbin III, and Naveed M. Akhtar

| 68 | **Heart Failure With Preserved Ejection Fraction** 424
John Tremblay and Mikhail Torosoff

| 69 | **Heart Failure With Reduced Ejection Fraction** 435
John Tremblay and Mikhail Torosoff

| 70 | **Dilated Cardiomyopathy** 441
John Tremblay and Mikhail Torosoff

| 71 | **Hypertrophic Cardiomyopathy** .... 448 |

Robert L. Carhart, Mostafa Vasigh and Muhammad Malik

| 72 | **Restrictive Cardiomyopathy** .... 454 |

Robert L. Carhart, Subash Nepal, and Muhammad Malik

| 73 | **Myocarditis** .... 467 |

Hamza Oglat, William Alderisio, and Sulagna Mookherjee

| 74 | **Toxin-Induced Cardiomyopathies** .... 473 |

Robert L. Carhart and Teni Olatunde

| 75 | **Acute Heart Failure** .... 481 |

Matthew Derakhshesh and Dmitri Belov

| 76 | **Chronic Heart Failure Management** .... 492 |

Kellsey Peterson

| 77 | **Cardiac Resynchronization Therapy** .... 498 |

Phillip Olsen and Alfred M. Loka

| 78 | **Mechanical Circulatory Support** .... 505 |

Phillip Olsen and Dmitri Belov

SECTION 6: VASCULAR MEDICINE

| 79 | **Aortic Diseases** .... 513 |

Brian Conway and William Bachman

| 80 | **Peripheral Artery Disease** .... 523 |

Brian Conway and Neil Yager

| 81 | **Cerebrovascular Disease** .... 529 |

Brian Conway and William Bachman

| 82 | **Renal Artery Stenosis** .... 535 |

Brian Conway and Neil Yager

| 83 | **Mesenteric Arterial Disease** .... 541 |

Brian Conway and William Bachman

| 84 | **Venous Thromboembolism** .... 549 |

Hamza Oglat and Robert D. Millar

| 85 | **Pulmonary Embolism** .... 554 |

Hamza Oglat and Robert D. Millar

SECTION 7: CARDIOVASCULAR SURGERY

86   **Coronary Artery Bypass Surgery** 561
Mohammad El-Hajjar and Samuel Kim

87   **Aortic Valve Surgery** 567
Hamza Oglat and William Bachman

88   **Mitral Valve Surgery** 572
Hamza Oglat and William Bachman

89   **Thoracic Aortic Surgery** 577
Andrew J. Castellano

90   **Peripheral Arterial Surgery** 583
Samuel Kim and Neil Yager

91   **Carotid Endarterectomy** 591
Meet Patel

92   **Transplantation and Long-Term Implantable Mechanical Circulatory Support** 600
Phillip Olsen and Dmitri Belov

93   **Surgical Approach for Congenital Heart Disease** 607
Robert L. Carhart and Anderson C. Anuforo

94   **Chest Wall Infections Following Open Heart Surgery** 615
Robert L. Carhart, Monique Monita, and Hiba Zafar

SECTION 8: PREVENTIVE CARDIOLOGY

95   **Preventive Cardiology/Pathophysiology of Atherosclerosis** 621
Robert L. Carhart, Anojan Pathmanathan, and Niranjan Ojha

96   **Cardiovascular Disease Risk Assessment in Clinical Practice** 626
Jacqueline S. Coppola, Joshua Schulman-Marcus, and Sulagna Mookherjee

97   **Lifestyle Implementation for Cardiovascular Disease Prevention: A Focus on Smoking Cessation, Diet, and Physical Activity** 632
Jacqueline S. Coppola, Joshua Schulman-Marcus, and Sulagna Mookherjee

98   **Diabetes and Cardiometabolic Medicine** 637
Jacqueline S. Coppola, Joseph D. Sacco, and Sulagna Mookherjee

99 Lipid Disorders 643
Jacqueline S. Coppola, Joseph D. Sacco, and Sulagna Mookherjee

100 Hypertension 650
Robert L. Carhart, Sean Byrnes, Shweta Paulraj, and Subash Nepal

101 Cardiac Rehabilitation 654
Robert L. Carhart, Ronald Russo, Philip Chebaya, and Muhammad Malik

SECTION 9: ADULT CONGENITAL HEART DISEASE

102 Anatomic and Physiologic Classification of Congenital Heart Disease 659
Robert L. Carhart and Harneet Bhatti

103 Evaluation of Suspected and Known Adult Congenital Heart Disease 662
Kellsey Peterson

104 Pregnancy and Reproductive Health in Adult Congenital Heart Disease 668
Jacqueline S. Coppola, Joshua Schulman-Marcus, and Sulagna Mookherjee

105 Pharmacologic Therapy for Adult Congenital Heart Disease ... 675
Harneet Bhatti and Robert L. Carhart

106 Shunt Lesions 678
Samuel Kim and Joshua Schulman-Marcus

107 Left-Sided Obstructive Lesions 684
Anojan Pathmanathan, Niranjan Ojha, and Robert L. Carhart

108 Right-Sided Lesions 693
Atika Azhar, Meet Patel, and Robert L. Carhart

109 Complex Lesions 699
Ronald Russo, Philip Chebaya, and Robert L. Carhart

110 Pulmonary Arterial Hypertension Associated With Congenital Heart Disease 705
Nathan Centybear and Naveed M. Akhtar

111 Noncardiac Surgery in Those With Adult Congenital Heart Disease 711
Atika Azhar and Robert L. Carhart

Index 717

CONTRIBUTORS

Evan C. Adelstein, MD
Associate Professor of Medicine
Division of Cardiology
Department of Medicine
Albany Medical College
Albany, New York

Naveed M. Akhtar, MD, FACC
Assistant Professor of Medicine
Division of Cardiology
Department of Medicine
Albany Medical College
Albany, New York

William Alderisio, MD
Attending
Division of Cardiology
Department of Medicine
Albany Medical College
Albany, New York

Anderson C. Anuforo, MD
Fellow
Division of Cardiology
Department of Medicine
State University of New York Upstate
 Medical University
Syracuse, New York

Ashwini K. Ashwath, MBBS
Fellow
Division of Cardiology
Department of Medicine
State University of New York Upstate
 Medical University
Syracuse, New York

Atika Azhar, MD
Physician
Department of Internal Medicine
State University of New York Upstate
 Medical University
Syracuse, New York

Natasha Babar, MD
Fellow
Division of Cardiology
Department of Medicine
Albany Medical College
Albany, New York

William Bachman, MD
Assistant Professor of Medicine
Division of Cardiology
Department of Medicine
Albany Medical College
Albany, New York

Sanchari Banerjee, MD
Resident
Department of Internal Medicine
State University of New York Upstate
 Medical University
Syracuse, New York

Dmitri Belov, MD
Assistant Professor of Medicine
Division of Cardiology
Department of Medicine
Albany Medical College
Albany, New York

Harneet Bhatti, MD
Fellow
Division of Cardiology
Department of Medicine
State University of New York Upstate
 Medical University
Syracuse, New York

Sean Byrnes, MD
Fellow
Division of Cardiology
Department of Medicine
State University of New York Upstate
 Medical University
Syracuse, New York

Robert L. Carhart, MD
Associate Professor
Department of Medicine
State University of New York Upstate Medical University
Syracuse, New York

Andrew J. Castellano, DO
Cardiologist
Department of Cardiology
Ellis Medicine
Schenectady, New York

Nathan Centybear, MD, BS
Fellow
Division of Cardiology
Department of Medicine
Albany Medical College
Albany, New York

Philip Chebaya, MD, MSc
Fellow
Division of Cardiology
Department of Medicine
State University of New York Upstate Medical University
Syracuse, New York

Brian Conway, MD, MS
Fellow
Division of Cardiology
Department of Medicine
Albany Medical College
Albany, New York

Jacqueline S. Coppola, DO
Cardiologist
Division of Cardiology
Department of Medicine
Albany Medical College
Albany, New York

Matthew Derakhshesh, MD, BS
Fellow
Division of Cardiology
Department of Medicine
Albany Medical College
Albany, New York

Rohan Desai, MD
Resident
Department of Internal Medicine
Texas Tech University Health Sciences Center El Paso
El Paso, Texas

Mohammad El-Hajjar, MD
Associate Professor of Medicine
Division of Cardiology
Department of Medicine
Albany Medical College
Albany, New York

Steven A. Fein, MD
Professor
Division of Cardiology
Department of Medicine
Albany Medical College
Albany, New York

Jacqueline Kenitz, DO
Fellow
Division of Cardiology
Department of Medicine
Albany Medical College
Albany, New York

Alisha Khan, MD
Fellow
Board-Certified Internist
Division of Cardiology
Department of Medicine
State University of New York Upstate Medical University
Syracuse, New York

Ciril Khorolsky, MD
Fellow
Division of Cardiology
Department of Medicine
Albany Medical College
Albany, New York

Samuel Kim, MD
Fellow
Division of Cardiology
Department of Medicine
Albany Medical College
Albany, New York

Alfred M. Loka, MD
Assistant Professor
Division of Cardiology
Department of Medicine
Albany Medical College
Albany, New York

Radmila Lyubarova, MD
Associate Professor of Medicine
Division of Cardiology
Department of Medicine
Albany Medical College
Albany, New York

Rakhee Makhija, MD
Fellow
Department of Cardiology
Mount Sinai Hospital
New York, New York

Muhammad Malik, MD
Fellow
Division of Cardiology
Department of Medicine
State University of New York Upstate
 Medical University Hospital
Syracuse, New York

Robert D. Millar, MD, FACC
Attending Cardiologist
Division of Cardiology
Department of Medicine
Albany Medical College
Albany, New York

Monique Monita, MD, MPH
Chief Resident
Department of Internal Medicine
State University of New York Upstate
 Medical University
Syracuse, New York

Sulagna Mookherjee, MD, MS, FACC
Program Director, Cardiovascular Disease
 Fellowship Program
Associate Professor of Medicine
Division of Cardiology
Department of Medicine
Albany Medical College
Albany Med Health System
Albany, New York

Debabrata Mukherjee, MD, MS, FACC, FAHA, MSCAI
Professor and Chair
Department of Internal Medicine
Paul L. Foster School of Medicine
Texas Tech University Health Sciences
 Center El Paso
El Paso, Texas

Mohamed Khalid Munshi, MD, FACC
Physician
Department of Cardiology
Albany Stratton VA Medical Center
Albany, New York

Anthony Gerald Nappi, MD
Assistant Professor of Medicine
Division of Cardiology
Department of Medicine
Albany Medical College
Albany, New York

Subash Nepal, MD
Fellow
Division of Cardiology
Department of Medicine
State University of New York Upstate
 Medical University
Syracuse, New York

Hamza Oglat, MD
Fellow
Division of Cardiology
Department of Medicine
Albany Medical College
Albany, New York

Niranjan Ojha, MBBS
Fellow
Division of Cardiology
Department of Medicine
State University of New York Upstate Medical University
Syracuse, New York

Amole Ojo, MD
Assistant Professor of Medicine
Division of Cardiovascular Diseases
Department of Medicine
University of Rochester School of Medicine and Dentistry
University of Rochester Medical Center
Rochester, New York

Teni Olatunde, MD
Fellow
Division of Cardiology
Department of Medicine
State University of New York Upstate Medical University Hospital
Syracuse, New York

Phillip Olsen, MD
Cardiology Fellow
Division of Cardiology
Department of Medicine
Albany Medical College
Albany, New York

Marisa A. Orgera, MD
Staff Cardiologist
Department of Medicine
Albany Stratton VA Medical Center
Albany, New York

Joseph Cade Owens, MD
Fellow
Department of Internal Medicine
Albany Medical College
Albany, New York

Meet Patel, MD
Resident
Department of Internal Medicine
Interfaith Medical Center
One Brooklyn Health
Brooklyn, New York

Anojan Pathmanathan, MD
Fellow
Division of Cardiology
Department of Medicine
State University of New York Upstate Medical University
Syracuse, New York

Shweta Paulraj, MBBS
Clinical Assistant Instructor
Division of Cardiology
Department of Medicine
State University of New York Upstate Medical University
Syracuse, New York

Kellsey Peterson, MD, FACC
Senior Staff Cardiologist
Department of Cardiology
Henry Ford Hospital
Detroit, Michigan

Edward F. Philbin III, MD, FACC, FAHA
George Pataki Endowed Chair in Cardiology
Professor and Chair
Division of Cardiology
Department of Medicine
Albany Medical College
Albany, New York

Vishal Phogat, MBBS
Resident
Division of Cardiology
Department of Medicine
State University of New York Upstate Medical University Hospital
Syracuse, New York

Kim A. Poli, MD, FACC
Assistant Professor of Medicine
Division of Cardiology
Department of Medicine
Albany Medical College
Albany, New York

Ronald Russo, MD
Physician
Division of Cardiology
Department of Medicine
State University of New York Upstate Medical University
Syracuse, New York

Joseph D. Sacco, MD
Professor of Medicine
Division of Cardiology
Department of Medicine
Albany Medical College
Albany, New York

Karan Sarode, MD
Fellow
Department of Cardiology
Texas Tech University Health Sciences Center El Paso
El Paso, Texas

Joshua Schulman-Marcus, MD
Associate Professor of Medicine
Division of Cardiology
Department of Medicine
Albany Medical College
Albany, New York

Anshu Shridhar, MD
Staff Physician
Department of Cardiology
Veteran Affairs Medical Center
Syracuse, New York

Mandeep S. Sidhu, MD, MBA, FACC, FAHA
Associate Dean of Clinical Sciences and Research Affairs
Division of Cardiology
Department of Medicine
Albany Medical College
Albany, New York

Bilal Talha, MD
Resident
Department of Internal Medicine
State University of New York Upstate Medical University
Syracuse, New York

Mikhail Torosoff, MD
Professor of Medicine
Division of Cardiology
Department of Medicine
Albany Medical College
Albany, New York

John Tremblay, DO
Fellow
Division of Cardiology
Department of Medicine
Albany Medical College
Albany, New York

Bhavi Trivedi, MD
Resident
Department of Internal Medicine
Texas Tech University Health Sciences Center El Paso
El Paso, Texas

Mostafa Vasigh, MD
Fellow
Division of Cardiology
Department of Medicine
State University of New York Upstate Medical University
Syracuse, New York

Ravi Kiran Vuthoori, MD
Interventional Cardiologist
Division of Cardiology
Department of Medicine
Albany Medical College
Albany, New York

Casey White, MD
Fellow
Clinical Cardiac Electrophysiology Fellowship
Department of Cardiology
University of Rochester School of Medicine and Dentistry
University of Rochester Medical Center
Rochester, New York

Neil Yager, DO, MBA, FACC
Associate Professor of Medicine
Division of Cardiology
Department of Medicine
Albany Medical College
Albany, New York

Jeanwoo Yoo, DO
Fellow
Division of Cardiology
Department of Medicine
Albany Medical College
Albany, New York

Hiba Zafar, MD
Resident
Department of Internal Medicine
State University of New York Upstate
    Medical University Hospital
Syracuse, New York

Wen Qian (Jenny) Zheng, MD
Fellow
Division of Cardiology
Department of Medicine
Albany Medical College
Albany, New York

SECTION 1 CLINICAL CARDIOLOGY

CLINICAL CARDIOLOGY*

CHAPTER 1

John Tremblay, Mikhail Toroseff, and Sulagna Mookherjee

QUESTIONS

1.1 A 63-year-old female with a past medical history of hypertension, hyperlipidemia, myocardial infarction (MI) status post (s/p) percutaneous intervention, and ischemic cardiomyopathy presents for her yearly appointment. The patient states that over the last year, she has noticed vague symptoms of dyspnea and fatigue when walking briskly. She becomes mildly dyspneic when walking up two flights of stairs. The patient is comfortable at rest and denies any dyspnea or fatigue when performing her activities of daily living. What New York State Heart Association (NYHA) functional class does this patient fall under?

- **A.** NYHA Class I
- **B.** NYHA Class II
- **C.** NYHA Class III
- **D.** NYHA Class IV

1.2 A 68-year-old female was referred to the cardiology clinic for evaluation. The patient states she has been experiencing chest pain starting 3 months ago which is unchanged. Her chest pain is substernal in nature, relieved by nitroglycerin, and is exacerbated by a variety of activities. Which of the following is unlikely to be the cause of cheat pain in this patient?

- **A.** Emotional stress
- **B.** Exposure to cold
- **C.** Regurgitation of food
- **D.** Eating a meal

1.3 Which of the following is **NOT** a variable in determining the pretest probability of obstructive coronary artery disease using the Duke Clinical Score?

- **A.** Hypertension
- **B.** Smoking status
- **C.** Angina
- **D.** Previous MI
- **E.** Electrocardiogram (ECG) changes

---

*Questions and Answers are based on Chapter 1: The Patient History by Kazue Okajima and Richard A. Lange in Cardiovascular Medicine and Surgery, First Edition.

14 A 74-year-old woman presents to the clinic complaining of dyspnea. When prompted, the patient elaborates stating she "feels like she is suffocating while lying flat." Her symptoms improve when sitting up, and she has been sleeping in her recliner. The patient had initial blood work drawn from her primary care physician with her today which resulted in a hemoglobin of 15.5 g/dL. Her body mass index (BMI) is 27. Which of the following would be useful in determining this patient's etiology of dyspnea?
   A. Chest computed tomography
   B. Sleep study
   C. B-type natriuretic peptide (BNP)
   D. Echocardiogram
   E. All of the above

15 A 63-year-old male presents to the emergency department (ED) with syncope. The patient has a past medical history of hypertension, diabetes mellitus type 2, and coronary artery disease s/p percutaneous intervention to the proximal right coronary artery. His current home medications include metformin 500 mg bid, metoprolol succinate 50 mg bid, chlorthalidone 25 mg daily, aspirin 81 mg daily, and atorvastatin 80 mg HS. Which of the following does **NOT** fall under a diagnosis of cardiac syncope?
   A. Ventricular tachycardia
   B. Complete heart block
   C. Pulmonary hypertension
   D. Orthostatic blood pressure changes

16 Which of the following features will increase the probability of cardiac syncope?
   A. Male
   B. Symptoms with positional changes from supine to standing
   C. Prodrome of nausea or vomiting
   D. Frequent recurrence with a prolonged history

17 A 32-year-old male presents to your outpatient cardiology office complaining of palpitations. These palpitations last for a few moments and subside spontaneously. Associated symptoms include chest discomfort without dizziness, presyncope, or syncope. Patient drinks six cups of coffee a day and smokes 1 packs per day (ppd) for the last 10 years. What is the next **BEST** step in determining the etiology of the patients' palpitations?
   A. Thyroid-stimulating hormone (TSH)
   B. Basic metabolic panel (BMP)
   C. Anxiety screening
   D. 48-hour Holter monitor
   E. All of the above

18 A 52-year-old male with a past medical history of obesity (BMI 32 kg/m^2), hypertension, dyslipidemia, chronic kidney disease (CKD) stage III, and gastroesophageal reflux disease (GERD) presents to the office to establish care. The patient's family history is significant for coronary artery disease and MI in his father and paternal grandfather in their early 60s. The patient works as an accountant and lives a sedentary lifestyle. His New Year's resolution was to improve his health. The patient has started to exercise after work but complains of leg pain. When asked to describe his leg pain, he states his pain is located at the posterior buttock. The pain is worse with standing and is intermittent in nature. The pain is improved when the patient is at the grocery store pushing a shopping cart. Which of the following is the **MOST LIKELY** cause of the patient's leg pain?

A. Peripheral artery disease
B. Spinal stenosis
C. Nerve root compression
D. Venous claudication
E. Compartment syndrome

1.9 A 72-year-old male with a past medical history of obesity (BMI 38 kg/m²), polycystic kidney disease s/p renal transplant 12 years ago, CKD stage III, and deep vein thrombosis (DVT) presents to the clinic with leg pain. The patient is a retired pharmacist and spent most of his working days on his feet for 40 years. He has recently joined his son in a weight loss challenge and has started exercising but his exercise is limited by bilateral leg pain. The patient states that his pain is in the entire leg but is worse in the calf. His right calf seems more affected than his left. He describes the pain as a tight, bursting pain. The pain is worse after walking and slowly subsides with rest. He finds that the pain is improved with leg elevation. Which of the following is the **MOST LIKELY** cause of the patient's leg pain?

A. Peripheral artery disease
B. Spinal stenosis
C. Nerve root compression
D. Venous claudication
E. Compartment syndrome

1.10 A 67-year-old male with a past medical history of tobacco use, hypertension, and coronary artery disease who has undergone a lumbar spinal fusion after a motor vehicle accident 15 years ago presents to the clinic complaining of leg pain. The patient works as an architect and lives a mostly sedentary lifestyle until recently in the last 3 months has tried to improve his fitness. His exercise has been limited by leg pain. When asked about his leg pain, the patient states that he feels fatigue in the calf muscles that is exacerbated by exercise and is relieved within 10 minutes after rest. He experiences these symptoms in both calves, but his left causes more discomfort than his right. The discomfort is nonradiating, and the patient denies any recent trauma to the area. On physical examination, the skin is intact without any lower extremity ulcers; peripheral pulses are 1+ bilaterally with muscle atrophy noted in the lower extremity bilaterally. Which of the following is the **MOST LIKELY** cause of the patient's leg pain?

A. Peripheral artery disease
B. Spinal stenosis
C. Nerve root compression
D. Venous claudication
E. Compartment syndrome

ANSWERS

1.1 The correct answer is B:
Rationale: The NYHA is a classification system to assess the functional status of a patient with heart failure. This patient's current symptom description will classify her into NYHA class II. NYHA class II symptoms will include slight limitations due to symptoms of angina, fatigue, and dyspnea with physical activity. This patient is comfortable at rest but ordinary physical activity results in fatigue, palpitations, dyspnea, or anginal pain. Patients who present as NYHA class I are patients with cardiac disease but without any limitations in physical activity at rest or with exertion. NYHA class III symptom severity is classified as marked limitations with physical activity. Less than ordinary activity will cause these patients to experience symptoms of fatigue, palpitations, dyspnea, or anginal pain. Patients classified as NYHA class III will be asymptomatic at rest. Patients classified into NYHA class IV symptoms will experience symptoms of cardiac insufficiency or anginal syndrome even at rest. If any physical activity is undertaken, this will increase the patient's discomfort (**Table 1.1**).

TABLE 1.1 Activity Scales Used to Assess Functional Capacity

Class	New York Heart Association (NYHA)	Canadian Cardiovascular Society (CCS)	Specific Activity Scale
I	Patients with cardiac disease but without resulting limitations of physical activity. Ordinary physical activity does not cause undue fatigue, palpitation, dyspnea, or anginal pain.	Ordinary physical activity does not cause angina, such as walking and climbing stairs. Angina with strenuous or rapid or prolonged exertion at work or recreation	Patient can perform to completion any activity requiring 7 or more metabolic equivalents.
II	Patients with cardiac disease resulting in slight limitation of physical activity. They are comfortable at rest. Ordinary physical activity results in fatigue, palpitation, dyspnea, or anginal pain.	Slight limitation of ordinary activity. Walking or climbing stairs rapidly, walking uphill, walking or stair climbing after meals, or in cold, or in wind, or under emotional stress, or only during the few hours after awakening. Walking more than two blocks on the level and climbing more than one flight of ordinary stairs at a normal pace and in normal conditions	Patient can perform to completion any activity requiring 5 or more metabolic equivalents but cannot or does not perform to completion activities requiring 7 or more metabolic equivalents.
III	Patients with cardiac disease resulting in marked limitation of physical activity. They are comfortable at rest. Less than ordinary	Marked limitation of ordinary physical activity. Walking one to two blocks on the level and climbing one	Patient can perform to completion any activity requiring 2 or more metabolic equivalents but cannot or does

TABLE 1.1 Activity Scales Used to Assess Functional Capacity (continued)

Class	New York Heart Association (NYHA)	Canadian Cardiovascular Society (CCS)	Specific Activity Scale
	physical activity causes fatigue, palpitation, dyspnea, or anginal pain.	flight of stairs in normal conditions and at a normal pace	not perform to completion any activities requiring 5 or more metabolic equivalents.
IV	Patients with cardiac disease resulting in inability to carry on any physical activity without discomfort. Symptoms of cardiac insufficiency or of the anginal syndrome may be present even at rest. If any physical activity is undertaken, discomfort is increased.	Inability to carry on any physical activity without discomfort—anginal syndrome may be present at rest.	Patient cannot or does not perform to completion activities requiring 2 or more metabolic equivalents.

Data from Goldman L, Hashimoto B, Cook E, Loscalzo A. Comparative reproducibility and validity of systems for assessing cardiovascular functional class: advantages of a new specific activity scale. *Circulation.* 1981;64(6):1227-1234.

1.2 The correct answer is C.

Rationale: Stable angina can be precipitated by a variety of factors including physical exertion, emotional stress, eating a meal, and exposure to cold. Pain is usually relieved by resting and/or by nitroglycerin. The anginal episode typically lasts only a few minutes; fleeting discomfort for a few seconds or a dull ache lasting for hours is rarely angina. Chronic stable angina is the initial manifestation of coronary heart disease (CHD) in about half of the patients; the other half initially experience unstable angina, MI, or sudden death.

Regurgitation of food is most likely associated with gastrointestinal disease (**Tables 1.2** and **1.3**).

TABLE 1.2 Differential Diagnosis of Chest Pain

Diagnosis	Characteristics	Comments
Ischemic heart disease	Typical or atypical angina	Caused by diminished coronary blood flow and/or increased myocardial oxygen demand
Nonischemic heart disease	Palpitations or typical angina	Tachycardia
Arrhythmias	Typical angina, often exertional	Heart murmur present
Valvular heart disease	"Tearing" pain, often abrupt onset	Widened mediastinum, often with hypertension
Aortic dissection Pericarditis	Pleuritic pain, relieved by sitting up and leaning forward	Friction rub may be present; diffuse ST-segment elevation (PR-segment depression) on electrocardiogram

(continued)

TABLE 1.2 Differential Diagnosis of Chest Pain (continued)

Diagnosis	Characteristics	Comments
Pulmonary disease		
Pulmonary embolus	Pleuritic pain (sharp, worse with inspiration), associated dyspnea	Hypoxia/hypoxemia, pulsus paradoxus, and risk factors for thromboembolic disease
Pneumothorax	Acute onset, pleuritic pain, associated dyspnea	Hyperresonance; tension pneumothorax associated with distended neck veins, hypotension, and tachycardia
Pneumonia	Pleuritic pain, associated fever, and cough	Associated with fever and productive cough
Gastrointestinal disease		
Esophageal disease	May be indistinguishable from angina (ie, relieved with nitroglycerin), may note regurgitation of food and relief with antacids	Often diagnosed following a negative evaluation for ischemic heart disease
Gastritis, peptic ulcer disease	May be indistinguishable from angina	May be exacerbated by alcohol and aspirin and relieved by food and antacids
Biliary disease	Right upper quadrant pain that radiates to the back or scapula	Exacerbated by fatty foods
Pancreatitis	"Boring" epigastric pain, may radiate to the back	Typically worse following meals
Chest wall or dermatologic pain		
Costochondritis	Reproduced with palpation or movement	
Rib fracture	Point tenderness	
Herpes zoster	Point tenderness	Pain may precede rash.
Fibrositis	Follows a nerve distribution/dermatome Characteristic point tenderness	
Psychiatric disorders		
Anxiety disorders Affective disorders (eg, depression) Somatoform disorders Thought disorders (eg, fixed delusions) Factitious disorders (eg, Munchausen syndrome)	Nonexertional, often associated with anxiety, hyperventilation, perioral paresthesia, and "panic attacks"	Often diagnosed following a negative evaluation for angina Often associated with palpitations, sweating, and anxiety

TABLE 1.3	Classification of Chest Pain
Cardiac (definite)	Meets all three of the following characteristics: • Substernal chest discomfort of characteristic quality and duration • Provoked by exertion or emotional stress • Relieved by rest and/or nitrates within minutes
Possibly Cardiac	Meets two of the above-mentioned characteristics
Nonanginal chest pain	Lacks or meets only one or none of the above-mentioned characteristics

1.3 The correct answer is A.
Rationale: The Duke Clinical Score is used to determine the pretest probability of obstructive coronary artery disease and was adopted by the American College of Cardiology and the American Heart Association. Factors for the Duke Clinical Score include age, sex, angina, smoking status, dyslipidemia, diabetes, previous MI, and ECG changes. Hypertension is not a risk factor when calculating the Duke Clinical Score.

1.4 The correct answer is E.
Rationale: Cardiac and noncardiac etiology of dyspnea may share the same descriptors. Initial evaluation of BNP may aid the clinician in differentiating between cardiac and noncardiac causes of dyspnea. Obstructive sleep apnea and obesity hypoventilation syndrome have emerged as important causes of cardiopulmonary diseases reflecting the increase in obesity rates. Echocardiogram would certainly be helpful in terms of further evaluation of left ventricular systolic function, presence of significant pericardial effusion, and other valvular disorders that may be contributing to her symptoms.

1.5 The correct answer is D.
Rationale: Syncope is an abrupt, transient, complete loss of consciousness, associated with the inability to maintain postural tone, with subsequent rapid and spontaneous recovery. The mechanism of syncope is presumed to be cerebral hypoperfusion (excluding other forms of loss of consciousness such as seizures, trauma, or pseudosyncope). The causes of syncope can be broadly categorized as cardiac, reflex (neurally mediated), and orthostatic. Cardiac syncope includes (1) tachyarrhythmias (ventricular fibrillation and ventricular tachycardia), (2) bradyarrhythmias (advanced atrioventricular block and sinus node dysfunction), and (3) structural heart abnormalities (aortic stenosis, hypertrophic obstructive cardiomyopathy, atrial myxoma, cardiac tamponade, and great vessel disorder such as pulmonary embolism, acute aortic dissection, and pulmonary hypertension).

Orthostatic hypotension is another important cause of syncope, especially in the older population. Patients with hypovolemia or autonomic dysfunction experience fainting while standing because of decline in blood pressure. A history of positional (standing/sitting) syncope and orthostatic vital signs on physical examination are crucial to establishing this diagnosis.

1.6 The correct answer is A.
Rationale: A careful history must be taken from patients who present with syncope. Factors or descriptions that are more often associated with cardiac causes of syncope

include age greater than 60, male gender, presence of known ischemic or structural heart disease, brief prodrome (palpitations, sudden loss of consciousness without prodrome), low number of episodes (one or two), abnormal cardiac examination, family history of inheritable conditions or premature sudden cardiac death and known congenital heart disease. In addition, there are risk factors and findings that lower the probability of a cardiac cause of syncope. Factors associated with noncardiac causes of syncope include younger age, no known cardiac disease, syncope only in the standing position, positional changes from supine or sitting to standing, presence of prodrome (nausea, vomiting, feeling warmth), presence of specific triggers or situational triggers, frequent recurrence, and prolong history of syncope with similar characteristics.

1.7 The correct answer is E.
Rationale: Palpitations can result from a variety of arrhythmias including premature atrial contraction, premature ventricular contractions, nonsustained supraventricular or ventricular tachycardia. Abrupt onset is common for these palpitations secondary to pathologic arrhythmias. It is important to rule out noncardiac causes of palpitations including endocrine and metabolic abnormalities (thyroid, psychiatric disorders, and medication or substance use effects). Palpitations are common in healthy individuals who experience anxiety which can be discovered by a Generalized Anxiety Screening tool, GAD-7.

1.8 The correct answer is B.
Rationale: The patient's leg pain/cramping is most likely related to spinal stenosis. A few key characteristics include the location of the pain (bilateral buttock), improvement with spinal flexion (pushing a shopping cart), and variable relief with rest. Spinal stenosis may mimic claudication (pseudoclaudication). This patient does not have the classic symptoms of claudication. Venous claudication involves the entire leg and is worse in the calf. Nerve root compression will cause burning and numbness in a nerve distribution.

1.9 The correct answer is D.
Rationale: Many conditions can result in leg pain and claudication-like symptoms (**eTable 1.4**)[1]. Venous claudication typically involves the entire leg but is worse in the calf. The pain is typically described as a tight or busting pain. The pain is worse after working and subsides slowly and relieves with elevation. Venous claudication is typically seen in patients with a history of DVT. Peripheral artery disease can also cause claudication, but symptoms are typically relieved in 10 minutes. Nerve root compression typically presents with a burning unilateral pain in the nerve distribution. Spinal stenosis typically starts in the buttocks regions and improves with spinal flexion. In addition, it will have a variable relief pattern with rest.

1.10 The correct answer is A.
Rationale: Symptoms of peripheral arterial disease (PAD) are characterized as fatigue, discomfort, cramping, or pain of vascular origin consistently induced by exercise and relieved within 10 minutes with rest. About 40% of patients do not complain of leg symptoms at all and 50% of patients have atypical symptoms. Clinical findings suggestive of lower extremity PAD include abnormal lower extremity pulse examination, bruits, nonhealing lower extremity wound or arterial ulcerations, hair loss, shiny skin, and muscle atrophy.

---

[1] *This table can be accessed in the accompanying eBook. See inside front cover for access instructions.*

GENERAL CARDIOVASCULAR EXAMINATION

John Tremblay, Mikhail Torosoff, and Steven A. Fein

CHAPTER 2

QUESTIONS

2.1 A 21-year-old female is being evaluated in the cardiology clinic for a heart murmur evaluation after referral from her primary care provider. She recently moved from abroad and has never been evaluated by a health care professional until recently. The patient's physical examination reveals short stature with a short neck. Which of the following murmurs would **MOST LIKELY** be heard in this patient?

- A. Soft systolic murmur over the pulmonic area with fixed splitting of S_2
- B. Pansystolic murmur loudest in the left lower sternal border (LLSB)
- C. Decrescendo blowing diastolic murmur loudest at the LLSB
- D. Harsh-sounding murmur heard underneath the left collar bone

2.2 A 58-year-old male presents to the cardiology clinic to establish care. The patient has recently moved to the area and presents to the clinic at the request of his wife. The patient has never received medical care and has never followed up with any medical providers. He denies taking any medication, vitamins, or other supplements. When asked about his family history, the patient states he was adopted and does not know his family history. Patient underwent blood work including a lipid panel that is pending. Which of the following is/are associated with cutaneous manifestation(s) of hyperlipoproteinemia?

- A. Yellow macules/papules along the creases of the palm
- B. Tuberous yellow nodules located on the buttocks
- C. Erythematous yellow papules on the extensor surfaces
- D. Yellow cutaneous nontender lesions on the eyelids
- E. All of the above

2.3 An 85-year-old bedbound male is being evaluated for lower extremity edema. The patient has a past medical history of gastroesophageal reflux disease (GERD), hypertension (HTN), diabetes mellitus type 2 (DMT2), and gout. The patient, on examination, has bilateral lower limb edema. Pedal pulses are 2+ bilaterally and the limbs are warm. No clubbing or cyanosis is seen. Jugular venous distension (JVD) measures 3 cm above the angle of Louis.

Questions and Answers are based on Chapter 2: General Cardiovascular Exam by Timothy J. O'Connor, William H. Fennell, and John W. McEvoy in Cardiovascular Medicine and Surgery, First Edition.

Which of the following is the **MOST LIKELY** diagnosis?
- A. Right-sided heart failure
- B. Chronic venous insufficiency
- C. Venous thrombosis
- D. Lymphatic obstruction
- E. All of the above

2.4 A 67-year-old male with a past medical history of diet-controlled diabetes, HTN, and hyperlipidemia (HLD), presents to the emergency room for shortness of breath. When performing the physical examination, the patient is placed in the semireclined position with the head of the bed at 45°. The patient's head is turned slightly to the left and a pulsation is observed through the sternocleidomastoid muscle. Which of the following features are **MORE LIKELY** related to the jugular venous pulse versus the carotid pulse?
- A. Monophasic waveform
- B. Palpability
- C. Decreases with inspiration
- D. Not obliterated with gentle pressure

2.5 A 59-year-old female presents to the hospital with dyspnea. The patient has a past medical history of HTN, DMT2, obesity, HLD, atrial fibrillation, GERD, and asthma. The patient has recently lost her job and her health insurance, which has made it hard for her to afford her medications. Chest x-ray shows no acute intrathoracic abnormalities. Auscultation of the chest reveals tachycardia with irregular rhythm; no murmurs or rubs were appreciated. Which of the following abnormalities are **MOST LIKELY** to be observed when assessing jugular venous wave form?
- A. Absence of the X descent
- B. Prominent V wave
- C. Cannon A waves
- D. Loss of A waves

2.6 An 18-year-old male presents to the cardiology clinic referred by his pediatrician for abnormal heart sounds. The patient is adopted and has an unknown family history. The patient denies any chest pain, palpitations, or dyspnea. The patient's electrocardiogram (ECG) shows normal sinus rhythm, and heart rate is 62 bpm. On auscultation of the chest, an ejection systolic click followed by a systolic murmur is auscultated in the right upper parasternal area. When the patient is asked to stand, there is no change in the duration or quality of the murmur. Echocardiography will confirm which of the following valvular abnormalities?
- A. Mitral valve prolapse
- B. Mitral valve stenosis
- C. Bicuspid aortic valve stenosis
- D. Tricuspid stenosis

2.7 A 22-year-old female presents to the cardiology clinic for abnormal heart sounds auscultated by her primary care provider during a college sports physical. The patient is a Division 2 Collegiate soccer player and has been training for the start of her soccer season. The patient denies any chest pain, angina, dyspnea, or palpitations. The patient denies any family history of cardiac disease. On cardiac auscultation, a high-pitched, opening snap shortly after S_2 followed by a mid-diastolic lower pitch murmur is appreciated. Which of the following murmurs will **MOST LIKELY** be confirmed on follow-up echocardiography?

A. Aortic regurgitation
B. Mitral stenosis
C. Atrial tumor
D. Mitral regurgitation

2.8 A 38-year-old male presents to the cardiology clinic for initial evaluation. The patient is an ex-collegiate athlete, exercises daily, and tries to uphold a healthy lifestyle by following the DASH (Dietary Approaches to Stop Hypertension) diet. Patient denies any symptoms including chest pain, dyspnea, syncope, or palpitations. The patient requested to be evaluated by a cardiologist due to his concern of cardiogenic genetic disorders. Unfortunately, the patient is unsure of the details of his familial cardiac disease. On physical examination, a 3/6 mid-systolic murmur is appreciated. No thrill is palpable. The patient's murmur is dynamic and changes with position. On standing and during the Valsalva maneuver, the intensity of the murmur increases to a 4/6. Which of the following murmurs are **MOST LIKELY** identified in this patient?

A. Aortic stenosis
B. Aortic regurgitation
C. Pulmonary stenosis
D. Hypertrophic obstructive cardiomyopathy (HOCM)
E. Mitral regurgitation

CASE 1

A 26-year-old internal medicine resident presents to your clinic for cardiac evaluation. The patient was referred by her primary care physician (PCP) for concerns of an abnormal cardiac auscultation. An echocardiogram was ordered by her PCP but is currently pending. The patient has a family history of bicuspid aortic valve in her father. The patient participates in regular exercise including biking/running 20 to 30 miles per week. She denies any shortness of breath (SOB), dyspnea, chest pain, palpitations, or lower extremity edema. Her only medication is ibuprofen 400 mg twice a day, as needed, for joint pain.

2.9 For the patient in **Case 1**, on cardiac examination there is a late systolic murmur preceded by a mid-systolic click. The murmur is located over the fifth left midclavicular intercostal space. What anatomic location is the murmur **MOST LIKELY** to radiate toward?

A. Radiates to the neck
B. Radiates to the back
C. Radiates to the axilla
D. All of the above

2.10 Which of the following dynamic movements will increase the duration and the quantity of the murmur for the patient in **Case 1**?

A. Valsalva
B. Inspiration
C. Squatting
D. Standing

ANSWERS

2.1 The correct answer is D.

Rationale: The harsh-sounding murmur heard underneath the left collar bone is associated with coarctation of the aorta. The patient most likely has Turner syndrome based on her physical features of short stature, short neck, receding jaw, droopy eyelids, and short bones of the hands. Turner syndrome occurs in females who have a complete absence or partial deletion of one of the X chromosomes. Turner syndrome can have a variety of cardiac associations including aortic isthmus stenosis, bicuspid aortic valve, pulmonary valve stenosis, and coarctation of the aorta.

A soft systolic murmur heard over the pulmonic area with a fixed splitting of S_2 is associated with atrial septal defect (ASD). ASD can be related to Down syndrome, Holt-Oram syndrome, Wolf-Hirschhorn syndrome, Noonan syndrome, and Edwards syndrome. A pansystolic murmur heard loudest in the LLSB is associated with a ventricular septal defect (VSD). A VSD can be observed in patients with the following genetic disorders including Down syndrome, Holt-Oram syndrome, Wolf-Hirschhorn syndrome, or Edwards syndrome. A decrescendo blowing diastolic murmur loudest at the LLSB is associated with aortic insufficiency and is not associated with Turner syndrome (**Table 2.1**).

2.2 The correct answer is E.

Rationale: Lipid metabolism disorders from genetic disease or secondary etiologies are typically associated with xanthomas. Xanthomas are yellow cutaneous lesions at various body sites (choice D). Tendonous xanthomata typically indicate type IIa hyperlipoproteinemia (choice B). Yellow macules/papules along the creases of the palm are described as palmar xanthomata and are typically associated with type III familial hyperlipoproteinemia (choice A). Type IIa and III familial hyperlipoproteinemia are associated with tuberous and tuber eruptive xanthomata located on the buttocks, hands, and knees. Eruptive xanthomata are small erythematous yellow papules that appear on the extensor surfaces and are associated with type I and V (choice C). All of the these cutaneous manifestations can be associated with genetic disease or secondary causes of hyperlipoproteinemia.

2.3 The correct answer is B.

Rationale: Absence of JVD makes right-sided heart failure unlikely. Bilateral lower limb edema in a bedbound patient without JVD suggests diagnosis of chronic venous insufficiency. Chronic venous insufficiency is also supported by signs such as varicose veins, venous ulcerations, hyperpigmentation, and stasis dermatitis. The patient's swelling is bilateral, which makes venous thrombosis less likely. Unilateral swelling can be commonly seen in venous thrombosis or previous vein grafts. The patient's history is not suggestive of lymphatic obstruction.

TABLE 2.1 Cardiac Murmurs and How to Differentiate Them

Timing and Lesion	Site	Radiation/Dynamic Maneuvers	Helpful Hints
SYSTOLIC MURMURS			
Early systolic			
Acute mitral regurgitation (MR)	Apex	Radiates to the axilla when the regurgitant leaflet is the anterior mitral valve leaflet but may radiate to the cardiac base with posterior leaflet disease	• Loud early systolic murmur that increases with expiration and diminishes as the pressure gradient between the left ventricle and left atrium decreases in late systole
Acute tricuspid regurgitation	Left lower sternal border		• Increases in intensity during inspiration with a prominent "v" wave (or "c-v" wave) in jugular venous pressure (JVP)
Mid-systolic			
Aortic stenosis	Upper right sternal border (second intercostal space)	Radiates to carotids	• High-pitched murmur that is louder on expiration • Intensity is greatest in mid-systole and wanes in late systole—crescendo-decrescendo pattern. • Murmur preceded by an ejection click in young patients • S_2 variable and can be absent in severely calcified valve • Reverse splitting in severe aortic stenosis (P_2-A_2)
Pulmonary stenosis	Upper left sternal border (second intercostal space)	Can radiate slightly toward the neck and back	• Harsh and high-pitched murmur louder on inspiration • Similar crescendo-decrescendo pattern • Ejection click, delayed P_2 may be soft
Hypertrophic obstructive cardiomyopathy	Left lower sternal border	Louder and longer on standing and Valsalva maneuver	• Ejection crescendo-decrescendo murmur that can mimic aortic stenosis—differentiate with dynamic maneuvers (ie, Valsalva, squat) • A pansystolic murmur at the apex and radiating to axilla may occur in the presence of systolic anterior motion of the mitral valve. • Patients may present with an S_4 gallop and a reverse splitting of S_2.

(continued)

TABLE 2.1 Cardiac Murmurs and How to Differentiate Them (continued)

Timing and Lesion	Site	Radiation/Dynamic Maneuvers	Helpful Hints
Atrial septal defect	Left upper sternal border	Can radiate to the back	• Fixed splitting of A_2-P_2—interval is wide and remains constant throughout respiration.
Innocent murmur	All areas		• Soft murmur that can appear when cardiac output is high
Late systolic			
Mitral valve prolapse	Apex	Radiates to the axilla but also may go to the neck or back. Enhanced by Valsalva maneuvers and decreased by squatting	• Following a normal S_1, the valve prolapses, resulting in a mid-systolic click. Immediately after the click, a brief crescendo-decrescendo murmur is heard.
Pansystolic			
Chronic MR	Apex	Radiates to the axilla	• Mild MR is characterized by a systolic murmur plateau louder on expiration while moderate MR is accompanied by an S_3 gallop. Severe MR has an associated diastolic flow rumble.
Chronic tricuspid regurgitation	Left sternal border	Has a blowing quality and often associated with an S_3	• Increases in intensity during inspiration with a prominent "v" wave in JVP. Left parasternal heave may be present.
DIASTOLIC MURMURS			
Early diastolic			
Aortic regurgitation	Mid-left sternal border (third intercostal space)	Louder over left sternal border with patient sitting up and leaning forward on full expiration	• Begins directly after S_2 and has a blowing decrescendo quality
Mid-diastolic			
Mitral stenosis	Apex	Maximal intensity with patient in lateral decubitus position	• Soft rumbling diastolic murmur preceded by an opening snap and best heard with the bell of the stethoscope and patient in the lateral decubitus position • Useful mnemonic, "*Rup-t-t-eee.*" *Rup* (loud S_1)—*t* (S_2)—*t* (opening snap)—*eee* (diastolic murmur)
Atrial tumors	Apex		Rarely present Low-pitched sound that fluctuates with patient positioning as the tumor moves toward or away from mitral valve

2.4 The correct answer is C.
Rationale: Differentiating between the carotid and jugular venous pulse is a fundamental element to the cardiovascular examination. Increased jugular venous pressure (JVP) can be used to estimate the right arterial pressure in the absence of pulmonary disease. It is important to place the patient in the proper position to examine for JVD. This includes the head of the bed elevated to 45° and a slight rotation to the left with the chin extended. It is important to not over rotate the neck as this can compress the internal jugular vein. The jugular venous pulse and the carotid pulse have their own unique characteristics. In a patient in sinus rhythm, the jugular venous pulse has a biphasic wave form with two waves per cardiac cycle, is not palpable, decreases on inspiration, and is obliterated with gentle pressure at the base of the neck. The carotid pulse is monophasic, palpable, does not change with respirations, and is not obliterated with gentle pressure.

2.5 The correct answer is D.
Rationale: The morphology of the JVP wave form can be observed to inform clinical assessment. The "a" wave is the first positive deflection representing atrial contraction that occurs after the P wave on ECG. The "a" wave would be absent in this patient as she is currently in atrial fibrillation. Cannon "a" waves occur when the atria contract against the closed tricuspid secondary to atrioventricular dissociation in patients with complete heart block. Prominent "v" waves are observed in conditions such as tricuspid regurgitation or ASD. The "x" descent may be absent in significant tricuspid regurgitation.

2.6 The correct answer is C.
Rationale: Congenital bicuspid aortic stenosis with pliable aortic valve leaflets can result in an ejection systolic click followed by the ejection murmur heard over the aortic area. The systolic click is classically high pitched and is heard early in systole. This is due to abrupt doming of the abnormal valve early in systole and often disappears as the culprit valve loses pliability over time. An ejection click heard over the mitral area is related to mitral valve prolapse. The mitral prolapse click is heard after S_1 and may be followed by a systolic murmur. Mitral valve prolapse murmur is affected by positional changes. In mitral valve prolapse, when standing, ventricular preload and afterload decrease, resulting in the click moving closer to S_1. With squatting, ventricular preload and afterload increase, resulting in the click moving away from S_1. Mitral valve stenosis and tricuspid stenosis are diastolic murmurs.

2.7 The correct answer is B.
Rationale: The patient, on examination, has a high-pitched sound shortly after S_2, making her murmur a diastolic murmur. The mid-diastolic murmur with a lower pitch makes this murmur most likely mitral valve stenosis. Mitral valve stenosis is best heard at the apex with the patient lying in the left lateral decubitus position. Aortic regurgitation is a diastolic murmur classified as beginning directly after S_2 with a blowing decrescendo quality. Mitral flow obstruction by atrial tumors can sometimes be heard as an end-diastolic murmur. These murmurs are classified as low-pitched sounds that fluctuate with patient positioning as the tumor moves away or toward the mitral valve. Mitral regurgitation is a mid-systolic high-pitched murmur.

2.8 The correct answer is B.
Rationale: The patient is presenting with a mid-systolic murmur of HOCM. Mid-systolic murmurs, in general, are aortic stenosis, pulmonary stenosis, HOCM, ASDs, and innocent murmurs. This patient's murmur increases with standing and during the Valsalva maneuver. When a patient changes position and goes from squatting to standing, venous return and systemic resistance increases. This will cause an increase in left ventricular diastolic volume and arterial pressure. In aortic stenosis, squatting will increase the intensity of the murmur. Conversely, HOCM will become softer with squatting and louder with standing as the preload is decreased. Pulmonic stenosis is a right-sided murmur that can increase with changes in respiration. Aortic regurgitation is a diastolic murmur. Mitral regurgitation is classified as an early systolic murmur in acute mitral regurgitation or a pansystolic murmur in chronic mitral regurgitation (**Table 2.1**).

2.9 The correct answer is B.
Rationale: The patient's cardiac auscultation, which is characterized by a mid-systolic click followed by a late systolic murmur, is most likely the auscultation findings of mitral valve prolapse. In mitral valve prolapse, the mitral valve prolapsing into the left atrium results in the mid-systolic click. Immediately after the mid-systolic click, a brief crescendo-decrescendo murmur can be heard. Classically, it will radiate to the axilla but may also radiate to the neck or back. Murmurs that can also radiate to the neck include aortic stenosis and pulmonic stenosis. Murmurs that can radiate to the back include pulmonic stenosis and ASDs. Murmurs that radiate toward the axilla include mitral regurgitation and mitral valve prolapse (**Table 2.1**).

2.10 The correct answer is A.
Rationale: When the patient is asked to perform the Valsalva maneuver, the left ventricular diastolic volume, stroke volume, and arterial blood pressure falls. Most cardiac murmurs become softer. This will cause the late systolic murmur of mitral valve prolapse to occur earlier (due to the decreased left ventricular volume) and become longer and louder. Inspiration will increase the intensity of right-sided cardiac murmurs. Squatting will help differentiate HOCM from aortic stenosis as squatting will increase preload and systemic resistance will increase the intensity of aortic stenosis. Reversely, HOCM murmur will decrease in intensity while squatting because of the increase in left ventricular diastolic volume reduces the obstruction of the outflow tract.

CLINICAL PHARMACOLOGY

Niranjan Ojha, Anojan Pathmanathan, and Robert L. Carhart

CHAPTER 3

QUESTIONS

3.1 A 63-year-old male with a history of tobacco use and hypertension is evaluated for typical chest pain in a cardiologist's office. He has recently moved from New Zealand and mostly eats fast food. His medications include oral hydrochlorothiazide 12.5 mg daily. He had a positive stress echocardiography and is referred for cardiac catheterization. He is found to have mid right coronary artery stenosis and got stented with a drug-eluting stent. He was loaded with aspirin and Plavix and was subsequently started on aspirin 81 mg and Plavix 75 mg po daily. Which of the following will the patient benefit from?

  A. Screening for diabetes
  B. Screening for dyslipidemia
  C. VerifyNow P2Y12 testing is indicated.
  D. All of the above

3.2 A 65-year-old male presented to the emergency department with acute-onset retrosternal chest pain with radiation to the left jaw and shoulder. He recently moved to the United States from Nepal and is getting treatment for latent tuberculosis with daily rifampin. The electrocardiogram (ECG) showed nonspecific T-wave changes in anterior leads and his high-sensitivity troponin was 240 ng/L. He underwent cardiac catheterization and got a drug-eluting stent in the left anterior descending artery. Which of the following statements is **TRUE** regarding antiplatelet treatment?

  A. Monotherapy with aspirin is sufficient.
  B. Dual antiplatelet treatment with aspirin and Plavix is preferred.
  C. Dual antiplatelet treatment with aspirin and ticagrelor is preferred.
  D. Treatment with Plavix and Eliquis is preferred.

3.3 A 51-year-old White female smoker with a history of hypertension, well controlled on medication, and diabetes mellitus type 2, on oral hypoglycemic agent, had low-density lipoprotein (LDL) cholesterol of 130 mg/dL. Due to an intermediate atherosclerotic cardiovascular disease (ASCVD) risk score, the patient was previously started on atorvastatin, which she did not tolerate due to side effects. She also did not tolerate rosuvastatin in the past. She was prescribed Livalo, but her insurance rejected the prescription and suggested that Zypitamag be started, citing lower cost of the suggested drug despite both being pitavastatin. What principle of pharmacoeconomics is utilized in decision-making by an insurance company?

---

*Questions and Answers are based on Chapter 3: Clinical Pharmacology: Pharmacogenomics, Pharmacovigilance, Pharmacoepidemiology, and Pharmacoeconomics by Steven P. Dunn and Craig J. Beavers in Cardiovascular Medicine and Surgery, First Edition.

A. Cost-minimization analysis
B. Cost-benefit analysis
C. Cost-effective analysis
D. Cost-utility analysis

3.4 A 71-year-old male who has a history of coronary artery disease with multiple hospital admissions and multiple percutaneous coronary interventions (PCIs) is admitted again for chest pain and found to have elevated troponin. He ended up with a drug stent in one of the marginal branches of the left circumflex artery. His lipid panel showed LDL cholesterol of 98 mg/dL despite being on the maximum tolerable dose of atorvastatin and ezetimibe. He was subsequently started on a proprotein convertase subtilisin/kexin type 9 (PCSK-9) inhibitor by his cardiologist based on the American College of Cardiology/American Heart Association (ACC/AHA) Guidelines on the Management of Blood Cholesterol 2018, which suggested improved quality-adjusted life years (QALYs) with PCSK-9 inhibitors. What pharmacoeconomic principle is utilized by the ACC/AHA in decision-making?

A. Cost-minimization analysis
B. Cost-benefit analysis
C. Cost-effective analysis
D. Cost-utility analysis

3.5 A 51-year-old female with a history of hypertension and recently diagnosed diabetes mellitus type 2 presented with shortness of breath and weight gain. She reported orthopnea and bilateral lower extremity swelling. The patient's home medications include lisinopril 20 mg po nightly, metformin 1,000 mg po twice a day, and rosiglitazone 4 mg po. On examination, patient has 2+ bilateral pitting edema, basal crackles, and S_3 gallop. Echocardiography showed mild diffuse hypokinesis of the left ventricular (LV) wall with reduced LV function with ejection fraction of 40%. What would be an appropriate next step?

A. Diuresis and cardiac catheterization
B. Diuresis and stress testing
C. Medicine reconciliation and diuresis
D. Diuresis and repeat echocardiography

3.6 A 37-year-old female reported progressive shortness of breath. After extensive workup by her primary care physician, she was referred to a cardiologist for echocardiographic findings of increased right ventricular pressure. She underwent right heart catheterization and the findings were suggestive of World Health Organization (WHO) group 1 pulmonary artery hypertension (PAH). She was seen in the pulmonary hypertension clinic and the decision was made to start the patient on riociguat. What is **TRUE** regarding riociguat prescription?

A. Mandatory provider and pharmacy certification and education are needed.
B. Mandatory patient education and annual assessment of contraception are required.
C. Documentation of negative pregnancy status is required.
D. All of the above

ANSWERS

3.1 The correct answer is D.
Rationale: Risk factor modification is a key component in the management of ischemic heart disease. In addition, patient-specific drug metabolism is also an important factor. The effectiveness of clopidogrel depends on its conversion to an active metabolite, which is accomplished by the cytochrome P450 2C19 enzyme. Loss-of-function copies of the *CYP2C19* gene are classified as CYP2C19 poor metabolizers and have a reduced antiplatelet effect, causing the failure of the dual antiplatelet treatment. Incidence of poor metabolizers is highest among individuals of Oceanian descent, which includes Australasian, New Zealanders, and Pacific Islanders, so VerifyNow P2Y12 testing should be considered in such populations. Clopidogrel has the Food and Drug Administration (FDA; 2022) black box warning on CYP2C19 poor metabolizers.

3.2 The correct answer is C.
Rationale: Rifampin strongly induces CYP2C19, resulting in an increase in the level of the clopidogrel active metabolite and in platelet inhibition, which in particular might potentiate the risk of bleeding. As a precaution, we should avoid concomitant use of strong CYP2C19 inducers or use the alternative when available. Treatment with anticoagulants such as Eliquis also has shown increased risk of bleeding with no clinical benefit over dual antiplatelet treatment.

3.3 The correct answer is A.
Rationale: Cost-minimization analysis. The ingredient of the drug is the same, so the expected outcome is also the same, equal efficacy. The least expensive alternative is suggested by the insurance company. The cost of statin therapy will outweigh the cost of future hospitalizations associated with complications of hyperlipidemia, which is a cost-benefit ratio or a net cost/net benefit, whereas in cost-effective and cost-utility analyses, the outcome is measured in terms of natural health units and patient preference or quality of life or QALYs, respectively.

3.4 The correct answer is D.
Rationale: Cost-utility analysis is a form of cost-effective analysis in which two or more treatment alternatives or programs in which resources are measured in monetary terms and outcomes are expressed in patient preferences or quality of life or QALYs. The outcomes of this type of analysis determine the life years gained and then multiplied by the utility of that life year. In 2018, on the basis of the ACC Guidelines on the Management of Blood Cholesterol, authors suggested, based on mid-2018 medication list prices in the simulations, that PCSK-9 inhibitors had an incremental cost-effectiveness ratio from $141,700 to $450,000 per QALY added when used in secondary prevention in patients with ASCVD.

3.5 The correct answer is C.
Rationale: Pharmacovigilance is the science and activities related to the detection, assessment, understanding, and prevention of adverse effects or any other drug-related problem. The patient is taking rosiglitazone, which carries a black box warning for new or exacerbation of existing heart failure. The consideration has to be given to discontinue rosiglitazone and this drug is no longer available in the US market due to safety concerns. With advancement of cardiovascular medicine, there are many new drugs in the market. Surveillance, risk management, individual case reports, database analysis, premarket analysis, and postmarket clinical trials play an important role in pharmacovigilance and appropriation of the drug in health care.

3.6 The correct answer is D.
Rationale: Legislation change in 2008 allowed the FDA to more broadly require various actions by a company to mitigate risk to patients; these have become collectively known as Risk Evaluation and Mitigation Strategies (REMS) and can be used when the FDA determines that a risk to safety that is not sufficiently minimized by the standard product labeling is present. REMS for riociguat have the abovementioned strategies to minimize risk from the drug, which includes but is not limited to teratogenicity. Riociguat is a soluble guanylate cyclase stimulator that is approved for PAH and chronic thromboembolic pulmonary hypertension (CTEPH; after surgical treatment or inoperable CTEPH) to improve exercise capacity. This drug is available to females only through the restricted Adempas (riociguat) REMS program. All females, regardless of their reproductive potential, must be enrolled in the REMS program. Prescribers and pharmacies must also be enrolled in the program. It carries the US boxed warning: Do not administer to pregnant patients because it may cause fetal harm. All females of reproductive potential should have a negative pregnancy test result prior to beginning therapy, and testing should continue monthly during treatment and 1 month after discontinuing therapy. Effective contraception should be used during therapy and for 1 month following discontinuation of riociguat.

STABLE ISCHEMIC HEART DISEASE*

Samuel Kim, Radmila Lyubarova, Neil Yager, and Mandeep S. Sidhu

CHAPTER 4

QUESTIONS

4.1 What is the leading cause of death and morbidity in the United States?
- **A.** Cancer
- **B.** Pulmonary disease
- **C.** Coronary artery disease (CAD)
- **D.** Trauma

4.2 Of the noninvasive functional stress testing modalities, which test is the **MOST** sensitive?
- **A.** Exercise electrocardiography (ECG)
- **B.** Exercise stress echocardiography
- **C.** Exercise myocardial perfusion imaging
- **D.** All are equivalent.

4.3 A 42-year-old male with a past medical history of dyslipidemia presents to your clinic with complaints of 2 months of vague chest discomfort that appears to be stable. You are considering potential coronary artery etiology after completing your initial history and physical examination and thus wish to order a noninvasive ischemic evaluation. After confirming his ability to exercise and obtaining an ECG to ensure it is interpretable, which test would be **BEST** for this patient?
- **A.** Vasodilator myocardial perfusion imaging
- **B.** Cardiac magnetic resonance imaging (MRI) with dobutamine
- **C.** Exercise ECG
- **D.** Dobutamine echocardiography

4.4 A 52-year-old male with a past medical history of known CAD and hypertension is presenting to your clinic and reports chronic stable angina for the past several months. His blood pressure is 135/75 mm Hg, heart rate 82 beats per minute (bpm), and saturation 99% on room air. His current medication includes aspirin 81 mg and atorvastatin 80 mg. What further medication should be added at this time?
- **A.** Nitroglycerin sublingual
- **B.** Metoprolol succinate
- **C.** Isosorbide dinitrate
- **D.** Both A and B

---

*Questions and Answers are based on Chapter 4: Stable Ischemic Heart Disease by Gharibyan Rosie Jasper and James C. Blankenship in Cardiovascular Medicine and Surgery, First Edition.

4.5 Which of the following is **FALSE** regarding ranolazine?
   A. It is a selective late sodium channel inhibitor.
   B. It is metabolized and excreted only through the gastrointestinal (GI) system.
   C. It is more potent in patients with diabetes.
   D. It should be used with extreme caution in patients with severe kidney disease.

4.6 A 55-year-old male with known past medical history of hypertension and dyslipidemia presents as a postdischarge follow-up after undergoing percutaneous coronary intervention (PCI) with a drug-eluting stent for unstable angina. He reports no complaints currently and admits to continuing to smoke tobacco. His medication on discharge included aspirin 81 mg once daily, clopidogrel 75 mg once daily, metoprolol succinate 25 mg once daily, lisinopril 20 mg once daily, and rosuvastatin 10 mg daily. His blood pressure today is 125/60 mm Hg with a heart rate of 62 bpm. You review his hospital labs that included a lipid panel as follows: total cholesterol of 158, triglyceride of 140, high-density lipoprotein (HDL) of 40, and low-density lipoprotein (LDL) of 110. In addition to providing smoking cessation counseling, you discuss with the patient regarding cholesterol-lowering options. What is the **BEST** lipid-lowering strategy in this patient?
   A. Increase rosuvastatin dose.
   B. Add niacin.
   C. Add ezetimibe.
   D. Add proprotein convertase subtilisin/kexin type 9 (PCSK-9) inhibitor.

4.7 A 54-year-old male with a past medical history of stable CAD, hypertension, and heart failure with ejection fraction of 35% presents to your clinic for follow-up and with no complaints. His vitals today are similar to his previous, with a blood pressure of 135/84 mm Hg and heart rate of 65 bpm. His current medication includes aspirin 81 mg once daily, carvedilol 25 mg twice daily, atorvastatin 40 mg once daily, and nitroglycerin sublingual as needed. Which of the following medications would you consider adding to his current regimen?
   A. Amlodipine
   B. Lisinopril
   C. Chlorthalidone
   D. No change in regimen

4.8 In the same patient from **Question 4.7**, what would the target blood pressure be?
   A. Less than 130/80 mm Hg
   B. Less than 140/90 mm Hg
   C. Less than 120/70 mm Hg
   D. 150/80 mm Hg

4.9 In which of the following scenarios would revascularization to improve survival in stable ischemic heart disease **NOT** be recommended?
   A. Left main disease 50% or greater
   B. Proximal left anterior descending (LAD) stenosis 70% or greater with one other major CAD
   C. Significant disease 70% or greater in two major coronary arteries with severe or extensive myocardial ischemia (eg, high-risk criteria on stress testing, abnormal fractional flow reserve [FFR], or >20% perfusion defect by myocardial perfusion stress imaging)
   D. 70% or greater disease in left circumflex coronary artery

4.10 A 63-year-old male with a past medical history of hypertension, diabetes mellitus, and CAD who was recently hospitalized for unstable angina and status post drug-eluting stent placement approximately 1 year ago presents to your clinic for his annual follow-up. He had an echocardiogram prior to discharge and was overall unremarkable. He has no complaints today and no recurrence of symptoms that includes chest discomfort. His blood pressure is 125/70 mm Hg and his heart rate is 63 bpm. His current medication includes aspirin 81 mg once daily, ticagrelor 90 mg twice daily, rosuvastatin 40 mg once daily, metoprolol succinate 50 mg once daily, and lisinopril 40 mg. In addition to basic blood work of complete blood count (CBC) and comprehensive metabolic panel (CMP), what additional workup would you consider for him today?

- **A.** Annual stress test
- **B.** Echocardiogram
- **C.** Lipid panel and HbA$_{1c}$
- **D.** No additional testing is needed at this time.

ANSWERS

4.1 The correct answer is C.
Rationale: CAD is the leading cause and continues to be the number one cause of death in the United States (even more than due to all cancers and pulmonary diseases combined). It accounts for one in three deaths and overall CAD prevalence is 6.7% (18.2 million) in US adults older than 20 years of age. The lifetime risk of developing CAD in those 40 years and older is predicted to be greater than 40% in men and greater than 30% in women.

4.2 The correct answer is C.
Rationale: Exercise myocardial perfusion imaging has a sensitivity of detecting obstructive CAD of 82% to 88% and is recommended for intermediate- to high-risk patients (American College of Cardiology Foundation/American Heart Association [ACCF/AHA] 2012 and European Society of Cardiology [ESC] 2013 Ib recommendation), especially if accompanied with a baseline interpretable ECG (ACCF/AHA 2012 and ESC 2013 class IIa recommendation). It is, however, important to remember that the severity of ischemia may be underestimated in multivessel or left main CAD that results in balanced flow reduction.

Exercise ECG sensitivity is reported to be 61% and carries a class I recommendation (ACC/AHA 2012 and ESC 2013) for intermediate-risk patients who are able to exercise adequately with baseline interpretable ECG (class III if patients are unable to exercise, using digoxin, or have an uninterpretable ECG).

The exercise stress echocardiography has a sensitivity of 70% to 85% with a specificity of 77% to 89% and has a class Ib recommendation for intermediate- to high-risk patients with an uninterpretable ECG. It allows one to assess the systolic and diastolic left ventricular (LV) function and its response to stress (**Table 4.1**).

TABLE 4.1 Noninvasive Functional Stress Testing Modalities and Guideline Recommendations

Testing Modality	Sensitivity and Specificity for Obstructive CAD	Benefits and Pitfalls	Guideline Recommendations ACCF/AHA 2012 and ESC 2013
Exercise electrocardiography	Sensitivity: 61%[a] Specificity: 70%-77%[b] *Performs well in low- to intermediate-risk group (risk 10%-60%).*	Prognostic findings: Exercise duration Chronotropic incompetence, HR recovery Angina Arrhythmias Blood pressure drop with exercise Extent and duration of ST changes	**Class I** for intermediate-risk patients **Class IIa** for low-risk patients **Class III** for patients who are unable to exercise, using digitalis or have uninterpretable ECG *Rated the same for ACCF and ESC guidelines.*
Exercise echocardiography	Sensitivity: 70%-85% Specificity: 77%-89%	Assessment of systolic and diastolic left ventricular function and response to stress	**Class Ib** for intermediate- to high-risk patients and uninterpretable ECG **Class IIa** (ESC) symptomatic patients with prior revascularization and to assess functional severity of intermediate coronary lesions
Dobutamine echocardiography	Sensitivity: 85%-90% Specificity: 79%-90%	Assesses viability better than exercise, favorable when there is resting wall motion abnormality	**Class Ia** for intermediate- to high-risk patients and unable to exercise **Class III** not recommended if patient is able to exercise and has interpretable ECG

TABLE 4.1   Noninvasive Functional Stress Testing Modalities and Guideline Recommendations (*continued*)

Testing Modality	Sensitivity and Specificity for Obstructive CAD	Benefits and Pitfalls	Guideline Recommendations ACCF/AHA 2012 and ESC 2013
Exercise myocardial perfusion imaging	Sensitivity: 82%-88% Specificity: 70%-88%	Balanced flow reduction may lead to underestimation of extent of ischemia in multivessel or left main coronary disease. Transient ischemic dilation, reduced poststress ejection fraction, and increased uptake in lung field can help identify severe CAD.	**Class Ib** for intermediate- to high-risk patients **Class IIa** for intermediate- to high-risk patients and interpretable ECG **Class III** for low-risk patients
Vasodilator[c] myocardial perfusion imaging	Sensitivity: 88%-91% Specificity: 75%-90%	Balanced flow reduction may lead to underestimation of extent of ischemia in multivessel or left main coronary disease.	**Class Ia** for intermediate to high risk and unable to exercise **Class III** not recommended if patient is able to exercise and has interpretable ECG
Cardiac magnetic resonance imaging with dobutamine or perfusion stress	Sensitivity: 88% Specificity: 72% Cardiac magnetic resonance angiography has shown good correlation with FFR measurements.	Not widely used	No recommendations

ACCF, American College of Cardiology Foundation; AHA, American Heart Association; CAD, coronary artery disease; ECG, electrocardiogram; ESC, European Society for Cardiology; FFR, fractional flow reserve; HR, heart rate.
[a]Valid in patients with normal electrocardiogram (ECG).
[b]Lower in women.
[c]Adenosine, regadenoson, or dipyridamole.
Compiled with data from Fihn SD, Gardin JM, Abrams J, et al. 2012 ACCF/AHA/ACP/AATS/PCNA/SCAI/STS Guideline for the diagnosis and management of patients with stable ischemic heart disease: a report of the American College of Cardiology Foundation/American Heart Association Task Force on Practice Guidelines, and the American College of Physicians, American Association for Thoracic Surgery, Preventive Cardiovascular Nurses Association, Society for Cardiovascular Angiography and Interventions, and Society of Thoracic Surgeons. *J Am Coll Cardiol*. 2012;60(24):e44-e164 and Montalescot G, Sechtem U, Achenbach S, et al. 2013 ESC guidelines on the management of stable coronary artery disease: The Task Force on the management of stable coronary artery disease of the European Society of Cardiology. *Eur Heart J*. 2013;34(38):2949-3003.

43. The correct answer is C.

Rationale: This is an intermediate-risk patient given his age and gender and, thus, consideration for CAD assessment can be with a noninvasive approach. In patients who can exercise adequately, functional stress testing is preferred as it provides additional information about prognosis based on threshold for ischemia, reproduction and correlation of symptoms, as well as exercise tolerance/capacity.

Vasodilator myocardial perfusion imaging and dobutamine echocardiography are not recommended if the patient is able to exercise and has an interpretable ECG (ACCF/AHA 2012 and ESC 2013 class III recommendation).

Cardiac MRI with dobutamine also would be preferred for those who cannot exercise but has limited availability.

44. The correct answer is B.

Rationale: All patients with stable CAD should be prescribed sublingual nitroglycerin or nitroglycerin spray for immediate anginal relief (class Ib recommendation). Beta-blockers are the first-line therapy for relief of ischemic symptoms in stable patients with CAD (class I recommendation) with titration for goal heart rate of 55 to 60 bpm. According to the Clinical Outcomes Utilizing Revascularization and Aggressive Drug Evaluation (COURAGE) trial, patients with greater than 70% CAD based on angiography and received a beta-blocker reported 22% improvement in their anginal symptoms. Abrupt discontinuation of beta-blockers is not recommended as it can worsen angina and precipitate acute coronary syndrome (ACS).

Long-acting nitrate formulations are offered and recommended after the maximum tolerated beta-blocker is not effective in providing anginal relief. The most common cause of failure of nitrate therapy is due to nitrate tolerance. Depending on the nitrate formulation, a 10- to 14-hour nitrate-free interval is indicated.

45. The correct answer is B.

Rationale: Ranolazine is metabolized within the liver and intestines and excreted through the kidney primarily, as well as through the GI system in the feces.

Ranolazine is a selective late sodium channel inhibitor and reduces sodium-dependent calcium currents within the ischemic myocardium and has antianginal efficacy when used as monotherapy or in combination with first- and second-line antianginal agents. It does have more potent effects in patients with elevated HbA_{1c}.

46. The correct answer is A.

Rationale: As per ACCF/AHA 2018 guidelines, patients with CAD should be treated with high-intensity statin therapy to reduce serum LDL cholesterol concentration by greater than 50% (class Ia recommendation). Rosuvastatin 10 mg is considered moderate-intensity statin, so the dose should be increased to a high-intensity dose, which is 20 mg or 40 mg daily.

In very high-risk patients (multiple major cardiovascular events or one major event with multiple high-risk conditions such as diabetes mellitus, smoking, chronic kidney disease, etc) who have serum LDL cholesterol greater than 70 mg/dL despite high-intensity statin therapy, addition of nonstatin therapy (class IIa recommendation, such as ezetimibe and PCSK-9 inhibitor) is reasonable.

4.7 The correct answer is B.
Rationale: In patients with stable CAD, addition of angiotensin-converting enzyme inhibitors (ACEIs) was found to reduce overall mortality, nonfatal myocardial infarction (MI), and heart failure by 20% to 28%. Given these findings, in adults with stable CAD who have systolic heart failure, hypertension, or diabetes mellitus, therapy with ACEI carries a class Ia recommendation.

Angiotensin receptor blocker (ARB) therapy is recommended for patients who are intolerant to ACEI (class Ia recommendation). Simultaneous use of ACEI and ARB is not recommended due to the high incidence of adverse outcomes.

4.8 The correct answer is A.
Rationale: According to the 2017 ACCF/AHA and 2018 ESC guidelines, patients with stable CAD should have a target of a systolic blood pressure less than 130 mm Hg and a diastolic blood pressure less than 80 mm Hg. Beta-blockers, ACEIs, and ARBs are class I antihypertensive therapeutic options for these patients and thus should be the initial choices.

4.9 The correct answer is D.
Rationale: A survival benefit with coronary revascularization has been apparent in the following cases with class Ia recommendation: (1) left main diameter stenosis 50% or greater, (2) proximal LAD stenosis 70% diameter stenosis or more plus one other major coronary artery, (3) three-vessel disease with significant 70% diameter stenosis or greater. It is reasonable with class IIa recommendation to revascularize for survival benefit in cases of two major coronary arteries with 70% diameter stenosis or greater with extensive myocardial ischemia as well.

Revascularization to improve survival is not recommended (class III recommendation) in cases of single-vessel disease of the left circumflex or right coronary artery without proximal LAD involvement with a small area of viable myocardium or ischemia.

4.10 The correct answer is C.
Rationale: This is a patient who has a medical history that includes hospitalization for ACS, which resulted in the placement of a drug-eluting stent. Clinical evaluation is recommended every 4 to 6 months during the first year and at least annually thereafter, with a focus on continuing evidence-based medical management, implementing risk factor modifications, assessing adherence and effectiveness of prescribed therapies, and monitoring symptoms and assessing progression of disease. An annual evaluation should include ECG, HbA_{1c} measurement, lipid panel, basic metabolic panel as well as hepatic panel, and administration of annual influenza vaccine.

An echocardiogram should be considered after revascularization to assess LV function, which this patient has completed. Routine echocardiography is not recommended for stable patients with no change in clinical status.

Routine stress testing at an interval less than 2 years after PCI and less than 5 years after coronary artery bypass graft (CABG) is not recommended with class III. Thereafter, noninvasive testing should be guided depending on clinical suspicion and the patient's risk profile.

UNSTABLE ANGINA, NON–ST-ELEVATION MYOCARDIAL INFARCTION–ACUTE CORONARY SYNDROME*

Natasha Babar, Ravi Kiran Vutheeri, and Anthony Gerald Nappi

CHAPTER 5

QUESTIONS

5.1 In which of the following patients with chest pain would it be appropriate to take an early conservative approach?
- A. A 75-year-old male smoker with hypertension who presents with substernal chest pain, electrocardiogram (ECG) showing horizontal ST-segment depression of 2 mm in the anterior leads, and hs-troponin I level above reference range.
- B. A 55-year-old man with hypertension that has been well controlled, never smoker, who presents with one episode of chest pain that occurred approximately 6 hours prior. The ECG is without ST-segment changes and hs-troponin I levels are within normal range.
- C. A 65-year-old female with poorly controlled diabetes who presents with recurrent nausea, vomiting, and epigastric pain for 3 days. ECG shows sinus bradycardia and ST-segment depression in inferior leads. Blood pressure is 90/54 mm Hg.
- D. An 80-year-old male with a 30 pack-year smoking history presents in respiratory distress, with soft blood pressures, and a continuous murmur over the third left intercostal space that radiates to the axilla. An ECG shows q waves in the inferior leads. He reports an episode of intermittent anterior chest pain 3 days prior to presentation.

5.2 Which of the following is **NOT** a part of the Thrombolysis in Myocardial Infarction (TIMI) risk stratification tool for non–ST-elevation myocardial infarction (NSTEMI)?
- A. ST depression on ECG
- B. Elevated cardiac biomarkers
- C. More than one anginal equivalents in the past 24 hours
- D. Use of aspirin in the past 7 days

5.3 When compared to clopidogrel, which of the following characteristics is/are unique to prasugrel?
- A. Absence of genetic polymorphisms in the cytochrome P450 enzyme responsible for conversion to the active drug
- B. Prodrug that requires conversion through the cytochrome P450 enzyme system to its active metabolite
- C. Lower risk of cardiovascular death and nonfatal myocardial infarction
- D. Both A and C are correct.
- E. All the following are correct.

*Questions and Answers are based on Chapter 5: Unstable Angina, Non–ST-Elevation Myocardial Infarction-Acute Coronary Syndrome by Talal T. Attar and Rebecca Miller in Cardiovascular Medicine and Surgery, First Edition.

CHAPTER 5 | Unstable Angina, Non–ST-Elevation Myocardial Infarction

5.4 In which of the following situations should prasugrel be avoided?
   A. In patients with a history of cerebrovascular accidents
   B. In patients who present with an acute coronary syndrome (ACS) who are being managed with an early conservative approach
   C. In patients older than 75 years of age
   D. In patients that weigh less than 60 kg
   E. All of the above

5.5 Which of the following medications reversibly bind and inhibit the P2Y12 receptor on the surface of platelets?
   A. Clopidogrel
   B. Prasugrel
   C. Ticagrelor
   D. Cangrelor
   E. Both C and D are correct.

5.6 In which scenario should the use of nitroglycerin be avoided when treating an ACS?
   A. A patient with ST-segment elevations in leads II and III, blood pressure of 90/50 mm Hg, clear lungs, and distended neck veins on examination
   B. A male patient who admits to using tadalafil 36 hours prior
   C. A patient with at least 1 mm of ST-segment elevation in V4R on a right-sided ECG
   D. Both A and C are correct.
   E. All of the above

5.7 Early addition of the following intervention can lead to improved endothelial function, decreased coronary vascular inflammation, and reduced platelet aggregation?
   A. Aspirin
   B. P2Y12 inhibitor
   C. Statins
   D. Beta-blockers

5.8 A 55-year-old man with a long history of cigarette smoking and poorly controlled hypertension presents to the emergency department complaining of substernal chest pressure that started 2 hours prior while mowing his lawn. He denies a history of diabetes mellitus, kidney failure, or prior stroke. On examination, he appears mildly anxious, has a blood pressure of 150/90 mm Hg, heart rate of 90 bpm, clear lungs, and S_4 gallop is heard on auscultation. His ECG shows sinus rhythm with 1-mm ST-segment depressions in the inferolateral leads and serum hs-troponin I levels are just above the reference range. A diagnosis of an NSTEMI is made with plans to take the patient to the *catheterization* lab in the next hour. Which of the following treatment regimens is the most appropriate for this patient at the time of presentation?
   A. Aspirin 325 mg, ticagrelor 180 mg, heparin intravenous (IV), and metoprolol 25 mg twice daily
   B. Aspirin 325 mg, prasugrel 60 mg, heparin IV, and metoprolol 25 mg twice daily
   C. Aspirin 325 mg, clopidogrel 300 mg, tirofiban IV, heparin IV, and metoprolol 25 mg bid
   D. Aspirin 325 mg, clopidogrel 600 mg, tirofiban IV, heparin IV, and metoprolol 25 mg bid

5.9 The use of which of the following anticoagulants is considered appropriate in the setting of ACS?
  A. Low-molecular-weight heparin
  B. Unfractionated heparin
  C. Bivalirudin
  D. Fondaparinux
  E. All answer choices are correct.

5.10 As compared to patients with NSTEMI treated medically, those treated with early revascularization have the following advantage(s):
  A. Lower rates of recurrent hospitalization
  B. Lower rates of recurrent unstable angina
  C. Lower rates of myocardial infarction and death
  D. All of the above are true.

ANSWERS

5.1 The correct answer is B:
Rationale: An early conservative approach can appropriately be utilized for patients with limited coronary artery disease risk factors, with negative troponins, and in the absence of ECG changes. A single episode of chest pain that self-resolves and lasts many hours is reassuring as opposed to multiple episodes that are short-lived. Risk factors that increase the likelihood of ACS include hypertension, hyperlipidemia, and smoking history. It is important to remember that women with ACS may not always present with typical features of angina including substernal chest pain, radiation to the left arm, jaw pain, and diaphoresis; a high index of suspicion and thorough cardiac workup should be considered in such circumstances, particularly in women presenting with unexplained gastrointestinal symptoms. Late-presentation myocardial infarction should be suspected in any patient with respiratory distress with a new murmur and q waves on ECG. These patients can be prone to quick decompensation, and an early conservative approach would not be appropriate.

5.2 The correct answer is C:
Rationale: The TIMI risk stratification tool helps predict 30-day and 1-year mortality in patients with NSTEMI. It is 1-point scoring system based on a patient's risk factors used to determine timing of left heart catheterization in patients with NSTEMI. A single point is given for each of the following: (a) age older than 65; (b) greater than three risk factors for CAD; (c) history of CAD; (d) ST changes greater than 0.5 mm on ECG; (e) more than two episodes of angina within 24 hours; (f) use of aspirin within the past 7 days; and (g) elevated cardiac biomarkers. A cumulative score of 0 to 2 corresponds to low-risk, 3 to 4 with intermediate risk, and greater than 4 with high risk. Patients in the moderate- to high-risk category should be considered for early (within 24 hours) catheterization and intervention. A patient with multiple episodes of chest pain raise the suspicion for significant coronary artery disease and these patients can benefit from an early invasive versus delayed invasive approach (**Table 5.1**).

TABLE 5.1 TIMI Risk Score for NSTE-ACS

Present on Admission	Points
Age older than 65	1
Greater than three risk factors for coronary artery disease	1
Prior coronary artery disease	1
ST elevation on ECG	1
Greater than two angina events in the past 24 hours	1
Use of aspirin in the past 7 days	1
Elevated cardiac biomarkers	1
TOTAL POINTS	7 possible

ECG, electrocardiogram; NSTE-ACS, non–ST-elevation myocardial infarction-acute coronary syndrome; TIMI, thrombolysis in myocardial infarction.

5.3 The correct answer is D.
Rationale: Both clopidogrel and prasugrel are prodrugs that require conversion through the cytochrome P450 enzyme system to their active metabolites. Prasugrel has a faster onset of action as it is metabolized to the active form by esterases and the cytochrome P450 system during intestinal absorption, whereas clopidogrel is activated by the cytochrome P450 system in the liver, following intestinal absorption. Prasugrel also has greater antithrombotic effect than clopidogrel owing in part to genetic polymorphisms within the cytochrome P450 system responsible for clopidogrel's activation, which lead to variability in clopidogrel's antiplatelet response. Prasugrel has also been shown to carry a lower risk of cardiovascular death, nonfatal myocardial infarction, urgent target vessel revascularization, and stent thrombosis when compared to clopidogrel.[1] However, prasugrel carries a higher bleeding risk and should be avoided in certain high-risk populations. This includes patients with a history of cerebrovascular accident (with or without hemorrhage), patients older than 75 years, and patients with low body weight.

5.4 The correct answer is E.
Rationale: Prasugrel is contraindicated in patients with a history of any cerebrovascular accident/stroke whether hemorrhagic or not, in those older than 75 years, and those less than 60 kg as this group of patients has been shown to have lower clinical benefit of prasugrel and increased major bleeding risk.[1] Patients being managed with an early conservative approach should not be treated with prasugrel as its use is limited to cases where the anatomy is known (ST-elevation myocardial infarction) and when percutaneous intervention is planned. For this reason, prasugrel is often referred to as a *cardiac catheterization lab drug*.

5.5 The correct answer is E.
Rationale: Clopidogrel and prasugrel are two irreversible inhibitors of platelet P2Y12 receptors available in oral form. As such, patients treated with clopidogrel and prasugrel often require a 5- to 7-day "washout" period (the time it takes for platelets to turn over) prior to major surgery, including coronary artery bypass surgery. Cangrelor is an IV antiplatelet that acts as a reversible competitive inhibitor of P2Y12 receptors and has a very short half-life of 3 to 5 minutes, allowing for rapid cessation of action once the infusion is turned off. Ticagrelor is an oral P2Y12 inhibitor with reversible and noncompetitive inhibition of the P2Y12 receptor. Bentracimab, an IV medication, is now available for ticagrelor reversal. More widespread use of bentracimab is limited by the high cost associated with its use ($10,000-20,000 per dose).

5.6 The correct answer is E.
Rationale: Nitroglycerin and other nitrates should be avoided in cases of hypotension and where right-sided ventricular failure due to myocardial infarction is suspected (ST elevations on a right-sided ECG). These patients are preload dependent and nitrate-mediated venodilation can lead to severe hypotension and hemodynamic compromise. Use of nitrates is also contraindicated in patients taking phosphodiesterase 5 (PDE5) inhibitors including sildenafil, tadalafil, and vardenafil due to risk of severe hypotension. Importantly, sildenafil and vardenafil require a 24-hour washout period, whereas tadalafil requires a 48-hour washout period prior to the use of nitrates.

5.7 The correct answer is C.
Rationale: Early addition of statins should be considered in cases of ACS given their pleiotropic effects, including anti-inflammatory effect on coronary vasculature, improved endothelial function, and ability to reduce platelet aggregation. These pleiotropic characteristics of statins may allow for improved reflow after coronary vessel intervention, leading to a reduction in the no-reflow phenomenon.[2] In addition, the Pravastatin or Atorvastatin Evaluation and Infection Therapy–Thrombolysis In Myocardial Infarction 22 trial (PROVE IT-TIMI 22) showed that an aggressive approach with high-intensity statins (atorvastatin 80 mg) compared to moderate-intensity statins (pravastatin 40 mg) leads to a reduction in 30-day cardiac events including death, myocardial infarction, or rehospitalization in patients with ACS.[3]

5.8 The correct answer is A.
Rationale: Patients with NSTEMI can be appropriately loaded with the antiplatelets ticagrelor and clopidogrel. Prasugrel should only be used after the coronary anatomy is known such as in the case of ST-elevation myocardial infarction thus should not be used for treatment of NSTEMI. It is important to remember that anatomic localization of culprit lesions is not possible from surface ECGs unless ST elevations are present. Tirofiban and eptifibatide are GIIbIIIa inhibitors that prevent platelet-fibrinogen binding and are used when there is angiographic evidence of large thrombus burden or poor reflow following revascularization.

5.9 The correct answer is E.

Rationale: Although unfractionated heparin is often used for clinical management of ACS, low-molecular-weight heparin (eg, enoxaparin), and bivalirudin, (direct thrombin inhibitors), and fondaparinux (antithrombin III activator) are all forms of anticoagulation that can be used for treatment of ACS. Bivalirudin, argatroban, and fondaparinux should be considered in patients with ACS and a history of heparin-induced thrombocytopenia. Heparin products however are generally preferred over bivalirudin due to the latters higher price. Bivalirudin is also generally considered a cardiac catherterization lab drug and is reserved for patients. It is important to remember that when used as treatment for NSTEMI, low-molecular-weight heparin (and fondaparinux) must be continued for the duration of index hospitalization or until coronary angiogram/percutaneous coronary intervention is achieved. This is opposed to the use of unfractionated heparin, which is continued for 48 hours only.

5.10 The correct answer is D.

Rationale: In patients with NSTEMI, early revascularization therapy compared to medical management alone has shown lower rates of recurrent hospitalization, lower rates of unstable angina, and lower rates of myocardial infarction and death in randomized controlled trials and meta-analyses.[4] An early invasive approach is appropriate in patients with typical cardiovascular risk factors, with ST changes on ECG, with multiple episodes of chest pain within 24 hours and with troponin leak.

REFERENCES

1. Wiviott SD, Braunwald E, McCabe CH, et al. Prasugrel versus clopidogrel in patients with acute coronary syndromes. N Engl J Med. 2007;357(20):2001-2015. PMID: 17982182.
2. Iwakura K, Ito H, Kawano S, et al. Chronic pre-treatment of statins is associated with the reduction of the no-reflow phenomenon in the patients with reperfused acute myocardial infarction. Eur Heart J. 2006;27(5):534-539. PMID: 16401674.
3. Ray KK, Cannon CP, McCabe CH, et al. Early and late benefits of high-dose atorvastatin in patients with acute coronary syndromes: results from the PROVE IT-TIMI 22 trial. J Am Coll Cardiol. 2005;46(8):1405-1410. PMID: 16226162.
4. Bavry AA, Kumbhani DJ, Rassi AN, et al. Benefit of early invasive therapy in acute coronary syndromes: a meta-analysis of contemporary randomized clinical trials. J Am Coll Cardiol. 2006;48(7):1319-1325. PMID: 17010789.

ST-ELEVATION MYOCARDIAL INFARCTION*

Natasha Babar, Ravi Kiran Vutheeri, and Anthony Gerald Nappi

CHAPTER 6

QUESTIONS

6.1 Each of the following insults can present as acute ST-elevation myocardial infarction (STEMI) **EXCEPT**?

   A. Rupture or erosion of an unstable coronary plaque
   B. Air embolization
   C. Cocaine use
   D. Ascending thoracic aortic dissection
   E. All answer choices are correct

6.2 Which of the following electrocardiogram (ECG) patterns is concerning for significant left main coronary artery occlusion?

   A. New left bundle branch block
   B. Isolated ST depressions in leads V_1-V_3
   C. PR elevation in lead aVR (augmented vector right)
   D. Diffuse ST depression greater than 1 mm in multiple precordial leads with ST elevation in aVR

6.3 Fibrinolysis therapy for STEMI should **NOT** be considered in which of the following circumstances?

   A. Onset of symptoms at less than 12 hours
   B. In a patient with history of ischemic stroke 3 months ago
   C. Nearest percutaneous coronary intervention (PCI)-capable cardiac catheterization laboratory is more than 120 minutes away.
   D. In a patient with no history of intracranial hemorrhage

6.4 An 80-year-old male with a history of MI status post drug-eluting stent more than 10 years ago, type 2 diabetes, hypertension, and active tobacco use presents with substernal chest pain of several hours duration. ECG reveals 2-mm ST depressions in leads V_1-V_3 with tall R waves. The nearest PCI-capable facility is 4 hours away. Which of the following is the appropriate course of action?

---

*Questions and Answers are based on Chapter 6: ST-Elevation Myocardial Infarction by Ranjan Dahal and Debabrata Mukherjee in Cardiovascular Medicine and Surgery, First Edition.

- A. Administer aspirin 325 mg + clopidogrel 600 mg + fibrinolytic therapy + unfractionated heparin and transfer patient.
- B. Administer aspirin 325 mg + clopidogrel 75 mg + fibrinolytic therapy + unfractionated heparin and transfer patient.
- C. Administer aspirin 325 mg + clopidogrel 300 mg + fibrinolytic therapy + unfractionated heparin and transfer patient.
- D. Administer aspirin 325 mg + clopidogrel 75 mg + unfractionated heparin and transfer patient.

6.5 Which of the following indicates failure of thrombolytic therapy?
- A. Accelerated idioventricular rhythm within 2 hours of alteplase (tPA) administration
- B. A 25% reduction in the largest ST-segment elevation within 60 to 90 minutes
- C. Resolution of chest pain
- D. All of the above are correct

6.6 The following is an absolute contraindication to the use of prasugrel in patients requiring dual antiplatelet therapy?
- A. Active bleeding
- B. Prior stroke/transient ischemic attack (TIA)
- C. Hypersensitivity reaction
- D. Unknown coronary anatomy
- E. All of the above are correct.

6.7 **CORRECTLY** match the following clinical scenarios with the associated appropriate time frames for patients with STEMI:

Clinical Scenarios
1. Time to fibrinolysis response evaluation
2. Timing of left heart catheterization following successful thrombolysis
3. Door-to-balloon time in patients transferred without thrombolytic therapy
4. Door-to-balloon time at patient's first medical contact facility with PCI capability

Time Frames
A. 3 to 24 hours
B. 60 to 90 minutes
C. 90 minutes
D. 4 to less than 120 minutes

- A. 1-B, 2-A, 3-D, 4-C
- B. 1-A, 2-B, 3-C, 4-D
- C. 1-D, 2-C, 3-B, 4-A
- D. 1-C, 2-B, 3-A, 4-D

6.8 Which of the following is **TRUE** concerning the use of cangrelor?
- A. It is a reversible intravenous P2Y12 inhibitor.
- B. It should be considered during PCI when other P2Y12 inhibitors have not been administered and if the patient is not receiving a glycoprotein (GP)IIb/IIIa inhibitor.
- C. Its use should be limited to the cardiac catheterization laboratory.
- D. Its use requires switching to an oral P2Y12 inhibitor following PCI.
- E. All of the above are correct.

6.9 A 55-year-old female with no significant past medical history other than family history of premature coronary artery disease, collapses while running a 1K marathon. She is pulseless and bystander CPR is performed. EMS arrives within 10 minutes. An automated external defibrillator (AED) is placed, and the patient is found to be in ventricular tachycardia. Return of spontaneous circulation is achieved in approximately 30 minutes following collapse after 2 shocks were delivered from the AED. Post-arrest EKG reveals 3mm ST elevations in the lateral leads with reciprocal ST depressions in the inferior leads. The post-arrest vital sign check reveals hypotension to 65/40 mmHg. Norepinephrine drip is started to maintain mean arterial pressure >65 mmHg. She is intubated (and sedated) for airway protection and is transferred to the nearest percutaneous coronary intervention (PCI) capable hospital. What is the next best course of action?

A. Admit to cardiac intensive care unit (ICU) and start targeted temperature management. Perform PCI only if purposeful brain activity returns after 24 hours of cooling.
B. Perform urgent revascularization in the setting of postarrest STEMI and cardiogenic shock.
C. Admit to cardiac ICU and wean sedation daily. Perform PCI during index hospitalization only if purposeful brain activity is noted off sedation.
D. Given current mental status and shock state, treat medically with aspirin and antiplatelet load and continuous heparin infusion. Perform PCI only if shock state resolves and mental status improves.

6.10 A 39-year-old female with a past medical history of hypertension and active tobacco use (quarter pack of cigarettes a day) presents to the emergency department with 3 hours of substernal chest pressure with associated nausea, vomiting, and diaphoresis. ECG reveals 1-mm ST elevation in leads II, III, and aVF. High-sensitivity troponin is elevated at 600 ng/L. She is loaded with aspirin and clopidogrel and started on heparin infusion. An urgent left heart catheterization is performed and reveals 30% occlusion of proximal right coronary artery. What is the **MOST LIKELY** diagnosis?

A. Cardiac syndrome X
B. MI with nonobstructive coronary artery (MINOCA) disease due to coronary artery dissection
C. MINOCA disease due to coronary artery vasospasm
D. All of the above are possible.

ANSWERS

6.1 The correct answer is E.
Rationale: A common etiology for acute STEMI includes rupture of unstable coronary artery plaque. Plaques that are less calcified and thus less stable are more prone to rupture compared to plaques that have higher calcium content. Lesser known causes of STEMI include air embolization from instrumentation such as during or following diagnostic left heart catheterization, coronary artery vasospasm in the setting of cocaine use (a vasoactive drug), ascending aortic dissection with proximal extension to the level of the coronary arteries, and SCAD. Although treatment may differ depending on etiology of STEMI, prompt diagnostic left heart catheterization is indicated in the setting of any STEMI.

6.2 The correct answer is D.
Rationale: Diffuse ST depressions with ST elevation in aVR on a 12-lead ECG should raise concern for either left main coronary artery disease or multivessel coronary artery disease and should prompt further ischemic evaluation. New left bundle branch block was previously considered a STEMI equivalent but current practice does not support this ideology. A new left bundle branch block with other evidence of ischemia by history or examination raises suspicion for significant coronary artery disease but not does not specifically correspond to left main involvement. Isolated ST depressions in the anterior lead cannot be localized to a certain coronary artery distribution as localization is only possible with ST elevations on a surface ECG. An isolated elevation in the PR interval in lead aVR can be seen in the case of acute pericarditis but does not correspond with ischemia in the left-sided coronary system (**Table 6.1**).

TABLE 6.1 Electrocardiographic Criteria for ST-Elevation Myocardial Infarction

- New ST-segment elevation at the J point in two contiguous leads with the cutoff point as >0.1 mV in all leads other than V_2 or V_3.
- In leads V_2-V_3, the cutoff point is ST-segment elevation >0.2 mV in men older than 40 y and >0.25 in men younger than 40 y, or >0.15 mV in women.

Left bundle branch block
- ST-segment elevation of ≥1 mm that is concordant with (in the same direction as) the QRS complex
- ST-segment depression of ≥1 mm in leads V_1, V_2, or V_3
- ST-segment elevation of ≥5 mm that is discordant with (in the opposite direction) the QRS complex

Ventricular-paced rhythm
Left bundle branch block (LBBB) pattern seen during isolated right ventricular (RV) pacing. Same diagnostic criteria as LBBB may be helpful.

Isolated posterior myocardial infarction
Isolated ST depression ≥0.5 mm in V_1-V_3 and ST-segment elevation ≥0.5 mm in posterior leads V_7-V_9

Ischemia owing to left main coronary artery occlusion or multivessel disease
ST-segment depression ≥1 mm in multiple leads along with ST elevation in aVR (augmented vector right)

Right ventricular infarction
ST-segment elevation ≥1 mm in right precordial leads V_3R and V_4R

6.3 The correct answer is B.

Rationale: Every patient who presents with a STEMI at a presenting center that is not capable of PCI should be considered for lytic therapy in the absence of certain contraindications if the nearest PCI-capable center is more than 120 minutes away. Absolute contraindications for the use of lytic therapy includes ischemic stroke within 3 months (except for acute stroke within 4.5 hours in which lytics can be used therapeutically), active bleeding or history of bleeding disorders, significant facial trauma or closed head trauma within 3 months, presence of malignant intracranial neoplasm, and cerebral vascular malformations such as arteriovenous malformations. Relative contraindications include blood pressures greater than 180/100, dementia, noncompressible vascular punctures, and pregnancy (**Figure 6.1**).

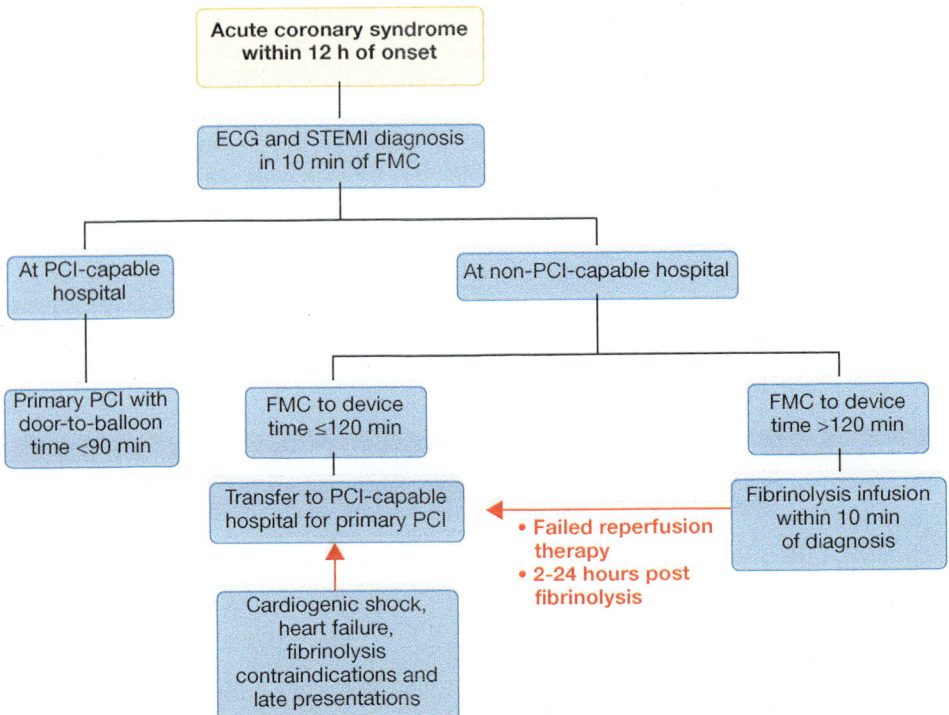

Figure 6.1 Management strategies for patients with STEMI. ECG, electrocardiogram; FMC, first medical contact; PCI, percutaneous coronary intervention; STEMI, ST-elevation myocardial infarction.

6.4 The correct answer is B.

Rationale: This patient with anterior ST depressions and tall R waves is likely having a posterior STEMI that can be additionally accessed with a posterior ECG. Patients who present with STEMI at a non-PCI-capable facility should receive lytic therapy prior to transfer if a PCI-capable laboratory is more than 120 minutes away. The following recommendations are based on age. For patients younger than 75 years of age, an aspirin load of 325 mg with clopidogrel 300 mg is recommended along with initiation of full-dose anticoagulation (whether low-molecular weight heparin, unfractionated heparin, or direct thrombin inhibitors). For patients 75 years of age or older, a Plavix load of 75 mg should be used with the remainder of recommendations as above.

6.5 The correct answer is B.
Rationale: ECG evidence for successful thrombolysis after lytic therapy includes greater than 50% reduction in the largest ST-segment elevation within a response time of at least 90 minutes. An accelerated idioventricular rhythm, which is often confused for a slow wide complex tachycardia, is also a marker of successful reperfusion in patients who have received lytic therapy. This rhythm should not be confused with monomorphic ventricular tachycardia, which can be seen in cases of ischemia or infarction. In patients with STEMI who have successfully responded to lytic therapy, a cardiac catheterization should be considered within 3 to 24 hours to assess coronary anatomy and further need for percutaneous intervention.

6.6 The correct answer is E.
Rationale: Prasugrel is from the thienopyridine drug class and acts as an irreversible antagonist of the platelet adenosine diphosphate (ADP) P2Y12 receptor, preventing platelet aggregation. Prasugrel carries an increased risk of hemorrhage and should be avoided in the case of active bleeding, prior stroke/TIA, known hypersensitivity, and when coronary artery anatomy is unknown such as in the case of non-STEMI. Prasugrel can be used in the setting of STEMI where ST changes on ECG are localized to specific coronary artery territories and thus correspond to known anatomy. In addition, prasugrel has been shown to increase risk of bleeding particularly in patients with prior stroke (not limited to hemorrhagic stroke), age older than 75 years, and body weight less than 60 mg and should be avoided in these populations.

6.7 The correct answer is A.
Rationale: The ideal door-to-balloon time in patients with STEMI in a PCI-capable facility is 90 minutes or less. Ideal door-to-balloon time in patients requiring transfer to a PCI-capable facility is less than 120 minutes. This timing is necessary in order to forgo administration of lytic therapy in patients with STEMI and lytic therapy becomes indicated if the nearest PCI-capable facility is more than 120 minutes away. The rule of "12s" is often used to recall the indications for lytic therapy including presentation within 12 hours of chest pain onset and timing of more than 120 minutes from nearest PCI-capable facility. Common fibrinolytic therapies used for treatment of STEMI include tenecteplase (TNK-PA), reteplase (rPA), and alteplase (tPA).

In patients who receive lytic therapy, response to therapy should be evaluated within 60 to 90 minutes of lytic administration and cardiac catheterization should be considered within 24 hours of positive response to lytics. If there is a failure in response to lytic therapy, urgent PCI needs to be arranged.

6.8 The correct answer is E.
Rationale: Cangrelor is an intravenous platelet P2Y12 receptor inhibitor. One of the benefits of cangrelor, unlike other commonly used P2Y12 inhibitors, is that it is reversible and has a short half-life of 3 to 5 minutes with an easy "on" and "off" use. Patients treated with cangrelor in the cardiac catheterization laboratory require switch to an oral P2Y12 following PCI either to ticagrelor, prasugrel, or

clopidogrel with appropriate loading doses. Patients should be loaded with prasugrel (60 mg) or clopidogrel (600 mg) immediately following discontinuation of cangrelor infusion, whereas ticagrelor (180 mg) can be loaded either during or after cangrelor infusion.

6.9 The correct answer is B.

Rationale: Postarrest STEMI and cardiogenic shock following STEMI are both indications for urgent and emergent revascularization, respectively. Although mental status is an important prognostic indicator following cardiac arrest, it should not delay cardiac catheterization in patients with out-of-hospital cardiac arrest who have shockable rhythms and STEMI on presentation. On the contrary, patients with out-of-hospital cardiac arrest with shockable rhythm, without STEMI can undergo delayed angiography. The Coronary Angiography After Cardiac Arrest (COACT) trial, published in *JAMA* (2020), was a randomized controlled trial on patients with out-of-hospital cardiac arrest with shockable rhythm without ECG evidence of STEMI. The COACT study revealed that delayed angiography was noninferior to early angiography in patients with cardiac arrest with shockable rhythm who did not present with ST elevations. Patients who underwent delayed revascularization (after neurologic recovery or move out of the ICU, on average 121 hours or ~5 days) were shown to have similar survival and cerebral recovery to patients who underwent early revascularization.

6.10 The correct answer is C.

Rationale: This patient likely has MI due to nonobstructive coronary artery disease, likely provoked due to coronary vasospasm from active smoking. Coronary artery dissection carries a high probability with increased risk in women and smokers; however, it is ruled out by invasive angiography. Cardiac syndrome X describes a syndrome most often seen in perimenopausal or postmenopausal women who present with anginal and, in some cases, atypical chest pain and are found to have no sign of coronary artery disease on invasive ischemic evaluation. The underlying pathology of cardiac syndrome X is thought to be due to microvascular disease. This patient has signs of nonobstructive coronary artery disease on her left heart.

SUGGESTED READINGS

Lemkes JS, Janssens GN, van der Hoeven NW, et al. Coronary angiography after cardiac arrest without ST segment elevation: one-year outcomes of the COACT randomized clinical trial. *JAMA Cardiol*. 2020;5(12):1358-1365. PMID: 32876654.

ACUTE MYOCARDIAL INFARCTION COMPLICATIONS*

Natasha Babar, Ravi Kiran Vuthoori, and Anthony Gerald Nappi

CHAPTER 7

QUESTIONS

7.1 A 56-year-old man with a history of hyperlipidemia presents to the emergency department with substernal chest pressure and shortness of breath that started 2 hours prior while he was at work. An electrocardiogram (ECG) shows an acute anterior wall myocardial infarction (MI) and an ST-segment elevation myocardial infarction (STEMI) code is activated. He is taken emergently to the laboratory where he is found to have an occluded proximal left anterior descending (LAD) artery. The remaining coronary arteries are widely patent. The LAD artery is successfully revascularized in the laboratory with placement of a drug-eluting stent to the vessel. The procedure is uncomplicated, and the patient has relief of his chest pain with resolution of the ST-segment elevations. A left ventriculogram shows akinesis of the anterior wall and apex with a left ventricular ejection fraction (LVEF) estimated to be 35%. He was then admitted to the coronary care unit and was given standard medical therapy including beta-blocker and statin. Within 30 minutes of the patient arriving at the unit, you get a call from the patient's nurse that he is having runs of a wide complex tachycardia at a rate of about 105 beats per minute (bpm). The blood pressure is 130/80 mm Hg, and the patient is not reporting recurrent chest pain. Which of the following interventions is recommended next?

A. Amiodarone intravenous (IV) bolus followed by a continuous drip
B. Emergent return to the cath lab for suspected acute stent thrombosis
C. Lidocaine IV bolus followed by a drip
D. Continued observation with no further intervention
E. Consult electrophysiology for urgent implantable cardioverter-defibrillator (ICD)

7.2 Acute mechanical complications of MI including ventricular free wall rupture, ventricular septal rupture, and papillary muscle rupture have which of the following bimodal presentations?

A. More than 24 hours and within 1 month of insult
B. 24 hours or less and within 1 week of insult
C. More than 48 hours and within 1 month of insult
D. More than 48 hours and within 1 week of insult

---

*Questions and Answers are based on Chapter 7: Acute Myocardial Infarction: Complications by Retesh Bajaj, Anantharaman Ramasamy, Vincenzo Tufaro, and Arjun K. Ghoshin in Cardiovascular Medicine and Surgery, First Edition.

73 Which of the following is a risk factor for cardiac free wall rupture?
A. Female sex
B. Age
C. First MI
D. No smoking history
E. All the above are correct.

74 All the following are true concerning papillary muscle rupture in the setting of acute MI **EXCEPT**:
A. The absence of a murmur heard on examination should not rule out the diagnosis.
B. It is most likely to occur in a patient with an anterior wall MI and occluded LAD artery.
C. This complication usually occurs between 2 and 7 days of the acute insult.
D. Resultant acute mitral regurgitation can present as severe respiratory compromise due to pulmonary congestion.

75 A 56-year-old female with a past medical history of hypertension, uncontrolled type 2 diabetes mellitus, and 20 pack-year smoking history presents with 1 week of severe nausea, epigastric pain, and dyspnea. ECG shows 2-mm ST elevations in leads V_1 to V_2. She is brought to the cardiac catheterization lab and an occluded LAD artery is successfully opened with placement of a drug-eluting stent. Two days later, she is noted to be hypotensive to 80/40 mm Hg with distant heart sounds, elevated jugular venous distension (JVD) and pulsus paradoxus. A bedside point-of-care ultrasound reveals a left-to-right ventricular shunt with a large circumferential pericardial effusion. Which of the following is the next **BEST** course of action?
A. Computed tomography (CT) scan of the chest
B. Urgent cardiac surgery consult for surgical intervention and possible ventricular septal defect patching
C. Repeat coronary angiogram to assess for possibility of coronary rupture
D. Urgent pericardiocentesis and placement of an intra-aortic balloon pump (IABP) in the cath lab

76 A 70-year-old man with no significant medical history presents with 1 month of severe substernal chest pressure at rest and worse with exertion that feels "like the weight of an elephant." His chest pain was rated a 9/10 2 weeks prior but has now subsided to a 1/10. ECG shows 2-mm ST elevations in leads V_1 to V_5 with deep Q waves. He is taken to the cardiac catheterization lab and is found to have nonobstructive coronary artery disease without evidence of significant stenosis. Which one of the following was likely seen on the left ventriculogram?
A. Normal ejection fraction
B. Globally reduced ejection fraction
C. Reduced ejection fraction with segmental wall motion abnormalities
D. Apical ballooning consistent with apical aneurysm with segmental anterior wall motion abnormality and reduced ejection fraction

7.7 CORRECTLY match the following arrhythmias with the likely ischemic territory involved in acute MI:

Arrhythmias
1. Complete heart block
2. Mobitz I heart block
3. Mobitz II heart block with narrow qrs
4. Mobitz II heart block with wide qrs

Ischemic Territory
A. Atrioventricular (AV) node
B. Bundle of His
C. Inferior MI
D. Distal His-Purkinje system (anterior MI)

A. 1-C, 2-A, 3-B, 4-D
B. 1-A, 2-B, 3-C, 4-D
C. 1-D, 2-C, 3-B, 4-A
D. 1-B, 2-A, 3-D, 4-C

7.8 Which of the following risk factors is associated with the greatest risk of developing atrial fibrillation in the setting of acute MI?
A. Male gender
B. Advanced age
C. Presence of advanced heart failure
D. Heart rate greater than 100 bpm on admission

7.9 In which scenario should a permanent pacemaker be considered following acute MI?
A. Persistent complete heart block following anterior MI.
B. Complete heart block in a patient presenting with acute inferior MI
C. Type I second-degree AV block in a patient with an occluded dominant right coronary artery (RCA)
D. Both A and C are correct.
E. All the above are correct.

7.10 A 57-year-old male is evaluated 2 days for chest pain following anterior wall MI for which he underwent percutaneous coronary intervention with a drug-eluting stent to the LAD artery. The pain is left sided, 10/10, worse with inspiration, and decreases in intensity when he leans forward. On examination, the patient has a low-grade fever T_{max} 99.9, tachycardia to 109 bpm, and no pericardial friction rub can be appreciated. An ECG shows diffuse ST depressions in the precordial and inferior leads as well as 1-mm PR elevation in lead aVR. Creatinine function is normal. What is the next **BEST** course of action?
A. Supportive care only with as-needed Tylenol for fever and fluid hydration
B. Start ibuprofen 600 mg every 8 hours and colchicine 1-mg load.
C. Start aspirin 750 mg every 8 hours for 1 to 2 weeks.
D. Start oral prednisone 0.5 mg/kg/day for 1 week and assess response.

ANSWERS

71. The correct answer is D.
Rationale: This patient's rhythm likely represents an accelerated idioventricular rhythm (AIVR), which is a benign reperfusion rhythm that can be seen 1 to 2 hours following successful revascularization in patients with STEMI. Although this patient has risk factors for wide complex tachycardia, including severe left ventricular dysfunction, the absence of hemodynamic compromise and slower heart rate (heart rate between 50 and 110 bpm) in the setting of recent revascularization make AIVR more likely. As AIVR is a benign rhythm, it requires observation only and no further intervention is needed. Amiodarone and lidocaine would be appropriate to use in the setting of ischemic ventricular tachycardia but not in the case of AIVR. An ICD should be considered in patients following MI with ejection fraction 40% or less, 40 days following MI without revascularization, or 90 days following MI with revascularization.

72. The correct answer is B.
Rationale: Patients with acute mechanical complications of MI usually present within 24 hours and 1 week of insult. A high index of suspicion should exist for patients with unexplained hypotension, new murmurs, and flash pulmonary edema after acute MI as these can be due to mechanical complications. Ventricular free wall rupture can present as severe hemodynamic compromise and cardiogenic shock. At other times, ventricular free wall rupture may be more localized and, in some cases, may auto-seal as in the case of low-pressure, right ventricular involvement. Ventricular septal rupture may present as a new ventricular septal defect with a harsh machine-like murmur. Papillary muscle rupture can present as flash pulmonary edema in the setting of acute severe mitral regurgitation. These patients often have severe decompensated heart failure as their atria and pulmonary vasculature cannot accommodate the high regurgitant volume from acute-onset severe mitral regurgitation.

73. The correct answer is E.
Rationale: Female sex, older age, no smoking history, and first MI are all risk factors for left ventricular free wall rupture. Prior MI is believed to be a protective factor against free wall rupture in the setting of acute MI due to scar formation. Importantly, smoking serves as a protective factor against mechanical complications of acute MI including free wall rupture as smokers tend to have coronary artery collateralization in the setting of prior occlusive coronary artery disease.

74. The correct answer is B.
Rationale: The anterolateral papillary muscle of the mitral valve receives dual blood supply from the LAD artery and the left circumflex artery, whereas the posteromedial papillary muscle receives blood supply from a single coronary artery, either the posterior descending artery OR the left circumflex artery, but not both. Therefore, the posteromedial papillary muscle is 10 times more likely to rupture compared to the anterolateral papillary muscle. Papillary muscle rupture may not always present with a new murmur as there is rapid equalization of ventricular and atrial pressures in the setting of acute severe mitral regurgitation, leaving the atria with little time to adjust to an increased volume load. This equalization of atrial and ventricular pressures results

in a faint murmur of mitral regurgitation compared to the holosystolic murmur that is often heard in chronic mitral regurgitation. Papillary muscle rupture usually occurs within 2 to 7 days of acute myocardial insult. The acuity of the severe mitral regurgitation and the inability of the left atrium to accommodate large volumes in the acute setting can lead to flash pulmonary edema and result in respiratory compromise.

75. The correct answer is B.
Rationale: Mechanical complications of STEMI, including new ventricular septal defect, ventricular free wall rupture, and acute mitral valve regurgitation due to papillary muscle rupture require urgent cardiothoracic surgery evaluation and intervention. A CT scan would further delay treatment of clinical tamponade and is not indicated in this patient's case. Urgent pericardiocentesis, although indicated in the setting of tamponade, would not address the underlying etiology, which is a ventricular septal defect with likely ventricular free wall rupture leading to tamponade. Coronary rupture is an extremely rare phenomenon (~0.1%-0.4% of cases) and is not a common complication of STEMI.

76. The correct answer is D.
Rationale: This patient is presenting after a month of ongoing anginal chest pain. His ECG is concerning for a completed MI as delineated by the presence of Q waves; however, no significant coronary artery disease is found on his left heart catheterization. The presence of deep Q waves along with ST elevations in leads V_1 to V_5 raises concern for left ventricular aneurysm likely resulting from a late presentation of an anterior MI. It is likely that this patient had spontaneous reperfusion of his coronaries prior to presentation.

77. The correct answer is A.
Rationale: Heart block can be seen as a rare complication of acute MI and the type of heart block observed varies by the ischemic territory involved. Complete heart block most commonly results from inferior MI with involvement of the RCA, which supplies the sinoatrial (SA) node and the AV node in a right dominant heart. Infarction at the level of the AV node can result in Mobitz I heart block, whereas infarction below the AV node (His-Purkinje involvement) results in Mobitz II heart block. His-Purkinje involvement will result in a wide (vs narrow) complex Mobitz II heart block and is often seen in the setting of anterior MI.

78. The correct answer is C.
Rationale: Male gender, advanced age, and elevated heart rates above 100 bpm on presentation all qualify as risk factors associated with the development of atrial fibrillation in the setting of acute MI. The presence of advanced heart failure, however, carries the highest risk in this category.

79. The correct answer is A.
Rationale: Complete heart block following an inferior MI should resolve within 5 to 7 days of the acute insult and a permanent pacemaker is usually not required. Patients with high-degree AV block and complete heart block following anterior MIs should be considered for permanent pacemaker placement. Type I second-degree AV block (or Mobitz I heart block) is a benign phenomenon that does not require intervention unless the patient is symptomatic.

7.10 The correct answer is C.

Rationale: Nonsteroidal anti-inflammatory drugs (NSAIDs) other than aspirin interfere with early myocardial healing and scar formation and thus should be avoided early on following MI. Aspirin is thus the recommended drug of choice for post MI pericarditis. Colchicine should be added for late (1-2 weeks) versus early (2-4 days) post MI pericarditis and in cases of early post MI pericarditis that is refractory to aspirin alone (per European Society of Cardiology guidelines). Prednisone should be avoided as there is an increased risk of recurrent pericarditis with prednisone as well as an increased risk of myocardial rupture with prednisone following acute MI.

REFRACTORY ANGINA*

Natasha Babar, Ravi Kiran Vutheori, and Anthony Gerald Nappi

CHAPTER 8

QUESTIONS

8.1 Which of the following is a characteristic of refractory angina?
- A. Established coronary artery disease
- B. Persistent angina for more than 3 months
- C. Not controlled by traditional medical therapy
- D. All of the above are correct.

8.2 A 58-year-old woman with a past medical history of nonobstructive coronary artery disease (last catheterization 1 year ago) on optimal medical therapy including aspirin, statin, and beta-blockers and diet-controlled type 2 diabetes presents with exertional chest pain for 3 months. An electrocardiogram (ECG) shows 1-mm ST depressions in the inferior leads. A stress echocardiogram is conducted and shows normal ejection without wall motion abnormalities. Which of the following is likely the origin of the patient's chest pain?
- A. Obstruction of the right coronary artery
- B. Obstruction of the posterior descending artery
- C. Prearteriolar microvascular obstruction
- D. Obstruction of multiple epicardial coronary arteries

8.3 A 65-year-old male with a history of coronary artery disease status post percutaneous intervention with a drug-eluting stent more than 10 years ago, hypertension, and hyperlipidemia previously lost to follow-up presents to the clinic with exertional chest pain ongoing for about 1 year. Laboratory work shows a microcytic anemia at 10.5 (previously >13 before 2 years). He is currently on aspirin, a lipid-lowering agent, and on maximal beta-blockers. An ECG is obtained and the finding is within normal limits. A nuclear stress test is conducted and the result shows no focal area of ischemia. What is the next **BEST** option for addressing this patient's chest pain?
- A. Start a long-acting nitrate.
- B. Start ranolazine.
- C. Schedule a left heart catheterization.
- D. Investigate and treat underlying anemia.

---

*Questions and Answers are based on Chapter 8: Refractory Angina by Anbukarasi Maran, Katrina A. E. L. Bidwell, and Valerian Fernandes in Cardiovascular Medicine and Surgery, First Edition.

8.4 Which of the following is a contraindication to the use of ranolazine?
   A. A patient with nonalcoholic steatohepatitis with liver function enzymes 3 times more than the upper limit of normal
   B. A patient with chronic kidney disease with creatinine above normal baseline
   C. Both A and B are correct.
   D. A patient with heart failure with reduced ejection fraction

8.5 All of the following qualify as appropriate interventions for persistent substernal chest pain in a patient with nonobstructive coronary artery disease (otherwise on appropriate guideline directed medical therapy) **EXCEPT**:
   A. 30 mg of nifedipine
   B. 0.6 mg of sublingual nitroglycerin
   C. 120 mg of diltiazem
   D. 500 mg of ranolazine twice a day

8.6 Which of the following can be considered in a patient with a history of coronary artery disease with persistent anginal pain despite use of appropriate medical therapy including antianginals?
   A. Percutaneous coronary intervention of epicardial vessels with chronic total occlusion
   B. Transmyocardial laser revascularization
   C. Intravascular ultrasound to assess for operable lesions in a patient with nonobstructive coronary artery disease
   D. All of the above are correct.

ANSWERS

8.1 The correct answer is D.
Rationale: Refractory angina is described as angina that persists for more than 3 months in a patient with known coronary artery disease despite adequate medical therapy, including, but not limited to, beta-blockade, calcium channel blockade, and long-acting nitrates. Angina is also considered refractory when it persists despite the use of two first-line antianginal agents. Ion channel inhibitors are commonly added as second-line agents for patients with refractory angina pectoris despite beta-blockade or calcium channel blockade and nitrate therapy. Commonly used ion channel inhibitors for treatment of refractory angina pectoris include ranolazine and ivabradine. Ranolazine and ivabradine cause negative inotropy by inhibiting ion channels involved in the cardiac action potential. It is important to remember that sublingual nitroglycerin is a short-acting nitrate and technically does not count as a long-acting agent for the treatment of angina pectoris. Long-acting nitrates such as isosorbide mononitrate and isosorbide dinitrate should also be added to the sublingual nitroglycerin given to patients who suffer from refractory angina.

8.2 The correct answer is C.

Rationale: A surface ECG with ST depressions with a normal stress echocardiogram is reassuring. Recall that only ST-segment elevations can help localize ischemia, making answer choices A and B incorrect. Although the patient has diabetes, obstruction of multiple epicardial coronary arteries in the setting of controlled diabetes and a negative cardiac angiogram within the past year is unlikely. Answer choice C best explains this patient's refractory angina despite optimal medical therapy as microvascular obstruction, often caused by subendocardial ischemia, is the likely culprit in the absence of obstructive epicardial disease.

8.3 The correct answer is D.

Rationale: Before considering medical therapy for resistant angina, it is important to work up and treat any underlying alternative causes of anginal chest pain including anemia, infection, metabolic disease (such as uncontrolled diabetes, lipidemia, or hypertension), and active smoking or other vasoactive drug use. Long-acting nitrates and ranolazine are appropriate therapies for chronic stable angina but treatment of other underlying factors should be considered prior to initiation of medical therapy. Given a high likelihood of alternative diagnosis that can be contributing to this patient's angina pectoris (anemia), and in the setting of a negative nuclear stress test finding, a left heart catheterization is not indicated at this time (**Figure 8.1**).

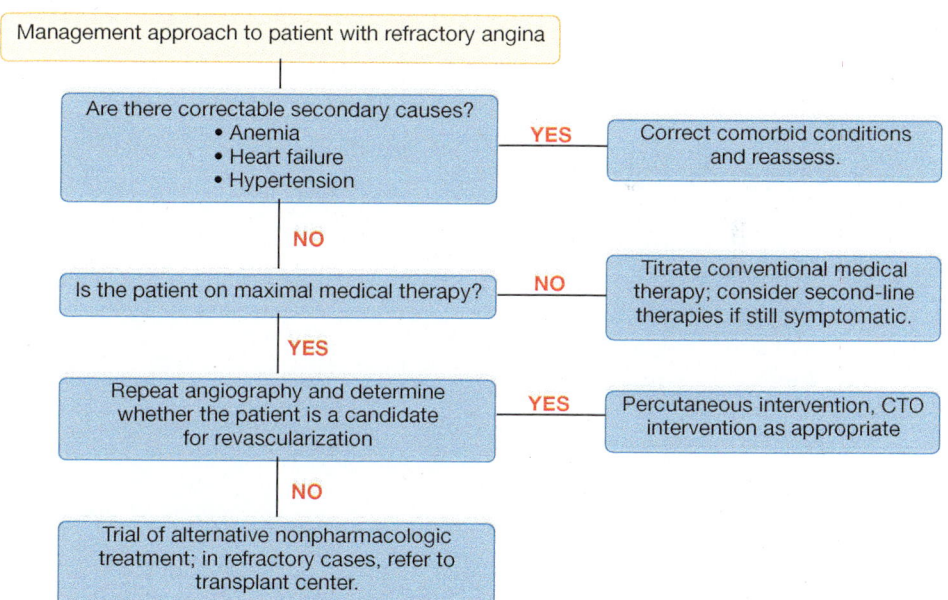

Figure 8.1 Approach to the patient with refractory angina. CTO, chronic total occlusion.

8.4 The correct answer is C.
Rationale: Ranolazine is contraindicated in patients with liver dysfunction and in patients with renal dysfunction with creatinine clearance less than 30. Use of ranolazine is not known to have implications in patients with heart failure.

8.5 The correct answer is B.
Rationale: Sublingual nitroglycerin is a short-acting nitrate. Optimal medical treatment for refractory angina includes long-acting nitrates such as isosorbide mononitrate or dinitrate, calcium channel blockers such as nifedipine, verapamil, and diltiazem, and ion channel inhibitors such as ranolazine and ivabradine.

8.6 The correct answer is D.
Rationale: Transmyocardial laser revascularization (TMLR) involves the surgical or thoracoscopic application of lasers to ischemic myocardium to open channels that allow for better perfusion and have been hypothesized to lead to possible angiogenesis and denervation of the myocardium, thus alleviating anginal symptoms. Clinical trials on the efficacy and safety of TMLR have mixed results and its use for refractory angina is an American Heart Association/American College of Cardiology (AHA/ACC) class 2b recommendation.

RHEUMATIC HEART DISEASE

Natasha Babar, Radmila Lyubarova, Sulagna Mookherjee, and Robert D. Millar

CHAPTER 9

QUESTIONS

9.1 Which of the following characteristics of group A beta-hemolytic streptococci (GAS) bacteria allows for the development of rheumatic heart disease?

  A. Ability to cause pharyngitis
  B. Formation of autoantibodies that attack joints and deep brain structures
  C. Ability to attach to tissues and organs via molecular mimicry
  D. None of the above is correct.

9.2 An 11-year-old female with no significant past medical history is evaluated in a remote Ugandan clinic for severe shortness of breath, abdominal distension, and orthopnea developing over the course of 2 weeks. There is a remote history of pharyngitis more than 6 weeks ago in the patient and her siblings. Examination reveals 1+ edema, a positive abdominal fluid wave, and a holosystolic murmur at the apex that radiates to the left axilla. Subcutaneous olecranon nodules are also noted. She is diagnosed with acute rheumatic fever. Which of the following is the **MOST LIKELY** affected cardiac structure?

  A. The myocardium
  B. The pericardium
  C. The mitral valve
  D. The tricuspid valve

9.3 The following are major criteria for the diagnosis of acute rheumatic fever **EXCEPT**:

  A. Fever higher than 38 °C
  B. Chorea
  C. Prolonged PR interval
  D. Subcutaneous nodules
  E. Both A and C are correct.

9.4 A 56-year-old immigrant from Pakistan who does not really follow up with doctors presents to the cardiology clinic to establish care for worsening dyspnea on exertion. An echocardiogram performed at an outside clinic raised concern for rheumatic mitral stenosis. Which of the following morphologic feature(s) are likely to be seen on this patient's echocardiogram?

  A. Mitral valve chordal thickening
  B. Restricted mitral valve leaflet motion
  C. Anterior mitral valve leaflet thickening
  D. All of the above are correct.

*Questions and Answers are based on Chapter 9: Rheumatic Heart Disease by Gbemiga Sofowora in Cardiovascular Medicine and Surgery, First Edition.

9.5 Which of the following is/are characteristic of rheumatic valve disease?
   A. The tricuspid valve is affected more commonly than the mitral and aortic valves.
   B. Stenotic lesions are more common than regurgitation.
   C. Thickening of leaflet tips is commonly seen.
   D. All of the above

9.6 How does the diagnosis of rheumatic heart disease differ from the diagnosis of acute rheumatic fever?
   A. Mitral valve disease is seen only in patients with rheumatic heart disease but not in those with acute rheumatic fever.
   B. The diagnosis of rheumatic heart disease does not require proof of prior GAS infection.
   C. Heart failure is not usually a presenting factor in acute rheumatic fever.
   D. Both B and C are correct.

9.7 An epidemiologic approach for treating and preventing rheumatic heart disease should involve which of the following interventions?
   A. Making treatment of GAS infection readily available for at-risk populations
   B. Providing adequate and safe housing without overcrowding
   C. Making access to care readily available for underserved populations
   D. All of the above are correct.

9.8 Which of the following is a contraindication to mitral valve balloon valvuloplasty in patients with symptomatic severe mitral valve stenosis?
   A. Presence of left atrial appendage thrombus
   B. Presence of concomitant severe mitral regurgitation
   C. Atrial fibrillation
   D. Both A and B are correct.

9.9 A 7-year-old male weighing 25 kg with no significant medical history is evaluated for acute onset of fever (T_{max} 38.3 °C) and difficulty swallowing for 2 days. There is no cough. Examination reveals tonsillar exudates and shotty anterior cervical chain lymphadenopathy. A rapid GAS antigen test result is positive. Chart review shows history of minimal rash with penicillin treatment previously. What is the **BEST** course of action to reduce this patient's risk of acute rheumatic fever?
   A. Oral penicillin V 250 mg 3 times a day for 10 days
   B. Intramuscular penicillin G 600,000 U for one dose
   C. Oral cefazolin 250 mg 3 times a day for 10 days
   D. Oral erythromycin 30 mg/kg/day for 10 days

9.10 An 18-year-old female with a history of childhood rheumatic heart failure at the age of 14 with mild mitral valve regurgitation presents to the outpatient cardiology clinic to establish care. She denies any symptoms and is euvolemic on examination. How would one approach secondary prophylaxis against rheumatic fever in this patient?
   A. Penicillin G injections every 4 weeks until 19 years of age
   B. Penicillin G injections every 4 weeks until 25 years of age
   C. Penicillin G injections every 4 weeks for life
   D. No further treatment is necessary in the absence of symptoms.

ANSWERS

9.1 The correct answer is C.
Rationale: GAS attach to tissues via an M-moiety that is similar in structure to cardiac myosin, tropomyosin, actin, and laminin. Over time, repeated infections with GAS bacteria lead to the development of antibodies against the M-moiety. Given their similarity to cardiac tissues, these antibodies can act as autoantibodies, attacking host cardiac tissues in a process known as molecular mimicry. Repeated insults of GAS infection over the years are thought to cause inflammation of heart valves, leading to the eventual development of rheumatic heart disease.

9.2 The correct answer is C.
Rationale: The mitral valve is the most common cardiac structure affected in acute rheumatic fever and mitral regurgitation is the most common valve lesion seen. Suspect mitral regurgitation and mitral valve valvulitis in young children from endemic areas presenting with symptoms of acute heart failure including weight gain, orthopnea, and lower extremity edema.

9.3 The correct answer is E.
Rationale: The diagnosis of acute rheumatic fever involves evidence of preceding GAS infection and two major or one major and two minor criteria (**Table 9.1**). Major criteria include carditis, polyarthritis, chorea, erythema marginatum, and subcutaneous nodules. Fever, arthralgia, elevated erythrocyte sedimentation rate (ESR) and C-reactive protein (CRP), and prolonged PR interval (in the absence of carditis) are minor criteria for the diagnosis of acute rheumatic fever.

9.4 The correct answer is D.
Rationale: All of the above features can be seen in rheumatic mitral valve disease. Anterior mitral valve thickening is age dependent and more than 3 mm is considered abnormal in young (younger than 20 years) patients, whereas more than 5 mm is considered abnormal in this patient's age group (older than 40 years). Restricted mitral valve leaflet motion caused by thickening of the anterior mitral valve leaflet with concomitant commissural fusion and distal tip restriction results in the pathognomonic "hockey stick" movement of the anterior mitral valve leaflet in the parasternal long axis.

9.5 The correct answer is C.
Rationale: In endemic regions, mitral regurgitation is often the most common lesion found, followed by mixed mitral valve disease or combined aortic and mitral valve disease noted depending on the region. Regurgitant lesions appear to be more frequent than stenotic lesions, and the order of valve involvement is mitral > aortic > tricuspid > pulmonic. Rarely are the right-sided valves involved in isolation without mitral valve involvement.

9.6 The correct answer is B.
Rationale: Mitral valve lesions are commonly seen in both rheumatic heart disease and acute rheumatic failure, with mitral regurgitation being the most common presenting valvular lesion as is presentation with acute decompensated heart failure symptoms. The correct answer is B. Diagnosis of rheumatic heart disease can be based solely on echocardiographic criteria without prior evidence of GAS infection.

TABLE 9.1 Revised Jones Criteria

A. FOR ALL PATIENT POPULATIONS WITH EVIDENCE OF PRECEDING GAS INFECTION	
Diagnosis: initial ARF	Two major manifestations or one major plus two minor manifestations
Diagnosis: recurrent ARF	Two major or one major and two minor or three minor

B. MAJOR CRITERIA	
Low-risk populations[a]	Moderate- and high-risk populations
Carditis[b] (clinical or subclinical)	Carditis (clinical or subclinical)
Arthritis (polyarthritis only)	Arthritis (monoarthritis, polyarthritis, or polyarthralgia)[c]
Chorea	Chorea
Erythema marginatum	Erythema marginatum
Subcutaneous nodules	Subcutaneous nodules

C. MINOR CRITERIA	
Low-risk populations[a]	Moderate- and high-risk populations
Polyarthralgia	Monoarthralgia
Fever (≥38.5 °C)	Fever (≥38 °C)
ESR ≥60 mm in first hour and/or CRP ≥3.0 mg/dL[d]	ESR ≥30 mm/h and/or CRP ≥3.0 mg/dL[d]
Prolonged PR interval, after accounting for age variability (unless carditis is a major criterion)	Prolonged PR interval, after accounting for age variability (unless carditis is a major criterion)

ARF, acute rheumatic fever; CRP, C-reactive protein; ESR, erythrocyte sedimentation rate; GAS, group A streptococcal infection.

[a]Low-risk populations are those with acute rheumatic fever (ARF) incidence 2 or less per 100,000 school-aged children or all-age rheumatic heart disease prevalence of 1 or less per 1,000 population per year.

[b]Subclinical carditis indicates echocardiographic valvulitis, as defined in another part of the original text.

[c]Polyarthralgia should only be considered as a major manifestation in moderate- to high-risk populations after exclusion of other causes. As in past versions of the criteria, erythema marginatum and subcutaneous nodules are rarely "stand-alone" major criteria. In addition, joint manifestations can only be considered in either the major or minor categories, but not both in the same patient.

[d]C-reactive protein (CRP) value must be greater than the upper limit of normal for laboratory. Also, because erythrocyte sedimentation rate (ESR) may evolve during the course of ARF, peak ESR values should be used.

Reprinted with permission Gewitz MH, Baltimore RS, Tani LY, et al. Revision of the Jones criteria for the diagnosis of acute rheumatic fever in the era of Doppler echocardiography: a scientific statement from the American Heart Association. *Circulation.* 2015;131:1806-1818. Copyright © 2015 American Heart Association, Inc.

9.7 The correct answer is D.

Rationale: From an epidemiologic standpoint, prevalence of rheumatic fever is related to overcrowding of individuals due to lack of safe and adequate housing; poor hygiene, which is associated with poor infrastructure; and reduced access to health care. System-level changes that focus on infrastructure, especially in developing countries, can be difficult to achieve. The focus of addressing the burden of rheumatic heart disease thus lies in primary prevention, with prompt treatment of GAS pharyngitis early on in its course.

9.8 The correct answer is D.

Rationale: The presence of a left atrial appendage thrombus is a contraindication for mitral valve balloon valvuloplasty due to risk of embolization. Balloon valvuloplasty can worsen mitral regurgitation and therefore is contraindicated in the setting of severe mitral regurgitation.

9.9 The correct answer is D.

Rationale: This patient has a penicillin allergy. Given the possibility of cross-reactivity between cephalosporins and penicillins, this patient should be treated with oral erythromycin using a pediatric formulation.

9.10 The correct answer is B.

Rationale: Options for secondary prophylaxis against rheumatic heart disease include penicillin G injections every 3 to 4 weeks or daily oral penicillin V or oral erythromycin. Indications for prophylaxis are the following:

1. Five years since the last episode of acute rheumatic fever until 18 years of age (whichever is longer) in the absence of any carditis
2. In the presence of mild or resolved carditis: 10 years since the last episode of acute rheumatic fever until 25 years of age (whichever is longer)
3. In the presence of severe carditis or previous requirement of surgical intervention: lifelong prophylaxis

This patient developed mild carditis from rheumatic fever at the age of 14. Prophylaxis will be required for at least 10 years (at the age of 24) or, in her case, at the age of 25 as this is longer.

MITRAL VALVE DISEASE

Matthew Derakhshesh and William Bachman

CHAPTER 10

QUESTIONS

10.1 All the following can lead to degenerative mitral valve regurgitation **EXCEPT**:
   A. Endocarditis
   B. Myxomatous mitral valve
   C. Dilated left ventricle
   D. Radiation
   E. Cabergoline

10.2 A 59-year-old male with a past medical history significant for persistent atrial fibrillation presents to the clinic with complaints of progressive shortness of breath over the past several months. He reports that his breathlessness is worse with exertion and with lying flat in the supine position. He has also noticed mild, bilateral leg swelling. A transthoracic echocardiogram performed that day reveals a dilated left atrium and pulmonary vein flow reversal with a peak tricuspid valve regurgitant velocity of 4.2 m/s. Continuous-wave Doppler through the mitral valve reveals a dense, triangular holosystolic jet. The mitral valve effective regurgitant orifice area is 0.45 cm². What is the **BEST** characterization of his mitral valve disease?
   A. Mild mitral regurgitation (MR)
   B. Mild to moderate MR
   C. Moderate MR
   D. Severe MR

10.3 A 47-year-old female with a past medical history significant for rheumatic fever presents to the clinic with shortness of breath with exertion that has worsened in the last year. She denies any accompanying chest pain, fatigue, or leg swelling. A transthoracic echocardiogram is arranged and performed. Which of the following echocardiographic parameters would be consistent with mild mitral stenosis?
   A. Mean gradient of 8 mm Hg
   B. Pulmonary artery pressure of 45 mm Hg
   C. Mitral valve area of 1.6 cm²
   D. Mean gradient of 11 mm Hg

---

*Questions and Answers are based on Chapter 10: Mitral Valve Disease by Nicholas S. Amoroso, Jessica Atkins, and Valerian Fernandes in Cardiovascular Medicine and Surgery, First Edition.

10.4 All of the following medications have been shown to be helpful in reducing the severity of functional MR **EXCEPT:**
A. Hydralazine
B. Isosorbide dinitrate
C. Lisinopril
D. Nifedipine
E. Valsartan

10.5 A 42-year-old female presents to the emergency department with 3 days of palpitations. She reports that the palpitations have been intermittent and associated with mild chest pressure along with dyspnea on exertion. Her medical history is significant for rheumatic mitral stenosis diagnosed a decade earlier. Her last transthoracic echocardiogram revealed moderate mitral stenosis with a dilated left atrium. An electrocardiogram is performed and shows new atrial fibrillation with a rate of 125 beats/min. What is the preferred management to reduce the risk of thromboembolism?
A. Warfarin
B. Apixaban
C. Left atrial appendage ligation
D. Dabigatran
E. Aspirin and clopidogrel

10.6 Which of the following patients with MR would **NOT** benefit from mitral valve repair or surgery?
A. A 67-year-old female with diabetes mellitus and symptomatic, severe, myxomatous MR
B. A 52-year-old male with asymptomatic, severe rheumatic MR and left ventricular end-diastolic diameter (LVESD) of 42 mm
C. A 59-year-old male with multivessel coronary artery disease and severe MR in the setting of dilated left ventricle (LV) undergoing evaluation for coronary artery bypass grafting
D. A 45-year-old female with hypertension and asymptomatic, severe MR due to mitral valve prolapse. Left ventricular ejection fraction (LVEF) is 65% and ESD is 38 mm.

10.7 Which valve anatomy confers the **BEST** outcome for percutaneous mitral valve commissurotomy (PTMC)?
A. Mobile, 6-mm-thick leaflets with scattered calcification and thickening extending to distal 1/3 chords
B. Restricted, 9-mm-thick leaflets with bright annular calcification, leaflet calcification and minimal subvalvular involvement
C. Mobile, mid-base 3-mm-thick leaflets with isolated, single area calcifications and minimal subvalvular involvement
D. Immobile, 10-mm-thick leaflets with extensive leaflet calcifications and thickening of distal 1/3 of chord length

10.8 A 54-year-old male with a history of rheumatic mitral stenosis presented to the clinic following a hospitalization for acute decompensated heart failure. At the time, he endorsed shortness of breath with mild exertion and orthopnea. Chest x-ray revealed bilateral pleural effusions. He was treated with diuretics with symptomatic improvement. Today, he notes that though his breathing has improved, he still experiences dyspnea with brisk walking. A transthoracic echocardiogram performed at this visit reveals a mitral valve area of 1.4 cm^2, a pressure half time of 170 milliseconds, a mean gradient of 13 mm Hg, a regurgitant fraction of 40%, an effective regurgitant orifice area of 0.29 cm^2, a pulmonary artery systolic pressure of 42 mm Hg, and a dilated left atrium. Assuming he is at low surgical risk, which of the following would be the **BEST** intervention for his mitral valve?

A. Reassurance and close monitoring
B. Percutaneous mitral balloon commissurotomy (PMBC)
C. Surgical mitral valve replacement
D. Transcatheter edge-to-edge mitral valve repair

10.9 When considering an intervention for a patient with severe mitral stenosis, mitral valve surgery is preferred compared to PMBC in all of the following **EXCEPT:**

A. Severe aortic stenosis
B. Mild MR
C. Left atrial clot
D. Three-vessel coronary artery disease
E. Wilkins score of 13

10.10 When considering the EVEREST, MITRA-FR, and COAPT trials, which patient would benefit the most from a MitraClip?

A. An 82-year-old female with normal left ventricular size and severe, symptomatic MR due to left atrial dilatation
B. A 73-year-old male with severe, symptomatic MR due to severely dilated cardiomyopathy
C. A 47-year-old male with progressive, symptomatic MR due to endocarditis
D. A 69-year-old female with severe, symptomatic MR due to extensive mitral annular calcification
E. A 55-year-old male with severe, asymptomatic MR due to myxomatous disease and an LVEF of 50% who is considered at low surgical risk

ANSWERS

10.1 The correct answer is C:
Rationale: Degenerative MR is due to inherent or acquired pathology of the valve leaflets, chordae tendinae, and papillary muscles. Leaflet degeneration can occur in the setting of endocarditis or in myxomatous mitral valve disease, the latter of which prevents adequate leaflet coaptation. Iatrogenic causes of leaflet destruction include radiation-induced and medication-induced (such as cabergoline) valve disease. A dilated LV can cause functional mitral valve regurgitation as it can disrupt the supporting valve apparatus while the leaflets and chordae tissue remain unaffected.

10.2 The correct answer is D.

Rationale: In severe mitral valve regurgitation, the continuous-wave Doppler reveals a dense, triangular jet during systole as opposed to a parabolic or faint jet with less severe regurgitation. Severe, chronic MR will contribute to left atrial dilatation, pulmonary vein flow reversal, and ultimately a significant tricuspid valve regurgitant velocity, as seen in this patient. Quantitatively, the effective regurgitant orifice area in severe MR is greater than 0.4 cm^2. All together, these echocardiographic parameters are indicative of severe mitral valve regurgitation.

10.3 The correct answer is C.

Rationale: According to the american society of echocardiography (ASE) Criteria for Evaluation of Mitral Stenosis, the mitral valve area is greater than 1.5 cm^2 in patients with mild mitral stenosis. The mean gradient is classically less than 5 mm Hg in mild mitral stenosis, between 5 and 10 mm Hg in moderate mitral stenosis, and greater than 10 mm Hg in severe mitral stenosis. Finally, a pulmonary artery pressure of 45 mm Hg is consistent with moderate mitral stenosis while a pulmonary artery pressure less than 30 mm Hg is associated with mild mitral stenosis.

10.4 The correct answer is D.

Rationale: In comparison to degenerative MR, functional MR can be greatly affected by medical therapy. As functional MR may be due to an underlying cardiomyopathy, guideline-directed medical therapy including angiotensin-converting enzyme inhibitors, aldosterone antagonists, and long-acting nitrates are typically used. Vasodilators such as hydralazine can be used for afterload reduction. Dihydropyridine calcium channel blockers have not been shown to be useful. For functional MR, patients should be treated with maximally tolerated heart failure medications for 3 months before reassessing the severity of regurgitation to determine if surgical intervention is required.

10.5 The correct answer is A.

Rationale: This patient likely has valvular atrial fibrillation in the setting of mitral stenosis secondary to rheumatic heart disease. Left atrial clot formation can occur due to several mechanisms including tissue inflammation and blood stasis (which can be illustrated by Virchow triad) due to a lack of atrial activity. To date, warfarin is the only approved anticoagulant for valvular atrial fibrillation. The direct oral anticoagulants such as dabigatran and apixaban have yet to be approved for valvular atrial fibrillation. Aspirin and clopidogrel are two antiplatelet agents that are not particularly effective in reducing the risk of thromboembolism. Finally, left atrial appendage ligation has not been approved for use in valvular atrial fibrillation because, in this condition, atrial thrombi are thought to be less isolated to the appendage.

10.6 The correct answer is D.

Rationale: In a patient with primary, severe MR in the setting of mitral valve prolapse or rheumatic disease which are both considered degenerative diseases, mitral valve surgery is a class I indication in those with an LVEF less than 60% or ESD greater than 40 mm (choice B). These criteria, however, are not fulfilled with choice D. Mitral valve surgery is also a class I indication in symptomatic, primary, severe MR (choice A). For patients with secondary severe MR undergoing coronary artery bypass grafting, mitral valve surgery is a class 2a indication (choice C) (**Figure 10.1**).

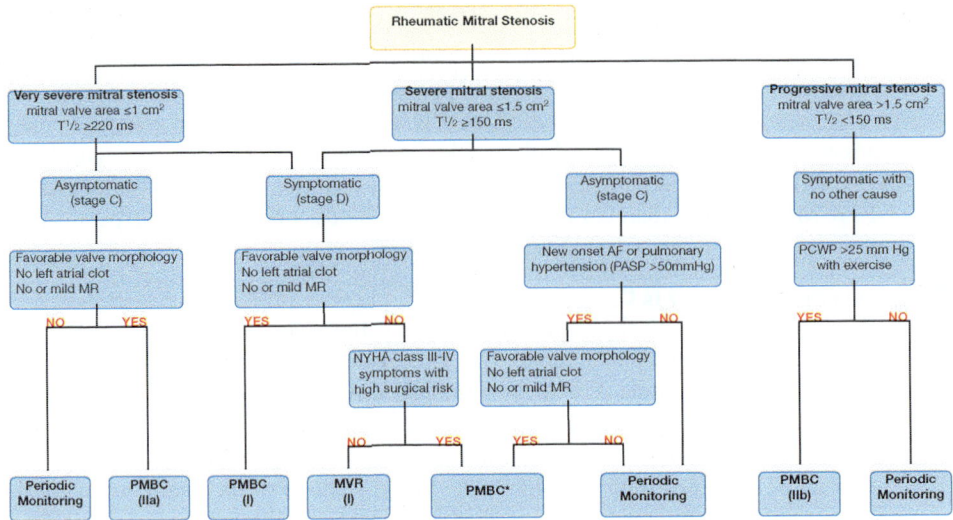

Figure 10.1 Indications for rheumatic mitral stenosis intervention. (Reprinted with permission from Otto CM, Nishimura RA, Bonow RO, et al. 2020 ACC/AHA guideline for the management of patients with valvular heart disease: executive summary: a report of the American College of Cardiology/American Heart Association Joint Committee on clinical practice guidelines. *Circulation.* 2021;143(5):e35-e71. ©2020 American Heart Association, Inc.)

10.7 The correct answer is C.
Rationale: The Wilkins score was the first and now the most frequently used score to predict the outcome of valve opening with PTMC. A score less than 8 suggests an optimal outcome while a score more than 12 suggests a poor outcome. According to the Wilkins score, the valve anatomy that has the lowest score and therefore corresponds to the best outcome is choice C. A mobile mid-base leaflet is 2 points, a 3-mm-thick leaflet is 1 point, an isolated area of calcification is 1 point, and minimal subvalvular involvement is 1 point for a total score of 5 points. Choices A and B have a total score of 9 points each, and choice D has a score of 15 points.

10.8 The correct answer is C.
Rationale: This patient continues to be symptomatic with New York Heart Association (NYHA) class II symptoms following his hospitalization for acute decompensated heart failure. The mitral valve area (by American College of Cardiology [ACC]/American Heart Association [AHA] criteria), pressure half time, and mean gradient are indicative of severe mitral stenosis, whereas the regurgitant fraction and effective regurgitant orifice area, along with a dilated left atrium, suggest moderate to severe MR. Taken together, severe mitral stenosis with at least moderate MR in a patient with NYHA class II symptoms is a class I indication for surgical mitral valve replacement. PMBC would be preferred if the MR is less than moderate. Close monitoring is not an appropriate option for severe, symptomatic mitral stenosis. Transcatheter edge-to-edge mitral valve repair is not the optimal choice in a patient with low surgical risk who would benefit from mitral valve replacement.

10.9 The correct answer is B.
Rationale: PMBC is a class I indication in patients with symptomatic, severe mitral stenosis even with concomitant mild MR. Mitral valve surgery is preferred in the presence of more severe MR. Mitral valve surgery is preferred in patients who have additional conditions that would benefit from surgery such as severe aortic stenosis (choice A) and multivessel disease (choice D). PMBC should also be avoided in individuals with left atrial clot (choice C). A Wilkins score above 12 predicts a poor outcome with PMBC, with mitral valve surgery being preferred in these scenarios.

10.10 The correct answer is A.
Rationale: The EVEREST, MITRA-FR, and COAPT trials have shown that the population who benefits most from transcatheter edge-to-edge mitral valve repair are those with functional MR. In choices C and D, these patients have degenerative, severe MR and therefore would not be the ideal candidates. These trials also demonstrated that patients with a less dilated LV (choice A) are more likely to benefit from MitraClips than those with severe LV dilatation (choice B).

AORTIC VALVE DISEASE

Matthew Derakhshesh and William Bachman

CHAPTER 11

QUESTIONS

11.1 A transthoracic echocardiogram (TTE) is performed after a crescendo-decrescendo systolic murmur is auscultated on a 66-year-old male with a history of hyperlipidemia. His TTE reveals an aortic valve mean gradient of 32 mm Hg, a peak velocity of 3.5 m/s, and an aortic valve area (AVA) of 1.3 cm^2 with a left ventricular ejection fraction (LVEF) of 55%. How would his aortic valve disease be graded?

A. Aortic valve sclerosis
B. Mild aortic valve stenosis
C. Moderate aortic valve stenosis
D. Severe aortic valve stenosis

11.2 A 57-year-old female with a history of ischemic cardiomyopathy has a surveillance TTE that reveals an LVEF of 35%, an aortic valve transvalvular mean gradient of 31 mm Hg, and an AVA of 0.9 cm^2. She has remained asymptomatic, denying any chest pain, shortness of breath, or syncopal episodes. Which of the following findings on dobutamine stress echocardiogram would support aortic valve intervention?

A. AVA 0.8 cm^2, mean gradient 40 mm Hg
B. AVA 1.2 cm^2, mean gradient 38 mm Hg
C. AVA 1.1 cm^2, mean gradient 43 mm Hg
D. AVA 1.3 cm^2, mean gradient 45 mm Hg

11.3 All of the following patients are suitable candidates for an aortic valve replacement **EXCEPT**:

A. A 79-year-old male with dyspnea on exertion, a V_{max} of 4.3 m/s, and an aortic transvalvular mean pressure gradient of 44 mm Hg
B. A 66-year-old female presenting with syncope and a TTE revealing an AVA of 1.4 cm^2, a V_{max} of 3.2 m/s, and an LVEF of 55%
C. A 62-year-old male with an abnormal exercise stress test and a TTE with an AVA of 0.9 cm^2 and a V_{max} of 4.9 m/s
D. A 72-year-old female who is asymptomatic, has an AVA of 0.8 cm^2, a mean pressure gradient of 42 mm Hg, a V_{max} of 4.1 m/s, and an LVEF of 45%

Questions and Answers are based on Chapter 11: Aortic Valve Disease by Laurie Bossory Goike, Antonios Pitsis, and Konstantinos Dean Boudoulas in Cardiovascular Medicine and Surgery, First Edition.

CHAPTER 11 | Aortic Valve Disease

11.4 A 43-year-old male with a history of bicuspid aortic valve undergoes a TTE showing severe aortic stenosis. As he is asymptomatic, he prefers to forego any valvular intervention at this time. When would be the most appropriate time to repeat a TTE for monitoring of his aortic valve disease?
  A. 12 months
  B. 24 months
  C. 3 years
  D. 4 years

11.5 A 45-year-old male with a history of severe aortic stenosis in the setting of a bicuspid aortic valve undergoes a mechanical aortic valve replacement. According to the American College of Cardiology (ACC)/American Heart Association (AHA) guidelines, what is the class I recommendation for this patient's antithrombotic therapy?
  A. Warfarin alone
  B. Warfarin and clopidogrel
  C. Warfarin and aspirin
  D. Apixaban

11.6 Which of the following is a potential complication following the transcatheter aortic valve replacement (TAVR) procedure?
  A. Paravalvular regurgitation
  B. Prosthesis-patient mismatch
  C. Complete heart block
  D. Prosthetic valve endocarditis
  E. All of the above

11.7 Which of the following is **NOT** a clinical sign of aortic regurgitation?
  A. Wide pulse pressure
  B. Mid-diastolic murmur
  C. Diastolic pulsation of the uvula
  D. Pistol shot sounds in femoral arteries on both systole and diastole
  E. Head bobbing with each heartbeat

11.8 A surveillance TTE is performed on a 47-year-old male with a known bicuspid aortic valve. On TTE, the left ventricular size is 51 mm. Analysis of the aortic valve reveals a pressure half time (PHT) of 320 milliseconds, a vena contracta of 0.4 cm, a regurgitant fraction of 38%, and an effective regurgitant orifice area (EROA) of 0.18 cm^2. How would one classify his aortic valve disease?
  A. No aortic regurgitation
  B. Mild aortic regurgitation
  C. Moderate aortic regurgitation
  D. Severe aortic regurgitation

11.9 A 62-year-old female has been referred by her primary care physician for an evaluation of a murmur. She denies any shortness of breath with exertion, chest pain, orthopnea, or paroxysmal nocturnal dyspnea. Examination of the aortic valve on TTE shows a vena contracta of 0.7 cm and an EROA of 0.4 cm^2. The regurgitant fraction is 60% and holodiastolic flow in the descending aorta is visualized. Which of the following additional findings would favor surveillance over intervention?

A. LVEF 40%, left ventricular end-systolic dimension (LVESD) 55 mm, and left ventricular end-diastolic dimension (LVEDD) 65 mm
B. LVEF 55%, LVESD 48 mm, and LVEDD 70 mm
C. LVEF 60%, LVESD 52 mm, and LVEDD 60 mm
D. LVEF 55%, LVESD 45 mm, and LVEDD 60 mm

11.10 A 46-year-old male with a history of cocaine abuse presents to the emergency department via emergency medical services with sudden-onset shortness of breath. His vitals include a blood pressure of 87/55 mm Hg, a heart rate of 130 beats per minute (bpm), and an SpO_2 of 82% with a nonrebreather mask. He appears tachypneic and is using accessory respiratory muscles. The decision is made to intubate. Once placed on a ventilator, he undergoes a computed tomography (CT) angiogram that does not show any pulmonary embolism or aortic dissection but does reveal moderate, bilateral pleural effusions. A TTE is subsequently performed, revealing an LVEF of 35%. Color flow Doppler of the aortic valve shows aortic regurgitation with a vena contracta of 0.8 cm and an EROA of 0.5 cm². What is the preferred, definitive management in this patient?

A. Intra-aortic balloon pump
B. Dobutamine
C. Aortic valve replacement
D. Norepinephrine

ANSWERS

11.1 The correct answer is C.
Rationale: In moderate aortic stenosis, the mean transvalvular gradient is 20 to 39 mm Hg, the peak velocity is between 3.0 and 3.9 m/s, and the AVA is between 1.1 and 1.5 cm².

11.2 The correct answer is A.
Rationale: This patient has low flow-low gradient severe aortic stenosis in the setting of poor left ventricle (LV) systolic function. Dobutamine stress echocardiography can help differentiate between patients with true, severe aortic stenosis and pseudoaortic stenosis. Unlike in pseudoaortic stenosis in which dobutamine increases the transvalvular gradient and leaflet excursion improves to augment AVA, in true aortic stenosis the increase in transvalvular gradient will not improve leaflet mobility and AVA will remain in the severely stenotic range. Of the choices listed, the only option for which the AVA remains severe is choice A, thereby warranting intervention.

11.3 The correct answer is B.
Rationale: Even with symptoms, aortic valve replacement is currently not indicated in patients with moderate aortic stenosis and preserved systolic function. When systolic function is reduced in the setting of moderate aortic stenosis, dobutamine stress echocardiography can be performed. If the AVA is less than 1.0 cm² and the

peak velocity is greater than 4 m/s, then there is a class IIa indication for aortic valve replacement (choice B). Aortic valve replacement is a class I indication in patients with symptomatic severe aortic stenosis (choice A) as well as with asymptomatic severe aortic stenosis with an LVEF less than 50% (choice D) (**Figure 11.1**).

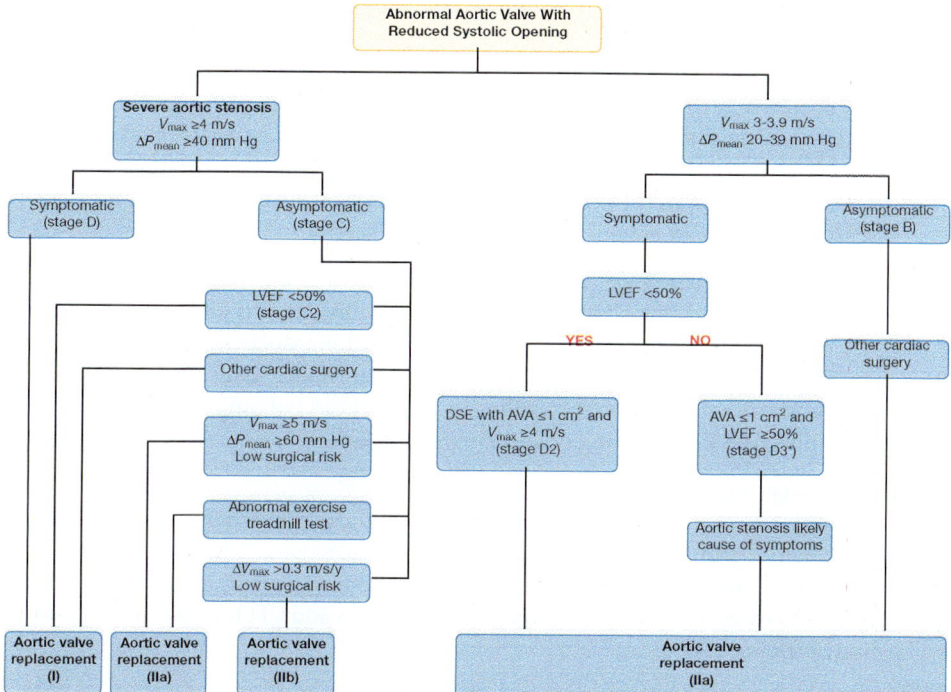

Figure 11.1 Indication of aortic valve replacement (AVR) in aortic stenosis. Stage B—patients with mild to moderate disease who are asymptomatic. Stage C—patients who have severe disease, but remain asymptomatic. Stage C1—patients have preserved left ventricular (LV) function. Stage C2—patients with decompensated LV function. Stage D—patients who are symptomatic because of severe valvular disease. *In stage D3 aortic stenosis, AVR should be considered if valve obstruction is likely the cause of symptoms, stroke volume index is <35 mL/m^2, and indexed AVA is 0.6 cm^2/m^2 (obtained when the patient is normotensive with a systolic blood pressure <140 mm Hg). AVA, aortic valve area; DSE, dobutamine stress echocardiography; LVEF, left ventricular ejection fraction; P_{mean}, mean pressure gradient; V_{max}, maximum velocity. (Adapted from Nishimura RA, Otto CM, Bonow RO, et al. 2014 AHA/ACC guideline for the management of patients with valvular heart disease: executive summary: a report of the American College of Cardiology/American Heart Association Task Force on Practice Guidelines. *J Am Coll Cardiol.* 2014;63(22):2438-2488. Copyright © 2014 American Heart Association, Inc., and the American College of Cardiology Foundation, with permission.)

11.4 The correct answer is A.

Rationale: In asymptomatic severe aortic stenosis that is not undergoing intervention, it is best to repeat a TTE every 6 to 12 months. A TTE can be repeated every 1 to 2 years for moderate aortic stenosis and every 3 to 5 years for mild aortic stenosis.

11.5 The correct answer is C.

Rationale: According to the ACC/AHA guidelines, the combination of aspirin and warfarin is a class I indication for the first 6 months following mechanical aortic valve replacement. Warfarin alone is not sufficient, and the combination of warfarin and aspirin is preferred over warfarin and a P2Y12 inhibitor. Apixaban has not been well studied.

11.6 The correct answer is E.

Rationale: Paravalvular regurgitation is a common complication following TAVR. Patient-prosthesis mismatch can occur when the prosthetic valve has been under-sized or when balloon dilatation is not performed. Complete heart block can occur in up to 30% of TAVR insertions due to mechanical strain of the annulus during the procedure, which can disturb the infranodal pathway. Finally, the chances of endocarditis increase with any prosthetic heart valve insertion.

11.7 The correct answer is C.

Rationale: Systolic, not diastolic, pulsation of the uvula, also known as the Muller sign, is a physical examination sign that is observed in association with aortic regurgitation. A wide pulse pressure, a mid-diastolic murmur, pistol shot sounds in the femoral arteries throughout the cardiac cycle, and head bobbing with each heartbeat are all observed in the setting of aortic regurgitation.

11.8 The correct answer is C.

Rationale: A vena contracta between 0.3 and 0.6 cm, PHT between 200 and 500 milliseconds, and a regurgitant fraction between 30% and 39% are consistent with moderate aortic regurgitation. In this clinical scenario, a regurgitant fraction of less than 30% to go along with the same vena contracta and PHT would correspond to mild aortic regurgitation.

11.9 The correct answer is D.

Rationale: In the case of asymptomatic, severe aortic regurgitation as is present in this patient (a vena contract >0.6 cm, an EROA >0.3 cm^2, and a regurgitant fraction >50%) if the LVEF is less than 50%, aortic valve replacement is indicated (choice A). In patients with preserved LV function, aortic valve replacement is indicated if the LVESD is greater than 50 mm (choice C) or the LVEDD is greater than 65 mm (choice B). Otherwise, periodic monitoring is preferred (choice D) (**Figure 11.2**).

11.10 The correct answer is C.

Rationale: The patient's symptoms are concerning for acute decompensated heart failure in the setting of new aortic regurgitation. The vena contracta of 0.8 cm and an EROA of 0.5 cm^2 are consistent with severe aortic regurgitation. Regardless of LV systolic function, symptomatic, severe aortic regurgitation is a class I indication for aortic valve replacement, which is the best and most definitive management in this clinical scenario. Insertion of an intra-aortic balloon pump is contraindicated in severe aortic regurgitation (choice A). Although dobutamine and norepinephrine can be used when cardiogenic shock is suspected as in this patient, these measures are only temporizing (choices B and D).

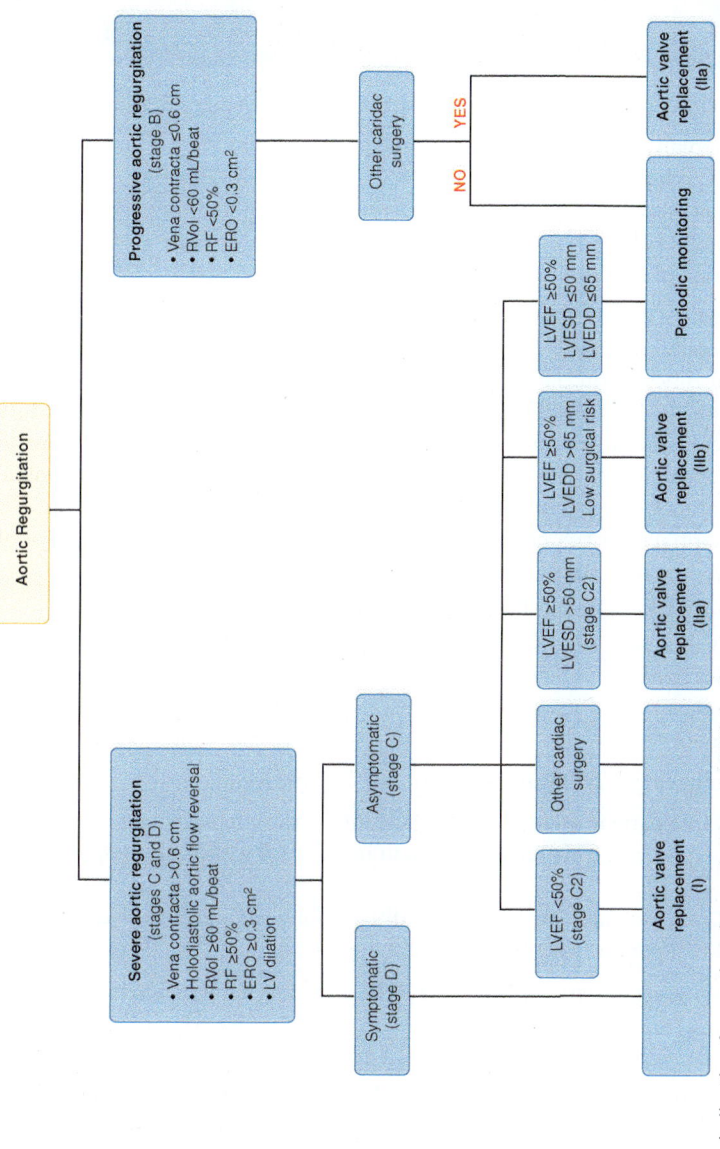

Figure 111.2 Indication for aortic valve replacement (AVR) in chronic aortic regurgitation (aortic regurgitation). Stage B—patients with mild to moderate disease who are asymptomatic. Stage C—patients who have severe disease, but remain asymptomatic. Stage C1—patients have preserved LV function. Stage C2—patients with decompensated LV function. Stage D—patients who are symptomatic because of severe valvular disease. ERO, effective regurgitant orifice; EROA, effective regurgitant orifice area; LV, left ventricular; LVEDD, left ventricular end-diastolic dimension; LVEF, left ventricular ejection fraction; LVESD, left ventricular end-systolic dimension; LVOT, left ventricular outflow tract; RF, regurgitant fraction; RVol, regurgitant volume. (Adapted from Nishimura RA, Otto CM, Bonow RO, et al. 2014 AHA/ACC guideline for the management of patients with valvular heart disease: executive summary: a report of the American College of Cardiology/American Heart Association Task Force on Practice Guidelines. *J Am Coll Cardiol.* 2014;63(22):2438-2488. Copyright © 2014 American Heart Association, Inc., and the American College of Cardiology Foundation, with permission.)

ADULT-ACQUIRED TRICUSPID AND PULMONARY VALVE DISEASE*

Matthew Derakhshesh and Mohamed Khalid Munshi

CHAPTER 12

QUESTIONS

12.1 Which of the following is a cause of secondary tricuspid valve regurgitation (TR)?
   A. Ebstein anomaly
   B. Carcinoid syndrome
   C. Eisenmenger syndrome
   D. Infective endocarditis
   E. Endomyocardial biopsies

12.2 A 39-year-old male with a history of polysubstance is admitted for 3 days of intermittent fevers and chills. His initial temperature was 39.05 °C. On examination, a holosystolic murmur is best appreciated in the left lower sternal border along with jugular venous distention to the mandible, hepatomegaly, and 2+ bilateral, lower extremity edema. Blood cultures show pan-sensitive methicillin-sensitive *Staphylococcus aureus* (MSSA) bacteremia. A transthoracic echocardiogram (TTE) shows a 1-cm mobile density on the anterior tricuspid valve (TV) leaflet. Color Doppler through the TV reveals a vena contracta of 0.8 cm along with an effective regurgitant orifice area of 45 mm^2. What is the next **BEST** step in management?
   A. Intravenous (IV) ampicillin for 6 weeks
   B. Furosemide boluses
   C. Urgent TV repair
   D. A and B only
   E. All of the above

12.3 Which of the following is **NOT** an indication for TV intervention?
   A. Severe TR in a patient undergoing surgical mitral valve replacement
   B. Severe TR with a tricuspid annulus of 2 cm in a patient without right-sided heart failure
   C. Severe TR in a patient with TV endocarditis and a flail anterior TV leaflet
   D. Severe TR in a patient with Ebstein anomaly

12.4 Which of the following statements is **NOT TRUE** regarding surgical TV replacements for severe TR?
   A. A bioprosthetic TV confers a higher mortality benefit than a mechanical TV.
   B. In patients who develop severe TR after orthotropic heart transplants and require valve replacement, a bioprosthetic tissue valve is preferred to a mechanical valve.
   C. A bioprosthetic TV has a lower thrombotic risk than a mechanical TV.
   D. The risk of complete heart block increases with TV replacements.

*Questions and Answers are based on Chapter 12: Adult-Acquired Tricuspid and Pulmonary Valve Disease by Maureen E. Cheung and Bryan A. Whitson in Cardiovascular Medicine and Surgery, First Edition.

12.5 Who is **MOST LIKELY** to experience recurrent severe TR following TV annuloplasty?
- A. A 48-year-old male with a left ventricular ejection fraction (LVEF) of 55% and mild TR following annuloplasty
- B. A 55-year-old female with moderate mitral regurgitation (MR) and a tricuspid annulus of 3 cm
- C. A 60-year-old male with a dual-chamber pacemaker and a right ventricular systolic pressure (RVSP) of 35 mm Hg
- D. A 53-year-old female with a dual-chamber pacemaker and a tricuspid annulus of 5 cm

ANSWERS

12.1 The correct answer is C.
Rationale: The most common cause of secondary TR is left-sided valvular pathology. Other secondary causes include other pathologies that can cause right ventricular dysfunction and dilation. Eisenmenger syndrome leads to progressive right ventricular dilation and tricuspid annular enlargement, which is in turn a secondary cause of TR. Ebstein anomaly, carcinoid syndrome, infective endocarditis, and endomyocardial biopsies all disrupt the structural components of the TV and therefore are primary causes of TR.

12.2 The correct answer is D.
Rationale: This gentleman has a fever above 38 °C, blood cultures that are positive for *Staphylococcus aureus*, a mobile density on his TV, and severe TR, which all favor a diagnosis of endocarditis (see Modified Duke criteria). The initial treatment will include antibiotics like ampicillin, which is an appropriate antimicrobial for pan-sensitive MSSA bacteremia as well as furosemide for his right-sided heart failure (choice D). TV repair does not need to be performed urgently, but nonurgent repair may still be an option due to the patient's heart failure symptoms and the size of the vegetation.

12.3 The correct answer is B.
Rationale: Surgical treatment of severe TR is a class I indication for those undergoing concomitant cardiac surgery such as mitral valve replacement. Surgery is also indicated in severe TR in the setting of a flail leaflet or conditions such as Ebstein anomaly as conservative management alone is unlikely to be reliable (choices A and C). There is also a class IIa recommendation for surgery in patients with severe TR and a tricuspid annulus size of 4 cm and/or right-sided heart failure but not with an annulus of 2 cm or without heart failure as in choice B.

12.4 The correct answer is A.
Rationale: Overall, a bioprosthetic TV confers no greater survival benefit than a mechanical TV (choice A). In patients who develop severe TR after orthotropic heart transplantation, which may occur due to repeat endomyocardial biopsies, a bioprosthetic valve is favored over a mechanical valve for multiple reasons including adequate durability in the lower pressure right heart and the ability to continue cardiac

surveillance with endomyocardial biopsies (choice B). A bioprosthetic tissue valve does have a lower thrombotic risk than a mechanical valve, which is why a mechanical valve requires lifelong anticoagulation. Finally, there is an underlying risk of bradycardia and complete heart block in patients undergoing TV interventions due to disruption of the conduction system, and as such, there is a low threshold for epicardial lead placement.

12.5 The correct answer is B.

Rationale: Risk factors for TR recurrence include pulmonary hypertension, left ventricular dysfunction, leaflet tenting, baseline regurgitant severity, presence of right ventricular device leads, and degree of annular dilation. Choice D has two risk factors that include the presence of a right ventricular lead and a large tricuspid annulus—larger than that of choice B. Recurrent, severe TR is also less likely when pulmonary hypertension (choice C) and TR (choice A) are mild (**Table 12.1**).

TABLE 12.1 Etiologies and Pathogenesis of Right-Sided Regurgitant Valve Lesions

Etiology	Pathogenesis
PRIMARY CAUSES (25%)	
Infectious endocarditis	Leaflet destruction
Trauma	Blunt or penetrating with disruption of structural components
Carcinoid syndrome	Fibrous tissue deposits on valve cusps
Rheumatic disease	Right- and/or left-sided valve thickening
Takayasu arteritis	Involvement of pulmonary arteries with pulmonary hypertension
Congenital causes (ie, Ebstein)	Tricuspid valve regurgitation
IATROGENIC	
Pacemaker/defibrillator leads	Direct interference with leaflet coaptation
Endomyocardial biopsies	Structural disruption—chordae or papillary muscle destruction/injury
SECONDARY CAUSES (75%)	
Left-sided valvular dysfunction	Pulmonary hypertension with progressive right ventricular dilation, tricuspid annular enlargement
Eisenmenger syndrome	Progressive right ventricular dilation, tricuspid annular enlargement
Primary pulmonary hypertension	Progressive right ventricular dilation, tricuspid annular enlargement
Right ventricular infarct	Papillary muscle dysfunction and/or regional wall motion abnormalities
Marfan syndrome and other myxomatous diseases	Mitral and tricuspid valve prolapse and/or chordae elongation or rupture
Dilated cardiomyopathy	Biventricular failure
Drug induced	

PROSTHETIC VALVE DYSFUNCTION*

Matthew Derakhshesh and Mohamed Khalid Munshi

CHAPTER 13

QUESTIONS

13.1 A 73-year-old male with a history of bioprosthetic mitral valve replacement performed 5 years ago, end-stage renal disease (ESRD), diabetes mellitus type 2, hypertension, and hyperlipidemia has undergone a transthoracic echocardiogram (TTE) after presenting with progressive shortness of breath. Which of the following would **NOT** increase his risk of bioprosthetic mitral valve degeneration?

- A. History of ESRD
- B. His age
- C. Positioning of the bioprosthetic valve
- D. History of diabetes
- E. History of hyperlipidemia

13.2 What risk factor is **NOT** associated with patient-prosthesis mismatch (PPM) in patients with prosthetic heart valves?

- A. Lower body surface area
- B. Small valve annulus
- C. Females
- D. Transcatheter aortic valve implantation (TAVI) without post-balloon dilation

13.3 A 58-year-old female presents to the emergency department (ED) with fatigue and shortness of breath with exertion. Her history is significant for a bioprosthetic aortic valve replacement 2 years prior to a diagnosis of severe aortic stenosis. Her hemoglobin is 7.5 g/dL and was previously 12.5 g/dL 6 months ago. A peripheral smear shows schistocytes. She undergoes an esophagogastroduodenoscopy along with a colonoscopy, both of which are unremarkable for any acute bleeding processes. A TTE is performed and reveals thickened aortic leaflets with decreased leaflet excursion. Spectral Doppler through the aortic valve shows an aortic valve peak velocity of 4 m/s, an effective orifice area (EOA) of 0.6 cm^2, and an acceleration time of 130 milliseconds. What is the **MOST LIKELY** pathogenesis and the most appropriate management for her condition?

- A. Lipid-mediated inflammation; frequent blood transfusions
- B. Immune response to residual xenoantigens; beta-blockers
- C. Calcification of glutaraldehyde coating; surgical valve replacement
- D. Small valve size; surgical valve replacement

---

*Questions and Answers are based on Chapter 13: Prosthetic Valve Dysfunction by Shuktika Nandkeolyar, Dmitry Abramov, Helme Silvet, and Purvi Parwani in Cardiovascular Medicine and Surgery, First Edition.

CASE 1

A 67-year-old male presents via emergency medical services (EMS) for acute-onset shortness of breath that required intubation on the field. His daughter who witnessed the episode is at his bedside. She states that he was sitting on his couch when he suddenly had difficulty breathing and quickly turned blue. He also has been unable to take his medications in the last 4 days because of diarrhea and vomiting. She notes that he did have a new valve placed about 6 months ago and that he takes "a blood thinner." However, she cannot recall any further details. Heart sounds are muffled, and there is no mechanical click on auscultation. Blood cultures taken on admission have been negative to date. A transesophageal echocardiogram (TEE) is performed and shows two, small echo bright densities with shadowing at both sides of the mitral annulus along with a 2-cm, mobile, slightly hypoechoic density that begins at the valvular ring.

13.4 In **Case 1**, what is the **MOST LIKELY** diagnosis for this patient's prosthetic valve dysfunction?

   A. Prosthetic valve endocarditis
   B. Pannus formation
   C. Prosthetic valve thrombosis
   D. PPM

13.5 For the patient from **Case 1**, which of the following is the **LEAST LIKELY** etiology for his prosthetic valve dysfunction?

   A. Subtherapeutic international normalized ratio (INR)
   B. Atrial fibrillation
   C. Low ejection fraction
   D. Atrial dilation

13.6 Chest x-ray shows moderate, bilateral effusions, and diuretics are administered for the patient in **Case 1**. Despite diuresis, he frequently becomes hypoxic on the ventilator and his mean arterial pressures have decreased to the 50s. What is the **BEST** management that would **MOST LIKELY** improve his clinical outcome?

   A. Unfractionated heparin
   B. Tissue plasminogen activator
   C. Streptokinase
   D. Surgical thrombus resection

13.7 Which of the following Doppler parameters are indicative of prosthetic heart valve stenosis?

   A. Tricuspid valve (TV): peak velocity 1.2 m/s, mean gradient 3 mm Hg, and a pressure half time (PHT) 150 milliseconds
   B. Aortic valve: peak velocity 3.8 m/s, EOA 0.55 cm^2, and Doppler velocity index (DVI) 0.2
   C. Pulmonic valve: peak velocity 1.5 m/s
   D. Mitral valve: peak velocity 1.5 m/s, mean gradient 6 mm Hg, and a PHT 140 milliseconds

13.8 Which of the following Doppler parameters are consistent with severe prosthetic heart valve regurgitation?

  A. TV: vena contract 0.4 cm, proximal isovelocity surface area (PISA) radius 0.6 cm, and no flow reversal in the hepatic vein
  B. Pulmonic valve: regurgitant width 35%, regurgitant volume 40 mL/beat, and PHT 170 milliseconds
  C. Mitral valve: regurgitant area 9 cm^2, effective regurgitant orifice area (EROA) 0.6 cm^2, and peak velocity 2.5 m/s
  D. Aortic valve: regurgitant width 45%, regurgitant volume 50 mL/beat, and PHT 350 milliseconds

13.9 A 62-year-old male with a history of mechanical aortic valve replacement and atrial fibrillation undergoes a TEE in anticipation of a cardioversion procedure. Although an atrial appendage clot is not visualized, a nonmobile density is seen on the posterolateral leaflet of the prosthetic valve. Which of the following would favor medical management over surgical removal of the thrombus?

  A. Suspected onset of thrombosis of less than 14 days
  B. Thrombus area 1.2 cm^2
  C. Patient is asymptomatic.
  D. Patient becomes unstable.

13.10 A 39-year-old female with a history of bioprosthetic TV replacement following an episode of TV endocarditis presents with subjective fevers and chills along with intermittent vomiting. Her temperature is 39.55 °C, and her heart rate is 52 beats per minute (bpm). A TTE reveals a mobile density on one of the leaflets of the bioprosthetic valve with new regurgitation concerning for a vegetation. Which of the following would favor medical management over debridement and valve replacement?

  A. Persistent bacteremia
  B. Vegetation size of 14 mm
  C. Annular abscess with high-degree atrioventricular (AV) block
  D. Severe right-sided heart failure
  E. *Streptococcus viridans* infection

ANSWERS

13.1 The correct answer is B.
Rationale: Risk factors for prosthetic heart valve degeneration include ESRD, which is associated with hypercalcemia (choice A), the position of the valve within the annulus—particularly the mitral valve (choice C), diabetes (choice D), and hyperlipidemia (choice E). Older patients such as those within this patient's age group experience lower rates of prosthetic heart valve degeneration compared to younger patients (choice B).

13.2 The correct answer is A.
Rationale: PPM occurs when the EOA or valve size is too small to accommodate uninterrupted blood flow across the valve. Smaller valve annulus (choice B) and lack of post-balloon dilation (choice D) during transcatheter valve insertion are risk factors associated with PPM. In terms of patient demographics, females (choice C) and those with larger, not smaller (choice A) body surface area are at higher risk for developing PPM.

13.3 The correct answer is C.
Rationale: Patient's symptoms, along with findings of anemia and schistocytes on peripheral smear, are suggestive of hemolytic anemia. Her echocardiogram shows a peak velocity and EOA consistent with severe, bioprosthetic aortic valve stenosis, which is likely the main driver of the hemolytic anemia. This degenerative stenosis can occur through lipid-mediated inflammation, calcification of the valve tissue, or immune responses to residual xenoantigens on the valve (choices A, B, and C). Small valve size is correlated with PPM, which this patient does not have (choice D). The best treatment for hemolytic anemia due to severe bioprosthetic aortic valve stenosis is surgical aortic valve replacement (choice C).

13.4 The correct answer is C.
Rationale: This patient's sudden onset of dyspnea is concerning for flash pulmonary edema, among other differentials. Though he does have a history of a recent valve replacement, both the type and location of the valve are uncertain through history alone. The echo bright densities with shadowing on both sides of the mitral annulus indicated that the valve is a mechanical mitral valve. The hypoechoic density beginning on the valvular ring could be a thrombus or a vegetation due to endocarditis. However, the absence of fever and positive blood cultures make prosthetic valve endocarditis less likely (choice A). A pannus typically takes time to form, is associated with progressive dyspnea, and is more echo bright on TEE (choice C). Echo densities are also not associated with PPM (choice D). This patient's inability to take his oral anticoagulant medication (which would have been warfarin) likely led to a subtherapeutic INR that predisposed him to develop prosthetic valve thrombosis (choice C).

13.5 The correct answer is C.
Rationale: As this patient's prosthetic heart valve is a mechanical mitral valve, a subtherapeutic INR is the most likely etiology of prosthetic valve thrombosis (choice A). Atrial fibrillation and atrial dilation can also lead to blood stasis with eventual thrombus formation that can migrate to the prosthetic, mitral valve (choices B and D). A low ejection fraction may lead to left ventricular (LV) thrombus formation, but it is unlikely that the thrombus would migrate to cause prosthetic, mitral valve thrombosis (choice C).

13.6 The correct answer is D.
Rationale: Surgical thrombus resection is emergently indicated in unstable patients with left-sided, prosthetic heart valves. This indication would apply to this patient who has a mechanical mitral valve thrombus and has frequent hypoxemic episodes on the ventilator despite diuretics (choice D). Medical therapy with unfractionated heparin, tissue plasminogen activator, or streptokinase (choices A, B, and C) is reasonable for left-sided prosthetic valve thrombosis in patients who are mildly symptomatic with a recent onset of thrombosis formation (<14 days) and a thrombus that is smaller in size (<0.8 cm^2).

13.7 The correct answer is B.

Rationale: An aortic valve peak velocity greater than 3 m/s with an EOA less than 0.65 cm^2 and DVI less than 0.25 is indicative of severe, prosthetic aortic valve stenosis (choice B). A peak velocity greater than 1.7 m/s, a mean gradient greater than 6 mm Hg, and a PHT greater than 230 milliseconds correspond to prosthetic, TV stenosis (choice A). A peak velocity greater than 2 m/s is seen in prosthetic, pulmonic valve stenosis (choice C). A mitral valve peak velocity greater than 2.5 m/s, a mean gradient greater than 10 mm Hg, and a PHT greater than 200 milliseconds correspond to prosthetic mitral valve stenosis.

13.8 The correct answer is C.

Rationale: A mitral valve regurgitant area greater than 9 cm^2, an EROA greater than 0.5 cm^2, and peak velocity greater than 1.9 m/s correspond to severe, prosthetic mitral valve regurgitation (choice C). In severe, prosthetic TV regurgitation, vena contracta is greater than 0.7 cm, the PISA radius is greater than 0.9 cm, and there is holodiastolic flow reversal in the hepatic vein (choice A). In severe, prosthetic pulmonic valve regurgitation, the regurgitant jet width is greater than 50%, the regurgitant volume is greater than 60 mL/beat, and the PHT is less than 100 milliseconds (choice B). In severe, prosthetic aortic valve regurgitation, regurgitant width is greater than 65%, a regurgitant volume is equal to or greater than 60 mL/beat, and a PHT is greater than 500 milliseconds (choice D) (**Table 13.1**).

TABLE 13.1 Doppler Parameters for Prosthetic Heart Valve (PHV) Regurgitation in Different Positions[a,b]

PHV Regurgitation	VC	Regurgitant Jet Width/ Area	PISA Radius (cm)	Rvol (mL/beat)	EROA (cm^2)	PHT (ms)	Other
Tricuspid Moderate Severe	0.3-0.69 cm VC >0.7 cm (or two moderate jets)		0.6-0.89 >0.9	>45	>0.4		Dense, early peaking, triangular CW signal; holodiastolic flow reversal in hepatic vein
Pulmonic[a]							
Mild		<25%		<30			
Moderate		25%-50%		30-60			Flow reversal in PA
Severe		>50%		>60		<100	
Mitral[b]							Peak velocity >1.9 m/s

(continued)

TABLE 13.1	Doppler Parameters for Prosthetic Heart Valve (PHV) Regurgitation in Different Positions (*continued*)						
PHV Regurgitation	VC	Regurgitant Jet Width/ Area	PISA Radius (cm)	Rvol (mL/ beat)	EROA (cm²)	PHT (ms)	Other
Mild	1-2 mm	<4 cm²			<0.2		DVI >2.5
Moderate	3-6 mm	4-8 cm²			0.2-0.50		Mean gradient
Severe	>6 mm	>8 cm²			>0.5		>5 mm Hg
Aortic							
Mild		<25%		<30		<500	
Moderate		25%-64%		30-59		200-500	
Severe		≥65%		≥60		>500	Holodiastolic reversal in aorta

CW, continuous wave; DVI, Doppler velocity index; EROA, effective regurgitant orifice area; PA, pulmonary artery; PHV, prosthetic heart valve; PHT, pressure half time; PISA, proximal isovelocity surface area; Rvol, regurgitant volume; VC, vena contracta.

^aParavalvular leak (PVL) is better predicted with flow reversal, and intravalvular regurgitation is better predicted with regurgitant jet width.
^bVC is more accurate for PVL, and regurgitant jet area is more accurate for intravalvular regurgitation.

13.9 The correct answer is A.

Rationale: Medical therapy is indicated for left-sided, prosthetic valve thrombosis, for which the suspected onset of thrombosis is less than 14 days (choice A). Surgical therapy is favored in patients who are either asymptomatic or unstable with a thrombus area greater than 0.8 cm² (choices B, C, and D).

13.10 The correct answer is E.

Rationale: In patients with suspected or confirmed endocarditis, persistent bacteremia despite antimicrobial treatment, a vegetation size greater than 10 mm, high-degree AV block in the setting of abscess formation, and severe right-sided heart failure are all indications for surgical intervention (choices A, B, C, and D). In terms of the organism type, fungi are the only pathogen that would require surgical intervention due primarily to the inability to clear fungi with medical therapy alone (choice E).

INFECTIVE ENDOCARDITIS

Matthew Derakhshesh and Mohamed Khalid Munshi

CHAPTER 14

QUESTIONS

14.1 Which of the following is **NOT TRUE** regarding the incidence of infective endocarditis (IE)?
- A. Rates of hospitalization for IE have increased between 2001 and 2012.
- B. It is more frequently seen in females.
- C. The most common valve involved is the tricuspid valve.
- D. The increasing use of cardiac devices has contributed to the rising incidence of IE.
- E. B and C

14.2 Which of the following is **TRUE** regarding the pathogenesis of IE?
- A. Endothelial disruption is not required for IE to occur.
- B. Vegetations classically form in the high flow areas of the valve, such as the ventricular side of the atrioventricular (AV) valves.
- C. Gram-negative pathogens are less likely to cause IE due to bactericidal activity in the blood.
- D. *Staphylococcus aureus* uses dextran to adhere to the platelet-fibrin matrix.

14.3 Which of the following is **NOT** considered a risk factor for IE?
- A. Mitral annular calcifications (MAC)
- B. Younger age
- C. Chronic dialysis
- D. HIV
- E. Ventricular septal defect

14.4 A 45-year-old female with a history of mitral valve prolapse is being evaluated for subjective fevers and chills that have been ongoing for the past week. Which of the following additional findings would help establish a definitive diagnosis for IE according to the modified Duke criteria?
- A. *S. aureus* seen on two blood cultures drawn 24 hours apart and a fever of 39 °C
- B. Transesophageal echocardiogram (TEE) showing a new mitral valve regurgitation and a 1.0-cm mobile density on the atrial side of the anterior mitral valve leaflet near the path of the regurgitant jet
- C. *Streptococcus viridans* seen on two blood cultures drawn 24 hours apart and a splenic infarct
- D. Osler nodes on physical examination and transthoracic echocardiogram (TTE) showing new, moderate mitral valve regurgitation

*Questions and Answers are based on Chapter 14: Infective Endocarditis by Jeffrey A. Dixson, Jeffrey Gaca, and Todd L. Kiefer in Cardiovascular Medicine and Surgery, First Edition.

Section 1: Clinical Cardiology

14.5 A 38-year-old male with a history of substance abuse presents with 3 days of frequent chills, nausea, and vomiting. He admits to using intravenous (IV) heroin daily for the last week. His temperature is 38.3 °C. His physical examination is a significant holosystolic murmur in the left lower sternal border without jugular venous distention or lower extremity edema. Four blood cultures drawn over a course of 24 hours grow methicillin-sensitive *Staphylococcus aureus* (MSSA). A TTE show mild tricuspid regurgitation and a TEE shows a 0.8-cm mobile density on the anterior tricuspid valve leaflet. What is the **BEST** overall management for this patient's suspected IE?

A. Ciprofloxacin and rifampin for 4 weeks
B. IV vancomycin for 2 weeks
C. Oral ampicillin for 8 weeks
D. Surgical intervention

14.6 When deciding on the duration of antibiotic treatment for IE, when would be considered the "start date" of treatment?

A. The moment that antibiotics are initiated
B. The time when the first blood cultures are positive
C. The time when the first blood cultures are negative after starting antibiotics
D. The moment a temperature of 38 °C is recorded

14.7 Which organism isolated on blood culture prompts surgical intervention in the setting of IE?

A. *S. viridans*
B. Methicillin-resistant *S. aureus*
C. *Candida albicans*
D. Vancomycin-resistant *Enterococcus*
E. *Aggregatibacter bacilli*

CASE 1

A 59-year-old male with a history of bioprosthetic aortic valve replacement presents to the emergency department (ED) with 1 week of intermittent fevers and chills along with shortness of breath. He is febrile to 39.2 °C with a heart rate of 52 beats per minute (bpm) and an O_2 saturation of 86%. Crackles are appreciated at the bases along with a soft diastolic murmur in the right upper sternal border. Labs show a white blood cell (WBC) count of 17×10^9/L. An electrocardiogram (ECG) shows second-degree Mobitz II AV block. A TTE shows moderate, prosthetic valve regurgitation and TEE reveals a 0.7-cm mobile density on the ventricular side of the noncoronary cusp along with a 2 × 2 cm paravalvular abscess. Blood cultures ultimately grow MSSA in three of the four bottles.

14.8 From **Case 1**, which of the following in the patient's presentation is **NOT** an indication for surgical intervention?

A. Vegetation size
B. Left-sided heart failure symptom
C. Second-degree Mobitz II AV block
D. Paravalvular abscess
E. A and D

14.9 From **Case 1**, what is the most appropriate timing for surgical intervention?
A. Less than 48 hours
B. Within 7 days
C. Within 2 weeks
D. Within 4 weeks

14.10 IE is suspected in a 66-year-old male with a dual-chamber permanent pacemaker. Blood cultures are positive for *Staphylococcus epidermidis* in four of the four bottles in a span of 24 hours. A TEE reveals several small mobile densities in the right ventricular lead. What is the **BEST** treatment for this patient's IE?
A. Antimicrobial therapy only
B. Removal of pacemaker leads only
C. Antimicrobial therapy for 4 to 6 weeks followed by removal of pacemaker leads
D. Removal of pacemaker leads along with antimicrobial therapy for 4 to 6 weeks

ANSWERS

14.1 The correct answer is E.
Rationale: Rates of hospitalization in the United States have increased from 11 per 100,000 to 15 per 100,000 between 2001 and 2012, according to a hospital database. The increasing incidence can in part be attributed to the increased use of cardiac devices, high rates of intravenous drug abuse (IVDU), and more prominent use of vascular access. IE is more frequently seen in males, with an estimated ratio of 1.2 to 2.7:1 when compared to females. The aortic valve, not the tricuspid, tends to be the most affected valve, with up to 38% of cases being identified, followed by the mitral valve.

14.2 The correct answer is C.
Rationale: Gram-negative bacteria are often eliminated by the complement system in the blood, thereby protecting against IE from gastrointestinal sources. Endothelial disruption is required for IE to occur as intact valvular endothelium effectively resists bacterial adhesion and colonization. When vegetations do begin to form, they classically occur on the "low flow" side of the valve, which includes the atrial side of AV valves. Streptococcus species, not *S. aureus* use dextran and other virulence factors to bind to the platelet-fibrin matrix. *S. aureus* binds to disrupted endothelial cells via species-specific clumping factors and has the ability to activate platelets via the von Willebrand receptor.

14.3 The correct answer is B.
Rationale: Older age is considered a risk factor for IE, especially since there is a greater incidence of degenerative valve lesions as the population ages. In that same token, autopsy studies have shown that MAC are commonly found in patients with endocarditis, suggesting that MAC may be a substrate for IE. Chronic hemodialysis is a risk factor for multiple reasons including the need for intravascular access, its association with calcific disease, and the ability to contribute to immune impairment. An altered immune response is also a reason why HIV and malignancy are risk factors for IE.

14.4 The correct answer is B.
Rationale: In order to establish a definitive diagnosis of IE in accordance with the modified Duke criteria, two major, one major and three minor, or five minor criteria must be fulfilled. Since the patient has a known mitral valve prolapse, one of the minor criteria for a predisposing heart condition has been fulfilled. The only choice that does establish a definitive diagnosis is choice B as the mobile density and the new mitral regurgitation fulfill two major criteria. For choices A and C, the presence of a typical microorganisms do fulfill a major criteria, but in combination with a fever of greater than 38 °C or the finding of a splenic infarct, only two minor criteria are achieved (when also considering the history of mitral valve prolapse). Only one major and two minor criteria are also fulfilled as Osler nodes are found in combination with mitral valve regurgitation and mitral valve prolapse (**Table 14.1**).

14.5 The correct answer is A.
Rationale: Multiple major criteria are fulfilled to diagnose this patient with IE including the MSSA bacteremia, vegetation on TEE, and new tricuspid valve regurgitation. Since he does not exhibit any signs of heart failure and his vegetation size is less than 10 mm, surgical intervention is not indicated. IV vancomycin would be more appropriate for methicillin-resistant *S. aureus*; 8 weeks of therapy is also excessive as the typical duration spans 4 to 6 weeks.

14.6 The correct answer is C.
Rationale: The official start date of antibiotic therapy for IE is when blood cultures are first found to be negative. Blood cultures are typically taken every 24 to 72 hours until they return negative. Though empiric antibiotics are usually initiated upon first suspicion of IE, the duration of treatment is not dictated by this timing as bacteremia may persist as evidenced by positive blood cultures. In turn, the start date of antibiotic therapy is also not dictated by when blood cultures first turn positive or by when a fever is recorded.

14.7 The correct answer is C.
Rationale: IE due to fungal infections is an indication for surgical intervention. Persistent fungemia tends to occur even with antimicrobial treatment. Peripheral embolization is also more likely with fungal compared to bacterial infections. Though there may be fewer antibiotic options available for vancomycin-resistant *Enterococcus* and methicillin-resistant *S. aureus*, they can still be cleared with medical therapy. *A. bacilli* is one of the haemophilus species, aggregatibacter actinomycetemcomitans, cardiobacterium hominis, eikenella corrodens, and kingella kingae (HACEK) organisms and is not taken into consideration when deciding between medical management and surgery.

14.8 The correct answer is A.
Rationale: Some of the indications for valve replacement include heart failure symptoms, conduction abnormalities including heart block and the presence of intracardiac abscess. Uncontrolled infections that can occur due to extension of paravalvular abscesses, fungal infections, or unresolved bacteremia for 5 to 7 days despite antibiotic treatment are also considered an indication for surgical intervention. According to the American College of Cardiology (ACC)/American Heart Association (AHA) guidelines, left-sided vegetation size of 10 mm or more can be considered for surgical intervention (class IIb) in order to reduce the risk of embolic events. The vegetation size in this case is 0.7 cm.

TABLE 14.1 Summary of Modified Duke Criteria for Infective Endocarditis

Modified Duke Criteria for Infective Endocarditis

MAJOR CRITERIA

Positive blood cultures	Typical microorganisms isolated from two separate blood cultures • Viridans streptococci • *Streptococcus bovis* • HACEK group • *Staphylococcus aureus* • Community-acquired enterococci
	Persistently positive blood culture from microorganisms consistent with IE • Two or more cultures drawn >12 h apart • Three or more cultures *or* a majority of four or more cultures with the first and last drawn at least 1 h apart
	Single culture positive for *Coxiella burnetii* or IgG Ab titer >1:800
Endocardial involvement (echocardiogram)	Vegetation (oscillating mass in the path of regurgitant jets without an alternative anatomic explanation) • TEE if prosthetic valve, "possible" IE, or complicated IE (eg, paravalvular abscess)
	Intracardiac abscess
	New prosthetic valve dehiscence
	New valve regurgitation

MINOR CRITERIA

Predisposition	Predisposing heart condition or IVDU
Fever	>38 °C
Vascular phenomena	Emboli, mycotic aneurysm, ICH, conjunctival hemorrhage
Immunologic phenomena	Glomerulonephritis, Osler nodes, Roth spots, rheumatoid factor
Microbiology *not* meeting major criteria	Positive blood cultures not meeting major criteria or serologic evidence of infection

INTERPRETATION

Definite endocarditis	• Two major criteria • One major + three minor • Five minor
Possible	• One major + one minor criterion • three minor
Rejected	• Firm alternative diagnosis • Resolution of IE syndrome with ≤4 d of antibiotics • Lack of pathologic evidence of IE with antibiotic therapy for ≤4 d • Does not meet "possible" criteria

ICH, intracranial hemorrhage; IE, infective endocarditis; IgG, immunoglobulin G; IVDU, intravenous drug abuse; TEE, transesophageal echocardiogram.

14.9 The correct answer is A:
Rationale: Intracardiac abscesses, conduction abnormalities, and fistula formation often confer a higher risk of decompensation. Therefore, more urgent surgical intervention is considered in these patient populations. Given that this patient has both a paravalvular abscess and a second-degree heart block, the risk of decompensation is high, and surgery within 48 hours is appropriate. Following a symptomatic stroke, surgery can be delayed 1 to 2 weeks in those without hemorrhagic conversion and 3 to 4 weeks in those with hemorrhagic conversion.

14.10 The correct answer is D:
Rationale: In patients with cardiac implantable electronic devices who develop endocarditis, the best treatment modality is to combine device removal (in this case, lead extraction) and treat with antibiotics (choice D). Treating with antimicrobial therapy alone and or extracting the pacemaker leads by without antimicrobial treatment is not appropriate (choices A and C).

PERICARDIAL DISEASE*

Ciril Khorolsky, Radmila Lyubarova, and Marisa A. Orgera

CHAPTER 15

QUESTIONS

15.1 A 41-year-old female from India presents to the emergency department for evaluation of dyspnea on exertion, orthopnea, and worsening fatigue over the past 2 months. She has no known past medical history and takes no medications. Physical examination is notable for blood pressure of 110/69 mm Hg, heart rate of 98 beats per minute (bpm), elevated jugular venous pressure, and presence of a high-pitched "scratchy" sound on cardiac auscultation. Electrocardiogram (ECG) shows normal sinus rhythm, and transthoracic echocardiogram (TTE) demonstrates a moderate size pericardial effusion. Laboratory evaluation reveals C-reactive protein (CRP) of 93.5 mg/L (0.0-8.0 mg/L) and creatinine of 1.5 mg/dL (0.80-1.4 mg/dL). What is the **MOST LIKELY** etiology of the pericardial effusion?

A. Idiopathic
B. Tuberculosis
C. Prior pericardiotomy
D. Uremia

15.2 A 59-year-old female recently diagnosed with metastatic breast cancer presents to the emergency department with dyspnea, dizziness, and chest discomfort. On examination, the patient is tachycardic with a heart rate of 120 bpm, blood pressure is 85/52 mm Hg, muffled heart sounds are heard, and increased jugular venous pressure is noted. An ECG shows sinus tachycardia with decreased QRS voltage. Which of the following is the most appropriate initial diagnostic tool for this patient?

A. Chest computed tomography (CT) angiography
B. Right heart catheterization
C. Cardiac magnetic resonance imaging (MRI)
D. TTE
E. Transesophageal echocardiogram (TEE)

15.3 Which of the following statements regarding the treatment of acute pericarditis is **TRUE**?

A. Treatment with low-dose once-daily ibuprofen or aspirin is recommended for patients with a history of peptic ulcer disease.
B. Corticosteroids can be used in combination with nonsteroidal anti-inflammatory drugs (NSAIDs) as the initial treatment of viral or idiopathic pericarditis.
C. Low-dose colchicine can be used initially in combination with NSAIDs therapy or added at a later time.
D. When used, colchicine therapy should be continued for at least 12 months.
E. Competitive athletes can return to participation in competitive sports after 1 month of being symptoms free.

Questions and Answers are based on Chapter 15: Pericardial diseases by Yaquta Kaka and Brent C. Lampert in Cardiovascular Medicine and Surgery, First Edition.

15.4 A 39-year-old male presents to the emergency department with 3 days of chest pain, fevers, and fatigue. He describes a pleuritic chest pain that is worse when lying down and less intense when sitting up. He has no known past medical history but reports having an upper respiratory tract infection 2 weeks ago. His blood pressure is 105/70 mm Hg, and his heart rate is 110 bpm. Physical examination is notable for a pericardial friction rub and is otherwise unremarkable. An electrocardiogram and echocardiogram are ordered. The electrocardiogram would **MOST LIKELY** demonstrate which of the following findings?

A. Diffuse convex ST elevation with associated PR-segment elevation
B. Diffuse concave ST elevation with associated PR-segment depression
C. ST elevation in augmented vector right (aVR) and presence of Q-waves
D. Reciprocal ST-segment depressions

15.5 A 55-year-old male is brought to the hospital because of worsening peripheral edema, abdominal distention, and fatigue over the past 3 to 4 months. Past medical history is unremarkable except for two episodes of recurrent pericarditis in the last 8 months successfully treated with ibuprofen and colchicine. Vital signs show blood pressure is 115/71 mm Hg with a heart rate of 95 bpm. Physical examination is notable for an elevated jugular venous pressure that persists during inspiration, abdominal distention, and lower extremity edema. Chest x-ray is unremarkable, and laboratory data demonstrate CRP of 3.0 mg/L (0.0-8.0 mg/L), aspartate transferase of 120 IU/L (5-45 IU/L), and alanine transaminase 139 IU/L (5-60 IU/L). Which of the following would be the most appropriate treatment?

A. Corticosteroid
B. NSAIDs and colchicine
C. Beta-blockers
D. Pericardiocentesis
E. Pericardiectomy

15.6 Which of the following statements about effusive-constrictive pericarditis (ECP) are **TRUE**?

A. Most common causes of ECP are iatrogenic such as postsurgical pericardial disease, postradiation, and prior chemotherapy.
B. ECP is defined as failure of the right atrial pressure to drop to a level below 10 mm Hg or to decrease by greater than or equal to 50% following pericardiocentesis.
C. Pericardiocentesis alone is often adequate to successfully treat ECP.
D. Kussmaul sign and pulsus paradoxus may both be present in patients with ECP.
E. Both B and D are correct.

15.7 You are evaluating a patient with suspected constrictive pericarditis (CP) or restrictive cardiomyopathy (RCM). The presence of which of the following hemodynamic findings would favor the diagnosis of CP?

A. Ventricular interdependence with discordant inspiratory effects on ventricular systolic pressures
B. Diastolic dip and plateau ("square root" sign) waveform pattern on ventricular pressure tracing at end diastole
C. Elevated right ventricular (RV) and left ventricular (LV) filling pressures with LV end-diastolic pressure that is greater than 5 mm Hg higher than the RV end-diastolic pressure
D. Systolic area index (SAI) of 0.9
E. Both A and B

15.8 When differentiating between CP and RCM, which of the following echocardiographic findings one would expect in a patient with CP?
   A. Hepatic vein diastolic flow reversal during inspiration
   B. Increase in mitral inflow velocity (mitral E-wave) by greater than or equal to 25% during expiration
   C. Increase in tricuspid valve (TV) inflow velocity (tricuspid E-wave) by greater than 40% during expiration
   D. Decreased mitral annular velocity (e′)
   E. All of the above

15.9 A 71-year-old male presents to the emergency department with worsening dyspnea, unintentional weight loss, and generalized fatigue. He has a past medical history of advanced metastatic lung cancer and a prior pericardial effusion, successfully drained via pericardiocentesis 3 months ago. He is currently on palliative chemotherapy. Physical examination is notable for blood pressure of 121/78 mm Hg, heart rate of 89 bpm, and distant heart sounds. A TTE demonstrates a large pericardial effusion. What is the most appropriate next step in management?
   A. Drain the pericardial fluid via pericardial window.
   B. Drain the pericardial fluid via pericardiocentesis.
   C. Treat medically with diuretics and anti-inflammatory agents.
   D. Schedule an outpatient follow-up echocardiogram in 1 month.
   E. Nonemergent pericardiectomy

15.10 Which of the following is **NOT** part of the clinical diagnostic criteria of acute pericarditis?
   A. Pericardial friction rub
   B. Typical sharp, pleuritic chest pain
   C. Fever with leukocytosis
   D. ECG with widespread ST elevation with PR-segment depression
   E. New or worsening pericardial effusion

ANSWERS

15.1 The correct answer is B.
Rationale: This case illustrates a patient from a developing country that presents with tuberculous pericarditis complicated by subacute pericardial effusion. There are many different etiologies of pericardial effusion that can be broadly divided into two categories: inflammatory and noninflammatory. Tuberculosis is the most common cause of pericardial effusions in developing countries, whereas in developed countries, the most common etiology is idiopathic (up to 50%). Most patients with pericardial effusions are asymptomatic, being discovered either on routine chest x-ray showing a globular shape to the heart or on TTE done for unrelated reasons. The clinical history does not suggest a history of prior pericardiotomy or pericardial injury. Uremia is a known cause of inflammatory pericardial effusion that may present with the classic uremic pericardial friction rub if concomitant pericarditis is present. However, uremic pericardial effusion is unlikely in this patient, given her mild acute kidney injury (AKI) and no known history of severe renal impairment.

15.2 The correct answer is D.
Rationale: This patient has pericardial effusion with evidence of cardiac tamponade based on the clinical exam and ECG findings. The recently diagnosed metastatic lung cancer is most likely the etiology of the effusion, as malignancies such as lung, breast, and lymphoma are known to cause pericardial effusion. TTE is the most appropriate initial diagnostic tool for patients with high clinical suspicion of tamponade. TTE can provide important information about the size, location, and hemodynamic effects of the effusion. Some common findings of tamponade on TTE include swinging or rocking of the heart within the pericardium, right atrial late diastolic collapse, RV early diastolic collapse, exaggerated respiratory variation with tricuspid and mitral inflow on Doppler, and abnormal ventricular septal motion. A right heart catheterization can provide additional insight into the patient's hemodynamic status and evaluate for the presence of other contributory cardiac pathologies, but it is not the first-line diagnostic modality. Although some of the patient's clinical findings may also be seen in cases of pulmonary embolism (PE), the presence of muffled heart sounds and decreased voltage on the ECG is more suggestive of pericardial effusion with tamponade, rather than PE. Cardiac MRI can show the presence and size of a pericardial effusion; however, it is both time-consuming and costly. The use of a TEE is more invasive and is generally not necessary for diagnosing cardiac tamponade.

15.3 The correct answer is C.
Rationale: Low-dose colchicine is used to prevent recurrence and relapses and can be used initially in combination with NSAIDs or added later if the individual is not responding to NSAID therapy. High-dose NSAID therapy such as ibuprofen 600 to 800 mg every 8 hours or aspirin 750 to 1,000 mg every 8 hours is the recommended dose for the treatment of viral, idiopathic, or inflammatory pericarditis. Corticosteroids have been shown to cause recurrences with pericarditis and therefore are not generally recommended unless there is a specific rheumatologic indication, pregnancy, or contraindication to NSAIDs. Colchicine therapy is usually continued for at least 3 months, not 12 months. Competitive athletes should not participate in competitive sports for at least 3 months following symptom resolution, not 1 month (**Figure 15.1**).

15.4 The correct answer is B.
Rationale: This patient has acute pericarditis, a condition that often presents with characteristic ECG changes. Typical findings on ECG include diffuse ST elevation with PR-segment depression and ST depression in aVR. The ST-segment elevations are usually concave, not convex, and generally do not exceed 5 mm in amplitude. Additionally, reciprocal ST-segment depressions, QRS widening, and Q-waves are not present.

15.5 The correct answer is E.
Rationale: The patient's presentation is most consistent with CP with a positive Kussmaul sign and the presence of right-sided heart failure symptoms. The definitive treatment of CP is surgical pericardiectomy, which can potentially be curative if done in a timely manner. Treatment with NSAIDs or corticosteroids and colchicine can be considered for asymptomatic patients with transient CP or CP that is associated with elevated inflammatory markers. This is not the most appropriate treatment choice, given the patient's significant symptoms and normal CRP. Beta-blocker therapy is unlikely to be effective, and there is no indication for pericardiocentesis based on this clinical scenario.

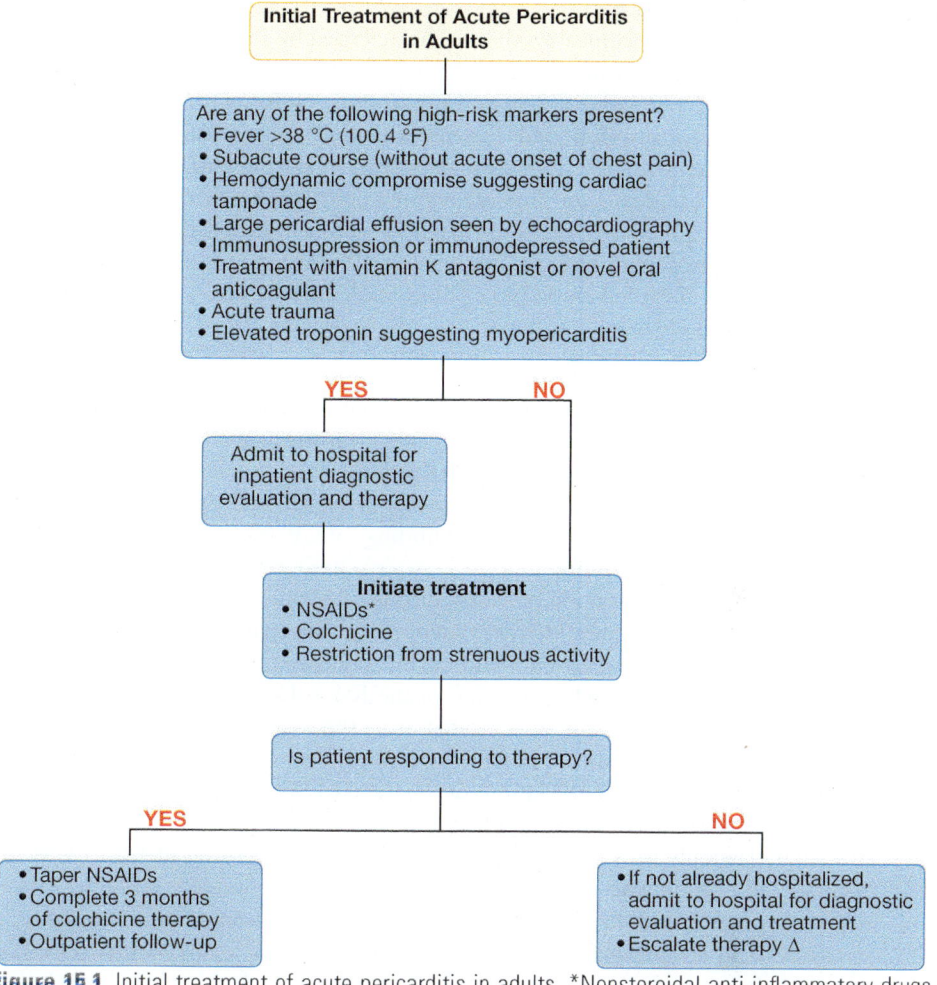

Figure 15.1 Initial treatment of acute pericarditis in adults. *Nonsteroidal anti-inflammatory drugs (NSAIDs) are the preferred anti-inflammatory for nearly all patients with acute idiopathic or viral pericarditis. Glucocorticoids should be used for initial treatment of acute pericarditis only in patients with contraindications to NSAIDs or for specific indications (ie, systemic inflammatory diseases, pregnancy, renal failure), and should be used at the lowest effective dose. (Reproduced with permission from Imazio M. Acute pericarditis: treatment and prognosis. In: Connor RF, ed. *UpToDate*. Wolters Kluwer; 2024. Copyright © 2024 UpToDate, Inc. and/or its affiliates. All rights reserved.)

15.6 The correct answer is E.
Rationale: ECP is a rare clinical syndrome characterized by a range of clinical manifestations that fall between true effusive tamponade and chronic CP. The most common causes of ECP are idiopathic (58%) and tuberculosis (38%), with postradiation and postsurgery occasionally identified. Patients with ECP can present with clinical features of pericardial effusion, CP, or both and may have the presence of both Kussmaul sign and pulsus paradoxus on physical examination. Invasive hemodynamic assessment is usually required to confirm the diagnosis of ECP, which is defined as failure of the right atrial pressure to drop to a level below 10 mm Hg or to decrease by greater than or equal to 50% following pericardiocentesis that reduces the intrapericardial pressure to 0 mm Hg.

15.7 The correct answer is E.
Rationale: CP and RCM can be present in a similar way and are often challenging to differentiate. The use of invasive hemodynamic assessment is frequently required to confirm the hemodynamic profile and establish the correct diagnosis. The following hemodynamic findings can help distinguish between CP and RCM: Ventricular interdependence is one of the most specific findings of CP due to the stiff pericardium that restricts ventricular filling and leads to enhanced ventricular interaction with discordant LV and RV systolic pressures during respiration. In RCM, on the other hand, there is no ventricular interdependence, and the ventricular systolic pressures are concordant during respiration. Ventricular interdependence can also be quantified by the SAI, which is defined as the ratio of the RV to LV pressure-time area during inspiration and expiration and is calculated using the area under the ventricular pressure curves. SAI greater than 1.1 is highly sensitive and specific for CP. Another typical finding with CP is the dip and plateau (or square root) sign on the ventricular pressure tracing that occurs due to the abrupt halt of ventricular filing by the stiff pericardium. Although classically seen in CP, the square root sign may also occur with RCM. In both CP and RCM, the ventricular filling pressures are elevated; however, in CP, the left ventricular end-diastolic pressure (LVEDP) and right ventricular end-diastolic pressure (RVEDP) are close to equal (<5 mm Hg), whereas in RCM the LVEDP is greater than 5 mm Hg compared to the RVEDP (**Table 15.1**).

15.8 The correct answer is B.
Rationale: Echocardiography is often the initial diagnostic test used to evaluate CP and can be very helpful in differentiating between CP and RCM. The following echocardiographic findings are typically noted in patients with CP: increase in mitral inflow velocity (mitral E-wave) by greater than or equal to 25% during expiration, increase in TV inflow velocity (tricuspid E-wave) by greater than 40% during inspiration, hepatic vein diastolic flow reversal in expiration, and normal to elevated mitral annulus velocity. In patients with RCM, on the other hand, there is no change in mitral and tricuspid inflow respiratory variation, hepatic vein diastolic flow reversal occurs during inspiration, and the mitral annulus velocity is normal to reduced.

15.9 The correct answer is A.
Rationale: This patient has a large pericardial effusion; however, he does not appear to be in clinical tamponade as evidenced by his hemodynamic stability. The most appropriate next step in management is to drain the pericardial fluid via pericardial window,

TABLE 15.1 Echocardiographic Parameters of Constrictive Pericarditis and Restrictive Cardiomyopathy

Septal bounce	Yes	No
MV inflow respiratory variation	≥25%	None
TV inflow respiratory variation	>40%	None
MVDT	≤160 ms	<160 ms
Hepatic vein reversal	Diastolic reversal with expiration	None
IVRT	Decrease with expiration Increase with inspiration	Unchanged
TR duration	Increased	Normal
Mitral annulus velocity (ie, early diastolic Doppler tissue velocity e′ at mitral annulus)	Normal or increased (≥8 cm/s)	Normal or decreased (<8 cm/s)
Strain analysis (absolute global longitudinal strain)	>16%	≤10%

IVRT, isovolumic relaxation time; MV, mitral valve; MVDT, mitral valve deceleration time; TR, tricuspid regurgitation; TV, tricuspid valve.
Adapted with data from Mookadam F, Jiamsripong P, Raslan SF, Panse PM, Tajik AJ. Constrictive pericarditis and restrictive cardiomyopathy in the modern era. *Future Cardiol.* 2011;7(4):471-483.

which is the preferable drainage method for effusions that are more likely to reaccumulate, such as malignant effusions. Pericardiectomy is the treatment of choice for CP, and it may be indicated in the future if there is evidence of constriction; however, it is not indicated at this time. Anti-inflammatory therapy is used for acute pericarditis and has no role in this case, and diuretics are generally not recommended in large pericardial effusions because they can decrease the preload and precipitate development of clinical tamponade. Scheduling an outpatient follow-up echocardiogram in 1 month is not appropriate, as the patient has a large symptomatic pericardial effusion and is at risk of progressing to clinical tamponade if not drained.

15.10 The correct answer is C.

Rationale: The clinical diagnosis of acute pericarditis requires at least two of the following criteria: (1) typical sharp, pleuritic chest pain; (2) pericardial friction rub; (3) ECG changes (widespread ST elevation with PR-segment depression); and (4) new or worsening pericardial effusion. Additional clinical findings such as elevated inflammatory markers or pericardial inflammation on CT or MRI are supportive of the diagnosis but are not part of the clinical diagnostic criteria.

PULMONARY HYPERTENSION

Ciril Khorolsky and Mohammad El-Hajjar

CHAPTER 16

QUESTIONS

16.1 Which of the following statements regarding the hemodynamic classification of pulmonary hypertension (PH) is **CORRECT**?
  A. PH is defined by a mean pulmonary artery pressure (mPAP) greater than or equal to 25 mm Hg.
  B. Precapillary PH is defined as mPAP greater than 20 mm Hg, pulmonary capillary wedge pressure (PCWP) less than or equal to 15 mm Hg, and pulmonary vascular resistance (PVR) greater than or equal to 3 Wood units.
  C. Combined PH is defined as mPAP greater than 20 mm Hg, PCWP greater than 15 mm Hg, and PVR less than 3 Wood units.
  D. Postcapillary PH is defined as mPAP greater than 20 mm Hg, PCWP greater than 15 mm Hg, and PVR greater than or equal to 3 Wood units.
  E. None of the above

16.2 In patients with PH, which of the following clinical factors is the most important determinant of clinical outcomes and survival?
  A. Response to invasive vasoreactivity testing
  B. Baseline blood pressure
  C. Pulmonary artery pressure (PAP)
  D. Right ventricular (RV) function
  E. PVR

16.3 Which of the following is the **CORRECT** pair of the PH group and its subgroup?
  A. PH group I: idiopathic pulmonary arterial hypertension (PAH)
  B. PH group II: obstructive lung disease
  C. PH group III: valvular heart disease
  D. PH group IV: pulmonary veno-occlusive disorder
  E. Both A and D are correct.

16.4 A 45-year-old female with a known history of PAH presents to the cardiology clinic for follow-up. She reports worsening dyspnea on exertion over the past 3 months. A transthoracic echocardiogram demonstrates moderate tricuspid regurgitation and an estimated RV systolic pressure of 55 mm Hg. You refer her for a right heart catheterization (RHC) with vasoreactivity testing. Which of the following would be considered a positive response to invasive vasoreactivity testing?

---

*Questions and Answers are based on Chapter 16: Pulmonary Hypertension by Saurabh Rajpal, Jeremy Slivnick, William H. Marshall V, and Zachary Garrett in Cardiovascular Medicine and Surgery, First Edition.

A. Reduction in mPAP by greater than or equal to 15 mm Hg to a level less than 50, with increased or unchanged cardiac output (CO)
B. Reduction in mPAP by greater than or equal to 15% to a level less than 50 mm Hg, with increased or unchanged CO
C. Reduction in mPAP by greater than or equal to 10 mm Hg to a level less than 40, with increased or unchanged CO
D. Reduction in mPAP by greater than or equal to 10% to a level less than 40 mm Hg, with increased or unchanged CO
E. None of the above

16.5 A 39-year-old female with PAH presents to the cardiology clinic for evaluation of 2 months of exertional dyspnea. She recently underwent genetic testing and was found to have a mutation in the gene encoding for bone morphogenetic protein receptor type 2. Physical examination is notable for blood pressure of 130/75 mm Hg, heart rate of 89 beats per minute (bpm), and a high-pitched, holosystolic murmur at the left lower sternal border that increases with inspiration. There is no jugular venous distention, no peripheral edema, and the lungs are clear. Basic labs are unremarkable, and a transthoracic echocardiogram demonstrates a left ventricular ejection fraction (LVEF) greater than 55%, moderate tricuspid regurgitation, and an estimated RV systolic pressure of 59 mm Hg. You refer her for an RHC, which reveals an mPAP of 48 mm Hg, PCWP of 11 mm Hg, PVR of 4 Wood units, and CO of 5 L/min. Following administration of inhaled nitric oxide, the mPAP is reduced to 35 mm Hg and CO is increased to 6 L/min. The patient tolerates the invasive vasoreactivity testing without any complications. Which of the following would be the most appropriate next step in management?

A. Initiate diuretics.
B. Repeat RHC with vasoreactivity testing using a different vasoreactivity agent.
C. Obtain high-resolution computed tomography (CT) and pulmonary function testing (PFT).
D. Initiate dual oral therapy with an endothelin receptor antagonist and phosphodiesterase-5 inhibitor.
E. Initiate high-dose calcium channel blockers (CCBs).

16.6 Which of the following statements is **TRUE** regarding the treatment of patients with PAH?

A. Bosentan is the only oral monotherapeutic agent that has demonstrated mortality benefit in nonvasoreactive PAH.
B. Intravenous epoprostenol is the only PAH medication with a demonstrated survival benefit.
C. High-dose CCBs is the preferred first-line treatment in nonvasoreactive PAH.
D. De-escalation of therapy in responders should be considered, given the increased risk of severe side effects with prolonged use.
E. The combination of sildenafil and riociguat is recommended if PAH-specific monotherapy is unsuccessful.

16.7 A 62-year-old male presents to the cardiology clinic for evaluation of worsening dyspnea and fatigue over the past 3 months. He has a history of hypertension, hyperlipidemia, and a pulmonary embolism a year and a half ago, which was successfully treated with 6 months of Eliquis. Vital signs show a blood pressure of 135/75 mm Hg, resting oxygen saturation of 90%, and a heart rate of 98 bpm. Physical examination is notable for an elevated jugular venous pressure, an accentuated P2 on cardiac auscultation, and bilateral lower extremity edema. You refer the patient for an RHC, which demonstrates an mPAP of 37 mm Hg, PCWP of 13 mm Hg, and PVR of 5 Wood units. Which of the following tests would be the most appropriate next step in the diagnostic evaluation of this patient?

A. CT pulmonary angiography
B. Magnetic resonance angiography
C. PFTs
D. Ventilation-perfusion (V̇/Q̇) imaging

16.8 All the following statements regarding group II PH due to left heart disease (LHD) are **TRUE EXCEPT**:

A. PH due to LHD is the least common of the five clinical groups of PH.
B. PH due to LHD is defined hemodynamically by RHC as an mPAP greater than 20 mm Hg and PCWP greater than 15 mm Hg.
C. No PAH-specific therapies have been shown to be beneficial in this condition.
D. The treatment of PH due to LHD is primarily focused on the management of the underlying heart disease.

16.9 You are reviewing the results of a recent RHC of one of your patients with heart failure with suspected PH. The mPAP is 33 mm Hg and the PCWP is 19 mm Hg. Which of the following hemodynamic parameters would be most consistent with the group II PH subclassification termed as combined postcapillary and precapillary PH?

A. PVR less than 3 Wood units, transpulmonary gradient (TPG) greater than 12 mm Hg, and diastolic pulmonary gradient (DPG) less than 7 Wood units
B. PVR greater than or equal to 3 Wood units, TPG less than 12 mm Hg, and DPG greater than 7 Wood units
C. PVR greater than or equal to 3 Wood units, TPG greater than 12 mm Hg, and DPG greater than 7 Wood units
D. PVR less than 3 Wood units, TPG less than 12 mm Hg, and DPG less than 7 Wood units

16.10 Which of the following statements regarding PH in patients with sickle cell disease is **TRUE**?

A. PH is present in up to 25% of patients with sickle cell disease.
B. PH due to sickle cell disease is a subgroup of PAH.
C. Phosphodiesterase-5 inhibitor is a safe and effective treatment option for PH in patients with sick cell disease.
D. Endothelial receptor antagonists are contraindicated.
E. Decreased bioavailability of nitric oxide because of hemolysis and oxidative stress contributes to the development of PH.

ANSWERS

16.1 The correct answer is B.
Rationale: The classification system and definition of PH have changed over time as there has been an increased recognition of outcomes and treatment options through efforts by the National Institutes of Health and the World Society of Pulmonary Hypertension (WSPH). In the past, PH was defined as a mPAP of greater than or equal to 25 mm Hg; however, in the sixth WSPH held in 2018, PH definition was updated to an mPAP greater than 20 mm Hg. Precapillary PH is defined as an mPAP greater than 20 mm Hg, PCWP less than or equal to 15 mm Hg, and PVR greater than or equal to 3 Wood units. Postcapillary PH is defined as an mPAP greater than 20 mm Hg, PCWP greater than 15 mm Hg, and PVR less than 3 Wood units. Combined PH is defined as an mPAP greater than 20 mm Hg, PCWP greater than 15 mm Hg, and PVR greater than or equal to 3 Wood units.

16.2 The correct answer is D.
Rationale: The outcome of patients with PH depends on the function of the right ventricle. The right ventricle is thin walled, crescent shaped, and has smaller myocytes in a more circumferential arrangement as compared to the left ventricle. Under normal physiologic conditions, the right ventricle facilitates venous return into the low-impedance pulmonary vasculature, with one-fourth of the stroke work of the left ventricle. PH leads to RV pressure overload, causing RV hypertrophy, flattening of the interventricular septum, and eventually progressive RV dilation and dysfunction. Elevations in PAPs and PVR contribute to RV dysfunction; however, at the early stages, the RV may be able to compensate for the high PAPs and PVR without the presence of significant symptoms.

Patients with a positive response to invasive vasoreactivity testing have improved survival; however, this test is only indicated for patients with precapillary PH. It is not uncommon for patients with PH to have low blood pressure, especially if they are on vasodilators. Although this may contribute to decreased survival over time, RV function is a stronger predictor of outcomes and survival.

16.3 The correct answer is A.
Rationale: There are five clinical groups of PH that are further categorized into subgroups based on etiology, pathophysiology, and response to treatment (**Table 16.1**).

16.4 The correct answer is C.
Rationale: Vasoreactivity testing with inhaled nitric oxide, intravenous adenosine, or intravenous prostacyclin is recommended in all group I patients with precapillary PH, with a positive response defined as a decrease in mPAP by 10 mm Hg or more to 40 mm Hg or less with an increased or unchanged CO.

TABLE 16.1 Sixth WSPH Clinical Classifications of Pulmonary Hypertension

PH Groups	Subgroups

Group I: PAH	1.1 Idiopathic PAH
	1.2 Heritable PAH
	1.3 Drug or toxin-induced PAH
	1.4 PAH associated with:
	    Connective tissue disease
	    HIV
	    Portal hypertension
	    Congenital heart disease
	    Schistosomiasis
	1.5 PAH responsive to calcium channel blockers
	1.6 Pulmonary veno-occlusive disorder
	1.7 Persistent PH of the newborn syndrome

Group II: PH due to left heart disease	2.1 With preserved LVEF 2.2 With reduced LVEF 2.3 Due to valvular heart disease 2.4 Left-sided due to congenital heart disease
Group III: PH due to lung disease	3.1 Obstructive lung disease 3.2 Restrictive lung disease 3.3 Mixed obstructive/restrictive lung disease 3.4 Hypoxemia without lung disease 3.5 Congenital lung disorders
Group IV: PH due to pulmonary artery obstruction	4.1 Chronic thromboembolic PH 4.2 Other chronic pulmonary obstructions, for example, tumors, congenital (Alagille syndrome)
Group V: PH of unclear or multifactorial mechanism	5.1 Hematologic disorders 5.2 Systemic and metabolic disorders 5.3 Others 5.4 Complex congenital heart disease

HIV, human immunodeficiency virus; LVEF, left ventricular ejection fraction; PAH, pulmonary arterial hypertension; PH, pulmonary hypertension; WSPH, World Society of Pulmonary Hypertension.
(Reproduced with permission of the © ERS 2024: Simonneau G, Montani D, Celermajer DS, et al. Haemodynamic definitions and updated clinical classification of pulmonary hypertension. *Eur Respir J.* 2019;53(1):1801913.)

16.5 The correct answer is E.
Rationale: This patient has heritable PAH with a positive acute response to vasoreactivity testing defined as a decrease in mPAP by 10 mm Hg or more to 40 mm Hg or less with an increased or unchanged CO. For patients with a positive response, called super responders, high-dose CCBs are the treatment of choice and are associated with improved survival. There is no role for diuretics in this patient with normal PCWP and no evidence of hypervolemia or RV failure. There is no indication to repeat RHC with vasoreactivity testing as there is nothing to suggest faulty or

erroneous results of the invasive vasoreactivity testing. Obtaining high-resolution CT and PFT would be indicated if there is a high suspicion for the presence of pulmonary veno-occlusive disease (PVOD). Patients with PVOD usually develop pulmonary edema in response to vasoreactivity testing, which did not occur in this patient. Dual oral therapy with an endothelin receptor antagonist and phosphodiesterase-5 inhibitor is the recommended initial therapy in low-to-intermediate risk nonvasoreactive PAH.

16.6 The correct answer is B.
Rationale: In patients with high-risk disease, defined as 1-year mortality greater than or equal to 10% or persistent intermediate- to high-risk symptoms despite dual oral therapy, treatment with intravenous prostacyclin or its analogues should be considered. Intravenous epoprostenol, a synthetic analogue of prostacyclin, is the only PH medication with a demonstrated survival benefit. In nonvasoreactive PH, numerous oral agents have demonstrated benefits in 6-minute walk test distance, quality of life, disease progression rates, or reduction in PH-related events in randomized studies. However, no oral monotherapeutic agent has currently demonstrated mortality benefit. High-dose CCBs are the treatment of choice in patients with a positive response to vasoreactivity testing but not in nonvasoreactive PAH. De-escalation of therapy in responders is generally not recommended, given the progressive nature of PH. The combination of sildenafil and riociguat should be avoided due to the risk of hypotension.

16.7 The correct answer is D.
Rationale: This case illustrates a patient with group IV PH—chronic thromboembolic pulmonary hypertension (CTEPH). The gold standard imaging modality for the evaluation of CTEPH is $\dot{V}/\dot{Q}$ imaging due to its high sensitivity (90%-100%) and specificity (94%-100%). A normal or low-probability $\dot{V}/\dot{Q}$ scan essentially excludes CTEPH. CT pulmonary angiography and magnetic resonance angiography also may provide evidence of chronic thromboembolic PH; however, the diagnosis of CTEPH requires the presence of a perfusion mismatch on a $\dot{V}/\dot{Q}$ scan. PFTs would be more helpful in the evaluation of underlying airway and parenchymal lung diseases such as emphysema and interstitial lung disease but would not be as helpful in the diagnosis of CTEPH (**Table 16.2**).

16.8 The correct answer is A.
Rationale: PH due to LHD is the most common of the five clinical groups of PH and is associated with a high morbidity and mortality. In the sixth WSPH recommendation, PH due to LHD is defined hemodynamically by RHC as an mPAP greater than 20 mm Hg and PCWP greater than 15 mm Hg. The treatment of PH due to LHD is primarily focused on the management of the underlying heart disease itself, as no PAH therapies have been shown to be beneficial in this condition.

TABLE 16.2 Testing Modalities in Pulmonary Hypertension

Testing Modality	Common Findings
Electrocardiography	Right axis deviation, right ventricular strain or hypertrophy, right bundle branch block, P-pulmonale, and QTc prolongation. Findings are more commonly found in the setting of severe disease.
Chest x-ray	Central pulmonary arterial dilation with pruning of peripheral vessels. Right atrial and ventricular enlargement in advanced disease. Concomitant lung disease may be seen.
Pulmonary function testing and blood gases	Evaluates for underlying airway and parenchymal lung disease including emphysema and interstitial lung disease. Most patients with PAH have a low DLCO and include pulmonary veno-occlusive disease, scleroderma-associated PAH, and parenchymal lung disease. A DLCO <45% predicted is associated with poor outcomes. Combined emphysema and interstitial disease may present with normal spirometry (pseudonormalization) but a low DLCO and decreased lung volumes.
Echocardiography	Echocardiography is used for screening, differential diagnosis, follow-up, and prognostication of patients with PH. It can estimate portions of the PVR including PA systolic pressure using the tricuspid regurgitant velocity and estimated right atrial pressure, PCWP using the transmitral Doppler inflow velocity (E) to mitral annular tissue Doppler velocity (e') ratio, and cardiac output using the aortic velocity time integral and left ventricular outflow tract dimensions. Mean PA pressure can also be estimated from the right ventricular outflow tract acceleration time and pulmonary valve regurgitant velocity. These parameters can also help in the initial differentiation of precapillary versus postcapillary forms of PH. Echocardiogram can also show further evidence of PH including right atrial or ventricular dilation, right ventricular systolic dysfunction, a flattened interventricular septum, dilation of the IVC, and notching of the spectral pulse-wave Doppler of the right ventricular outflow tract. Echocardiography can also evaluate for left heart disease, intracardiac shunts, and congenital heart disease. Several echocardiographic parameters like right atrial size and the presence of pericardial effusion are important prognostic factors for pulmonary hypertension.
Ventilation-perfusion scan	Gold standard imaging modality for the evaluation of chronic thromboembolic PH due to its high sensitivity (90%-100%) and specificity (94%-100%). A normal or low-probability V̇/Q̇ scan essentially excludes chronic thromboembolic PH.

TABLE 16.2 Testing Modalities in Pulmonary Hypertension (*continued*)

Testing Modality	Common Findings
Computed tomography	CT can reveal indirect evidence of PH, such as PA enlargement or right ventricular dilation, and help detect underlying causes, such as pulmonary or vascular disease. A PA diameter >29 mm or a ratio to the ascending aorta diameter greater than 1 should raise concern for PH in symptomatic patients. Evidence of pulmonary veno-occlusive disease can also be seen on CT, including diffuse ground glass opacities, pulmonary edema, and thickened interlobar septa. Nonspecific ground glass opacities might also be seen in up to one-third of patients with PAH. With angiography, CT can also show evidence of chronic thromboembolism with complete pulmonary obstruction of arteries, bands, webs, and intimal irregularities. CT pulmonary angiography can also be used to assess vasculitis and arteriovenous fistulas.
Cardiac magnetic resonance	CMR can accurately assess right ventricular size, mass, and function as well as hemodynamics including cardiac output and stroke volume. CMR may also be useful if underlying congenital heart disease is suspected but not well evaluated with echocardiography. MR angiography provides an accurate assessment of pulmonary vasculature, which is particularly useful in suspected chronic thromboembolic PH when CT angiography is precluded due to either pregnancy or the presence of contraindications to iodinated contrast.
Blood testing	Chemistry, hematology, and thyroid function testing should be obtained in all patients with confirmed or suspected PH. Liver function tests and hepatitis serologies should also be considered in patients with PH to evaluate for underlying liver disease related to high central venous pressures and in cases where endothelin receptor antagonist therapy is considered. Thyroid disease is commonly associated with PAH or may develop during disease and should be considered if there is an abrupt clinical worsening. Markers for connective tissue disease, systemic scleroderma, hepatitis serologies, and HIV should also be assessed. Limited scleroderma may have a positive ANA, anticentromere, dsDNA, anti-Ro, U3-RNP, B23, Th/To, and U1-RNP, whereas diffuse scleroderma is usually associated with U3-RNP. All patients with chronic thromboembolic PH should be evaluated for hypercoagulability disorders including antiphospholipid antibodies, anticardiolipin antibodies, and lupus anticoagulants. BNP and NT pro-BNP are useful markers for diagnosis and prognostication of PH.
Ultrasonography	Abdominal ultrasonography can be used to evaluate for portal hypertension.
Six-minute walk test	Useful for assessing disease progression and response to treatment. A 6-min walk distance over 500 m indicates a good prognosis, whereas less than 300 m indicates a poor prognosis.

(continued)

TABLE 16.2 Testing Modalities in Pulmonary Hypertension (continued)

Testing Modality	Common Findings
Cardiopulmonary exercise testing	Cardiopulmonary exercise testing should be used after diagnosis of PH to assess the severity of exercise limitation related to PH and response to therapies. It can also be utilized to better define the predominant cardiopulmonary pathophysiology, resulting in symptoms and PH.
Right heart catheterization	RHC is required to confirm the diagnosis and assess the severity of PH. Left heart catheterization should also be considered in select patients when there are risk factors for coronary disease or HFpEF. RHC may also be considered to assess treatment effect of drugs, evaluate congenital cardiac shunts to support decisions on correction, and in patients planning to undergo transplantation. If the accuracy of measurements obtained during RHC is in question, then a left ventricular end-diastolic pressure should be directly measured. RHC for the evaluation of PH should be performed in expert centers. Pressures should be zeroed at the midthoracic line halfway between sternum and bed at the level of the left atrium. The PCWP should be measured as the mean of three measurements at the end of normal expiration. Full oximetry testing—in all right heart chambers, both vena cava and the PAs—should be done if PA oxygen saturation is >75% or if a left-to-right shunt is suspected. Vasoreactivity testing is used to evaluate the response of pulmonary pressures to calcium channel blocker therapy but should only be performed in expert centers. A positive response is a reduction in mean PA pressure ≥10 mm Hg to reach an absolute mean PA pressure <40 with increased or unchanged cardiac output. The PCWP can be reduced <15 mm Hg with diuretics, and some institutions have administered a 500-mL saline bolus to help distinguish PAH from left ventricular dysfunction; however, this is not routine practice. A transpulmonary gradient and PVR should be calculated. PVR is sensitive to changes in flow and filling pressures and may not represent the pulmonary circulation at rest. The diastolic pulmonary gradient (ie, difference between diastolic PA diastolic and mean PCWP) is less affected by flow and filling pressures. Hemodynamic sensors implanted during RHC may be used for long-term monitoring of PA pressures to guide management.

ANA, antinuclear antibody; BNP, brain natriuretic peptide; CMR, cardiac magnetic resonance; CT, computed tomography; DLCO, diffusing capacity of the lung for carbon monoxide; dsDNA, double-stranded DNA; HFpEF, heart failure with preserved ejection fraction; HIV, human immunodeficiency virus; IVC, inferior vena cava; MR, magnetic resonance; NT, natriuretic; PA, pulmonary artery; PAH, pulmonary arterial hypertension; PCWP, pulmonary capillary wedge pressure; PH, pulmonary hypertension; PVR, pulmonary vascular resistance; RHC, right heart catheterization; RNP, ribonucleoprotein; V̇/Q̇, ventilation-perfusion.

16.9 The correct answer is C.

Rationale: PH due to LHD can be further classified as isolated postcapillary PH (Ipc-PH) or combined postcapillary and precapillary PH (Cpc-PH). The term "Ipc-PH" describes those patients whose PH is merely because of passive pulmonary venous congestion. A minority of patients subject to long-standing elevated left-sided heart filling pressures undergo structural and functional pathophysiologic changes in the precapillary vasculature, including remodeling and vasoconstriction, resulting in mPAP disproportionately elevated relative to the PCWP. Such patients are described as having Cpc-PH. Additional hemodynamic parameters can be used to differentiate between these two subgroups and include TPG (difference between mPAP and PCWP) and DPG (difference between PA diastolic pressure and mean PCWP). In Ipc-PH, the PVR less than 3 Wood units, DPG less than 7 Wood units, and TPG less than 12 mm Hg. In Cpc-PH, on the other hand, the PVR is greater than or equal to 3 Wood units, TPG greater than 12 mm Hg, and DPG greater than 7 Wood units.

16.10 The correct answer is E.

Rationale: PH is present in 6% to 11% of patients with sickle cell disease and is categorized as group V PH. The etiology of PH in sickle cell disease appears to be multifactorial; however, the decreased bioavailability of nitric oxide because of hemolysis and oxidative stress likely contributes to the development of PH in these patients. Treatment with phosphodiesterase-5 inhibitors is contraindicated because of an increased risk of vaso-occlusive crisis; however, if precapillary PH is present, select patients can be treated with a prostacyclin agonist or endothelial receptor antagonist.

ADULT CONGENITAL HEART DISEASE

Harneet Bhatti and Robert L. Carhart

CHAPTER 17

QUESTIONS

17.1 A 42-year-old male with a known history of aorta coarctation repair presents to the clinic for follow-up. His blood pressure (BP) is noted to be 156/97 mm Hg, and his heart rate is 97 beats per minute (bpm). Physical examination demonstrates clear lung sounds, normal S1 and S2, with no murmurs appreciated. What would be the next **BEST** step in management?

   A. Prescribe lisinopril.
   B. Obtain transthoracic echocardiogram.
   C. Prescribe hydralazine.
   D. Prescribe isosorbide dinitrate.

17.2 A 28-year-old male presents to the clinic for follow-up. He recently underwent an atrial septal defect (ASD) repair. He denies any shortness of breath or chest pain and reports good exercise capacity. What is the next **BEST** step in management?

   A. Obtain transthoracic echocardiogram.
   B. Obtain transesophageal echocardiogram.
   C. Obtain chest x-ray.
   D. Obtain computed tomography angiography (CTA) thorax.

17.3 A 25-year-old male presents to the clinic for a new patient visit. He reports a history of left ventricle hypoplasia and underwent surgery at the age of 3 months, although he does not remember any details. He has not had follow-up with a physician for many years. He denies having any shortness of breath, chest pain, or palpitations, and is not currently taking any medications. His vitals in the clinic include BP of 136/86 mm Hg and heart rate of 87 bpm. Given his history of left ventricular hypoplasia, which of the following procedures is **MOST LIKELY** to have been performed on this patient?

   A. Fontan procedure
   B. Bentall procedure
   C. Patent ductus arteriosus (PDA) ligation
   D. Coarctation of aorta repair

---

*Questions and Answers are based on Chapter 17: Adult Congenital Heart Disease by Benjamin S. Hendrickson, Marc V. Lee, Jennifer DeSalvo, and Elisa A. Bradley in Cardiovascular Medicine and Surgery, First Edition.

CHAPTER 17 | Adult Congenital Heart Disease

17.4 A 19-year-old male presents to emergency department with worsening pain in bilateral lower extremities while walking. He has no known medical history. On presentation, his BP is 150/92 mm Hg, and his heart rate is 93 bpm. Lungs are clear to auscultation, with normal S1 and S2 heart sounds. Femoral pulse is present but diminished compared to the brachial pulse. BP in the right lower extremity is noted to be 90/52 mm Hg. Which of the following is the **MOST LIKELY** diagnosis?

A. Peripheral vascular disease
B. Coarctation of the aorta
C. Aortic stenosis
D. ASD

17.5 A 22-year-old female presents to the clinic with complaints of worsening shortness of breath on exertion over the past couple of months. Physical examination reveals significant clubbing of bilateral lower extremities. A systolic murmur is heard on the left side of the sternum at the second intercostal space. What is the **MOST LIKELY** diagnosis?

A. Right-to-left shunt across a PDA
B. Left-to-right shunt across a PDA
C. Right-to-left shunt across an ASD
D. Right-to-left shunt across a ventricular septal defect

17.6 A 22-year-old male presents to the emergency department with complaints of sudden onset of chest pain that started while he was exercising. He describes the chest pain as sharp and radiating to his back. On presentation, BP is 122/87 mm Hg in the right upper extremity and 100/85 mm Hg in the left upper extremity. The patient exhibits a tall body habitus with long extremities and digits. Kyphosis is also noted. What is the next **BEST** step in management?

A. CTA thorax and abdomen
B. Transthoracic echocardiogram
C. Troponin level
D. Electrocardiogram

ANSWERS

17.1 The correct answer is A.
Rationale: Hypertension and hyperlipidemia in patients with adult congenital heart disease should be managed the same way they are managed in all adult patients.

17.2 The correct answer is A.
Rationale: It is important to establish a baseline after any congenital heart disease repair. The aim should be to monitor these patients with serial testing over time to detect late manifestations prior to the development of any symptoms.

173. The correct answer is A.
Rationale: This patient likely had a Fontan procedure to help divert deoxygenated blood directly to the pulmonary artery. The Bentall procedure is used during the repair of an aortic dissection. This patient did not have a PDA or coarctation of the aorta.

174. The correct answer is B.
Rationale: This patient likely has undiagnosed coarctation of the aorta. This congenital vascular lesion can result in upper extremity hypertension and lower extremity claudication. Discrepancy in BP is often noted when comparing upper and lower extremities, depending on the location of the coarctation. It is unlikely that he has severe peripheral vascular disease given his age and lack of other risk factors. Aortic stenosis and an ASD are unlikely to cause lower extremity claudication.

175. The correct answer is A.
Rationale: This patient likely has a PDA given the differential cyanosis. A right-to-left shunt through a PDA will deliver deoxygenated blood to the aorta distal to the left subclavian artery, resulting in lower extremity hypoxia while the upper extremities are spared. Gibson in 1906 described PDA continuous systolic and diastolic murmur, that is, machinery murmur. With Eisenmenger syndrome, elevated pulmonary pressures cause reversal of the shunt to right-to-left, resulting in the loss of the diastolic murmur and a presentation that can mimic primary pulmonary hypertension.

176. The correct answer is A.
Rationale: This patient likely has Marfan syndrome given the physical examination findings. The discrepancy of greater than 20 mm Hg in systolic pressure in the upper extremities, along with complaints of sudden onset of chest pain, suggests an aortic dissection as the etiology of the patient's clinical presentation. Patients with Marfan syndrome are at a higher risk for developing aortopathy, including aortic root and thoracic aortic aneurysms placing them at risk for dissections.

REFERENCE:
Gibson. *A Clinical Lecture on Persistent Ductus Arteriosus.* Medical Press and Circular; 1906.

PREGNANCY AND HEART DISEASE

Wen Qian (Jenny) Zheng, Joshua Schulman-Marcus, Radmila Lyubarova, and Sulagna Mookherjee

CHAPTER 18

QUESTIONS

18.1 What is currently the most common form of cardiac disease encountered in pregnant women in the United States?

   A. Rheumatic heart disease
   B. Congestive heart disease
   C. Congenital heart disease
   D. Ischemic heart disease

18.2 Which of the following are known risk factors for peripartum cardiomyopathy?

   A. History of hypertension
   B. History of preeclampsia
   C. Family history of cardiomyopathy
   D. All the above

18.3 Which of the following is **NOT** a physiologic change that occurs during pregnancy?

   A. Increase in hematocrit
   B. Decrease in systolic blood pressure
   C. Increase in cardiac output
   D. Increase in heart rate

18.4 A 32-year-old female with no past medical history at 30th week gestation presents to the clinic for a follow-up visit. On the last visit 3 weeks ago, her blood pressure measured in the clinic was 145/95, and repeat measurement was 150/95. She has taken her blood pressure daily at home and the values range from 140 to 155/88 to 95. She has no symptoms such as chest pain, headaches, or dyspnea. She asks you if her blood pressure readings are considered elevated. What is the cutoff for diagnosis of hypertension in a pregnancy?

   A. 130/80 or more
   B. 140/90 or more
   C. 135/85 or more
   D. 150/90 or more

18.5 The same patient from **Question 18.4** is diagnosed with gestational hypertension after a thorough workup. Her blood pressure on the current visit is 150/100. Which of the following pharmacologic agents is considered first-line treatments?

   A. Hydrochlorothiazide
   B. Labetalol
   C. Atenolol
   D. Diltiazem

*Questions and Answers are based on Chapter 18: Pregnancy and Heart Disease by Alice Chan, Ayesha Salahuddin, Diana Wolfe, and Ali N. Zaidi in Cardiovascular Medicine and Surgery, First Edition.

18.6 A 38-year-old female with a history of hypertension, mixed dyslipidemia, and premature family history of myocardial infarction comes to your clinic to establish care. She is feeling well and is contemplating pregnancy in the next year. She is afebrile, her blood pressure is 110/70, and her heart rate is 75. Her current medications include atorvastatin 20 mg daily, hydrochlorothiazide 25 mg daily, and lisinopril 10 mg daily along with a prenatal vitamin. What is the next step in management (Table 18.1)?

- A. Continue current medications.
- B. Stop hydrochlorothiazide, continue lisinopril and atorvastatin.
- C. Stop hydrochlorothiazide and lisinopril, and continue atorvastatin.
- D. Stop hydrochlorothiazide, lisinopril, and atorvastatin.

18.7 Which of the following cardiomyopathies is the most well tolerated during pregnancy?

- A. Hypertrophic cardiomyopathy (HCM)
- B. Dilated cardiomyopathy
- C. Ischemic cardiomyopathy
- D. Alcohol-induced cardiomyopathy

18.8 A 30-year-old female is postpartum day 1 from an elective Cesarean section. She is doing well and has no cardiac symptoms. What should be part of her routine postpartum care?

- A. Bed rest for the first 24 hours
- B. Elastic leg stockings
- C. Oral anticoagulation for venous thromboembolism (VTE) prophylaxis
- D. Breastfeeding after 24 hours

18.9 There are many hemodynamic changes that occur throughout pregnancy. How is central venous pressure affected by pregnancy?

- A. It tends to increase.
- B. It tends to decrease.
- C. It tends to stay the same.
- D. It cannot be determined.

18.10 In general, regional anesthesia is preferable to general anesthesia during fetal delivery. In which of the following patients would general anesthesia be preferable?

- A. A 35-year-old female with pulmonary arterial hypertension who is having an elective C-section at 37-week gestation
- B. A 25-year-old female with dilated cardiomyopathy who is having an elective C-section at 37-week gestation
- C. A 30-year-old female on therapeutic anticoagulation for recent pulmonary embolism with a planned elective C-section at 37-week gestation
- D. A 33-year-old female with Marfan syndrome with a dilated aorta of 40 mm with planned elective C-section at 37-week gestation

18.11 Based on the CARPREG (CARdiac disease in PREGnancy) II risk score, which of the following is **NOT** a predictor of adverse cardiovascular events in pregnancy?

- A. History of arrhythmias
- B. Mild pulmonary/aortic valve regurgitation
- C. Mechanical valve prosthesis
- D. Left heart obstruction (pressure gradient >10 mm Hg or aortic valve area of less than 2 cm^2)

ANSWERS

18.1 The correct answer is C:
Rationale: Recently, congenital heart disease has become the most common form of heart disease complication in pregnancy in the United States. Rheumatic heart disease is the most common form of cardiac disease encountered in pregnant women and continues to be prevalent in developing countries.

18.2 The correct answer is D:
Rationale: All the options have been identified as risk factors for peripartum cardiomyopathy and increased risk of cardiac morbidity and mortality in pregnancy.

18.3 The correct answer is A:
Rationale: The hematocrit level decreases during pregnancy because of a disproportionate increase in plasma volume that exceeds the rise in red cell mass. Systolic blood pressure decreases during pregnancy by 10 to 15 mm Hg due to decrease in systemic vascular resistance. Cardiac output increases by 30% to 50% above baseline during normal pregnancy. Heart rate increases by 10 to 15 beats per minute (bpm) during pregnancy.

18.4 The correct answer is B:
Rationale: Pregnant women with a systolic blood pressure of 140 mm Hg or more and/or diastolic blood pressure of 90 mm Hg or more are considered hypertensive. Patients with elevated blood pressure may have chronic hypertension, gestational hypertension, or newly diagnosed preeclampsia. It is important to address hypertension timely during pregnancy as it is associated with both maternal and fetal morbidities.

18.5 The correct answer is B:
Rationale: Labetalol is considered one of the first-line treatments for this scenario along with nifedipine and methyldopa. Atenolol, diltiazem, and hydrochlorothiazide should all be used with caution during pregnancy due to possible teratogenic effects (**Table 18.1**).

TABLE 18.1 Cardiac Medications in Pregnancy

Medications	FDA Category	Pregnancy	Lactation
Adenosine	C	Safe	Use with caution
Alpha-methyldopa	B	Safe	Safe
Amiodarone	D	Contraindicated	Contraindicated
Amlodipine	C	Use with caution	Use with caution
Argatroban	B	Use with caution	Unknown
Aspirin	C	Use with caution	Use with caution
Atenolol	D	Contraindicated	Use with caution
Carvedilol	C	Safe	Unknown

(continued)

TABLE 18.1 Cardiac Medications in Pregnancy (*continued*)

Medications	FDA Category	Pregnancy	Lactation
Clonidine	C	Use with caution	Unknown
Clopidogrel	B	Use with caution	Use with caution
Digoxin	C	Safe	Safe
Diltiazem	C	Use with caution	Unknown
Dobutamine	B	Safe	Unknown
Dopamine	C	Safe	Unknown
Enoxaparin	B	Safe	Safe
Epoprostenol	B	Use with caution	Unknown
Flecainide	C	Use with caution	Use with caution
Furosemide	C	Safe	Use with caution
Heparin	C	Safe	Safe
Hydralazine	C	Use with caution	Safe
Hydrochlorothiazide	B	Use with caution	Safe
Isosorbide dinitrate	C	Use with caution	Unknown
Labetalol	C	Safe	Use with caution
Lidocaine	B	Safe	Safe
Metolazone	B	Use with caution	Unknown
Metoprolol	C	Safe	Use with caution
Nifedipine	C	Safe	Safe
Nitroglycerin	C	Use with caution	Unknown
Nitroprusside	C	Use with caution	Use with caution
Norepinephrine	C	Safe	Unknown
Procainamide	C	Use with caution	Use with caution
Propranolol	C	Safe	Use with caution
Sildenafil	B	Use with caution	Use with caution
Sotalol	B	Use with caution	Unknown
Ticagrelor	C	Use with caution	Unknown
Torsemide	B	Use with caution	Unknown
Treprostinil	C	Unknown	Unknown
Verapamil	C	Safe	Safe
Warfarin	D	Use with caution	Safe

Food and Drug Administration (FDA) Categories:
A, Human studies have not shown fetal risk; B, animal studies have not shown fetal risk; C, animal studies have shown fetal side effects (no human studies); D, human studies have shown side effects on the fetus, but medication can be used if there are potential benefits.

18.6 The correct answer is D.
Rationale: All three medications should be stopped as they have possible teratogenic side effects. Given her multiple risk factors of coronary heart disease, she needs close follow-up for blood pressure and lipid management throughout pregnancy.

18.7 The correct answer is A.
Rationale: HCM is generally well tolerated with a mortality of 0.5%. The risk of premature birth in these women is increased, but stillbirth and spontaneous abortion rates are similar to that of women without HCM. Dilated cardiomyopathies can be a result of many etiologies (toxin or drug, ischemia, viral infection, etc). These patients often do not tolerate pregnancy well and may have worsening ventricular function.

18.8 The correct answer is B.
Rationale: Early ambulation, elastic stockings, and meticulous leg care all decreased the risk of VTE during the postpartum period. VTE prophylaxis can be considered with enoxaparin or heparin during pregnancy, but oral anticoagulation is typically not used. Lastly, early breastfeeding promotes uterine contraction and is important to initiate before the first 24 hours.

18.9 The correct answer is C.
Rationale: Although changes in blood volume during pregnancy affect right ventricular afterload, central venous pressure remains unchanged during pregnancy. This is due to the reduction in cardiac afterload induced by substantial decreases in both systemic vascular resistance and pulmonary vascular resistance.

18.10 The correct answer is C.
Rationale: Patients who are on therapeutic anticoagulation should aim to avoid regional anesthesia during delivery because it increases the release of catecholamines which increase heart rate and blood pressure and pose a higher risk of postpartum hemorrhage due to uterine atony. The other scenarios (pulmonary arterial hypertension, dilated cardiomyopathy, and Marfan syndrome with aortic dilation) would have overall lower risk with regional anesthesia compared to general anesthesia during the delivery period.

18.11 The correct answer is B.
Rationale: Different risk estimation scores and algorithms have been developed based on large population–based studies. The CARPREG (CARdiac disease in PREGnancy) risk score includes four predictors. Women with a score of 0 and no lesion-specific risks are considered low risk, whereas women with a risk of 1 or more require a comprehensive evaluation. The CARPREG II risk index added more predictors. ZAHARA (Zürich assessment of the risk of pregnancy in women with a congenital heart defect) investigators assessed pregnancy-related complications in women with congenital heart disease and developed a weighted risk score which includes eight predictors with each quintile of score assigning a maternal risk of cardiovascular complications during pregnancy ranging from 2.9% to 70%. The most widely used risk classification system which is recommended by the European Society of Cardiology is a modified World Health Organization (mWHO)

classification. The mWHO classification categorizes patients into four risk classes, classes I–IV (see later) (**Tables 18.2-18.5**).

Based on the CARPREG II risk score, moderate/severe (not mild) pulmonary atrioventricular valve regurgitation is a predictor of adverse cardiovascular events with a weighted score of 0.75 (**Table 18.3**).

TABLE 18.2 CARPREG Risk Score

Predictors of Adverse Cardiovascular Events	Points
• Prior cardiac event (heart failure, transient ischemic attack) • Infarction before pregnancy or arrhythmia	1
• NYHA functional class at baseline >II or cyanosis	1
• Left heart obstruction (mitral valve area <2.0 cm^2) • Aortic valve area <1.5 cm^2 • Left ventricular outflow tract gradient >30 mm Hg	1
• Reduced systolic ventricular function (ejection fraction <40%)	1

CARPREG, Cardiac Disease in Pregnancy; NYHA, New York Heart Association.

TABLE 18.3 CARPREG II Risk Score

Predictors of Adverse Cardiovascular Events	Weighted Score
History of arrhythmias	1.5
Cardiac medications before pregnancy	1.5
NYHA functional class before pregnancy ≥II	0.75
Left heart obstruction (PG >50 mm Hg or AVA <1 cm^2)	2.5
Systemic atrioventricular valve regurgitation (moderate/severe)	0.75
Pulmonary atrioventricular valve regurgitation (moderate/severe)	0.75
Mechanical valve prosthesis	4.25
Cyanotic heart disease (corrected/uncorrected)	1.0

AVA, aortic valve area; CARPREG, Cardiac Disease in Pregnancy; LVEF, left ventricular ejection fraction; NYHA, New York Heart Association; PG, pressure gradient.

TABLE 18.4 ZAHARA Risk Score

Predictors of Adverse Cardiovascular Events	Points
• Prior cardiac events or arrhythmias	3
• Baseline NYHA III-IV or cyanosis	3
• Mechanical valve	3
• Systemic ventricular dysfunction (LVEF <55%)	2
• High-risk valve disease or • LVOTO (AVA <1.5 cm^2, subaortic gradient >30 mm Hg or moderate-to-severe mitral regurgitation, mitral stenosis <2.0 cm^2)	2
• Pulmonary hypertension • RVSP >49 mm Hg	2
• Coronary artery disease	2
• High-risk aortopathy	2
• No prior cardiac intervention	1
• Late pregnancy assessment	1

AVA, aortic valve area; LVEF, left ventricular ejection fraction; LVOTO, left ventricular outflow tract obstruction; NYHA, New York Heart Association; RVSP, right ventricular systolic pressure; ZAHARA, Zwangerschap bij vrouwen met een Aangeboren HARtAfwijking (Zürich assessment of the risk of pregnancy in women with a congenital heart defect).

TABLE 18.5 Modified World Health Organization (mWHO) Classification of Pregnancy Risk Classes

WHO Classification		
I	Uncomplicated small or mild PS PDA Mitral valve prolapse Successfully repaired simple lesions (ASD, VSD, PDA, PAPVC)	No detectable increased risk of maternal mortality and no/mild increase in morbidity
II	Unrepaired ASD or VSD Unrepaired tetralogy of Fallot	Small increase in maternal risk mortality or moderate increase in morbidity
II-III	Mild left ventricular impairment Hypertrophic cardiomyopathy Native or tissue valvular heart disease not considered WHO I or IV Marfan syndrome without aortic dilation Aorta <45 mm in association with BAV Repaired coarctation	Small-to-moderate increase in maternal risk mortality or moderate increase in morbidity

(continued)

TABLE 18.5 Modified World Health Organization (mWHO) Classification (continued)

WHO Classification		
III	Mechanical valve Systemic right ventricle Fontan circulation Unrepaired cyanotic heart disease Other complex congenital heart disease Aortic dilation 40-45 mm in Marfan syndrome Aortic dilation 45-50 mm in BAV	Significantly increased risk of maternal mortality or severe morbidity. Expert counseling required. If pregnancy is decided upon, intensive specialist cardiac and obstetric monitoring needed throughout pregnancy, childbirth, and the puerperium.
IV (Conditions in which pregnancy contraindicated)	PAH of any cause Severe systemic ventricular dysfunction (LVEF <30%, NYHA functional class III-IV) Previous peripartum cardiomyopathy with any residual impairment of left ventricular function Severe MS, severe asymptomatic AS Marfan syndrome with aorta dilated >45 mm Aortic dilation of >50 mm in aortic disease associated with BAV Native severe coarctation	

AS, aortic stenosis; ASD, atrial septal defect; BAV, bicuspid aortic valve; LVEF, left ventricular ejection fraction; LVOTO, left ventricular outflow tract obstruction; MS, mitral stenosis; NYHA, New York Heart Association; PAH, pulmonary arterial hypertension; PAPVC, partial anomalous pulmonary venous connection; PDA, patent ductus arteriosus; PS, pulmonary stenosis; VSD, ventricular septal defect; WHO, World Health Organization.

Data compiled from Regitz-Zagrosek V, Roos-Hesselink JW, Bauersachs J, et al. 2018 ESC Guidelines for the management of cardiovascular diseases during pregnancy: the Task Force for the Management of Cardiovascular Diseases During Pregnancy of the European Society of Cardiology (ESC). *Eur Heart J.* 2018;39:3165-3241; Thorne S, MacGregor A, Nelson-Piercy C. Risks of contraception and pregnancy in heart disease. *Heart.* 2006;92:1520-1525.

WOMEN AND HEART DISEASE*

Wen Qian (Jenny) Zheng, Kim A. Poli, Sulagna Mookherjee, and Radmila Lyubarova

CHAPTER 19

QUESTIONS

19.1 A 67-year-old female is seeing you in clinic to establish care. Her medical history includes rheumatoid arthritis, asthma, obesity, and hypothyroidism. She feels well, and her vitals are stable. Which of her past medical conditions is considered a nontraditional risk factor for cardiovascular disease?

- A. Rheumatoid arthritis
- B. Asthma
- C. Hypothyroidism
- D. Obesity

19.2 A 56-year-old female with a history of breast cancer (previously completed a course of trastuzumab and radiation therapy) 1 year ago and currently in remission, presents with dyspnea on exertion progressing over the last month. She is afebrile, with a blood pressure (BP) of 140/80 mm Hg, regular pulse of 90 beats per minute (bpm), respiratory rate (RR) of 22 breaths per minute, and oxygen saturation of 90% on room air. Physical examination reveals crackles in bilateral lung bases and elevated jugular venous pressure. What is the **MOST LIKELY** diagnosis?

- A. Pulmonary embolism
- B. Pneumonia
- C. Heart failure
- D. Atrial fibrillation

19.3 A 28-year-old female with a history of fibromuscular dysplasia, who is postoperative day 3 from an uncomplicated cesarean section, develops sudden-onset substernal chest pressure at rest. She also develops diaphoresis and dyspnea with minimal exertion. Her vitals are as follows: afebrile, BP 100/70 mm Hg, heart rate (HR) 105 bpm, RR 22 breaths per minute, and oxygen saturating 95% on room air. She appears uncomfortable, but her cardiac and pulmonary examination is otherwise unremarkable. Her troponin I is elevated at 2.5 ng/mL. An electrocardiogram (ECG) shows ST elevations in leads V2 to V4. What is the **MOST LIKELY** diagnosis?

- A. Microvascular dysfunction
- B. Pulmonary embolism
- C. Spontaneous coronary artery dissection
- D. Acute coronary syndrome from plaque rupture/atherosclerosis

*Questions and Answers are based on Chapter 19: Women and Heart Disease by Kelly Paschke and Dipti Itchhaporia in Cardiovascular Medicine and Surgery, First Edition.

19.4 After undergoing coronary catheterization, the same patient described in **Question 19.3** is found to have focal spontaneous coronary artery dissection (SCAD) in the mid segment of the left anterior descending artery. What is the next step in management?

A. Percutaneous coronary intervention with drug eluting stents
B. Balloon angioplasty
C. Medical therapy with intravenous (IV) heparin for 48 hours
D. Medical therapy with aspirin and beta-blockers

19.5 Which of the following are risk factors for development of heart failure with preserved ejection fraction in women?

A. Hypertension
B. Obesity
C. Atrial fibrillation
D. All of the above

19.6 Which of the following reasons account for why women have higher mortality within 1 year and 5 years post-myocardial infarction than men?

A. Women are younger at initial presentation of coronary artery disease.
B. Women are more likely to develop heart failure post-myocardial infarction.
C. Women are more likely to participate in cardiac rehabilitation.
D. Women are less likely to present with atypical symptoms, which may delay diagnosis of coronary artery disease.

19.7 What is the recommendation for BP target in men and women according to the systolic blood pressure intervention trial (SPRINT) trial?

A. Target for men: greater than 130/80 mm Hg; target for women: greater than 140/90 mm Hg
B. Target for men: greater than 140/90 mm Hg; target for women: greater than 130/80 mm Hg
C. Target for men: greater than 130/80 mm Hg; target for women: greater than 130/80 mm Hg
D. Target for men: greater than 140/90 mm Hg; target for women: greater than 140/90 mm Hg

19.8 Hyperlipidemia is a recognized modifiable risk factor of coronary artery disease. Which of the following is typically **TRUE** when comparing lipid panels between men and women?

A. Women have higher high-density lipoprotein cholesterol (HDL-C) levels than men.
B. Women have lower total cholesterol levels than men.
C. Women have higher low-density lipoprotein cholesterol (LDL-C) levels than men.
D. Women have higher triglyceride levels than men.

19.9 A 35-year-old female is presenting to the office to establish care. She has a history of migraines and deep vein thrombosis 2 years ago, which occurred after prolonged immobilization following ankle surgery. She is an active smoker with a 5-pack-year history. She does not drink alcohol or use any recreational drugs. You advise smoking cessation. Continued tobacco use can increase the risk of which of the following:

A. Myocardial infarction
B. Cerebrovascular accidents
C. Thromboembolism
D. All of the above

ANSWERS

19.1 The correct answer is A.
Rationale: Traditional risk factors for heart failure with preserved ejection fraction include age, hypertension, diabetes mellitus/metabolic syndrome, hyperlipidemia, and smoking/obesity. Nontraditional risk factors for women include rheumatologic disorders, breast cancer treatment, pregnancy-related complications, and depression. Rheumatologic disorders increase cardiovascular disease risk due to their inflammatory nature, which has been shown to increase mortality (**Figure 19.1**).

19.2 The correct answer is C.
Rationale: Women with a history of breast cancer, especially those who have been treated with anthracycline-based chemotherapy, trastuzumab, or radiation, are at higher risk of developing heart failure. It is recommended that women undergoing treatment for breast cancer undergo further assessment for cardiovascular risk factors. They should be monitored closely during and after breast cancer treatment for development of signs and symptoms of heart failure, such as dyspnea, orthopnea, or weight gain. Pulmonary embolism usually presents with sudden symptoms of dyspnea, tachycardia, and hypoxia. Atrial fibrillation is not typically associated with trastuzumab.

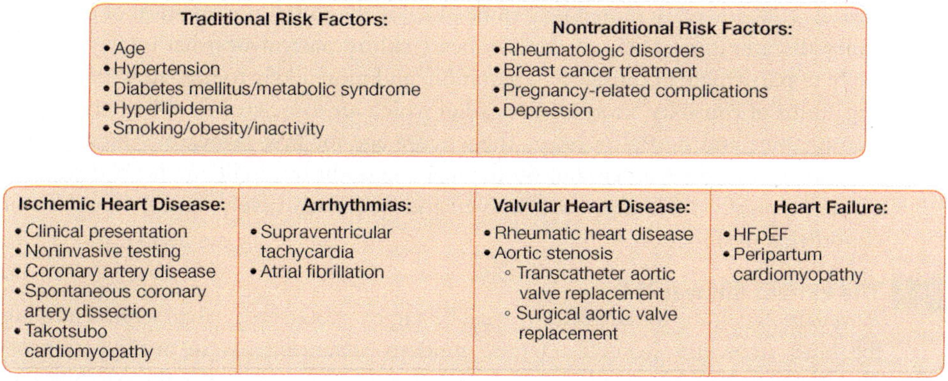

Traditional Risk Factors:	Nontraditional Risk Factors:
• Age • Hypertension • Diabetes mellitus/metabolic syndrome • Hyperlipidemia • Smoking/obesity/inactivity	• Rheumatologic disorders • Breast cancer treatment • Pregnancy-related complications • Depression

Ischemic Heart Disease:	Arrhythmias:	Valvular Heart Disease:	Heart Failure:
• Clinical presentation • Noninvasive testing • Coronary artery disease • Spontaneous coronary artery dissection • Takotsubo cardiomyopathy	• Supraventricular tachycardia • Atrial fibrillation	• Rheumatic heart disease • Aortic stenosis 　◦ Transcatheter aortic valve replacement 　◦ Surgical aortic valve replacement	• HFpEF • Peripartum cardiomyopathy

Figure 19.1 Cardiovascular disease in women: chapter overview. HFpEF, heart failure with preserved ejection fraction.

19.3 The correct answer is C:

Rationale: This patient has significant risk factors for SCAD, including postpartum state and a history of fibromuscular dysplasia. SCAD is characterized by the dissection of the coronary artery wall, resulting in the creation of a false lumen and subsequent intramural hematoma, which can lead to acute myocardial infarction. The presentation of SCAD varies in the degree of severity and may present with acute heart failure and/or cardiogenic shock. SCAD occurs mostly in young women; however, recent data suggest an increasing numbers of postmenopausal women presenting with SCAD. It is important to screen women with SCAD for fibromuscular dysplasia, with computed tomography (CT) imaging of the brain, chest, abdomen, and pelvis. Microvascular and pulmonary embolism typically do not present with sudden-onset chest pain, and acute coronary syndrome from plaque rupture is less likely given her age.

19.4 The correct answer is B:

Rationale: The treatment of SCAD with percutaneous intervention can be challenging and is generally not recommended in most cases due to the potential to worsen coronary dissection. Instead, medical therapy with aspirin, beta-blockers, and cardiac rehabilitation is recommended. Statin therapy should be considered if hyperlipidemia is present. Long-term surveillance is essential as recurrence of SCAD occurs in up to 10% of individuals. Systemic anticoagulation with heparin should be avoided after the diagnosis of SCAD.

19.5 The correct answer is D:

Rationale: All of the above are known risk factors for heart failure with preserved ejection fraction (HFpEF). HFpEF is nearly 2 times more common in women compared to men. In the presence of hemodynamic stress, the myocardium in women is more likely to remodel in a concentric pattern compared to men, who tend to experience eccentric hypertrophy. Risk factors for developing HFpEF include hypertension, obesity, and atrial fibrillation. Female patients should be educated on risk reduction strategies and undergo aggressive BP and weight control to prevent HFpEF.

19.6 The correct answer is B:

Rationale: Women are more likely to be older at the initial presentation of coronary artery disease, more likely to develop heart failure post-myocardial infarction, less likely to participate in cardiac rehabilitation, and more likely to present with atypical symptoms of coronary artery disease, all of which are associated with higher hospital readmissions and mortality rates. The average age for first myocardial infarction is 72 years of age for women and 65 for men. In addition, ischemic heart disease in women typically differs from that in men and frequently involves microvascular and endothelial dysfunction.

19.7 The correct answer is C:

Rationale: According to the SPRINT trial, BP targets should be less than 130/80 mm Hg for both men and women. Despite modern advancements in antihypertensive agents, mortality associated with hypertension has increased over the past decade. Nearly one in three individuals with hypertension are unaware of their diagnosis. However, women tend to have better awareness of their hypertension diagnosis, receive treatment, and have better BP control compared to men. It is estimated that improving hypertension management could lead to a 38% reduction in cardiovascular disease mortality among women.

19.8 The correct answer is A.
Rationale: Women typically have higher total cholesterol and HDL-C levels compared to men, but they have lower LDL-C and triglyceride levels. The advent of cholesterol-lowering agents, especially statins, has led to a significant reduction in hypercholesterolemia within the population. Despite baseline gender differences in cholesterol and triglycerides, treatment recommendations remain the same for both men and women. The 2019 ACC/AHA guidelines on primary prevention of cardiovascular disease include recommendations for statin therapy based on atherosclerotic risk scoring and consideration of associated risk factors.

19.9 The correct answer is D.
Rationale: Tobacco use significantly increases the risk of myocardial infarction, stroke, and thromboembolism, making it imperative to strongly discourage smoking during each visit. Smoking remains the most significant cause of preventable death worldwide. Although approximately 13.5% of women are tobacco users, they represent a smaller proportion of the smoking population compared to men. Additionally, up to 7.2% of women continue to smoke during pregnancy, which may increase the overall risk of pregnancy-associated hypertension and preterm birth. Complete smoking cessation is important given the increased risk of cardiovascular disease, even with reduced tobacco use. Younger tobacco users and e-cigarette users should be warned about the potential unknown cardiovascular effects of newer nicotine and tobacco agents.

OLDER ADULTS AND HEART DISEASE*

Wen Qian (Jenny) Zheng, Sulagna Mookherjee, and Radmila Lyubarova

CHAPTER 20

QUESTIONS

20.1 Which of the following biologic changes occur in the cardiovascular system with age?
- A. Increase in angiotensin II levels
- B. Increase in nitric oxide production
- C. Decrease in matrix metalloproteinase concentration
- D. Decrease in collagen and elastase levels

20.2 A 70-year-old male with a history of hypertension, mixed dyslipidemia, and coronary artery disease (CAD) is presenting to the office for a blood pressure (BP) follow-up. His BPs at home have been between 150-160 mm Hg systolic and 90-100 mm Hg diastolic range. He is taking aspirin 81 mg daily, metoprolol succinate 50 mg daily, atorvastatin 40 mg daily, and hydrochlorothiazide 25 mg daily. He does not have any chest pain, palpitations, dyspnea with exertion, or lightheadedness while standing. His vitals in the office are as follows: BP of 155/92 mm Hg, heart rate of 74 beats per minute (bpm), and oxygen saturation of 95% on room air. His last echocardiogram shows an ejection fraction (EF) of 40% to 45% with global hypokinesis. His last basic metabolic panel showed a normal potassium level and creatinine of 0.90 According to the American College of Cardiology and the American Heart Association (ACC/AHA) 2017 guidelines, what is the next **BEST** step in management?
- A. Increase dose of hydrochlorothiazide.
- B. Add another antihypertensive agent.
- C. Continue ambulatory BP monitoring.
- D. Continue the same medication regimen.

20.3 For the same patient described in **Question 20.2**, what is the **BEST** medication to add for BP management?
- A. Carvedilol
- B. Valsartan
- C. Spironolactone
- D. Doxazosin

20.4 A 75-year-old male presents for evaluation of worsening chest pressure on exertion for the past month. He has bilateral knee arthritis and has difficulty walking up more than one flight of stairs due to pain. His resting electrocardiogram (ECG) shows sinus rhythm with right bundle branch block. Which of the following choices would be indicated for further risk stratification?

---

*Questions and Answers are based on Chapter 20: Elderly and Heart Disease by Madhan Shanmugasundaram and Toshinobu Kazui in Cardiovascular Medicine and Surgery, First Edition.

A. Exercise stress electrocardiography
B. Coronary angiography
C. Pharmacologic myocardial perfusion imaging
D. Coronary computed tomography (CT) angiography

20.5 A 77-year-old man with no past medical history walks into the emergency room with 2 hours of substernal chest pain at rest associated with diaphoresis and dyspnea. Rest ECG reveals ST elevations in inferior leads with reciprocal ST depressions in the lateral leads. The nearest cath lab is 30 minutes away. What is the **MOST** appropriate step in management?

A. Aspirin, clopidogrel, intravenous (IV) heparin, and fibrinolytic therapy
B. Aspirin, clopidogrel, and IV heparin
C. Fibrinolytics and reassess with close monitoring in intensive care unit (ICU) setting
D. Load with aspirin, clopidogrel, IV heparin, and transport immediately to nearest cath lab

20.6 A 70-year-old man is presenting to the hospital with heart failure (HF) exacerbation and is found to have systolic dysfunction with a left ventricular EF of 35% to 39%. An ischemic workup reveals no CAD. He improves with IV diuretics and medical therapy. He is being prepared for discharge and has normal renal function, stable electrolytes, and stable vital signs. Which of the following is the **BEST** long-term medical therapy for this patient?

A. Beta-blocker, angiotensin-converting enzyme inhibitor (ACEi), and mineralocorticoid receptor antagonist (MRA)
B. Beta-blocker, angiotensin receptor blocker (ARB), and MRA
C. Beta-blocker, angiotensin receptor blocker/neprilysin inhibitor (ARNI), and MRA
D. Beta-blocker, ACEi, ARB, and MRA

20.7 The same patient from **Question 20.6** improved with rate control and diuresis. An ischemic evaluation reveals nonobstructive coronary disease. He is discharged on guideline-directed medical therapy. Six months later, he follows up in clinic and feels well and can tolerate moderate activity. His vitals are as follows: BP 104/70 mm Hg, HR 74 bpm, saturating well on room air. His repeat left ventricular ejection fraction (LVEF) is 30%. Renal function is normal. The ECG shows atrial fibrillation (AF) with left bundle branch block (LBBB) (QRS >150 ms) with a ventricular rate of 52 bpm. What is the next **BEST** step in management?

A. Increase dose of metoprolol
B. No change in medical management; follow for additional 6 months
C. Refer to electrophysiology (EP) for consideration of cardiac resynchronization therapy with implantable cardioverter-defibrillator (ICD)
D. Workup for cardiac transplantation

20.8 For the patient in **Question 20.6**, which of the following is a potential benefit of ICD therapy?

A. Primary prevention of sudden cardiac death
B. Secondary prevention of sudden cardiac death
C. Decreasing episodes of flash pulmonary edema
D. Normalizing his EF

20.9 What is the **MOST** common valve disease in older adults in the United States?
   A. Aortic stenosis
   B. Mitral regurgitation
   C. Aortic regurgitation
   D. Mitral stenosis

20.10 An 86-year-old man with hypertension presents with new-onset AF and decompensated HF. He is found to have pulmonary edema, elevated jugular venous pressure, and lower extremity edema. His vitals are as follows: afebrile, BP 132/80 mm Hg, HR 135 bpm, saturating at 90% on 1.5 L supplemental O_2. The ECG shows AF with a ventricular rate of 138 bpm. Echocardiography reveals an LVEF of 25% to 30% with global hypokinesis. Pertinent laboratory data include hemoglobin of 12.5 g/dL, potassium of 4.4 mmol/L, and creatinine of 2.2 mg/mL, with a creatinine clearance of 30 mL/min. In addition to diuresis, what is the **MOST** appropriate first step in the management of his AF?
   A. Rate control and anticoagulation
   B. Pharmacologic rhythm control and anticoagulation
   C. Electrical cardioversion and anticoagulation
   D. Coronary angiography to evaluate for ischemic heart disease

ANSWERS

20.1 The correct answer is A.
Rationale: One of the most important changes seen in old individuals is increased arterial stiffness and decreased compliance. With advancing age, there is an increase of matrix metalloproteinase, angiotensin II, and transforming growth factor, leading to endothelial dysfunction, decreased nitric oxide production, and impaired vasodilatation. These changes lead to isolated systolic hypertension in old people, characterized by increased systolic pressure, decreased diastolic pressure, and widened pulse pressure.

20.2 The correct answer is B.
Rationale: This patient would benefit from improved BP management with the addition of another agent. According to the ACC/AHA 2017 guidelines, the target BP should be less than 130/80 mm Hg. Ambulatory monitoring has consistently shown elevated BP, and there are no signs of orthostatic hypotension. Increasing hydrochlorothiazide is unlikely to significantly decrease his BP. The Systolic Hypertension in the Elderly Program (SHEP) and the Hypertension in the Very Elderly Trial (HYVET) confirmed the benefits of antihypertensive therapy in patients 80 years or older, showing a significant reduction in fatal and nonfatal stroke, all-cause mortality, and cardiovascular death.

The Systolic Blood Pressure Intervention Trial (SPRINT) randomized over 9,000 patients with hypertension to intensive treatment or standard therapy, demonstrating significant reduction in the composite outcome of myocardial infarction (MI), stroke, HF, and cardiovascular death in the intensive treatment arm. These benefits of intensive BP lowering were also seen in older adults (≥75 years).

20.3 The correct answer is B.
Rationale: Valsartan, an ARB, would be the best choice of the options listed, given that the patient's history of CAD and mild cardiomyopathy, for which optimal guideline-directed medical therapy is recommended. Since the patient is already taking metoprolol, adding a second beta-blocker would not be appropriate. While spironolactone is a possible option, it is less potent compared to valsartan for BP control and would not be the next best choice, though it should be considered in the future, particularly if LVEF worsens. Doxazosin, an alpha-blocker, is not the best choice for BP management, especially in older patients, due to its propensity for orthostasis.

20.4 The correct answer is C.
Rationale: Risk stratification with stress testing would be the ideal next step. However, performing an exercise stress ECG would be challenging in this patient given his inability to walk due to knee pain. Coronary angiography would be premature at this time, considering that percutaneous coronary intervention (PCI) is associated with a greater risk of complications in older adults than in younger patients, including acute kidney injury, bleeding, stroke, death, and periprocedural MI. The Clinical Outcomes Utilizing Revascularization and Aggressive Drug Evaluation (COURAGE) trial revealed that there was no significant difference in outcomes among patients with stable CAD treated with optimal medical therapy (OMT) versus those treated with PCI and OMT. Therefore, PCI should be reserved for patients with refractory symptoms despite maximally tolerated medical therapy for stable CAD. Coronary CT angiography may be less specific in older patients due to the higher prevalence of coronary calcifications.

20.5 The correct answer is D.
Rationale: Given that this older patient is presenting with an inferior ST-segment elevation myocardial infarction (STEMI) and is nearby a PCI-capable center (first medical contact to balloon time of <90 minutes), he should be promptly transferred for PCI. Fibrinolytic therapy, while an alternate treatment, poses an increased risk of bleeding, including intracranial hemorrhage, in the older population. Therefore, it is reserved for patients who do not have access to expeditious PCI. A study comparing PCI to thrombolytic therapy in patients over 75 years old was stopped prematurely because there was a significant reduction in death, MI, or stroke with PCI.

20.6 The correct answer is C.
Rationale: Beta-blockers and MRAs have been shown to lead to significant reductions in death or HF hospitalization in older patients. ARNI therapy is more beneficial over ACEi in preventing all-cause mortality, cardiovascular mortality and HF-related hospitalizations among patients with reduced left ventricular systolic function, with benefits extending to older adults, as demonstrated in Determine Impact on Global Mortality and Morbidity in Heart Failure trial (PARADIGM-HF).

ACEi significantly reduce mortality in HF hospitalizations in patients older than 60 years, as demonstrated in a meta-analysis of 27 trials. Subgroup analyses of large randomized, controlled ARB trials confirm a significant reduction in cardiovascular outcomes in older patients with HFrEF treated with ARBs compared to placebo.

ARBs were evaluated in older patients with HFrEF and shown to be equally effective as ACEi in preventing HF-related hospitalizations and mortality. However, ARBs and ACEi should not be administered concomitantly because patients receiving both have increased risk of mortality and morbidity.

Aldosterone antagonists were evaluated in three trials: the Randomized ALdactone Evaluation Study (RALES), the Eplerenone Post-acute myocardial infarction Heart failure Efficacy and Survival Study (EPHESUS), and the Eplerenone and Mild Patient's Hospitalization and Survival Study and Heart Failure (EMPHASIS-HF).

Subgroup analyses of the RALES and EMPHASIS studies showed a significant reduction in death or HF hospitalization in older patients treated with an aldosterone antagonist compared to placebo. However, the EPHESUS subgroup failed to show this benefit.

Hyperkalemia was common in patients with significant renal insufficiency, who were excluded from these studies. While diuretics are indicated to reduce symptoms, they have not been shown to improve outcomes.

20.7 The correct answer is C:
Rationale: This patient has persistent LBBB and an LVEF that has not improved with medical therapy. Since the heart rate is already well controlled, there is no indication to increase his beta-blockade. Cardiac resynchronization therapy (CRT) in combination with an ICD has been shown to improve mortality, symptoms, and reduce HF hospitalizations in patients with HFrEF. These devices have been shown to be beneficial for the older patients as well. Currently, there are no clinical indications for cardiac transplant.

20.8 The correct answer is A:
Rationale: ICD placement in this patient is indicated given his LVEF of 30% despite receiving guideline-directed medical therapy for approximately 6 months. Since he has not had an episode of ventricular arrhythmia, the ICD would not be placed for secondary prevention. The Multicenter Automatic Defibrillator Implantation Trial (MADIT II) did show a significant reduction in mortality in older patients who received an ICD for primary prevention. It is important to note that although age alone should not be the sole factor in deciding whether a patient receives an ICD, it is recognized that older adults (>80 years) are underrepresented in ICD trials. Current guidelines recommend against implanting an ICD in patients with less than 1 year of expected survival.

20.9 The correct answer is A:
Rationale: Aortic stenosis is the most common valvular heart disease in geriatric population, with an estimated prevalence of 4% in those older than 70 years. In older adults, calcific degeneration of the trileaflet aortic valve is the most common etiology; bicuspid valves present a decade earlier.

20.10 The correct answer is A:
Rationale: AF is the most common arrhythmia in older adults, and its prevalence increases with age. Rate control with anticoagulation should be addressed acutely in this setting. Rhythm control and EP referral may certainly be considered during this hospitalization, given the patient's presentation with concomitant HF. Coronary angiography is reasonable to consider during the hospital stay once the patient's status has stabilized and his renal function improves.

CARDIAC MANIFESTATION OF SYSTEMIC DISEASES

Wen Qian (Jenny) Zheng, Joshua Schulman-Marcus, and Sulagna Mookherjee

CHAPTER 21

QUESTIONS

21.1 In patients with systemic lupus erythematosus (SLE), which of the following is **TRUE** with regards to coronary artery disease risk?

  A. Patients with SLE have elevated levels of total cholesterol and low-density lipoprotein concentrations.
  B. Coronary artery calcifications are less common in patients with SLE than unaffected individuals.
  C. Patients with SLE have a lower risk of cardiovascular disease and mortality than unaffected patients.
  D. Patients with SLE have a lower prevalence of proinflammatory form of high-density lipoprotein than unaffected individuals.

21.2 A 30-year-old female with recently diagnosed rheumatoid arthritis presents to your clinic to establish care. She feels well and is taking nonsteroidal anti-inflammatory drugs (NSAIDs) daily for her symptoms. She is at increased risk of which of the following conditions?

  A. New-onset hypertension
  B. Valvular stenosis
  C. Atrioventricular block
  D. Myocarditis

21.3 A 40-year-old man with a history of systemic sclerosis presents with an episode of syncope at home. You are evaluating him in the emergency room. For which of the following is he at risk?

  A. Atrial flutter
  B. Atrioventricular block
  C. Ventricular arrhythmias
  D. All of the above

21.4 A 45-year-old woman is presenting to the emergency room with multiple weeks of worsening palpitations and is diagnosed with new-onset atrial fibrillation with rapid ventricular response. As part of her workup, her thyroid-stimulating hormone (TSH) is noted to be 0.05 mIU/L (normal range is 0.5-5.0 mIU/L) with a free T4 of 3.5 ng/dL (normal range is 0.8-1.8 mIU/L). What other long-term cardiac sequelae is she at risk for if untreated?

---

*Questions and Answers are based on Chapter 21: Cardiac Manifestations of Systemic Diseases by Toniya Singh, Ijeoma Isiadinso, Gina P. Lundberg, and Nidhi Madan in Cardiovascular Medicine and Surgery, First Edition.

A. Mitral regurgitation
B. Left ventricular (LV) hypertrophy
C. Atrioventricular block
D. Sick sinus syndrome

21.5 For the same patient described in **Question 21.4**, which of the following hemodynamic changes can occur?

A. Decreased cardiac output
B. Decreased blood volume
C. Decreased heart rate
D. Decreased systemic vascular resistance (SVR)

21.6 A 32-year-old female presents to the emergency room with 2 days of worsening lower left extremity swelling and pain. She is diagnosed with left leg deep vein thrombosis, which is her second recurrence. On hypercoagulable workup, she is diagnosed with antiphospholipid syndrome (APS). Which of the following cardiac conditions is she at highest risk for?

A. Coronary artery disease
B. Libman-Sacks endocarditis
C. Pulmonary hypertension
D. LV thrombi formation

21.7 A 75-year-old man presents with worsening dyspnea on exertion and lightheadedness upon standing for many months. He has also noticed worsening lower extremity edema and bilateral upper extremity numbness. He has normal vital signs. His electrocardiogram shows sinus rhythm with low voltage. What is the **MOST LIKELY** finding on his echocardiogram?

A. Small bilateral atria
B. Reduced LV ejection fraction
C. LV hypertrophy
D. Mitral stenosis

21.8 For the same patient described in **Question 21.7**, which of the following is he at risk for developing?

A. Diastolic heart failure
B. Complete heart block
C. Pericardial effusion
D. All of the above

21.9 A 66-year-old man with a history of pulmonary sarcoidosis presents to the office with intermittent lightheadedness for several months. His vital signs are stable, and his electrocardiogram reveals normal sinus rhythm. An echocardiogram is also unremarkable. A cardiac MRI is ordered. In which region is he **MOSTLY LIKELY** to exhibit focal sarcoid infiltration?

A. LV apex
B. LV basal septum
C. LV lateral wall
D. Right ventricle

21.10 Which of the following valvular conditions is **MOST** common in Marfan syndrome?
A. Mitral valve prolapse
B. Aortic stenosis
C. Mitral stenosis
D. Pulmonary regurgitation

ANSWERS

21.1 The correct answer is A.
Rationale: SLE is a chronic multisystem inflammatory disease. It is estimated that 50% of patients have cardiac abnormalities. Although death due to SLE has decreased because of advances in medical therapies, cardiovascular disease remains the leading cause of mortality, accounting for more than one-third of deaths in these patients. Premature atherosclerosis is a major contributing factor to the increased rate of ischemic heart disease in patients with SLE. Patients with SLE have a pro-atherogenic lipid profile consisting of elevated total cholesterol, triglycerides, and low-density lipoprotein cholesterol, whereas high-density lipoprotein cholesterol is reduced. They also have increased levels of coronary artery calcifications compared to those unaffected, as well as a higher risk of cardiovascular disease and mortality. The proinflammatory form of high-density lipoprotein is also higher in patients with SLE (**Figure 21.1**).

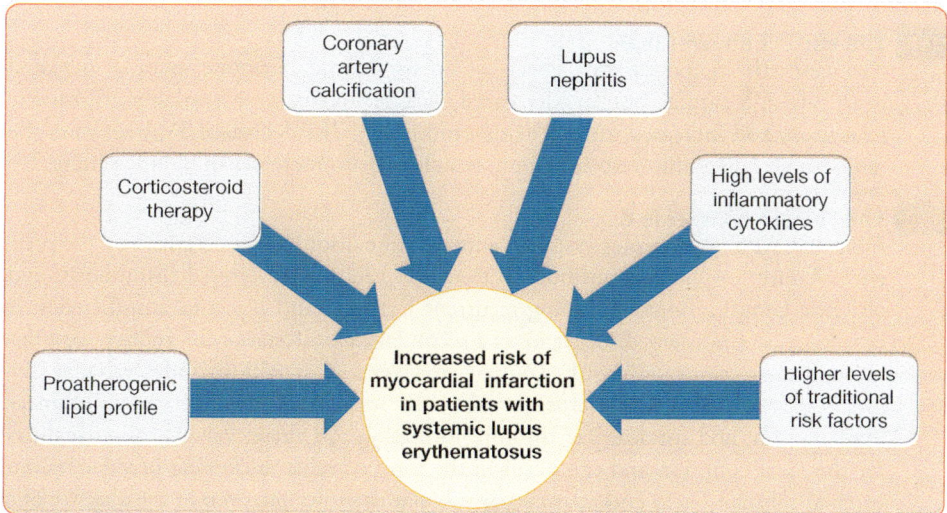

Figure 21.1 Increased risk of myocardial infarction among patients with systemic lupus erythematosus.

212 The correct answer is A.

Rationale: NSAIDs can precipitate new-onset hypertension and worsen blood pressure control in those with a diagnosis of hypertension. Patients with rheumatoid arthritis have a higher morbidity and mortality from cardiovascular disease compared to control populations, with this risk is nearly 2-fold compared to the general population. Premature atherosclerosis in patients with rheumatoid arthritis is one of the factors that leads to an increased risk of coronary artery disease. Rheumatoid arthritis itself can also increase the frequency of valvular regurgitation, heart failure, pericardial effusions, and ventricular arrhythmias.

213 The correct answer is D.

Rationale: Systemic sclerosis is a diffuse multisystem connective tissue disorder of unknown etiology characterized by systemic inflammation, fibrosis of organs and skin, and vascular dysfunction. Patients with systemic sclerosis have an increased risk of atherosclerosis because of endothelial dysfunction and inflammation, resulting in the release of proinflammatory markers. In addition, systemic sclerosis is responsible for a wide range of conduction abnormalities, including supraventricular tachycardia such as atrial fibrillation or flutter, premature ventricular contractions, and heart block.

214 The correct answer is B.

Rationale: This patient has hyperthyroidism. Hyperthyroidism is associated with increased risk of coronary artery disease, atrial fibrillation, heart failure, and cardiac-related mortality. The hemodynamic findings of excess thyroid hormone include an increased heart rate and cardiac output, decreased SVR secondary to arterial smooth muscle relaxation, and increased nitrous oxide production. Thyroid hormone also regulates intracellular calcium levels that lead to enhanced myocyte calcium cycling and contractility. These alterations lead to an increase in cardiac output, which can be 50% to 300% higher than normal in patients with symptomatic hyperthyroidism. This increased cardiac workload may eventually lead to LV hypertrophy and heart failure (**Table 21.1**).

215 The correct answer is D.

Rationale: The hemodynamic effects of excess thyroid hormone include increased heart rate and cardiac output, decreased SVR secondary to arterial smooth muscle relaxation, and increased nitrous oxide production. The decreased SVR activates the renin-angiotensin-aldosterone system, which leads to increases in blood volume.

216 The correct answer is B.

Rationale: APS is a complex systemic autoimmune disorder characterized by the presence of antiphospholipid antibodies, recurrent venous and arterial thrombosis, and obstetric complications, including recurrent fetal loss and placental insufficiency. It can occur as a primary disorder or as a secondary manifestation of another autoimmune disease, commonly SLE. Cardiac involvement in APS includes valvular disorders, accelerated atherosclerosis, CAD, MI, myocardial dysfunction, pulmonary hypertension, and intracardiac thrombi formation. Of these, valvular abnormalities are the most common and can occur in the form of valve thickening or valve lesions (such as Libman-Sacks endocarditis) or valvular dysfunction, even in the absence of a history of rheumatic fever or infective endocarditis. The valve lesions typically involve the mitral valve, followed by aortic valve, and are characterized by valve thickening of more than 3 mm involving the proximal or middle portions of the valve leaflets, or

TABLE 21.1 Cardiac Manifestations of Endocrine Disorders

Disorder	Coronary Arteries	Myocardium	Valves	Conduction	Pericardium
Hypothyroidism	Hypercholesterolemia Hyperlipidemia	Decreased contractility and cardiac output Heart failure		Sinus bradycardia	Pericardial effusion
Hyperthyroidism	Systolic hypertension	LVH secondary to increased cardiac output Heart family		SVT Atrial fibrillation	
Acromegaly	Endothelial changes Increased arterial stiffness Atherosclerosis	Ventricular dilatation LVH Heart failure	Aortic regurgitation Mitral regurgitation	Atrial fibrillation Ectopic beats SVT	
Pheochromocytoma	Catecholamine-induced vasospasm Vascular wall thickening	LVH Cardiomyopathy Ischemic heart disease Heart failure		Sinus tachycardia SVT VT Sick sinus syndrome	
Carcinoid		Plaque-like, fibrous endocardial thickening Heart failure	Tricuspid and pulmonary regurgitation		Pericardial effusions
Neurofibromatosis		Hypertrophic cardiomyopathy	Pulmonary stenosis Mitral regurgitation		

LVH, left ventricular hypertrophy; SVT, supraventricular tachycardia; VT, ventricular tachycardia.

as irregular nodules on the atrial side of mitral valve or vascular surface of the aortic valve. In about 4% to 6% of patients with APS with valvular abnormalities, severe valvular regurgitation can occur, requiring surgical intervention.

21.7 The correct answer is C.

Rationale: This patient most likely has cardiac amyloidosis. Amyloidosis refers to a group of protein-folding disorders characterized by the deposition of these proteins in tissues throughout the body. The deposition of these proteins in the heart carries a worse prognosis than the involvement of any other organ. The two subtypes of amyloidosis that account for 95% of all cardiac amyloidosis include light-chain amyloidosis (AL), which is the most common subtype, and transthyretin amyloidosis (ATTR). There are two subtypes of ATTR: a noninherited wild-type ATTR and inherited mutant ATTR. Both of these types result from a misfolding of the protein transthyretin, which is produced in the liver. These misfolded proteins combine to form amyloid fibers, which deposit in the interstitial space of the myocardium.

Cardiac manifestations of amyloidosis include heart failure and arrhythmias. AL, also known as primary amyloidosis, is the most serious form of the disease, with an untreated survival rate of less than 6 months in patients who present with heart failure. The deposition of amyloid proteins throughout the myocardial tissue leads to ventricular hypertrophy, decreased cardiac output, atrial dilatation, and atrial fibrillation. Cardiac amyloidosis can present with diastolic heart failure with preserved ejection fraction, dilated cardiomyopathy, or atrial fibrillation.

218. The correct answer is B:
Rationale: Cardiac manifestations of amyloidosis include heart failure and arrhythmias. AL, also known as primary amyloidosis, is the most serious form of the disease, with an untreated survival rate of less than 6 months in patients who present with heart failure. The deposition of amyloid proteins throughout the myocardial tissue leads to ventricular hypertrophy, decreased cardiac output, atrial dilatation, and atrial fibrillation. Patients with cardiac amyloidosis are also at risk for developing conduction diseases such as bundle branch blocks, dilated cardiomyopathy, and angina without coronary artery disease.

219. The correct answer is B:
Rationale: Sarcoidosis is a multisystem disease of unknown etiology characterized by the formation of granulomas in many organs, predominantly the lungs and intrathoracic lymph nodes. Approximately 5% of patients with sarcoidosis will exhibit symptoms of cardiac involvement, with an additional 20% to 25% having asymptomatic cardiac involvement. Clinical symptoms of cardiac sarcoidosis are commonly the disease's presenting symptoms, as two-thirds of patients with cardiac sarcoidosis have no other systemic signs of the disease. Cardiac sarcoidosis can present with ventricular arrhythmias, conduction abnormalities, or heart failure. Sarcoid infiltrations are common at the base of the septum, which can lead to heart block, ventricular tachyarrhythmias, and an increased risk of sudden death. Infiltrations can also affect the mitral valve, leading to regurgitation. Dilated cardiomyopathy, pericarditis, and LV aneurysms can also be seen in cardiac sarcoidosis.

220. The correct answer is A:
Rationale: Marfan syndrome is an autosomal dominant inherited connective tissue disorder caused by mutations in the extracellular matrix protein fibrillin (FBN1). The common cardiovascular (CV) manifestations involve aortic aneurysm, aortic valve regurgitation, aortic dissection, mitral valve prolapse (MVP), and dilated cardiomyopathy. These CV manifestations form a large proportion of the morbidity and mortality in patients with Marfan syndrome. The most prominent CV finding in many of these patients is the dilatation of the aortic root, particularly at the level of the sinus of Valsalva. Bicuspid valve may be present. This aortic dilatation can further evolve into an aneurysm formation, dissection, or rupture. Aortic regurgitation has also been observed to occur as a consequence of the dilatation at the aortic root. In about 10% to 20% of patients with Marfan syndrome, dilatation of the descending and abdominal aorta can also occur, leading to a type B aortic dissection. MVP is another important CV feature of Marfan syndrome. However, surgical intervention for MVP is required in only a small number of patients. MVP can cause severe mitral regurgitation that can, in turn, result in heart failure and pulmonary hypertension. The tricuspid valve may also be affected, resulting in tricuspid valve prolapse and tricuspid regurgitation.

SUBSTANCE ABUSE AND THE HEART*

Wen Qian (Jenny) Zheng, Joshua Schulman-Marcus, and Sulagna Mookherjee

CHAPTER 22

QUESTIONS

22.1 A 55-year-old man with a history of alcohol use and no other medical history conditions presents to the emergency room with palpitations and lightheadedness. He drank six beers approximately 4 hours ago. His electrocardiogram (ECG) shows atrial fibrillation with a rapid ventricular rate of 132 beats per minute (bpm). He is admitted overnight and spontaneously converts to sinus rhythm. What is the probability that his atrial fibrillation will recur if he were to drink heavily again?

   A. 1/3
   B. 1/4
   C. 1/2
   D. 1/6

22.2 For the same patient described in **Question 22.1**, what other adverse outcome is he **MOST LIKELY** to have due to alcohol use?

   A. Thromboembolism
   B. Diabetes mellitus
   C. Pulmonary hypertension
   D. Hyperlipidemia

22.3 A 30-year-old female is presenting with 2 weeks of dyspnea on exertion and orthopnea. She has no past medical history otherwise. Her vitals are as follows: HR 105 bpm, BP 130/80 mm Hg, RR 24 breaths per minute, and saturating 90% on 2 L nasal cannula. She has elevated jugular venous distension (JVD) and bilateral pulmonary crackles and is unable to lay flat. Her echocardiogram is showing a left ventricular ejection fraction (LVEF) of 30% to 35% with global hypokinesis and moderate mitral regurgitation. ECG reveals sinus tachycardia. What is the next step in the management of this patient?

   A. Cardiac catheterization
   B. D-dimer
   C. Urine toxicology screen
   D. Stress testing

22.4 The same patient described in **Question 22.3** tests positive for methamphetamine on her urine toxicology screen. Which of the following is a proposed mechanism of methamphetamine-associated cardiomyopathy?

---

*Questions and Answers are based on Chapter 22: Substance Abuse and the Heart by Janet Ma and Isac C. Thomas in Cardiovascular Medicine and Surgery, First Edition.

A. Decrease in free radical formation
B. Left ventricular concentric remodeling
C. Direct injury to the sarcoplasmic reticulum
D. Interstitial fibrosis and inflammatory cellular infiltrate

22.5 Regarding the same patient described in **Question 22.3**, what outcome is methamphetamine-induced cardiomyopathy associated with?

A. Increased frequency of comorbidities such as psychiatrist disorders
B. Lower 5-year heart failure readmission rates
C. Higher 10-year total mortality than a heart failure cohort who did not use methamphetamines
D. Lower risk for severity of heart failure and cardiomyopathy

22.6 The same patient described in **Question 22.3** comes for a follow-up in the office 2 years later and has made a full recovery from her heart failure episode. Unfortunately, she is still using methamphetamine and has developed gradual dyspnea on exertion over the past 1 year. Her vitals are stable, her lungs are clear with no elevation of JVD. There is some mild lower extremity edema. She says that she cannot climb more than one flight of stairs without having to stop and catch her breath. What is the next step in workup?

A. Echocardiography
B. Stress testing
C. Right heart catheterization
D. Computed tomography (CT) angiography

22.7 A 45-year-old man with a history of active cocaine use presents with worsening chest pain for the past 2 days. Vitals are as follows: afebrile, BP 160/90 mm Hg, HR 120 bpm, RR 20 breaths per minute, and saturating 97% on room air. He is diaphoretic on examination and anxious. His troponin-I is 1.2, and ECG is showing ST depressions in inferior leads with new Q waves. What is the next **BEST** step in management?

A. Start oral metoprolol succinate.
B. Start intravenous esmolol.
C. Start lorazepam and nitroglycerin.
D. Start oral carvedilol.

22.8 The same patient described in **Question 22.7** presents to the hospital 40 days later with left lower extremity weakness and is diagnosed with an ischemic stroke. He is still actively using cocaine. What is the **MOST LIKELY** etiology of his stroke?

A. Vasospasm induced
B. Cardioembolic induced from atrial fibrillation
C. Atherosclerotic disease
D. Cardioembolic induced from infective endocarditis

22.9 A 29-year-old male presents with fever and worsening dyspnea on exertion for the past week. He has a history of intravenous heroin use but no other cardiac history. His vitals are as follows: temperature of 38.2 °C, BP 100/70 mm Hg, HR 126 bpm, RR 26 breaths per minute, saturating 91% on 3 L nasal cannula. On examination, he is uncomfortable and tachypneic. He has crackles at the bases of both lungs; cardiac examination reveals tachycardia without murmur. He has mildly elevated JVD and bilateral pitting lower extremity edema. Electrocardiography shows sinus tachycardia with a rate of 120 bpm. Blood cultures are drawn, and he is started on broad-spectrum antibiotics and diuretic therapy. Which of the following is the next **BEST** step in management?

A. Transthoracic echocardiography
B. Transesophageal echocardiography
C. CT angiography
D. Cardiac surgery consultation

ANSWERS

22.1 The correct answer is B.
Rationale: Atrial fibrillation has been shown to occur even in infrequent and non-drinkers after a binge. Although atrial fibrillation typically terminates after 24 hours, it recurs in about a quarter of patients with subsequent binges.

22.2 The correct answer is A.
Rationale: Patients with heavy alcohol use were also more likely to have adverse outcomes such as thromboembolism, even after adjusting for anticoagulation use and $CHAD_2VASc$ score.

22.3 The correct answer is C.
Rationale: This patient, with no cardiac history, is in clinical heart failure and has a newly diagnosed cardiomyopathy. Given her age and absence of ischemic ECG changes, coronary artery disease is less likely. She is unable to lay flat and is in active heart failure, thus it would not be the optimal time to perform cardiac catheterization. D-dimer is often nonspecific and can be elevated in acute settings. While pulmonary embolism is a possible diagnosis, it typically does not present with left-sided heart failure, which this patient has, making it less likely to be the unifying diagnosis. Urine toxicology screen can help rule out other nonischemic sources of acute cardiomyopathy—such as alcohol and/or acute drug ingestion. Stress testing is not advised in a patient in active heart failure.

22.4 The correct answer is D.
Rationale: Multiple theories have been proposed about the mechanism of methamphetamine-associated cardiomyopathy, including an increase in radical formation, left ventricular dilatation, direct injury to cardiomyocytes and mitochondria, interstitial fibrosis, and inflammatory cellular infiltrates (**Table 22.1**).

22.5 The correct answer is A.
Rationale: Methamphetamine-induced cardiomyopathy indeed has an increased frequency of comorbidities such as psychiatrist disorders and social issues like homelessness. In addition, methamphetamine use is an independent risk factor for exacerbating the severity of cardiomyopathy and heart failure. It is also associated

TABLE 22.1 Suggested Considerations for Specific Substances and Associated Cardiovascular Effects

Substance	Cardiovascular Effects	Special Considerations
Tobacco smoking/e-cigarettes	Atherosclerotic disease	Preliminary data show that vaping and e-cigarette use have less harm compared to traditional cigarettes but still confer risk of myocardial infarction and lung disease.
Alcohol	Dilated cardiomyopathy Atrial fibrillation Hypertension	Moderate consumption has traditionally been thought to confer a cardioprotective effect; however, recent data challenge this notion.
Methamphetamine	Dilated cardiomyopathy Pulmonary hypertension	The incidence of methamphetamine-associated cardiomyopathy has grown in the past decade. It should be considered in individuals with nonischemic cardiomyopathy and a history of methamphetamine use.
Cocaine	Acute coronary syndrome Stroke Dilated cardiomyopathy	Avoid beta-blockers acutely in cocaine-associated myocardial infarction. Consider using bare mental stents due to increased risk of stent thrombosis.
Marijuana	Acute coronary syndrome	Abstinence from marijuana smoking is advisable for patients with preexisting cardiac disease.
Opioids	None established	More research is needed.

with higher rates of heart failure readmissions within 5 years but lower mortality rate at 10 years compared to their heart failure counterparts who did not use methamphetamines.

22.6 The correct answer is C.
Rationale: This patient likely has methamphetamine-induced pulmonary arterial hypertension. The best next step would be to perform a right heart catheterization to assess the severity of the disease and differentiate between the types of pulmonary hypertension. Coronary artery disease and pulmonary embolism are less likely given the insidious onset of symptoms.

22.7 The correct answer is C.
Rationale: The 2014 American College of Cardiology and the American Heart Association (ACC/AHA) guidelines reissued a class III recommendation against the use of beta-blockers in patients with myocardial infarction and active cocaine use, a reversal of previous recommendations. A class IIa recommendation was issued for using benzodiazepine alone or in combination with nitroglycerin for managing hypertension and tachycardia in these patients.

22.8 The correct answer is C.
Rationale: Cocaine can increase the risk of both ischemic and hemorrhagic stroke, though the exact mechanisms remain unclear. One study examined underlying stroke etiologies in hospitalized patients who were actively or formerly using cocaine and found that the likely etiology was due to underlying atherosclerosis.

22.9 The correct answer is A.
Rationale: This patient with a history of IV heroin use is presenting with fever and heart failure and is at very high risk for endocarditis. The first step in management would be to perform a transthoracic echocardiography to evaluate valvular function, visible vegetations, and LVEF. If there is suspicion of vegetation or valvular dysfunction, proceeding with transesophageal echocardiography would be reasonable to further evaluate the size of vegetation or valvular anatomy. Cardiac surgery consultation would be premature without an initial workup.

CHAPTER 23

CARDIAC TRAUMA

Nathan Gentybear and Mohamed Khalid Munshi

QUESTIONS

23.1 A 25-year-old male with no prior medical history is struck in the chest during a football game, after which he collapses on the field in cardiac arrest. Cardiopulmonary resuscitation (CPR) is started immediately, and he is found to be in ventricular fibrillation. Which of the following is **TRUE** about his condition?

A. It is associated with impacts greater than 40 miles per hour.
B. It occurs when the impact falls during ventricular depolarization.
C. It is associated with structural heart disease.
D. It is more commonly associated with males.

23.2 What is the **MOST** common site of cardiac injury in blunt chest trauma?

A. Right ventricle
B. Left ventricle
C. Right atrium
D. Left atrium

23.3 A 28-year-old male is brought to the emergency room (ER) following a collision while skiing. Aside from bruising to his chest and face, his examination and history are unremarkable. A troponin is checked due to concern for blunt cardiac injury and is mildly elevated. Which of the following is **MOST** appropriate in the management of this patient?

A. Perform a focused cardiac ultrasound, and if normal, discharge the patient home.
B. Perform an electrocardiogram (ECG), and if normal, discharge the patient home.
C. Perform a focused cardiac ultrasound and ECG, and if both are normal discharge, the patient home.
D. Admit the patient to the hospital and check serial troponins.

23.4 What are the most commonly injured valves in blunt cardiac trauma?

A. The tricuspid and mitral valves
B. The tricuspid and pulmonary valves
C. The aortic and pulmonary valves
D. The aortic and mitral valves

---

*Questions and Answers are based on Chapter 23: Cardiac Trauma by Debabrata Mukherjee in Cardiovascular Medicine and Surgery, First Edition.

23.5 A 50-year-old woman is brought to the ER following a motor vehicle collision. Chest x-ray is significant for first, second, and third rib fractures. Initial ECG and troponin are normal. She has numerous bruises on her face and torso but is hemodynamically stable. Which of the following is the **MOST** appropriate management of this patient?

    A. Cardiac computed tomography (CT)
    B. Consult cardiovascular surgery.
    C. Admit to the hospital for 24 hours and discharge with pain medications if repeat troponins are negative, her transthoracic echo is normal, and she does not have any arrhythmias.
    D. Perform a cardiac ultrasound and discharge with pain medications if normal.

23.6 A 49-year-old man presents to the ER following a motor vehicle collision. Chest x-ray shows a widened mediastinum. He is hemodynamically stable. Which of the following is the **MOST** appropriate management of this patient?

    A. CT angiography of the chest
    B. Cardiovascular surgery consult
    C. Transthoracic echocardiography
    D. Check a troponin level, and, if positive, consult cardiovascular surgery.

23.7 Which of the following is the **MOST** common site of injury to the aorta during blunt chest injury?

    A. Ascending thoracic aorta
    B. Aortic root
    C. Proximal descending thoracic aorta
    D. Distal descending thoracic aorta

23.8 What is the **MOST** common rhythm noted in blunt cardiac injury?

    A. Sinus tachycardia
    B. Atrial fibrillation
    C. Ventricular tachycardia
    D. Ventricular fibrillation

23.9 Which of the following is **TRUE** about cardiac concussion?

    A. Troponin will be elevated without wall-motion abnormalities.
    B. It is defined by new conduction abnormalities with normal wall motion.
    C. It results in segmental wall-motion abnormalities.
    D. It is defined by cardiogenic syncope resulting from chest trauma.

23.10 A man is stabbed in the chest in a bar fight, penetrating his left ventricle. Which of the following statements about his mortality is the **MOST** accurate?

    A. It is 91% to 100%.
    B. It is 81% to 90%.
    C. It is 70% to 80%.
    D. It is similar to a penetrating injury to the right ventricle.

ANSWERS

23.1 The correct answer is B.
Rationale: Commotio cordis is caused by low-impact blunt trauma during cardiac repolarizing and is associated with males and individuals without structural heart disease. The risk of ventricular fibrillation with low-impact blunt trauma is related to the cardiac cycle—impacts occurring in the early ventricular repolarization phase (typically within 20-40 milliseconds of the upslope of the T wave) are associated with ventricular fibrillation. Impacts under 40 mph have an increased chance of causing ventricular fibrillation, whereas impacts greater than 40 mph may cause cardiac contusion.

23.2 The correct answer is A.
Rationale: Because of its anterior location, the right ventricle is the most common site of injury. The severity of cardiac injury may range from minor, asymptomatic myocardial concussion (segmental wall-motion abnormality without biomarker evidence of myocardial injury) to ventricular rupture.

23.3 The correct answer is D.
Rationale: Although performing an ECG and cardiac ultrasound are appropriate, discharging the patient home when he has an elevated troponin is not. The 2012 practice management guidelines from the Eastern Association for the Surgery of Trauma (EAST) recommend that all patients with suspected cardiac injury should have an ECG and plasma troponin level measured. Patients with suspected blunt cardiac trauma and an initial positive troponin should be admitted for monitoring and further workup.

23.4 The correct answer is D.
Rationale: Despite the anterior location of the tricuspid and pulmonic valves, the aortic and mitral valves are most affected by blunt trauma because of high mural pressures. Traumatic valve rupture can cause rapid heart failure and usually presents with dyspnea, orthopnea, and new murmur.

23.5 The correct answer is A.
Rationale: This patient presented with a high-risk mechanism for cardiac trauma and has an abnormal chest x-ray. The first and second ribs are less prone to injury, so first and second rib fractures are indicative of severe chest trauma, warranting further evaluation with CT. Depending on the results of the CT scan, cardiovascular surgery consultation may be warranted.

23.6 The correct answer is A.
Rationale: Chest x-ray is often used as a primary screening tool after trauma due to its availability and ease of performing. The presence of a widened mediastinum on a chest x-ray, which our patient has, suggests aortic disruption with about 53% sensitivity and 59% specificity. This should prompt further evaluation with CT angiography or transesophageal echocardiogram without waiting for troponin results. On the other hand, a normal chest x-ray has close to a 90% negative predictive value (**Figure 23.1**).

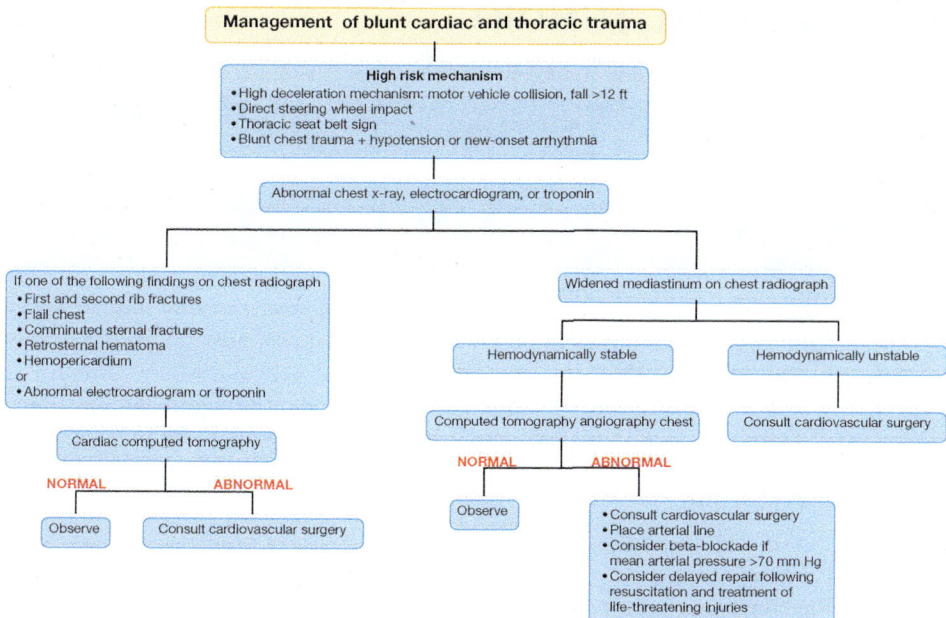

Figure 23.1 Clinical algorithm for management of patients presenting with cardiac trauma. (Adapted from Wu Y, Qamar SR, Murray N, et al. Imaging of cardiac trauma. *Radiol Clin North Am.* 2019;57(4):795-808. Copyright © 2019 Elsevier, with permission.)

23.7 The correct answer is C.

Rationale: Aortic injury can result from either blunt or penetrating trauma. However, aortic injuries are most often caused by blunt trauma—typically deceleration injuries from motor vehicle accidents or falls from height. Injury to the aorta most commonly occurs at the isthmus, approximately 90% of the time. This is the portion of the proximal descending thoracic aorta between the origin of the left subclavian artery and the ligamentum arteriosum.

23.8 The correct answer is A.

Rationale: Sinus tachycardia is the most commonly noted heart rhythm after cardiac injuries, followed by atrial fibrillation. Although ventricular arrhythmias can occur, their incidence is less common.

23.9 The correct answer is C.

Rationale: Cardiac concussion is defined by segmental wall abnormalities without biomarker evidence of myocardial injury. On the other hand, cardiac contusions represent actual myocardial cell injury leading to myocardial necrosis and elevation of cardiac enzymes.

23.10 The correct answer is A.

Rationale: The right ventricle is the most common site of entry in a penetrating cardiac injury (62% of penetrating cardiac injuries) due to its anterior location. Although the left ventricle is less affected with penetrating injuries, it is associated with a significantly higher mortality rate at 98%.

CHAPTER 24

CARDIAC TUMORS

Ciril Khorolsky and Robert D. Millar

QUESTIONS

24.1 A 45-year-old male presents to the emergency department with sudden onset right arm weakness and dysarthria. He has no known past medical history. Computed tomography (CT) of the head shows an acute ischemic stroke without evidence of intracranial bleeding and a transthoracic echocardiogram demonstrates a small mobile mass with a shimmering border that appears to be moving independently from neighboring structures. Which of the following is the **MOST LIKELY** diagnosis?

- A. Papillary fibroelastoma
- B. Cardiac myxoma
- C. Rhabdomyoma
- D. Fibroma

24.2 In which of the following benign primary cardiac tumors (PCTs) may surgical resection **NOT** be required?

- A. Papillary fibroelastoma
- B. Cardiac myxoma
- C. Rhabdomyoma
- D. Fibroma
- E. Both A and D are correct.

24.3 A 41-year-old female presents to the emergency department with fatigue, unintentional weight loss, and intermittent fevers over the past 2 months. She has no known past medical history and takes no medications. Her vital signs are stable. Physical examination is notable for an abnormal early diastolic sound but is otherwise unremarkable. A transesophageal echocardiogram is shown in **Figure 24.1**. Which of the following statements about this patient and the echocardiographic finding is **CORRECT**?

- A. Antibiotic therapy should be initiated as soon as possible.
- B. This lesion is known to be associated with Carney complex.
- C. Surgical resection is rarely indicated.
- D. This lesion primarily develops in the right atrium.
- E. Both A and C are correct.

*Questions and Answers are based on Chapter 24: Cardiac Tumors by Avirup Guha, Abdallah Mughrabi, and Zeeshan Hussain in Cardiovascular Medicine and Surgery, First Edition.

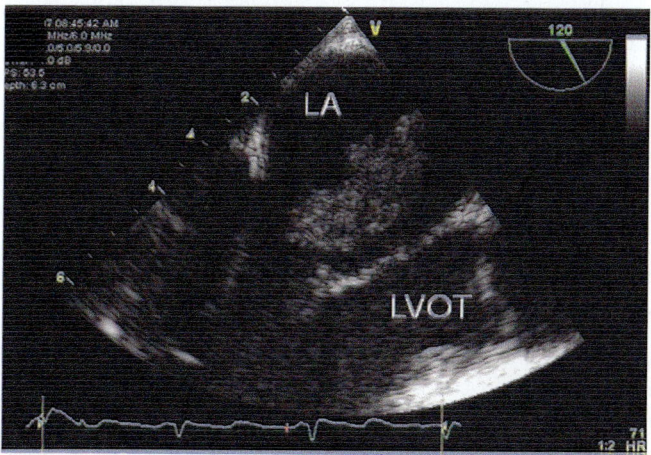

Figure 24.1 LA, left atrium; LVOT, left ventricular outflow tract.

24.4 A 60-year-old male with a recent history of acute myocardial infarction 2 months ago presents with sudden onset left-sided weakness and slurred speech. His blood pressure is 140/90 mm Hg, heart rate is 90 beats per minute (bpm), and respiratory rate is 18 breaths/min. On physical examination, he has weakness in the left upper and lower extremities with mild facial droop. CT scan of the head shows no evidence of intracranial hemorrhage. Echocardiography shows an irregularly shaped, mass-like structure in the left ventricle. Which of the following is the most appropriate management for this patient?

A. Surgical removal of the left ventricular mass-like structure
B. Observation with serial imaging
C. Direct oral anticoagulant (DOAC) therapy
D. Anticoagulation with warfarin with a target international normalized ratio (INR) of 2 to 3
E. Aspirin therapy

24.5 All of the following statements regarding malignant PCTs are **TRUE EXCEPT:**

A. Malignant PCTs represent only 5% to 6% of all PCTs.
B. Sarcomas are the most common.
C. Right-sided malignant PCTs usually grow outward.
D. Metastasis on presentation is seen in more than 50% of the cases.
E. Cardiac lymphomas are the most common malignant PCTs.

24.6 A 67-year-old male presents to the emergency department for evaluation of recurrent syncope, dyspnea on exertion, and unintentional weight loss over the past 10 weeks. Physical examination is notable for blood pressure of 110/70 mm Hg, heart rate of 100 bpm, elevated jugular venous pressure, and distant heart sounds. An electrocardiogram (ECG) shows sinus tachycardia with decreased QRS voltage and a transthoracic echocardiogram demonstrates a mild-to-moderate pericardial effusion with a mass-like structure in the left atrium. Which of the following imaging modalities would be most useful in differentiating between benign and malignant cardiac tumors?

A. Contrast echocardiography
B. Cardiac magnetic resonance (CMR)
C. Positron emission tomography (PET) with CT
D. Cardiac computed tomography (CCT)

24.7 You are evaluating a patient with a suspected PCT. All of the following imaging findings favor the diagnosis of malignant PCTs rather than benign PCTs **EXCEPT:**

A. Absence of late gadolinium enhancement
B. Wide base
C. Large mass greater than 5 cm
D. Mass arising from the right side or pericardium
E. Presence of first-pass perfusion

24.8 Which of the following malignancies is the **MOST LIKELY** to metastasize to the heart?

A. Breast cancer
B. Lung cancer
C. Lymphoma
D. Leukemia

24.9 A 57-year-old male with a known history of lung cancer presents to the emergency department with chest discomfort, dyspnea, and orthopnea. He recently completed his last cycle of chemotherapy with a favorable response. Physical examination is notable for blood pressure of 110/70 mm Hg, heart rate of 99 bpm, elevated jugular venous pressure, and a holosystolic murmur on cardiac auscultation. An ECG shows atrial fibrillation and a transthoracic echocardiogram shows a large mass in the left atrium with associated severe mitral valve regurgitation (MR). What is the most appropriate next step in management?

A. Refer the patient for palliative radiotherapy.
B. Arrange for a transesophageal echocardiogram and direct-current cardioversion.
C. Refer the patient for surgical resection of the cardiac mass.
D. No further intervention is needed, as the patient is in the terminal stages of their disease and management should be focused on comfort care.

24.10 Which of the following statements regarding pericardial cysts (PCs) is **CORRECT**?

A. Patients with PCs are most commonly males.
B. The majority of PCs are iatrogenic due to cardiac surgery.
C. Treatment with serial percutaneous aspirations is recommended in large or recurring PCs.
D. Asymptomatic lesions are usually followed by CCT or CMR every 1 to 2 years.

ANSWERS

24.1 The correct answer is A.

Rationale: This patient most likely has a papillary fibroelastoma. Patients are typically middle-aged and can present with embolic complications, particularly cerebral due to the tumor's predilection for left-sided valves. Papillary fibroelastoma can be diagnosed on echocardiography as a solitary mass in the middle part of the valve's leaflet, with a characteristic shimmering border vibrating independently from neighboring structures. Although cardiac myxoma may also cause embolic events and appear as a mobile mass on echocardiography, the echocardiographic finding of a shimmering border is more consistent with a fibroelastoma than myxoma. Rhabdomyoma and fibroma typically present during the first year of life, not in middle-aged adults (**Figure 24.2**).

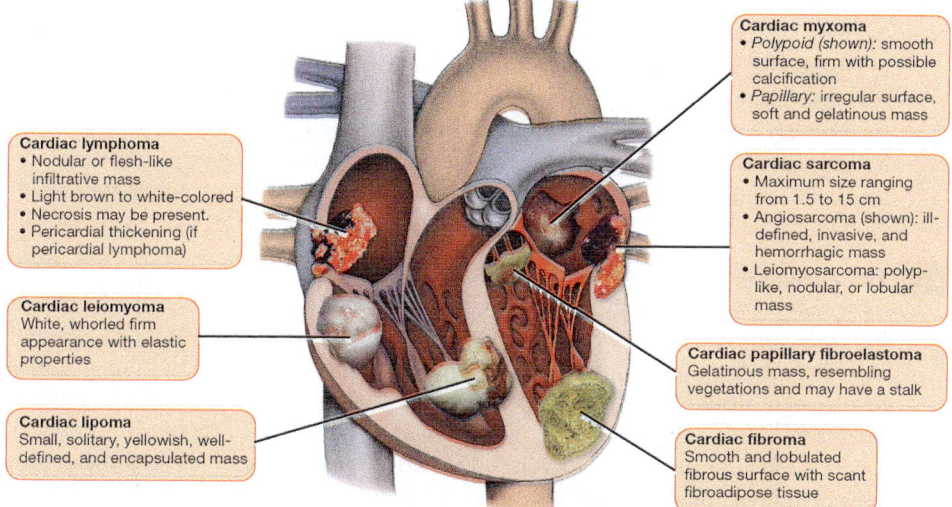

Figure 24.2 Gross appearance of different pathologic subtypes of primary cardiac tumors. Note the predilection for specific anatomic locations. Cardiac myxoma and sarcoma predominantly affect the left atrium. Papillary fibroelastoma affects valve leaflets and papillary muscles. Lipoma may involve any chamber and arises from subendocardium or intramyocardium. Cardiac lymphoma affects the right heart predominantly. Mesothelioma and paraganglioma (not shown) affect the pericardium.

24.2 The correct answer is C.

Rationale: Rhabdomyoma is the most prevalent pediatric PCT and typically presents during the first year of life as either a single mass or as multiple tumors in different cardiac chambers. In general, surgical resection is not required for most cases of rhabdomyoma due to spontaneous tumor regression. However, if there is significant cardiac flow limitation or electrophysiologic complications, surgical removal should be considered. Fibroelastomas, myxomas, and fibromas, on the other hand, are less likely to spontaneously regress and most often require surgical resection due to the increased risk of complications.

24.3 The correct answer is B.

Rationale: This patient's clinical presentation and echocardiographic finding are most consistent with left atrial myxoma. Although most cardiac myxomas are sporadic, the association with Carney complex is well established. Myxomas are morphologically classified into polypoid and papillary. The former, when large, may present with obstructive symptoms, with a "tumor plop" (early diastolic sound) being occasionally heard on auscultation. By contrast, papillary myxoma tends to cause embolic events. In both variants, constitutional symptoms such as fatigue, fever, and weight loss may be present. Surgical resection is the treatment of choice and is often indicated due to the risk of complications. Although this patient presents with intermittent fevers, clinical presentation is not suggestive of infective endocarditis; therefore, there is no indication for antibiotics.

24.4 The correct answer is B.

Rationale: The patient presents with symptoms suggestive of an acute ischemic stroke, and echocardiography reveals a mass-like structure in the left ventricle, which is highly suggestive of left ventricular thrombus (LVT). LVT is commonly seen after acute myocardial infarction with ventricular dysfunction and is highly embolic, leading to acute ischemic stroke in close to 12% of patients. Management of LVT involves anticoagulation with vitamin K antagonists such as warfarin, with a target INR of 2 to 3, for a duration tailored according to the patient's bleeding risk and the precipitating event. Use of DOACs for LVT is off-label and should be undertaken with caution due to the higher risk of stroke or systemic embolism reported in clinical studies compared with warfarin use. Surgical removal of the LVT is not recommended as it carries a high risk of morbidity and mortality. Observation with serial imaging is not appropriate as LVT is associated with a high risk of embolization, which can lead to devastating complications with mortality as high as 31.8%. Aspirin therapy alone is not sufficient for LVT management.

24.5 The correct answer is E.

Rationale: Malignant tumors are extremely rare and represent only 5% to 6% of PCTs. Sarcomas are most common (64.8%), followed by lymphomas (27%) and then mesotheliomas (8%). Clinical presentation is determined by the site of tumor involvement. Right-sided malignancies tend to grow outward and present only when the mass is large, with heart failure occurring at a later stage. Metastasis on presentation is seen in over half of the cases. Left-sided malignancies tend to present with early hemodynamic complications of systemic outflow obstruction and heart failure. Other clinical findings include malignant effusions and tamponade.

24.6 The correct answer is C.

Rationale: PET-CT has very high sensitivity in differentiating malignancies from benign entities. In addition, PET-CT can estimate the grade of tumor and screen for metastasis. Contrast echocardiography is often used as the initial imaging tool; however, there are not enough data to support its role in differentiating malignant from benign tumors. Compared to its role in benign tumor evaluation, CMR is less reliable in further subclassification of malignant tumors. This is because of the differences malignant tumors exhibit in terms of vascularity, water content, and differentiation among patients. CCT is useful in the localization of the mass and determining its relationship with adjacent structures; however, PET-CT is superior.

24.7 The correct answer is A.

Rationale: Echocardiography and CMR can be very helpful in differentiating between benign and malignant PCTs. On echocardiography, benign PCTs usually arise from the left atrial septal wall or valves and have a narrow base, while malignant PCTs more often arise from the right side or pericardium, have a wide base and absent stalk. On CMR, benign PCTs are usually smaller (<5 cm), less likely to have late gadolinium enhancement (only 41% of benign PCTs), and less likely to have contrast first-pass perfusion (47% of benign PCTs). Whereas malignant PCTs on CMR are usually larger (>5 cm), frequently positive for late gadolinium enhancement (92% of malignant PCTs), and frequently have contrast first-pass perfusion (84% of malignant PCTs). Additional findings on CMR that favor the diagnosis of malignant PCT are the presence of necrosis, calcification, high vascularity, infiltration of adjacent tissues, peritumorous edema, and pleural/pericardial effusions (**Table 24.1**).

TABLE 24.1 Role of Echocardiography and Cardiac Magnetic Resonance in Distinguishing Benign and Malignant Primary Cardiac Tumors

Modality and References	Benign Cardiac Tumors	Malignant Cardiac Tumors
Echocardiography	• Arises from left atrial septal wall or valves • Narrow base	• Arises from right side (50% chance of malignancy) or pericardium • Wide base, absent stalk • Invasive
Cardiac magnetic resonance	Smaller (<5 cm) Less associated with late gadolinium enhancement (41% of tumors) Less associated with contrast first-pass perfusion (47% of tumors)	• Larger (>5 cm) • More associated with late gadolinium enhancement (92% of tumors) • More associated with contrast first-pass perfusion (84% of tumors) Other characteristics: multiple, infiltration of adjacent tissues, necrosis, calcification, high vascularity, peritumorous edema, pleural/pericardial effusions

24.8 The correct answer is B.
Rationale: Secondary cardiac tumors (SCTs) are much more common than PCTs. In general, any malignant tumor may spread to the heart; however, certain malignancies are much more likely to do so. Lung cancer is the most common primary cancer to metastasize to the heart, accounting for 36% to 39% of cases of SCTs, followed by breast cancer (10%-12%) and hematologic malignancies such as lymphomas and leukemias (10%-21%).

24.9 The correct answer is C.
Rationale: Cardiac metastasis usually occurs in the late stages of the primary disease. However, management should be individualized and directed toward the primary tumor. In select conditions, surgical resection may be indicated, such as for patients with intracavitary metastases resulting in significant hemodynamic complications progressing to cardiac decompensation, or for patients with solitary cardiac disease when the primary tumor is controlled and a good prognosis is expected. In this case, the patient has a large mass in the left atrium with associated severe MR, which is causing hemodynamic complications and progression to cardiac decompensation. Moreover, the patient appears to have a good prognosis given his favorable response to his last chemotherapy cycle. Therefore, the most appropriate management in this patient would be to perform surgical resection of the cardiac mass. Transition to comfort care would not be appropriate in this patient with a good prognosis.

Palliative radiotherapy may not be sufficient in managing the patient's condition. Arranging for direct-current cardioversion would not be advisable in a patient with a large intracardiac mass as it may lead to embolic complications (**Figure 24.3**).

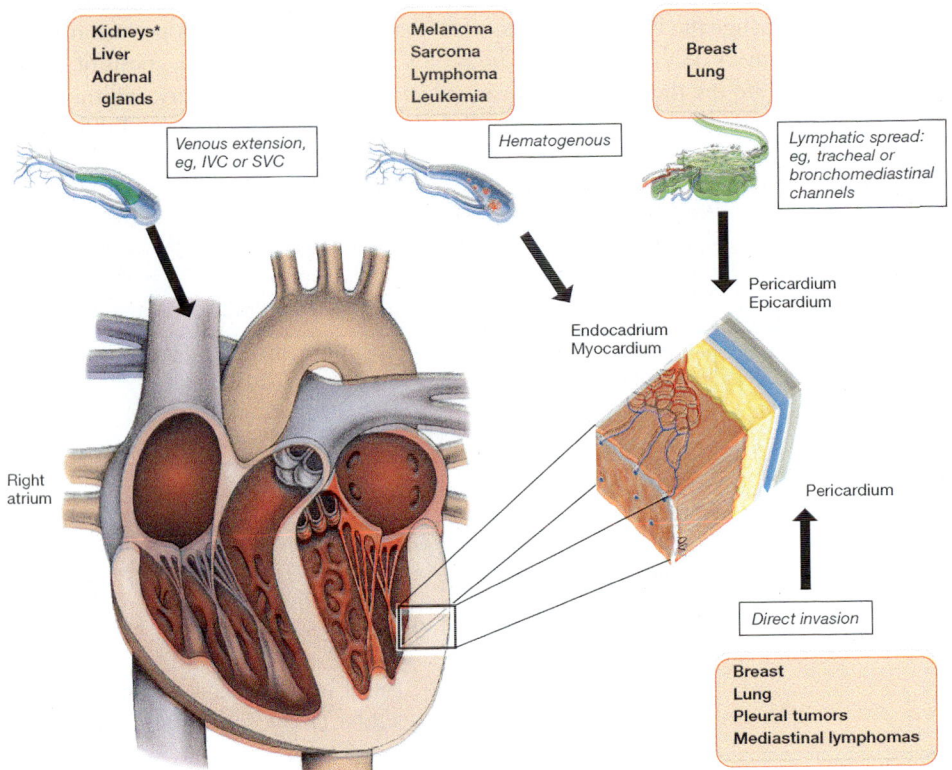

Figure 24.3 Different primary tumors utilize different routes for cardiac metastasis. *Cases of renal cell carcinoma that don't use the direct IVC route are also documented. IVC, inferior vena cava; SVC, superior vena cava.

24.10 The correct answer is B.

Rationale: PCs are single-layered, fluid-filled cavities arising from the outer layer of the heart. PCs are very rare and are seen in 1 per 100,000 individuals. PCs are mostly congenital (due to failure of pericardial lacunae fusion during embryologic development) but may also be acquired (ie, postsurgery) or infectious (eg, echinococcosis or tuberculosis). Patients are most commonly females with a mean age of 49 ± 16. Chest radiography and echocardiography are often the first modalities to detect a PC; however, CCT or CMR is the recommended modality to confirm the diagnosis. PCs are managed according to the clinical presentation. Asymptomatic lesions are usually followed by CCT or CMR every 1 to 2 years. Intervention by percutaneous aspiration with possible ethanol sclerosis is recommended in symptomatic cysts. However, observational evidence suggests that this strategy is associated with high recurrence rates. Surgical resection may be necessary if the cyst is large or recurring, when imaging is insufficient for definitive diagnosis and malignancy is suspected, or in cysts with a high propensity for rupture.

CARDIAC EVALUATION FOR NONCARDIAC SURGERY*

Teni Olatunde and Robert L. Carhart

CHAPTER 25

QUESTIONS

25.1 A 68-year-old female with a history of hypertension, hyperlipidemia, and lupus presents to your office for a preoperative risk stratification for an upcoming endoscopy for dysphagia. Apart from dysphagia, she reports occasional ankle swelling at the end of the day, which improves with leg elevation.

Her blood pressure in the office is 150/80 mm Hg, heart rate 70 beats per minute (bpm), with a body mass index (BMI) of 32. On physical examination: no audible murmurs on cardiac examination, lungs are clear to auscultation, and no lower extremity edema is noted. Her electrocardiogram (ECG) performed in the office showed sinus rhythm with an isolated premature atrial complex.

What further testing, if any, would you recommend prior to an endoscopic procedure?

- A. 2D echocardiogram
- B. Holter monitor
- C. Exercise stress testing
- D. No further testing required prior to procedure

25.2 A 52-year-old man presents to your office for preoperative risk stratification for abdominal hernia repair. He has a history of hypertension, type 2 diabetes, chronic kidney disease, and osteoarthritis with chronic back pain. His medications include amlodipine 10 mg daily, insulin, and acetaminophen as needed for pain. He lives a sedentary lifestyle and is able to perform activities of daily living; however, ambulation is limited by back pain. He is unable to walk half a block or up a flight of stairs.

His blood pressure is 150/82 mm Hg, with a heart rate of 72 bpm, S_4 gallop without murmurs audible on cardiac auscultation, lungs clear to auscultation bilaterally, and no lower extremity edema.

ECG performed was abnormal showing sinus rhythm with prominent Q waves in leads II, III, and aVF and criteria for left ventricular hypertrophy (LVH) met.

How would you proceed with further evaluation/management prior to surgery?

- A. No further testing prior to surgery
- B. Pharmacologic stress testing
- C. Medical management with aspirin and statin
- D. Exercise stress echocardiogram

25.3 A 62-year-old man with a history of coronary artery disease (CAD) with prior stents, hypertension, poorly controlled type 2 diabetes, and hyperlipidemia presents for a

---

*Questions and Answers are based on Chapter 25: Cardiac Evaluation for Noncardiac Surgery by Hugo Quinny Cheng in Cardiovascular Medicine and Surgery, First Edition.

colonoscopy. He takes lisinopril 40 mg, atorvastatin 40 mg daily, metformin, and insulin nightly. He denies angina, palpitations, orthopnea, paroxysmal nocturnal dyspnea, or lower extremity edema. During preprocedural assessment, the nurse asks the anesthesiologist for the patient's alcohol septal ablation (ASA).

What is his ASA classification?

A. ASA class I
B. ASA class II
C. ASA class III
D. ASA class IV

25.4 A 65-year-old male, with a medical history of hyperlipidemia and hypertension with a recent diagnosis of lung cancer, who is planned for a thoracotomy with resection of the right lower lobe presents for surgical preoperative risk classification. He reports a month of dyspnea on exertion, orthopnea, and lower extremity edema without angina or palpitations.

Vital signs revealed blood pressure 128/70 mm Hg, heart rate 75 bpm, jugular venous distension, S_3 gallop on cardiac examination, bibasilar rales on lung examination, hepatomegaly, and 2+ bilateral pitting edema.

What would you do next?

A. Perform a transthoracic echocardiogram (TTE).
B. Check pro-brain natriuretic peptide (proBNP) levels.
C. Perform a chest x-ray.
D. Proceed with surgery.

25.5 A 56-year-old female with a history of CAD with one stent placed 2 years ago, hypertension, and hyperlipidemia presents for cardiac preoperative risk stratification prior to an elective myomectomy for uterine fibroids. Her medications include aspirin 81 mg daily, carvedilol 6.25 mg twice a day, and atorvastatin 80 mg daily. She denies any angina, palpitations, dyspnea on exertion, orthopnea, or lower extremity edema.

Vital signs are stable. Physical examination did not reveal any heart murmurs, extra heart sounds, or signs of hypervolemia. A cardiac preoperative risk stratification is completed and it is decided that the patient can proceed with surgery without further testing, but the gynecology team would like to know specifically how to manage the patient's medication pre- and postsurgery.

What do you advise should be done?

A. Continue atorvastatin only perioperatively.
B. Discontinue all medication perioperatively and restart 24 to 48 hours postoperatively.
C. Continue carvedilol, and atorvastatin perioperatively but may discontinue aspirin prior to surgery.
D. Continue all medications perioperatively.

25.6 A 50-year-old female with a history of newly diagnosed breast cancer, CAD status post (s/p) myocardial infarction (MI) with a drug-eluting stent (DES) to the right coronary artery (RCA) 3 months ago, hypertension, and hyperlipidemia presents for surgical clearance prior to lumpectomy. She is on dual antiplatelet therapy (DAPT) with aspirin and clopidogrel, lisinopril 20 mg daily, rosuvastatin 40 mg daily, and metoprolol succinate 25 mg daily.

She denies any angina, palpitations, orthopnea, or lower extremity edema. Her vital signs are within normal limits; ECG showed old inferior wall MI with Q waves in II, III, and aVF; and the most recent echocardiogram from 1 month ago showed normal LVEF 55% with resolution of prior wall motion abnormality.

The surgeons would like some advice on preoperative and postoperative management of DAPT considering the patient recently had a stent placed. What would you advise them?

A. Discontinue clopidogrel prior to surgery but continue aspirin and restart clopidogrel as soon as possible postsurgery.
B. Discontinue DAPT prior to surgery and restart as soon as possible postsurgery.
C. Continue DAPT in the perioperative period.
D. Delay surgery until 6 months post percutaneous coronary intervention (PCI).

25.7 A 55-year-old female presents to the emergency department with sharp chest pain with radiation to her back. She has a history of uncontrolled hypertension, abdominal aortic aneurysm measuring 5.2 cm on computed tomography (CT) scan performed a year prior and non-insulin-dependent diabetes. Blood pressure on arrival is 90/60 mm Hg with heart rate (HR) 120 bpm on the right arm, and 70/50 with HR 130 bpm on the left arm. She is volume resuscitated and computed tomography angiography (CTA) thorax and abdomen showed a ruptured aneurysm.

Prior to surgery, which of the following should be performed?

A. 2D echocardiogram
B. ECG
C. Coronary angiography
D. No further testing; take patient straight to surgery.

25.8 A 60-year-old man with a history of atrial fibrillation, hypertension, and osteoarthritis is planned for a knee replacement surgery. He is seen at your office for preoperative surgical clearance prior to the procedure.

He denies angina, palpitations, peripheral edema, or orthopnea. He takes carvedilol 12.5 mg bid for rate control and apixaban 5 mg bid for anticoagulation, as well as naproxen as needed for pain.

What do you recommend for management of his anticoagulation?

A. Discontinue apixaban the day prior to surgery.
B. Discontinue apixaban 2 days prior to surgery but bridge with heparin.
C. Discontinue apixaban 2 days prior to surgery.
D. Discontinue apixaban 5 days prior to surgery.

CASE 1

A 50-year-old male with a history of bicuspid aortic valve and moderate to severe aortic stenosis and morbid obesity is sent for cardiac preoperative risk stratification prior to bariatric surgery. His last echocardiogram was a year-and-a-half ago. He denies any shortness of breath at rest or exertion or angina, orthopnea, paroxysmal nocturnal dyspnea, or lower extremity edema.

> But he reports occasional dizziness and lightheadedness. Vital signs reveal blood pressure 132/70 bpm, heart rate 82 bpm, no jugular venous distension seen, and grade 3 systolic murmur is heard in the second right intercostal space with radiation to carotids and other heart areas. S_2 is not audible. He has greater than 4 METs (metabolic equivalents) for physical activity. He asks if he can proceed with his planned procedure without further testing.

25.9 For the patient in **Case 1**, what do you recommend?
   A. Proceed with surgery.
   B. Obtain a 2D echocardiogram prior to surgery.
   C. Obtain a transesophageal echocardiogram (TEE).
   D. Obtain a low-dose dobutamine stress echocardiogram.

25.10 A TTE is performed for the patient in **Case 1**, which reveals left ventricular ejection fraction (LVEF) 55%, V_{max} 4.2 m/s, mean gradient 44 mm Hg, and aortic valve area 0.9 cm². He is diagnosed with severe aortic stenosis.

What is the next course of action?
   A. Proceed with elective surgery.
   B. Perform TEE.
   C. Defer elective surgery and refer patient for valve replacement surgery/procedure.
   D. Perform a low-dose dobutamine stress echocardiogram.

ANSWERS

25.1 The correct answer is B.
Rationale: Patient is planned for a low-risk procedure for cardiac complications: endoscopy. She does not require any further testing. On physical examination, she has no signs of volume overload and no audible murmurs that require further evaluation with an echocardiogram. Her ECG showed an isolated premature atrial contraction (PAC) that does not warrant a Holter monitor prior to planned procedure as the patient does not report any symptoms concerning for unstable arrhythmias. Although she has risk factors for CAD—hypertension, hyperlipidemia, and obesity—a stress test is not needed prior to the procedure especially in the absence of angina symptoms.

KEY POINTS

✓ The risk of perioperative cardiac complications depends on both patient-related risk factors and the risk of the procedure. Minimally invasive procedures, endoscopic cases, or procedures performed on the skin or eye have a very low risk of cardiac complications. Patients undergoing low-risk procedures generally do not require an in-depth preoperative cardiac evaluation.

25.2 The correct answer is B.

Rationale: This patient has less than 4 METs of activity as he is mostly sedentary but is able to perform activities of daily living (ADLs). Patients with limited exercise capacity are at increased risk for major adverse cardiovascular events (MACE). Per the Revised Cardiac Risk Index (RCRI) scoring system, he has three risk factors: diabetes, on insulin; chronic kidney disease (CKD) with creatinine (Cr) higher than 2, and signs of ischemic heart disease with evidence of old inferior wall MI on ECG. These factors per the RCRI risk calculator increase his risk for MACE; therefore, he should undergo noninvasive stress testing. Due to his physical limitation from back pain, pharmacologic stress testing is preferred.

KEY POINTS

- Guidelines from the American College of Cardiology/American Heart Association (ACC/AHA) and the European Society of Cardiology and European Society of Anesthesiology (ESC/ESA) identify patients who have both multiple RCRI predictors and poor functional capacity (<4 METS) who are undergoing major surgery as the most appropriate population for noninvasive stress testing.

25.3 The correct answer is C.

Rationale:

ASA I: normal, healthy individual
ASA II: patient with mild systemic disease (mild lung disease, well controlled hypertension)
ASA III: patient with severe systemic disease (stable CAD, poorly controlled diabetes)
ASA IV: patient with severe systemic disease that is a constant threat to life (eg, recent acute coronary syndrome, sepsis)
ASA V: moribund patient not expected to survive without surgery (eg, ruptured aortic aneurysm, intracranial hemorrhage with mass effect)

This patient has stable CAD and poorly controlled diabetes.

KEY POINTS

- Determine the patient's ASA physical classification.

25.4 The correct answer is A.

Rationale: Patient is exhibiting signs and symptoms of heart failure, which should be investigated further with a TTE. The guidelines from ACC/AHA and ESC/ESA are ambivalent about the utility of measuring preoperative biomarker levels. In this case, the patient is hypervolemic and in decompensated heart failure based on physical examination. He will benefit from heart failure therapy prior to surgery; therefore, you should not advise him to proceed with surgery. A chest x-ray will demonstrate pulmonary edema but will not provide a definite diagnosis such as an echocardiogram.

KEY POINTS

✔ Patients with new or suspected heart failure diagnosis without a prior TTE should undergo this study before surgery.

25.5 The correct answer is C.

Rationale: Surgical site bleeding is more common in aspirin-treated patients. Given the planned myomectomy that has increased risk of bleeding, aspirin may be held prior to surgery in this patient and restarted when the patient is stable and no longer bleeding per surgeon's assessment post the procedure. Her PCI was more than 1 year ago; therefore, discontinuation of aspirin temporarily is reasonable with a goal to resume 24 hours after surgery if there is no excessive bleeding. The hypothesis is that statins stabilize coronary plaque and prevent rupture and vascular injury that would lead to postoperative MI; therefore, in this patient with known CAD, statins should be continued perioperatively and postoperatively. Indications for beta-blockers in the perioperative period are limited; however, patients taking beta-blockers should continue perioperatively and postoperatively if there is hemodynamic stability.

KEY POINTS

✔ Understand perioperative management of cardiovascular medications. Individualize management of antiplatelet agents based on risks of bleeding and MACE. Beta-blockers should be continued perioperatively and postoperatively if there is hemodynamic stability. In patients with known CAD, statins should be continued perioperatively and postoperatively.

25.6 The correct answer is A.

Rationale: The ACC/AHA recommends the following guideline for management of DAPT.

Patients who had very recent PCI (within 4-6 weeks) with either bare metal stent (BMS) or DES should continue DAPT if at all possible due to the high risk of stent thrombosis. If a patient on DAPT must stop the P2Y12 receptor inhibitor prior to surgery, aspirin should be continued if possible and the P2Y12 receptor inhibitor restarted as soon as possible postsurgery. They also recommend delaying elective surgery at least 30 days after BMS implantation and 6 months after DES implantation, but if the operation is time sensitive as in this case, a delay of 3 months can be considered. This patient is past the 3-month mark; therefore, the time-sensitive surgery can be performed and clopidogrel held prior to surgery while continuing aspirin.

KEY POINTS

✔ The benefit of continuing DAPT is greater in patients with recent prior PCI. Continuing DAPT is strongly indicated within 4 to 6 weeks of BMS and 3 months of DES implantation. If a patient on DAPT must stop the P2Y12 receptor inhibitor prior to surgery, aspirin should be continued if possible and the P2Y12 receptor inhibitor restarted as soon as possible postsurgery.

25.7 The correct answer is D.

Rationale: An aortic aneurysm rupture is a surgical emergency and the patient should be taken straight to surgery. Obtaining an ECG is reasonable; however, findings would not change management. An echocardiogram can be considered if there is a need for it postsurgery, but not before this emergent surgery. Despite the patient having risk factors for CAD, there is no indication for coronary angiography prior to surgery.

KEY POINTS

✔ Preoperative risk stratification is not necessary prior to emergency surgery.

25.8 The correct answer is C.

Rationale: Direct oral anticoagulants (DOACs) should be discontinued 2 days prior to surgery for low-bleeding-risk procedures, but 3 days for high-bleeding-risk procedures. Bridging with heparin is not needed in atrial fibrillation. If hemostasis is adequate, they should be resumed 24 hours post the procedure for a low-bleeding-risk procedure and 48 to 72 hours after a high-bleeding-risk procedure.

KEY POINTS

✔ DOACs should be discontinued 2 days prior to surgery for low-bleeding-risk procedures but 3 days for high-bleeding-risk procedures.

25.9 The correct answer is B.

Rationale: This patient has a history of moderate to severe aortic stenosis and now has symptoms of dizziness and lightheadedness. An echocardiogram should be performed to assess progression of his disease. He should not proceed with surgery. A TTE should be performed prior to TEE. A low-dose dobutamine stress echocardiogram is performed to diagnose low-flow, low-gradient aortic stenosis, which is not the case in this patient.

KEY POINTS

✔ Patients with a murmur or other findings that raise concern for serious valvular heart disease (particularly aortic stenosis) should be evaluated with TTE. Patients with established moderate to severe valvular disease should undergo surveillance echocardiography if not performed in the prior year or if cardiovascular symptoms have worsened.

25.10 The correct answer is C.

Rationale: This patient has severe symptomatic aortic stenosis based on the echocardiogram findings; therefore, he should optimally undergo valve replacement and his elective surgery should be deferred. Since severe aortic stenosis has been confirmed on TTE, a TEE is not necessary. A low-dose dobutamine stress echocardiogram is not necessary as there is no low-flow, low-gradient aortic stenosis.

KEY POINTS

- Patients with independent indications for percutaneous or surgical treatment of valvular heart disease should have the procedure performed before elective noncardiac surgery, if possible. Patients with stenotic valvular disease (especially critical or symptomatic aortic stenosis) are at particularly high risk for cardiovascular complications from noncardiac surgery.

CARDIO-ONCOLOGY

Robert L. Carhart and Anojan Pathmanathan

CHAPTER 26

QUESTIONS

26.1 A 63-year-old male with recently diagnosed multiple myeloma and a history of hypertension, heart failure with preserved ejection fraction, and hyperlipidemia presents to the cardiology clinic for evaluation. He is to be initiated on carfilzomib and would like to know how to decrease his risk of cardiotoxicity. Which one of the following statements is **NOT** part of the ABCDE model approach for cardiovascular risk assessment?

  A. Diet rich in fruit, vegetables, whole grain
  B. Awareness of cardiovascular signs and symptoms
  C. Monthly echocardiogram
  D. Blood pressure less than 130/80 mm Hg

26.2 A 57-year-old female with a history of hyperlipidemia, hypertension, and hypothyroidism was recently diagnosed with ovarian cancer. She presents to the cardiology office as a new referral prior to her initiation of anthracycline therapy. She denies any complaints today but would like to know how to reduce her risk of cardiomyopathy. Which of the following statements is **NOT TRUE** about treatment with anthracycline?

  A. Lower doses prevent anthracycline-associated cardiomyopathy.
  B. Female sex is a risk factor for cardiotoxicity.
  C. Dexrazoxane can be used for patients with a higher risk of cardiotoxicity and who receive more than 300 mg/m^2 of doxorubicin.
  D. Anthracycline cardiotoxicity typically occurs within 1 to 2 years of exposure.

26.3 A 57-year-old male with recently diagnosed renal cell carcinoma is referred to the cardiology clinic for evaluation prior to chemotherapy. He currently has no complaints, and his lab studies are within normal limits. The echocardiogram shows a left ventricular ejection fraction (LVEF) of 55%, with no regional wall motion abnormalities or valvulopathies. He is being planned for chemotherapy with axitinib. Which of the following statements is **NOT TRUE** about vascular endothelial growth factor (VEGF) tyrosine kinase inhibitors (TKIs)?

  A. Liver toxicity is the primary major side effect in this class of therapy.
  B. Axitinib carries a black box warning for torsades de pointes.
  C. Patient risk factors for cardiotoxicity include hypertension and underlying pulmonary hypertension.
  D. VEGF-TKI use can result in dose-dependent elevations in blood pressure.

*Questions and Answers are based on Chapter 26: Cardio-Oncology by Courtney M. Campbell, Ajay Vallakati, Daniel Addison, and Ragavendra R. Baliga in Cardiovascular Medicine and Surgery, First Edition.

26.4 A 65-year-old male with Hodgkin lymphoma, hypertension, and coronary artery disease presents to the cardiology clinic prior to initiation of radiation therapy. He has no complaints today other than mild shortness of breath. Which of the following statements is **TRUE** about radiation-induced cardiotoxicity?

A. Early complications of radiation therapy include damage to slowly proliferating tissue such as the lung or heart.
B. Late complications of radiation therapy can be reversible.
C. In patients with Hodgkin lymphoma, the incidence of coronary artery disease was associated with rising mean heart radiation dose.
D. Valvular heart disease is usually seen within 5 years postradiation therapy.

26.5 A 76-year-old female with a known history of breast cancer presents to the cardiology clinic for continued evaluation. She has a history of hypertension and coronary artery disease. She was initiated on daunorubicin therapy 3 months ago. She is currently asymptomatic. Her echocardiogram prior to chemotherapy demonstrated an LVEF of 60% with no regional wall motion abnormalities. A repeat echocardiogram today shows an LVEF of 55% and a 20% decrease in global longitudinal strain (GLS). Which of the following statements is **TRUE**?

A. Asymptomatic cardiomyopathy requires no further management.
B. The patient should be initiated on beta-blocker and angiotensin blockade.
C. This patient is at low risk for cardiotoxicity.
D. Echocardiogram is not warranted 10 years posttreatment for this patient.

26.6 A 70-year-old male was recently diagnosed with multiple myeloma. He was started on carfilzomib-based treatment. He came in for 3 months follow-up. His blood pressure and heart rate were acceptable. The echocardiography showed LVEF of 55%, with no regional wall motion abnormalities. The echocardiography prior to treatment initiation was 60%. Which of the following statement is **TRUE**?

A. Patient's age of 70 years puts him at increased risk of cardiotoxicity.
B. Carfilzomib dose greater than 45 mg/m^2 is a risk factor.
C. GLS should be routinely performed in the monitoring of cardiotoxic chemotherapy.
D. All of the above

26.7 Which of the following statements **BEST** describes the cardiac toxicity associated with trastuzumab, a commonly used targeted therapy in breast cancer? Choose the **CORRECT** option:

A. Trastuzumab has no impact on cardiac function.
B. Cardiac toxicity is rare and occurs only in patients with preexisting heart conditions.
C. Trastuzumab may lead to cardiac dysfunction, and regular cardiac monitoring is recommended during treatment.
D. Cardiac toxicity is dose dependent and can be minimized by increasing the duration between trastuzumab infusions.

26.8 A 58-year-old female with a history of breast cancer is undergoing chemotherapy with anthracyclines for her malignancy. During treatment, she experiences mild symptoms of heart failure, including fatigue and dyspnea. What is the most appropriate management strategy for the cardiotoxicity associated with these chemotherapeutic drugs? Choose the **CORRECT** option:

A. Discontinuation of chemotherapy to prevent further cardiac damage
B. Initiation of angiotensin-converting enzyme (ACE) inhibitors or angiotensin II receptor blockers (ARBs) for cardioprotection
C. No specific intervention, as these symptoms are expected during cancer treatment
D. Immediate referral for cardiac surgery to address potential complications

ANSWERS

26.1 The correct answer is C.

Rationale: Prior to oncology treatment, a patient should be educated on ways to optimize their cardiotoxicity risk associated with chemotherapy. The ABCDE model is the current approach for risk assessment and comprises awareness of symptoms/signs; aspirin initiation; blood pressure less than 130/80 mm Hg; cholesterol management; cigarette cessation; diet rich in fruit, vegetables, and whole grain; and exercise. Although baseline echocardiogram testing should be obtained prior to initiation of oncology therapy, repeat testing during treatment varies per study. For high-risk patients, recommendations range from every 3 to 6 months. There is no justification for routine monthly echocardiograms.[1]

KEY POINTS

✔ The ABCDE model is the current approach for cardiotoxicity risk assessment and optimization regardless of oncology treatment modality.

26.2 The correct answer is A.

Rationale: Anthracycline cardiotoxicity typically occurs within 1 to 2 years of exposure. There is no safe dose of anthracyclines. Anthracycline cardiotoxicity can occur at doses below the suggested maximum thresholds. Therefore, careful monitoring for signs and symptoms of cardiomyopathy is required. High-risk factors for anthracycline cardiotoxicity include extremities of age, female sex, underlying cardiovascular disease, and prior irradiation of the mediastinum. Dexrazoxane is an iron chelation agent that can reduce cardiomyopathy in high-risk patients who receive more than 300 mg/m² of doxorubicin.[2,3]

KEY POINTS

✔ Anthracycline-associated cardiomyopathy can occur at doses below the suggested maximum thresholds.

26.3 The correct answer is B.
Rationale: VEGF-TKIs are used to treat a variety of cancers including renal cell carcinoma, hepatocellular carcinoma, thyroid cancer, endometrial cancers, and sarcomas. One drug in this class, vandetanib, carries a black box warning for QT prolongation, torsades de pointes, and sudden death. Cardiotoxicity with VEGF-TKIs most often manifests as hypertension from increased endothelin levels. This is a dose-dependent phenomenon and resolves upon therapy discontinuation.[4,5]

KEY POINTS

- Vandetanib is the only VEGF-TKI that carries a black box warning of QT prolongation, torsades de pointes, and sudden death.

26.4 The correct answer is C.
Rationale: Radiation to the heart is reported as mean heart dose. In patients with Hodgkin lymphoma, increasing mean heart doses correlate with an increased incidence of coronary artery disease. Overall, studies have shown that there is a 7.4% increased risk of coronary artery disease for every 1 Gy mean heart dose.

Late complications of radiation therapy involve small blood vessel damage that is not reversible. In the heart, the resulting cell loss and fibrosis can lead to atherosclerosis, cardiomyopathy, cardiac fibrosis, valvular fibrosis, pericarditis, pericardial effusions, constriction, and arrhythmias. Early complications occur in rapidly proliferating tissue such as the skin, gastrointestinal (GI) tract, and hematopoietic systems. Valvular heart disease usually occurs 22 to 25 years postradiation treatment.[6,7]

KEY POINTS

- Studies have shown that an increasing mean heart dose in radiation therapy increases a patient's risk for coronary artery disease.

26.5 The correct answer is B.
Rationale: Patients on anthracycline therapy require close monitoring for signs of cardiomyopathy. Although the value of GLS for cardio-oncology is still being established, meta-analysis studies are showing that patients benefit from treatment for cardiomyopathy when there is more than 15% decrease in GLS even if asymptomatic. Evidence of asymptomatic cardiomyopathy with a drop in LVEF should prompt initiation of a beta-blocker and angiotensin blocker.

With a history of hypertension, female gender, underlying coronary artery disease, and age, this patient is at high risk for cardiotoxicity with anthracycline therapy. Echocardiogram is warranted in high-risk patients with chemotherapy-induced cardiotoxicity 4 and 10 years posttreatment.[8,9]

KEY POINTS

- Initiation of guideline-directed medical therapy is critical for any patient with a drop in LVEF. Oncology patients with new cardiomyopathy should undergo testing for ischemic and other treatable causes of cardiomyopathy.

26.6 The correct answer is D.
Rationale: Potential risk factors include age, comorbidities, previous cardiotoxic therapies, and carfilzomib doses greater than 45 mg/m^2. Periodic monitoring of cardiac function with echocardiography with GLS is a routine practice in early recognition of cardiac toxicity from noncardiac cancer treatment.

26.7 The correct answer is C.
Rationale: Trastuzumab, a widely used targeted therapy for breast cancer, has been associated with potential cardiac toxicity, which is not dose dependent. Regular cardiac monitoring is crucial during trastuzumab treatment to detect and manage any cardiac dysfunction that may arise. This emphasizes the importance of close collaboration between oncologists and cardiologists to ensure the overall well-being of patients undergoing trastuzumab therapy. While cardiac impact is a consideration, the benefits of trastuzumab in treating HER2-positive breast cancer often outweigh the associated risks. Trastuzumab toxicity is not dose dependent and may be reversible with discontinuation of treatment and/or standard medical therapy for congestive heart failure.

26.8 The correct answer is B.
Rationale: Initiating ACE inhibitors or ARBs is a recommended strategy for managing chemotherapy-induced cardiotoxicity. These medications have shown efficacy in preventing further cardiac damage and preserving cardiac function during cancer treatment, providing cardioprotection for patients undergoing chemotherapy with agents like anthracyclines. This approach is part of a comprehensive strategy to minimize the impact of cardiotoxic effects on the cardiovascular health of patients with cancer.

REFERENCES

Arnett DK, Blumenthal RS, Albert MA, et al. 2019 ACC/AHA guideline on the primary prevention of cardiovascular disease: executive summary: a report of the American College of Cardiology/American Heart Association Task Force on clinical practice guidelines. *J Am Coll Cardiol.* 2019;74:1376-1414.

Henriksen PA. Anthracycline cardiotoxicity: an update on mechanisms, monitoring and prevention. *Heart.* 2018;104:971-977.

Kang Y, Assuncao BL, Denduluri S, et al. Symptomatic heart failure in acute leukemia patients treated with anthracyclines. *JACC: CardioOncology.* 2019;1:208-217.

Lenneman CG, Sawyer DB. Cardio-oncology: an update on cardiotoxicity of cancer-related treatment. *Circ Res.* 2016;118:1008-1020.

Hall PS, Harshman LC, Srinivas S, Witteles RM. The frequency and severity of cardiovascular toxicity from targeted therapy in advanced renal cell carcinoma patients. *JACC Heart Fail.* 2013;1:72-78.

Desai MY, Jellis CL, Kotecha R, Johnston DR, Griffin BP. Radiation-associated cardiac disease: a practical approach to diagnosis and management. *JACC Cardiovasc Imaging.* 2018;11:1132-1149.

van Nimwegen FA, Schaapveld M, Cutter DJ, et al. Radiation dose-response relationship for risk of coronary heart disease in survivors of Hodgkin lymphoma. *J Clin Oncol.* 2016;34:235-243.

Oikonomou EK, Kokkinidis DG, Kampaktsis PN, et al. Assessment of prognostic value of left ventricular global longitudinal strain for early prediction of chemotherapy-induced cardiotoxicity: a systematic review and meta-analysis. *JAMA Cardiol.* 2019;4(10):1007-1018.

Plana JC, Galderisi M, Barac A, et al. Expert consensus for multimodality imaging evaluation of adult patients during and after cancer therapy: a report from the American Society of Echocardiography and the European Association of Cardiovascular Imaging. *J Am Soc Echocardiogr.* 2014;27:911-939.

CARDIAC DISEASE IN HUMAN IMMUNODEFICIENCY VIRUS INFECTION*

Anshu Shridhar

CHAPTER 27

QUESTIONS

27.1 What is the cumulative lifetime cardiovascular disease (CVD) risk in patients with HIV infection?

A. 5%
B. 10%
C. 15%
D. 20%

27.2 What is the relative risk of acute myocardial infarction (MI) in patients with HIV infection as compared to non-HIV-infected patients?

A. 0.5 to 1
B. 1 to 1.4
C. 1.4 to 2
D. 2 to 2.5

27.3 What are the potential mechanistic factors in increased cardiovascular burden in patients with HIV infection?

A. Conventional risk factors, such as smoking, hypertension, obesity, dyslipidemia, insulin resistance, and diabetes
B. HIV-related immune dysfunction, systemic inflammation, disruption of lipid metabolism, hepatitis C coinfection, low CD4+ T-cell counts, high viral ribonucleic acid (RNA) levels
C. Antiretroviral drug effects
D. All of the above

27.4 What systemic inflammatory markers are strong predictors of mortality and patients with HIV infection?

A. Interleukin-6 (IL-6)
B. D-dimer
C. Both IL-6 and D-dimer
D. None of the above

---

*Questions and Answers are based on Chapter 27: Cardiac Disease in Human Immunodeficiency Virus Infection by Timir K. Paul and Sukhdeep Bhogal in Cardiovascular Medicine and Surgery, First Edition.

CHAPTER 27 | Cardiac Disease In Human Immunodeficiency Virus Infection

27.5 What type of plaques are more prevalent in patients with HIV infection compared with controls on computed tomography angiography (CTA)?
- A. Calcified plaque
- B. Noncalcified plaque
- C. Both calcified and noncalcified plaques
- D. None of the above

27.6 What is the most common clinical presentation of CVD in patients with HIV infection?
- A. ST-segment elevation myocardial infarction (STEMI)
- B. Non–ST-segment elevation myocardial infarction (NSTEMI)
- C. Unstable angina
- D. Congestive heart failure

27.7 Which ART (antiretroviral therapy; protease inhibitor) treatment for HIV is **NOT** associated with increased risk of MI?
- A. Lopinavir
- B. Indinavir
- C. Saquinavir
- D. Amprenavir/fosamprenavir

27.8 Which is the most common cardiac tumor in patients with HIV infection?
- A. Non-Hodgkin lymphoma
- B. Leiomyosarcoma
- C. Kaposi sarcoma (KS)
- D. Rhabdomyosarcoma

27.9 Which statins should **NOT** be used to treat CVD in patients with HIV?
- A. Atorvastatin
- B. Rosuvastatin
- C. Simvastatin
- D. Pravastatin

27.10 What is **NOT** recommended for primary prevention in patients with HIV?
- A. Aspirin
- B. Lifestyle changes with regular physical activity
- C. Counseling on smoking cessation
- D. Better management of concomitant comorbid diseases including diabetes and hypertension

ANSWERS

27.1 The correct answer is D.
Rationale: A cohort analysis has reported that cumulative lifetime CVD risk was estimated to be at 20.5% in persons infected with HIV versus 12.8% in the general U.S. population.

212. The correct answer is C.
Rationale: Study by Kaiser Permanente California Medical Group showed that patients who are HIV positive are at high risk for MI (adjusted RR 1.4 [95% CI 1.3-1.7; P <.001]) as compared to HIV-negative population. Data on 28,000 Veterans Administration (VA) patients showed a significantly increased risk of acute MI in patients with HIV infection with an adjusted hazard ratio (HR) of 1.94 (95% CI 1.58-2.37) as compared to non–HIV-infected patients.

213. The correct answer is B.
Rationale: Mechanistic factors in increased cardiovascular burden in patients with HIV infection include, in addition to conventional risk factors of smoking, hypertension, obesity, dyslipidemia, insulin resistance, and diabetes, HIV-related immune dysfunction, systemic inflammation, disruption of lipid metabolism, hepatitis C coinfection, low CD4+ T-cell counts, high viral RNA levels, and antiretroviral drug effects (**Figure 27.1**).

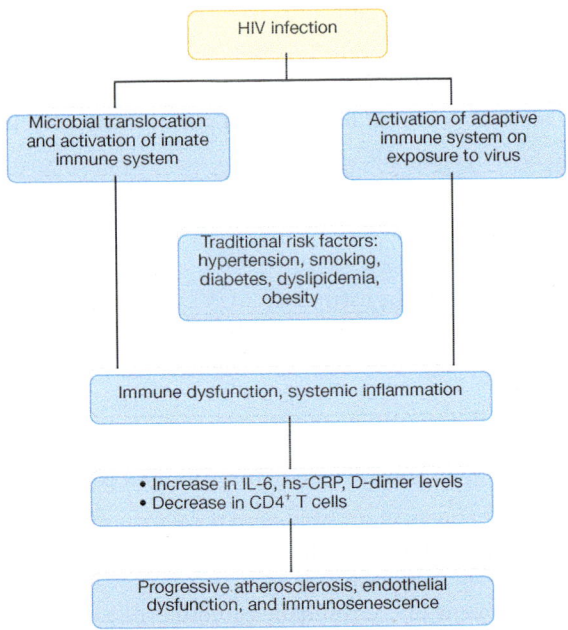

Figure 27.1 HIV and cardiovascular risk factors. HIV, human immunodeficiency virus; hs-CRP, high-sensitivity C-reactive protein; IL-6, interleukin-6.

214. The correct answer is C.
Rationale: The analysis of the Strategies for Management of Antiretroviral Therapy (SMART) trial confirmed that IL-6 and D-dimer are both strong predictors of mortality in these patients.

275. The correct answer is B.
Rationale: Observational studies have shown more prevalence of noncalcified soft plaques in HIV status compared to controls. Another meta-analysis of nine studies also showed a similar burden of coronary artery stenosis and calcified plaques compared to controls but higher rates of noncalcified plaques among individuals with HIV infection. These noncalcified plaques have a lipid-rich, inflammatory core and are prone to rupture that may be an explanation for younger age of presentation with acute coronary syndrome (ACS) among patients with HIV compared to the general population.

276. The correct answer is A.
Rationale: The clinical presentation of CVD in patients with HIV infection could range from silent ischemia to ACS. The most common presentation was STEMI, followed by NSTEMI, and unstable angina. Patients with HIV tend to be on average a decade younger than the uninfected individuals and are more likely to be young men (<50 years), smokers, having dyslipidemia, with lengthier duration (>8 years) of HIV, and taking ART. Angiographically, patients with HIV are more likely to have single-vessel disease than three-vessel disease and primarily underwent percutaneous coronary intervention (PCI) followed by coronary artery bypass grafting. HIV also poses an increased risk of heart failure independent of MI which could manifest even decades earlier than would be expected in the general population.

277. The correct answer is C.
Rationale: Among the choices listed, saquinavir has not been associated with an increased risk of MI. Nelfinavir, efavirenz, and nevirapine are also not associated with an increased risk of MI (**Table 27.1**).

278. The correct answer is C.
Rationale: The commonest cardiac tumor noted in patients with HIV infection is KS.

279. The correct answer is C.
Rationale: Statins should be considered because they significantly reduce major adverse cardiovascular events (MACE) in patients even with low levels of low-density lipoprotein cholesterol (LDL-C) (<130 mg/dL) and elevated markers of inflammation such as high-sensitivity C-reactive protein (hs-CRP). Statins that metabolized through the cytochrome P-450 system (CYP3A4 pathway), such as simvastatin and lovastatin, should be avoided in patients with HIV as protease inhibitors inhibit the CYP3A4 system, whereas nucleoside reverse transcriptase inhibitors induce it.

Low-dose atorvastatin, pitavastatin, pravastatin, and rosuvastatin are generally considered safe in these patients.

TABLE 27.1 Antiretroviral Drugs and Their Associated Cardiovascular Risk

Drugs	Cardiovascular Risk Based on Available Data (Observational)
Protease inhibitors	
Lopinavir	Increased CVD risk based on DAD and FHDH study
Indinavir	Increased CVD risk based on DAD study
Amprenavir	Increased CVD risk based on FHDH study, although it was underpowered
Fosamprenavir	Increased CVD risk based on FHDH study, although it was underpowered
Saquinavir	Not associated with MI
Darunavir	Increased risk of CVD based on 2018 DAD data
Atazanavir	Not associated with increased risk of CVD based on 2018 DAD data
Ritonavir	Not used alone, used as a booster with other PIs
Nelfinavir	Not associated with MI
Nonnucleoside reverse transcriptase inhibitor (NNRTI): efavirenz, nevirapine	Not associated with MI
Nucleoside reverse transcriptase inhibitors (NRTIs)	Abacavir and Didanosine have been linked with an increased risk for MI based on DAD data but discrepant results based on other studies.

CVD, cardiovascular; DAD, data collection on adverse events on anti-HIV drugs; FHDH, French Hospital Database on HIV; MI, myocardial infarction; PIs, protease inhibitors.

27.10 The correct answer is A.

Rationale: There is no study that directly evaluated the effect of aspirin in reducing CVD in patients with HIV. Based on American College of Cardiology (ACC)/American Heart Association (AHA) guidelines in the general population, aspirin is not recommended in these patients for primary CVD prevention. The primary intervention starts with adherence to lifestyle changes with regular physical activity. A randomized trial on patients with HIV who are sedentary and are at high risk for CVD demonstrated standardized group sessions focusing on behavioral lifestyle modification and was successful in reducing body weight and carbohydrate consumption, although it did not increase physical activity and no consensus on diet in patients with HIV and adherence to ACC/AHA dietary guidelines is recommended.

SUGGESTED READINGS

Boccara F, Lang S, Meuleman C, et al. HIV and coronary heart disease: time for a better understanding. *J Am Coll Cardiol*. 2013;61(5):511-523.

Chastain DB, Stover KR, Riche DM. Evidence-based review of statin use in patients with HIV on antiretroviral therapy. *J Clin Transl Endocrinol*. 2017;8:6-14.

D'Ascenzo F, Cerrato E, Calcagno A, et al. High prevalence at computed coronary tomography of non-calcified plaques in asymptomatic HIV patients treated with HAART: a meta-analysis. *Atherosclerosis*. 2015;240(1):197-204.

Fitch KV, Lo J, Abbara S, et al. Increased coronary artery calcium score and noncalcified plaque among HIV-infected men: relationship to metabolic syndrome and cardiac risk parameters. *J Acquir Immune Defic Syndr*. 2010;55(4):495-499.

Freiberg MS, McGinnis K, Butt A, et al. HIV is associated with clinically confirmed *myocardial infarction* after adjustment for smoking and other risk factors. Program and Abstracts of the 18th Conference on Retroviruses and Opportunistic Infections; February 27-March 2, 2011; Boston, MA.

Garg H, Joshi A, Mukherjee D. Cardiovascular complications of HIV infection and treatment. *Cardiovasc Hematol Agents Med Chem*. 2013;11(1):58-66. PMID: 22946901.

Klein D, Leyden WA, Xu L, et al. Contribution of immunodeficiency to CHD: cohort study of HIV+ and HIV− Kaiser Permanente members. Program and Abstracts of the 18th Conference on Retroviruses and Opportunistic Infections; February 27-March 2, 2011; Boston, MA.

Kuller LH, Tracy R, Belloso W, et al. Inflammatory and coagulation biomarkers and mortality in patients with HIV infection. *PLoS Med*. 2008;5(10):e203.

Losina E, Hyle EP, Borre ED, et al. Projecting 10-year, 20-year, and lifetime risks of cardiovascular disease in persons living with human immunodeficiency virus in the United States. *Clin Infect Dis*. 2017;65(8):1266-1271.

O'Brien MP, Hunt PW, Kitch DW, et al. A randomized placebo controlled trial of aspirin effects on immune activation in chronically human immunodeficiency virus-infected adults on virologically suppressive antiretroviral therapy. *Open Forum Infect Dis*. 2017;4(1):ofw278.

Varriale P, Saravi G, Hernandez E, Carbon F. Acute myocardial infarction in patients infected with human immunodeficiency virus. *Am Heart J*. 2004;147(1):55-59.

Webel AR, Moore SM, Longenecker CT, et al. Randomized controlled trial of the system CHANGE intervention on behaviors related to cardiovascular risk in HIV+ adults. *J Acquir Immune Defic Syndr*. 2018;78(1):23-33.

DYSAUTONOMIA*

Atika Azhar and Robert L. Carhart

CHAPTER 28

QUESTIONS

28.1 Which of the following tests is used to evaluate the parasympathetic nervous system and carotid sinus baroreceptors?

   A. Transthoracic echocardiogram
   B. Valsalva maneuver
   C. Tilt-table test
   D. Carotid sinus massage (CSM)
   E. Heart rate variability

28.2 Which of the following tests is most commonly used to evaluate autonomic function in patients?

   A. Transthoracic echocardiogram
   B. Repeat computed tomography (CT) scan
   C. Heart rate variability
   D. CSM
   E. Valsalva maneuver

28.3 A 38-year-old man presents to the emergency department with a history of recurrent episodes of syncope. He reports experiencing transient loss of consciousness associated with diaphoresis, warmth, and nausea in situations that cause emotional stress. His symptoms are followed by fatigue. On examination, his blood pressure is 118/74 mm Hg, and heart rate is 62 beats per minute (bpm). Which of the following is the most appropriate initial management for this patient's condition?

   A. Lifestyle modifications and avoidance of triggers
   B. Tilt-table test
   C. Metoprolol therapy
   D. Midodrine therapy
   E. Dual-chamber pacing

28.4 A 29-year-old woman presents to the clinic with a history of recurrent episodes of lightheadedness and palpitations upon standing. She reports a significant increase in heart rate (>30 bpm) within 30 seconds of assuming an upright position. The patient denies orthostatic hypotension. On examination, she has normal blood pressure in

---

Questions and Answers are based on Chapter 28: Dysautonomia by Salvatore Savona and Ralph Augostini in Cardiovascular Medicine and Surgery, *First Edition.*

both supine and standing positions. Which of the following is the most appropriate initial management for this patient's condition?

A. Nonpharmacologic lifestyle modifications
B. Skin biopsy for intraepidermal nerve fiber density
C. Water and salt intake optimization
D. Midodrine therapy
E. Propranolol therapy

28.5 A 67-year-old man presents to the clinic with a chief complaint of dizziness and frequent falls. He also reports constipation and urinary dysfunction. On examination, he has orthostatic hypotension along with signs of neurogenic dysfunction. Which of the following tests would be most useful in differentiating multiple system atrophy (MSA) from other synucleinopathies in this patient?

A. Cardiac iodine-131-meta-iodobenzylguanidine (MIBG) scintigraphy
B. Quantitative sudomotor axon reflex test (QSART)
C. Thermoregulatory sweat test (TST)
D. Levodopa challenge test
E. Pedunculopontine nucleus stimulation

28.6 A 42-year-old man presents to the clinic with complaints of palpitations and occasional lightheadedness. His symptoms are more pronounced after meals and during rest. Electrocardiogram (ECG) reveals atrial fibrillation. On further evaluation, his episodes of atrial fibrillation are preceded by sinus bradycardia and lower heart rates. Which of the following interventions may be considered for the management of his atrial fibrillation?

A. Beta-blockers
B. Vagal nerve stimulation
C. Ganglion plexus ablation
D. Renal sympathetic denervation
E. Surgical left cardiac sympathetic denervation

28.7 A 65-year-old man with a history of heart failure presents to the clinic with complaints of excessive daytime sleepiness and witnessed episodes of cessation of breathing during sleep. Last echocardiogram 2 months ago revealed a left ventricular ejection fraction of 30%. His cardiac symptoms have been worsening and he has worsening bilateral lower extremity edema. Which of the following interventions is contraindicated in the management of his sleep apnea?

A. Adaptive servoventilation (ASV)
B. Transvenous phrenic nerve stimulation
C. Neurostimulation of the vagal nerve
D. Valsalva maneuver

28.8 A 40-year-old woman presents to the clinic with complaints of dizziness, tachycardia, palpitations, and syncope. She is a cancer survivor and has received treatment with vinca alkaloids, alkylating agents, and radiation therapy to the thorax and neck. Which of the following should be performed to evaluate for autonomic dysfunction in this patient?

A. Heart rate deep breathing test
B. ECG
C. Complete blood count (CBC)
D. Liver function tests
E. Chest x-ray

ANSWERS

28.1 The correct answer is D.
Rationale: CSM is a diagnostic test used to evaluate the parasympathetic nervous system and carotid sinus baroreceptors. During CSM, unilateral compression of the carotid sinus is performed for 20 to 30 seconds, followed by releasing compression and repeating the procedure on the contralateral carotid sinus. The diagnosis of carotid sinus hypersensitivity can be made on the basis of the occurrence of asystole for more than 3 seconds, atrioventricular block, a significant drop in systolic blood pressure (≥ 50 mm Hg) indicating a vasodepressor response, or a mixed cardioinhibitory or vasodepressor response. CSM can also help determine the level of atrioventricular block in cases of second-degree atrioventricular block.

28.2 The correct answer is C.
Rationale: Heart rate variability is the most commonly used test to evaluate autonomic function. It measures beat-to-beat variation in the heart rate or the R-R interval on the ECG. Standardized breathing techniques are used to assess heart rate variability, and the changes are compared to standardized data accounting for age and gender. Heart rate variability is diminished in conditions such as parasympathetic dysfunction (eg, Parkinson disease [PD]) and cardiac disease states with sympathetic overdrive (eg, congestive heart failure). Transthoracic echocardiogram, repeat CT scan, and CSM are not directly related to evaluating heart rate variability and autonomic function. The Valsalva maneuver assesses both sympathetic and parasympathetic responses of the baroreflex but is not specifically used to evaluate heart rate variability.

28.3 The correct answer is A.
Rationale: This patient's clinical presentation is consistent with vasovagal syncope, which is characterized by a transient loss of consciousness associated with emotional stress, diaphoresis, and relative bradycardia. The initial management of vasovagal syncope includes conservative measures such as lifestyle modifications and avoidance of triggers. These measures may involve increasing salt/fluid intake and using counterpressure maneuvers or compression stockings. Recognition of prodromal symptoms and positioning the patient to a lying down position with legs elevated can also be beneficial. Medical therapy with beta-blockers, such as metoprolol, may be

considered in patients with more frequent or intolerable symptoms, particularly in those older than 40 years. Atenolol, however, should be avoided as it has been found to be no better than placebo. Midodrine therapy may be utilized in certain cases, but there is limited evidence supporting its use in this population. Dual-chamber pacing has shown benefit in patients older than 40 years with frequent severe symptoms and specific electrocardiographic criteria. It should be considered in patients who experience syncope accompanied by 3 seconds or more of asystole with syncope or 6 seconds or more of asystole without symptoms.

28.4 The correct answer is A.

Rationale: This patient's clinical presentation is suggestive of postural orthostatic tachycardia syndrome (POTS), characterized by symptoms of lightheadedness and palpitations upon standing, along with an increase in heart rate of 30 bpm or more within 30 seconds of assuming an upright position. The initial management of POTS involves nonpharmacologic lifestyle modifications. These include nonupright exercise, psychological treatment, and recreational therapy. Adequate hydration with a daily intake of 2 to 3 L of water and 10 to 12 g/day of salt is recommended. These measures help optimize blood volume and reduce symptoms. Pharmacologic therapy may be considered in refractory cases or for symptom control. Midodrine, an alpha-1 agonist that increases venous return, can be used during the daytime to alleviate symptoms. Propranolol, a beta-blocker, in low doses (10-20 mg orally) can be used to reduce tachycardia during standing. Skin biopsy for intraepidermal nerve fiber density may be utilized in certain cases to differentiate neuropathic POTS from non-neuropathic POTS, as it has implications for symptom severity and treatment approaches. However, it is not the initial step in management. Invasive therapies are not currently recommended for the treatment of POTS.

28.5 The correct answer is A.

Rationale: This patient's clinical presentation, including orthostatic hypotension, neurogenic dysfunction, and signs of autonomic failure, is consistent with a synucleinopathy, which is a spectrum of disorders including MSA, PD, dementia with Lewy bodies (LBD), and pure autonomic failure (PAF). Cardiac MIBG scintigraphy has been shown to be helpful in differentiating MSA from other synucleinopathies. The test evaluates cardiac autonomic impairment, especially in male patients with PD, and can provide insights into the underlying pathology. In patients with MSA, cardiac MIBG scintigraphy results are typically normal, while patients with PD, LBD, and PAF may show abnormalities. QSART measures sweat gland function and can help assess autonomic function, but it does not specifically differentiate MSA from other synucleinopathies. TST assesses sweat production and can be abnormal in MSA, but it is not specific to differentiating MSA from other synucleinopathies. Levodopa challenge test is used to evaluate motor symptoms in PD but does not have a primary role in differentiating synucleinopathies. Pedunculopontine nucleus stimulation has shown benefits in gait disorders associated with PD but is not directly related to differentiating MSA from other synucleinopathies.

28.6 The correct answer is C.

Rationale: This patient's clinical presentation is consistent with vagal-mediated atrial fibrillation, which occurs primarily in younger patients without structural heart disease. It is initiated during activities with higher vagal tone, such as after eating or during rest, and tends to recover with increased sympathetic tone. Vagal-mediated atrial fibrillation may be observed with esophageal stimulation or intake of cold beverages or large food boluses. The episodes are often preceded by sinus bradycardia and lower heart rates during atrial fibrillation. In the management of atrial fibrillation, autonomic nervous system modifications have been suggested, including ganglion plexus ablation. Ganglion plexus ablation aims to modify the autonomic influence on the heart by interrupting the ganglionated plexi located around the pulmonary veins. This procedure can help reduce excessive sympathetic and parasympathetic activity, thereby assisting in the management of atrial fibrillation. Beta-blockers, such as choice A, are commonly used to reduce sympathetic tone and assist in rate control in atrial fibrillation. Vagal nerve stimulation (choice B) is not a standard intervention for the management of atrial fibrillation. Renal sympathetic denervation (choice D) and surgical left cardiac sympathetic denervation (choice E) have been utilized in the management of refractory ventricular arrhythmias but are not specifically indicated for atrial fibrillation.

28.7 The correct answer is B:

Rationale: This patient with heart failure and central sleep apnea should not receive ASV as it has been associated with increased cardiac mortality despite improvements in the apnea-hypopnea index (AHI). Central sleep apnea in heart failure represents more advanced heart failure and is characterized by elevated cardiac sympathetic nerve activity, impaired heart rate variability, and an increased risk of nonsustained ventricular tachycardia. While positive airway pressure ventilation with continuous positive airway pressure (CPAP) is commonly used in obstructive sleep apnea, improvement in sleep apnea in patients with heart failure may be due to mixed central and obstructive sleep apnea. Transvenous phrenic nerve stimulation (choice C) has shown significant improvements in AHI, rapid eye movement sleep, and reduction of hypoxia during sleep in this population. Neurostimulation of the vagal nerve (choice D) has been evaluated in patients with heart failure, although its efficacy in improving left ventricular function is not consistent. The Valsalva maneuver (choice E) is generally avoided in patients with pulmonary arterial hypertension due to concerns about hemodynamic changes and autonomic dysfunction.

28.8 The correct answer is A:

Rationale: This patient, as a cancer survivor who has received treatments associated with causing autonomic dysfunction, should undergo comprehensive autonomic testing to evaluate for the presence of autonomic dysfunction. Common symptoms include dizziness, tachycardia, palpitations, and syncope. The heart rate deep breathing test is a component of comprehensive autonomic testing and is used to assess heart rate variability and autonomic function. Other tests may include the Valsalva maneuver, tilt-table test, and sudomotor testing. Recent research indicates that a high percentage of cancer survivors treated with certain chemotherapeutic agents and radiation therapy develop autonomic dysfunction, most commonly orthostatic hypotension, inappropriate sinus tachycardia, and POTS. Therefore, there should be a low threshold for evaluating cancer survivors presenting with autonomic symptoms to provide appropriate therapy.

ENVIRONMENTAL EXPOSURES AND CARDIOVASCULAR DISEASE*

CHAPTER 29

Nathan Centybear and Mohamed Khalid Munshi

QUESTIONS

29.1 A 30-year-old man develops dizziness and nausea 30 minutes after eating honey he bought from an online store. In the emergency room (ER), he is found to have hypotension, bradycardia, and heart block. This honey may have contained nectar from:

A. Areca palm
B. Rhododendron
C. Pink oleander
D. Aconitum

29.2 A man who lives in a city with high levels of smog wishes to reduce his cardiovascular (CV) risk from air pollutants by purchasing an air purifier. He should purchase one with a filter that removes particulate matter (PM) of what size?

A. PM 2.5
B. PM 5
C. PM 10
D. PM 20

29.3 A South Asian male is brought to the hospital with abdominal pain, vomiting, and bradycardia after having ingested pink oleander seeds. Treatment may include all of the following **EXCEPT**:

A. Activated charcoal
B. Antidigoxin fab
C. Temporary pacing
D. Hemodialysis

29.4 A 30-year-old female with no significant past medical history is brought to the emergency department with paresthesias, weakness, and vomiting. In the ER, she is found to be hypotensive, and ventricular arrhythmias are apparent on telemetry. Prior to symptom onset, she had taken a Chinese herbal supplement. Aconite poisoning is suspected. What primary mechanism is likely responsible for her ventricular arrhythmias?

A. Vasospasm-induced ischemia
B. Inhibition of sodium/potassium-adenosine triphosphatase (ATPase)
C. Inhibition of voltage-gated sodium and potassium channels
D. Activation of voltage-gated sodium and calcium channels

*Questions and Answers are based on Chapter 29: Environmental Exposures and Cardiovascular Disease by Ahmed Ibrahim and Richard A. Lange in Cardiovascular Medicine and Surgery, First Edition.

29.5 Researchers are investigating the unusually high incidence of cancer, cardiovascular disease (CVD), and diabetes in a population living on a Native American reservation. They found that in young inhabitants without CVD, there is also an elevated incidence of left ventricular hypertrophy. The researchers suspect that these findings are related to a contaminant in the drinking water. Which water contaminant is likely to be suspected?

   A. Cobalt
   B. Arsenic
   C. Organophosphates
   D. Chromium

29.6 You are seeing a patient in the office with a past medical history of rheumatoid arthritis. He tells you that he is receiving gold therapy for his arthritis. In counseling the patient about CV risks of gold therapy, you tell him it is associated with which of the following?

   A. Congestive heart failure
   B. Myocardial infarction (MI)
   C. Ventricular arrhythmias
   D. All of the above

29.7 Which of the following is **NOT** a potential risk for CVD with ingestion or exposure?

   A. Cadmium
   B. Chromium
   C. Copper
   D. Antimony

29.8 All of the following contain cardiac glycosides as active compounds **EXCEPT**:

   A. Foxglove
   B. Henbane
   C. Lily of the valley
   D. Squill

29.9 A teenager is brought to the ER with vomiting and headache after ingesting a skin lotion as part of a social media challenge. The type of skin lotion is unknown, but it is described as having a pleasant smell. He is noted to be tachycardic and an electrocardiogram (ECG) is ordered, which shows prolonged QRS and QTc intervals. Which of the following is **MOST LIKELY** to be an ingredient of the skin lotion?

   A. Dettol
   B. Yohimbe
   C. Camphor
   D. Limonene

29.10 Pyrethroid insecticides exhibit acute CV toxic effects through which mechanism?

   A. Inhibition of voltage-gated sodium and chloride channels
   B. Inhibition of acetylcholinesterase
   C. Inhibition of voltage-gated sodium and potassium channels
   D. Activation of voltage-gated sodium channels

ANSWERS

29.1 The correct answer is B.
Rationale: "Mad honey" contains nectar from the rhododendron flower. Grayanotoxin is a natural compound found in the leaves of various rhododendron species and in the honey derived from the nectar of this plant ("mad honey"). Mad honey has been used as an herbal medicine for the treatment of diabetes, gastrointestinal disorders, heart disease, hypertension, and sexual dysfunction; such usage has contributed to episodes of accidental poisoning. The rhododendrons associated with mad honey are found in the Black Sea region of Eastern Turkey as well as in North America. Grayanotoxin binds with the voltage-dependent sodium channels in their active state, thereby preventing inactivation; the channels remain in the state of depolarization. This effect on the vagus nerve leads to an increased parasympathetic tone, resulting in bradycardia, hypotension, and various degrees of atrioventricular (AV) block. Atrial fibrillation, asystole, and MI have also been observed. The most common side effects appear to be dizziness, nausea, presyncope, and ECG findings consisting of sinus bradycardia, AV block, ST elevation, and nodal rhythm.

29.2 The correct answer is A.
Rationale: PM less than 2.5 μm in diameter induces systemic inflammation through penetration of the pulmonary interstitium and is linked to premature CV death. The World Health Organization estimated that 58% of outdoor air pollution–related premature deaths were due to ischemic heart disease and stroke. A Japanese study showed an independent association between the increase in daily PM 2.5 concentration, even at lower levels and regulation-recommended standards and guidelines, and out-of-hospital cardiac arrest, especially in older individuals.

29.3 The correct answer is D.
Rationale: Cardenolides are naturally occurring cardiac glycosides found in plant species throughout the world. There are CV toxicity results from innovation of the Na+/K+ ATPase channel. Ingestion of cardenolides may lead to serious dysrhythmias including second- or third-degree heart block and cardiac arrest. Hemodialysis is ineffective because of the large volume of distribution of the toxin. The other choices may all be used in the treatment of cardenolide poisoning. Prolonged hospitalization is recommended after ingestion as dangerous dysrhythmias may be delayed up to 72 hours after ingestion. Patients who develop bradycardia arrhythmias may be medicated with atropine and isoprenaline or require a temporary pacemaker. Hemodialysis or hemoperfusion is ineffective in preventing toxicity because of the large volume of distribution of the toxin. In South Asia, cardenolide poisoning from pink, yellow, or white oleander is a leading cause of attempted suicide.

29.4 The correct answer is D.
Rationale: Aconite causes persistent activation of voltage-gated sodium and calcium channels. Because of the persistent activation of sodium channels, class I antiarrhythmic agents have been used to treat aconite-induced ventricular arrhythmias. Option B is the mechanism of action for digoxin.

29.5 The correct answer is B.
Rationale: The adverse health findings in this population are most consistent with arsenic poisoning. Arsenic has been found in high levels in drinking water on Native American reservations, which can be naturally occurring or a contaminant from mining and industrial operations. Arsenic is a contaminant of high concern because of its toxicity and probability of human exposure. Cobalt ingestion can cause a dilated cardiomyopathy that is reversible with normalization of cobalt levels. Organophosphates are used in pesticides and cause an acute hypercholinergic state. Chromium is a micronutrient that improves insulin sensitivity and reduces CV risk.

29.6 The correct answer is B.
Rationale: Gold therapy for rheumatoid arthritis has been associated with congestive heart failure (CHF), MI, and ventricular arrhythmias. In addition, gold-coated stents have been associated with allergic in-stent restenosis and thrombosis.

29.7 The correct answer is B.
Rationale: Chromium is a trace mineral that enhances glucose and lipid metabolism, thereby reducing CV risk. All other choices are associated with an increased CV risk when accumulated inside the body.

29.8 The correct answer is B.
Rationale: The active compounds in henbane are tropane alkaloids—atropine and scopolamine. All other choices contain cardiac glycosides (**Table 29.1**).

29.9 The correct answer is C.
Rationale: Camphor is a pleasant-smelling terpene used in skin lotions and in many Ayurvedic medicines intended for oral use as a termination agent/contraceptive, analgesic, antipruritic, antiseptic, and aphrodisiac. Ingestion of 2 g is enough to produce a toxic effect in adults. CV toxicities include tachycardia, prolonged QTc and QRS, AV conduction block, ST-segment changes, and myocarditis. Treatment is largely supportive and hemodialysis has not been shown to be of benefit. Dettol is a household disinfectant; hypotension and tachycardia and bradycardia arrhythmias have been described with Dettol poisoning. Yohimbe is an herbal supplement that can cause hypertension and tachycardia. Limonene, like camphor, is a pleasant-smelling terpene but is used in the food industry and does not have the toxic effects of camphor.

29.10 The correct answer is A.
Rationale: Pyrethroid insecticides inhibit voltage-gated sodium channels and chloride channels leading to sinus tachycardia, sinus arrest, and cardiomyopathy.

TABLE 29.1 Reported Cases of Heart Toxicity Related to Herbal Plant Consumption

Common Name	Scientific Name	Active Compounds	Uses	Side Effects (Cardiac)
Foxglove	*Digitalis lanata* / *Digitalis purpurea*	Cardiac glycosides	Congestive heart failure	Tachycardia, bradyarrhythmia, ventricular fibrillation, and death
Henbane	*Hyoscyamus niger*	Tropane alkaloids—atropine (hyoscyamine) and scopolamine (hyoscine)	Herbal therapy in most traditional medicines, stomach complaints, toothaches, ulcers, and tumors	Tachycardia, arrhythmia
Jin Bu Huan	*Lycopodium serratum*	*Levo*-tetrahydropalmatine; pyrrolizidine alkaloids	Traditional Chinese medicine used as a sedative, analgesic, and indigestion aid	Life-threatening bradycardia
Lily of the valley	*Convallaria majalis*	Cardiac glycosides	Arrhythmia, cardiac insufficiency, and "nervous heart" complaints	Arrhythmia, cardiac shock
Squill	*Urginea maritima*	Cardiac glycosides	Cardiac insufficiency, arrhythmia, "nervous heart" complaints; also bronchitis, asthma, whooping cough, and wounds	Arrhythmias, atrioventricular block, death
Yohimbe	*Pausinystalia yohimbe*	Yohimbine alkaloid	Erectile dysfunction and sports enhancement	Hypertension, tachycardia

AMYLOID CARDIOMYOPATHY

Ciril Khorolsky and Edward F. Philbin III

CHAPTER 30

QUESTIONS

30.1 A 71-year-old African American male presents to the cardiology clinic for evaluation of chest discomfort, dyspnea on exertion, and worsening fatigue over the past 2 months. On further questioning, the patient also reports numbness in his extremities, easy bruising, and postural lightheadedness. He has a history of hypertension, hyperlipidemia, and type 2 diabetes mellitus. Physical examination is notable for blood pressure of 127/71 mm Hg, heart rate of 86 beats per minute, elevated jugular venous pressure, and mild bruising around both eyes. An electrocardiogram (ECG) demonstrates normal sinus rhythm with a first-degree atrioventricular block and low voltage in the limb leads. Which of the following echocardiographic findings would one expect in this patient?

   A. Large pericardial effusion with right ventricular (RV) diastolic collapse
   B. Left ventricular hypertrophy (LVH)
   C. Normal diastolic function
   D. Apical sparing on longitudinal strain imaging
   E. Both B and D are correct.

30.2 All of the following statements regarding amyloid cardiomyopathy are **TRUE EXCEPT**:

   A. Light chain amyloidosis (AL) is more common in males, whereas transthyretin amyloidosis (ATTR) is more common in females.
   B. In AL, immunoglobulin light chains are secreted by monoclonal plasma cells in the bone marrow.
   C. In ATTR, the tetrameric transthyretin protein, primarily synthesized in the liver, dissociates and misassembles, resulting in amyloid fibrils that deposit in tissue.
   D. In both AL and ATTR, most patients are diagnosed after the age of 60.
   E. Among African Americans, 3% to 4% are estimated to carry a mutation that predisposes them to amyloidosis.

30.3 Which of the following statements regarding the clinical findings in cardiac amyloidosis is **TRUE**?

   A. Periorbital purpura is a pathognomonic sign in ATTR.
   B. Patients with cardiac amyloidosis rarely develop a significant reduction in peak stress myocardial blood flow.
   C. Atrial fibrillation rarely occurs in patients with amyloid cardiomyopathy.
   D. Troponin can be chronically mildly elevated in later stages of the disease.

Questions and Answers are based on Chapter 30: Amyloid Cardiomyopathy by Courtney M. Campbell, Rami Kahwash, and Ajay Vallakati in Cardiovascular Medicine and Surgery, First Edition.

CHAPTER 30 | Amyloid Cardiomyopathy

30.4 All of the following statements regarding autonomic dysfunction in patients with amyloidosis are **TRUE EXCEPT**:
A. Patients often present with profound hypotension and orthostatic symptoms such as syncope.
B. Orthostatic hypotension is a rare manifestation of autonomic neuropathy.
C. If a patient has underlying diabetes, the degree of neuropathy is often out of proportion and more rapidly progressive than otherwise anticipated.
D. Midodrine is frontline therapy for hypotension caused by autonomic dysfunction.

30.5 A 69-year-old male with suspected amyloid cardiomyopathy presents to the cardiology clinic for evaluation of fatigue, intermittent palpitations, and worsening dyspnea over the past month. He was recently diagnosed with paroxysmal atrial fibrillation (A-fib). Physical examination is notable for blood pressure of 135/70 mm Hg, heart rate of 86 bpm, elevated jugular venous pressure, and peripheral edema. ECG shows rate-controlled A-fib and a transthoracic echocardiogram performed in the office demonstrates left ventricular ejection fraction (LVEF) greater than 55%, LVH, and grade III diastolic dysfunction. Which of the following would be the most appropriate next step in the diagnostic evaluation of this patient?
A. Fat pad biopsy
B. Cardiac magnetic resonance imaging (MRI)
C. Serum free light chain quantification and both serum protein electrophoresis and immunofixation (SPEI) and urine protein electrophoresis and immunofixation (UPEI)
D. Nuclear technetium-99m pyrophosphate (PYP) scan

30.6 A 73-year-old male with suspected amyloid cardiomyopathy presents to the cardiology clinic with a 1-month history of dyspnea and fatigue. His vitals are stable and physical examination is unremarkable. A transthoracic echocardiogram shows LVH with a small pericardial effusion. Laboratory evaluation reveals B-type natriuretic peptide (BNP) of 192 (0.0-100.0 pg/mL) and a kappa-lambda ratio of 1.2 without paraproteinemia. You refer the patient for a PYP scan with single-photon emission computed tomography (SPECT) imaging. Which of the following statements regarding the PYP scan and diagnosis of ATTR is **TRUE**?
A. Heart/contralateral (H:CL) ratio less than 1 is equivocal for ATTR.
B. H:CL ratio greater than 1.5 and/or a visual grade of 2 to 3 is classified as ATTR positive.
C. Patients taking hydroxychloroquine may have a false-negative PYP scan finding.
D. An acute or recent myocardial infarction would not interfere with the results of a PYP scan.
E. H:CL ratio less than 1 and/or a visual grade 0 is indicative of an uninterruptible scan.

30.7 All of the following statements regarding the treatment of AL amyloid cardiomyopathy are **TRUE EXCEPT**:
   A. Treatment for AL is typically managed by hematologists.
   B. Treatment is aimed at suppression of light chain synthesis.
   C. Improvement in cardiac biomarkers is suggestive of good response to treatment.
   D. Liver transplantation is a viable treatment option in patients with poor response to chemotherapy and normal left ventricular (LV) systolic function.

30.8 A 68-year-old male with recently diagnosed ATTR cardiomyopathy presents to the cardiology clinic for postdischarge follow-up after he was briefly hospitalized for mildly decompensated heart failure 5 days ago. He was started on diuretics and reports feeling much better. His vitals are stable and there is no evidence of hypervolemia on examination. His most recent transthoracic echocardiogram demonstrated an LVEF greater than 55%, biventricular concentric hypertrophy, and grade II diastolic dysfunction. Which of the following would be the most appropriate treatment?
   A. Start patisiran (transthyretin RNA silencer therapy).
   B. Refer the patient for autologous stem cell transplant.
   C. Initiate a beta-blocker and angiotensin receptor/neprilysin inhibitor.
   D. Refer the patient for a heart transplant.
   E. Start tafamidis (transthyretin stabilizer therapy).

30.9 A 77-year-old male with recently diagnosed ATTR cardiomyopathy presents to the emergency room for worsening dyspnea and palpitations over the past 2 days. Physical examination is notable for blood pressure of 91/70 mm Hg, heart rate of 131 bpm, and bibasilar crackles. ECG demonstrates A-fib with rapid ventricular response (RVR). Which of the following statements regarding A-fib and amyloid cardiomyopathy is **TRUE**?
   A. A-fib is usually well tolerated in patients with amyloid cardiomyopathy.
   B. Digoxin is usually safe and effective in patients with amyloid cardiomyopathy.
   C. Patients with amyloid cardiomyopathy are more likely to develop intracardiac thrombus compared to other patient groups with atrial fibrillation.
   D. If considering cardioversion for A-fib in a patient with amyloidosis, a transesophageal echocardiogram should always be done to rule out left atrial thrombus regardless of anticoagulation status.

30.10 All of the following statements regarding the prognosis of amyloidosis are **TRUE EXCEPT**:
   A. Untreated amyloidosis has a very poor prognosis.
   B. Mortality is most directly correlated to the degree of cardiac involvement.
   C. The median survival of AL is 6 months when heart failure symptoms are present.
   D. The median survival of ATTR with significant cardiac involvement is less than 3 months.

CHAPTER 30 | Amyloid Cardiomyopathy

ANSWERS

30.1 The correct answer is E.

Rationale: This clinical case is most consistent with amyloid cardiomyopathy as evidenced by his symptoms, physical examination findings, and ECG findings. The echocardiogram is usually the initial imaging test ordered and may be normal in the very early stages of the disease. However, as the disease progresses, the heart develops concentric remodeling with LVH. Over time, the walls become thicker and the patient develops diastolic dysfunction. On longitudinal strain imaging, apical sparing can be present ("cherry red spot"). Next, the patient develops an infiltrative phenotype with biventricular concentric hypertrophy, valve thickening, interatrial septal thickening, and pericardial effusion. The pericardial effusion, if present, is usually not large in size and unlikely to progress to tamponade. Severe diastolic dysfunction with restrictive physiology ensues. Eventually, the patient develops systolic dysfunction with a nondilated left ventricle (**Figure 30.1**).

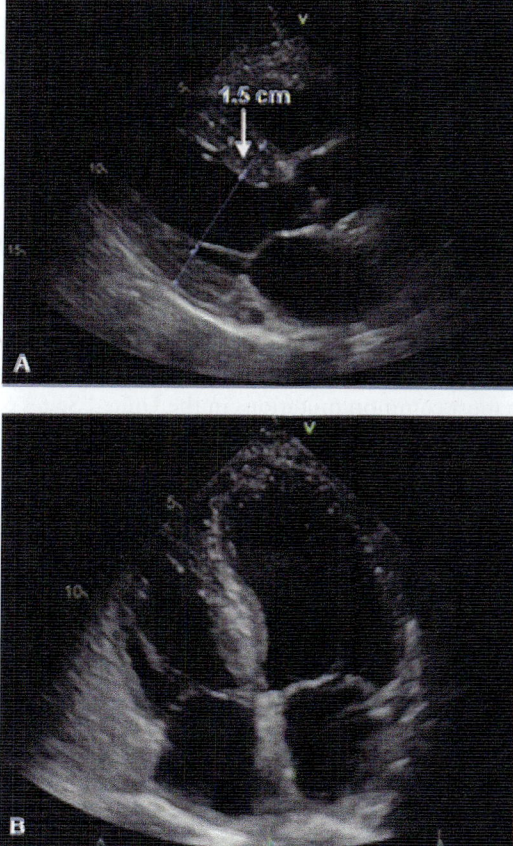

Figure 30.1 Transthoracic echocardiogram red flags in late amyloid cardiomyopathy. **A:** Parasternal long-axis view demonstrating thick right ventricular walls, thick left ventricular walls (1.5 cm), and granular sparkling appearance of the myocardium. **B:** Four-chamber view demonstrating thick mitral and tricuspid valves and thick interatrial septum. Pericardial effusion, another red flag, is not seen in this example.

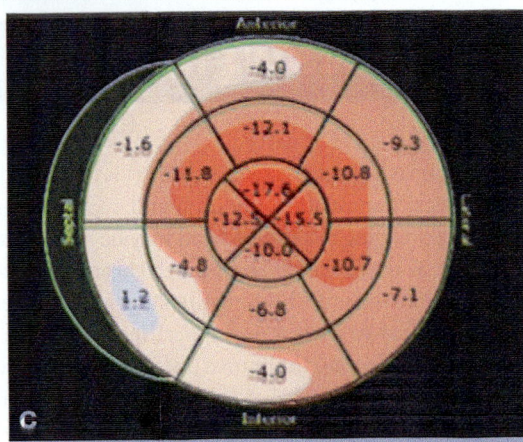

Figure 30.1 (*continued*) **C:** Global longitudinal strain demonstrating apical sparing, also known as "cherry on top" sign.

30.2 The correct answer is A:

Rationale: Amyloidosis occurs when proteins do not "fold" correctly and form amyloid fibrils, and then deposit in the body resulting in organ dysfunction. Two proteins are primarily responsible for amyloid cardiomyopathy: immunoglobulin light chains and transthyretin. Amyloid deposition of these proteins results in AL and ATTR, which is further unclassified to wild type (ATTRwt) or an inherited form (ATTRv) caused by pathogenic variants in the transthyretin gene. In AL, clonal immunoglobulin light chains are secreted by aberrant monoclonal plasma cells or B-cell dyscrasia from the bone marrow. In ATTR, however, the tetrameric transthyretin protein, primarily synthesized in the liver, dissociates and misassembles, resulting in amyloid fibrils that deposit in tissue. Both AL and ATTR are more common in men, with the majority of patients being older than 60 at the time of diagnosis. ATTRv is an inherited autosomal dominant disease and affects an estimated 50,000 people worldwide. The most common mutations in the United States occur in 3% to 4% of African Americans, which predisposes them to develop amyloidosis.

30.3 The correct answer is B:

Rationale: Troponin and N-terminal pro–B-type natriuretic peptide (NT-proBNP) are useful biomarkers in amyloid cardiomyopathy. In early stages, results of both tests are normal. As diastolic dysfunction develops, the NT-proBNP elevates commensurate with heart failure with preserved ejection fraction (EF). In later stages of the disease, the troponin can be persistently, mildly elevated with little change on repeat testing. Periorbital purpura is a pathognomonic sign in AL, not in ATTR. Almost all patients with cardiac amyloidosis (>95%) had significantly reduced peak stress myocardial blood flow (<1.3 mL/g/min). Atrial fibrillation is common in amyloid cardiomyopathy and can present in early or late stages of the disease.

30.4 The correct answer is B:

Rationale: When the autonomic nervous system is affected by amyloid deposition, patients often present with profound orthostatic hypotension and symptoms including dizziness and syncope. Nonpharmacotherapy approaches such as compression stockings, positional/physical therapy adjustments, and good hydration are important.

If a patient has diastolic heart failure, then volume balance is particularly difficult to maintain. Treatment requires close communication between physician and patient. For pharmacologic therapy of autonomic dysfunction, midodrine is the treatment of choice, titrated to the patient's needs. Direct treatment of underlying amyloidosis can mitigate and even improve autonomic dysfunction over the course of months to years. Patients with AL receiving effective light chain suppression treatment and those with ATTRv on RNA silencers can sometimes reduce or discontinue midodrine therapy.

30.5 The correct answer is C.

Rationale: In all suspected cases of amyloidosis, AL must be ruled out first before consideration of ATTR. This is because once cardiomyopathy develops in AL, the median survival is 6 months if left untreated. For AL, initial laboratory tests of choice are serum free light chain quantification, SPEI, and UPEI. In general, a kappa-lambda ratio greater than 1.7 with evidence of a monoclonal protein on SPEI or UPEI is indicative of AL. However, in the absence of monoclonal protein, a kappa-lambda ratio of up to 2.5 can be considered normal. Tissue diagnosis with either a fat pad biopsy or bone marrow biopsy is the final diagnostic step if the laboratory and clinical findings are consistent with AL. PYP scan should be obtained only after AL is ruled out. Cardiac MRI can be useful to detect the presence of cardiac amyloidosis or to evaluate for a different infiltrative process; however, it cannot differentiate between AL and ATTR and would not be appropriate as the initial test prior to lab analysis (**Figure 30.2**).

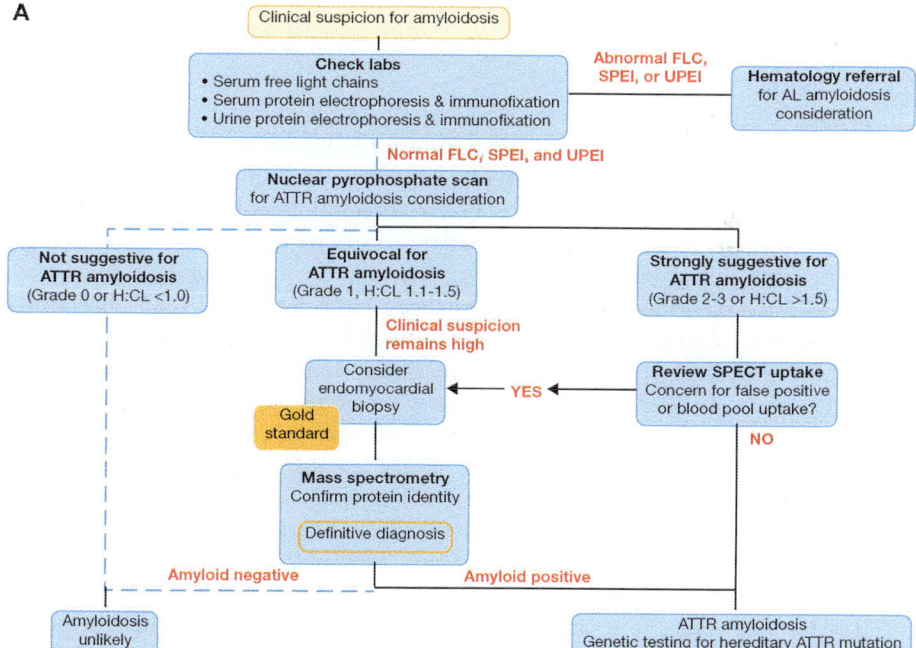

Figure 30.2 A and B: Diagnostic algorithm for evaluation of suspected cardiac amyloidosis. AL, light chain amyloidosis; ATTR, transthyretin amyloidosis; FLC, free light chain; H:CL, heart to contralateral lung; MGUS, monoclonal gammopathy of uncertain significance; SPECT, single-photon emission computed tomography SPEI, serum protein electrophoresis and immunofixation; UPEI, urine protein electrophoresis and immunofixation.

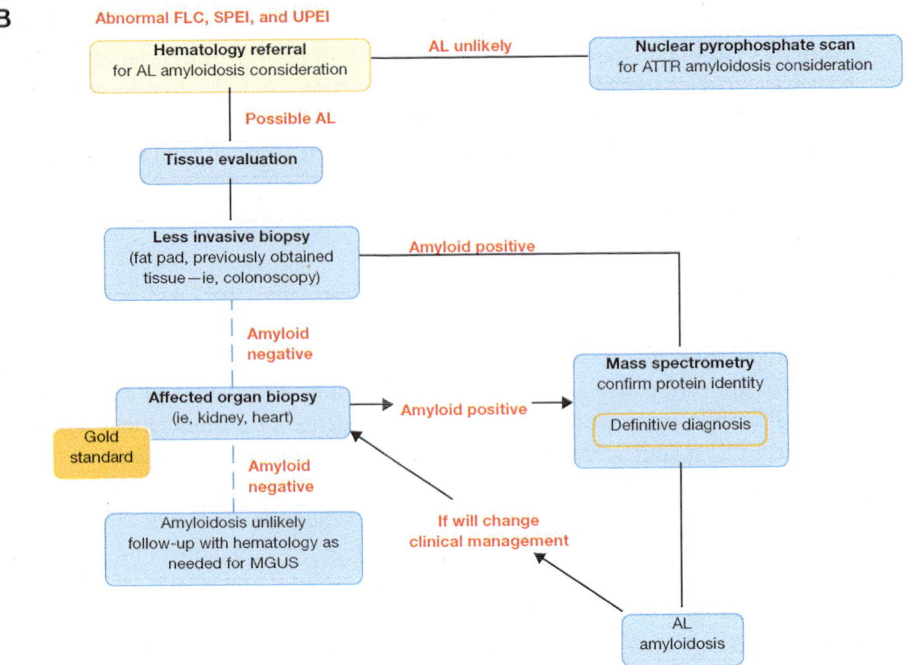

Figure 30.2 (continued)

30.6 The correct answer is B.

Rationale: Once AL is ruled out, screening for ATTR can be done with a PYP scan preferably in combination with SPECT imaging. Planar imaging is graded with a quantitative score at 1 hour and semiquantitative score at 3 hours. First, the cardiac uptake pattern is categorized as absent, focal, diffuse, or focal on diffuse. Then, planar imaging is used to calculate the H:CL ratio by comparing the mean counts in the respective regions of interest in the heart to the mean counts in contralateral bone (ie, the ribs) and is interpreted as follows: H:CL less than 1 is not suggestive of ATTR, H:CL 1 to 1.5 is equivocal for ATTR, and H:CL greater than 1.5 is strongly suggestive of ATTR. Then, at 3 hours, a planar and/or SPECT visual score is reported on the basis of the comparison between cardiac uptake and rib uptake on a scale of 0 to 3, which is interpreted as follows—Grade 0: Absent cardiac uptake is not suggestive of ATTR. Grade 1: Cardiac uptake less than rib uptake is equivocal for ATTR. Grade 2: Cardiac uptake equal to rib uptake is strongly suggestive of ATTR. Grade 3: Cardiac uptake greater than rib uptake is strongly suggestive of ATTR. Overall, an H:CL ratio greater than 1.5 at 1 hour and/or a visual grade of 2 to 3 is classified as ATTR positive, whereas an H:CL ratio less than 1 and/or a visual grade 0 is classified as ATTR negative. Certain clinical scenarios can generate false-positive or equivocal results. Positive planar uptake (grades 2-3) in the absence of SPECT uptake (grade 0) indicates blood pool and should be considered a nondiagnostic test. Patients taking hydroxychloroquine may have a false-positive PYP scan result. Focal uptake in the rib may represent a rib fracture and, in the heart, a recent myocardial infarction.

30.7 The correct answer is D.

Rationale: Treatment for AL is typically managed by hematologists with therapy aimed at suppression of light chain synthesis. Response to treatment is monitored by analysis of serum free light chains. Improvement in cardiac biomarkers of troponin and NT-proBNP can also signal good response. The first-line therapy includes a combination of steroids, alkylators, and proteasome inhibitors. The most common regimen is dexamethasone, cyclophosphamide, and bortezomib (aka CyBorD) infused on a monthly basis with hematologic response rates ranging from 60% to 94%. Liver transplantation is a possible treatment option in ATTR (abnormal protein is synthesized in the liver) but has no role in the treatment of AL (abnormal protein, ie, clonal immunoglobulin light chains are secreted by aberrant monoclonal plasma cells or B-cell dyscrasia from the bone marrow).

30.8 The correct answer is E.

Rationale: This patient would benefit most from initiation of tafamidis. It works by stabilizing the transthyretin tetramer, preventing dissociation and misfolding of the monomer units into amyloid fibrils. Tafamidis is U.S. Food and Drug Administration (FDA) approved for the treatment of both ATTRwt and ATTRv cardiomyopathy. In a randomized placebo-controlled trial (ATTR-ACT), patients with ATTR treated with tafamidis had lower all-cause mortality, fewer cardiovascular-related hospitalizations, and less decline in functional capacity/quality of life than placebo-treated patients. Improvements in biomarkers were noted starting at 9 months, and survival benefit was observed after 18 months. Patisiran is a small interfering RNA (siRNA) therapeutic agent that binds and promotes the degradation of transthyretin mRNA within the cytoplasm, stopping transthyretin protein production. However, it is currently only FDA approved for the treatment of hereditary amyloidosis polyneuropathy. The use of guideline-directed medical therapy (GDMT) is usually not well tolerated in patients with amyloid cardiomyopathy. It may be considered for patients with advanced amyloid cardiomyopathy with systolic dysfunction, if tolerated. Heart transplant could be considered in patients with refractory heart failure due to advanced cardiac amyloid deposition. Autologous stem cell transplant may be considered in patients with AL, not ATTR (**Table 30.1**).

30.9 The correct answer is C.

Rationale: Atrial fibrillation is common in amyloid cardiomyopathy, especially in the later stages of the disease. With underlying restrictive cardiomyopathy, atrial fibrillation is poorly tolerated and can lead to decompensated heart failure. Depending on the degree of cardiac involvement, beta-blockers may be poorly tolerated. Antiarrhythmics can be employed. Amiodarone is usually well tolerated in patients with amyloid cardiomyopathy. Digoxin has been considered contraindicated because of the potential for toxicity from its direct binding to amyloid fibrils. Multiple studies have demonstrated that patients with amyloid cardiomyopathy are more likely to develop an intracardiac thrombus than other patient groups with atrial fibrillation. All patients with amyloid cardiomyopathy

TABLE 30.1 Transthyretin Amyloidosis Therapy Details

Drug	Dose	Side Effects	Indication	Class	Status
Patisiran (Onpattro)	30 mg infused intravenously over 80 min every 3 wk	• Infusion reaction • Low serum vitamin A levels—supplement recommended	ATTRv neuropathy	RNA silencer	FDA approved
Inotersen (Tegsedi)	284 mg in 1.5 mL subcutaneous injection weekly	• Infusion reaction • Required monitoring for glomerulonephritis, thrombocytopenia	ATTRv neuropathy	RNA silencer	FDA approved
Tafamidis (Vyndaqel)	80 mg daily	• No significant effects seen in clinical trials	ATTR cardiomyopathy	Transthyretin stabilizer	FDA approved
Diflunisal	250 mg twice daily	• GI upset • Drowsiness • Dizziness	ATTR	Transthyretin stabilizer	Off-label; RCT supports use in ATTR neuropathy
Doxycycline	100 mg twice daily	• GI upset • Sun photosensitivity	AL or ATTR	Amyloid fibril inhibition	Off-label; ATTR phase II and observational studies
Ursodiol	250 mg up to 3 times daily	• GI upset • Dysuria • Itching	ATTR	Amyloid fibril inhibition	Off label; ATTR phase II
Green tea extract	1,200 mg daily—containing 600 mg EGCG	• Headache • GI upset • Dizziness	ATTRwt	Amyloid fibril inhibition	Off-label; single arm ATTRwt prospective study

AL, light chain amyloidosis; ATTR, transthyretin amyloidosis; ATTRv, transthyretin amyloidosis variant; ATTRwt, transthyretin amyloidosis wild type; EGCG, epigallocatechin gallate; FDA, U.S. Food and Drug Administration; GI, gastrointestinal; RCT, randomized controlled trial; RNA, ribonucleic acid.

with atrial fibrillation should be on long-term anticoagulation, regardless of their CHA_2DS_2-VASc score. If planning to perform a cardioversion for atrial fibrillation, all patients with amyloid cardiomyopathy should undergo a transesophageal echocardiogram to rule out atrial thrombus regardless of whether they have been on therapeutic anticoagulation.

30.10 The correct answer is D.

Rationale: The prognosis of amyloidosis is rapidly changing with evolving treatment modalities. Yet, untreated amyloidosis has a very poor prognosis. Although amyloid can deposit in different organ systems, mortality is most directly correlated to the degree of cardiac involvement. The median survival of AL is 6 months when heart failure symptoms are present. The median survival of ATTR with significant cardiac involvement is 20 months.

CARDIOVASCULAR IMAGING

Robert L. Carhart, Ashwini K. Ashwath, Sanchari Banerjee, and Hiba Zafar

CHAPTER 31

QUESTIONS

31.1 A 50-year-old male with a history of hypertension (HTN) and a family history of coronary artery disease (CAD) presents to the cardiology clinic with complaints of occasional chest pain during physical activity. He is concerned about his risk of CAD due to his family history and has been making lifestyle changes to improve his overall health. On examination, vital signs are within normal limits, and there are no signs of acute distress.

Given his family history and symptoms, you are considering further cardiac evaluations to assess the extent of his CAD.

In the evaluation of this patient with a family history of CAD and exertional chest pain, it is a universally true statement that anatomically obstructive lesions always equate to functionally significant lesions, as assessed by fractional flow reserve (FFR), an index of the physiologic significance of coronary stenosis.

A. True
B. False

31.2 A 47-year-old woman with HTN and a family history of significant heart disease presents to the cardiology clinic with recurrent chest pain episodes and exertional dyspnea. She has no prior history of cardiac conditions. Both the physical examination and baseline electrocardiogram (ECG) are unremarkable.

You decide that further cardiac evaluation is necessary, given her symptoms, risk factors, and family history. So, you want to order advanced cardiac imaging studies to assess her cardiac function and myocardial status.

In evaluating this patient with suspected cardiac pathology, which imaging technique is considered the gold standard for the following assessments in cardiology: volumetric assessment of ventricular function, measurement of myocardial mass, and detection of myocardial scarring?

A. Echocardiography
B. Cardiac computed tomography (CT)
C. Cardiac magnetic resonance imaging (MRI)
D. Positron emission tomography

*Questions and Answers are based on Chapter 31: Principles of Imaging Techniques by Mario J. Garcia and Kana Fujikura in Cardiovascular Medicine and Surgery, First Edition.

31.3 A 57-year-old male presents to the cardiology clinic with a history of recurrent chest pain, dyspnea, and significant peripheral edema. He reports that his symptoms have been gradually worsening over the past few months. Physical examination indicates jugular venous distension, hepatomegaly, and peripheral edema. The patient has a history of prior viral pericarditis.

Initial assessment includes an ECG and basic laboratory tests, which do not reveal acute coronary syndrome or significant abnormalities in electrolytes. To further evaluate the etiology of the patient's symptoms, you order advanced cardiac imaging studies.

In evaluating this patient, which imaging modality is considered the first-line choice for assessing anatomic and physiologic features?

A. Cardiac CT
B. Cardiac MRI
C. Transthoracic echocardiography with respirometric recording
D. Positron emission tomography

31.4 A 52-year-old male with HTN and hyperlipidemia presents to the primary care clinic for a routine checkup. He is currently asymptomatic, but he is concerned about his cardiovascular health due to his family history of heart disease.

His physical examination is noncontributory. He has been adhering to his antihypertensive and lipid-lowering medications. The patient is interested in additional tests to assess his cardiovascular risk beyond traditional risk factors.

In the evaluation of this asymptomatic patient with multiple cardiovascular risk factors and a family history of heart disease, which test has emerged as the most predictive single cardiovascular risk marker, capable of adding predictive information beyond traditional cardiovascular risk factors?

A. Stress echocardiography
B. Coronary angiography
C. Cardiac MRI
D. Coronary artery calcium (CAC) scoring

31.5 A 65-year-old male with a history of end-stage chronic kidney disease (CKD) on hemodialysis presents to the dermatology clinic with complaints of thickened, hyperpigmented skin and limited joint mobility. The symptoms started approximately 6 months ago and have progressively worsened, particularly in his lower extremities. He has been receiving regular hemodialysis treatments for several years. He also reports a shoulder injury 6 months ago, which was evaluated by MRI.

On examination, the patient's skin exhibits areas of thickening and darkening, especially in the lower limbs, and there is evidence of joint contractures. There are no signs of systemic illness.

In this patient with end-stage CKD and skin fibrosis, what is the potential cause of his condition?

A. Allergic reaction to a new medication
B. Exposure to asbestos in his workplace
C. Nephrogenic systemic fibrosis
D. Systemic sclerosis (scleroderma)

31.6 A 70-year-old male with a history of complete heart block and an implanted permanent pacemaker (PPM) presents to the emergency department (ED) with dizziness and palpitations. He mentions that he recently had an MRI of the lumbar spine for evaluation of back pain. The patient is concerned that the MRI may have caused his symptoms. His ECG shows a ventricular-paced rhythm with occasional premature ventricular contractions (PVCs).

In this patient with an implanted PPM who recently underwent an MRI of the lumbar spine, which of the following potential adverse effects is most concerning and could explain his symptoms of dizziness and palpitations?

A. Radiofrequency-induced heating of the lead tips
B. Transient reed switch activation
C. Changes in the capture threshold
D. Pacing inhibition/dysfunction

31.7 A 72-year-old female with a history of diabetes, HTN, and dyslipidemia presents with chest pain that lasts for a few seconds and then subsides. She denies any fevers, chills, cough, or shortness of breath. In the clinic, her vitals are within normal limits and the patient is asymptomatic at the time of evaluation. Considering the principles of cardiovascular imaging techniques, which modality is most appropriate as the initial noninvasive diagnostic test for evaluating CAD in this patient?

A. Coronary angiography
B. Stress echocardiography
C. Coronary computed tomography angiography (CCTA)
D. Single-photon emission computed tomography (SPECT) myocardial perfusion imaging

31.8 A 55-year-old patient presents for a routine transthoracic echocardiogram (TTE) to assess left ventricular function. He is asymptomatic on arrival, and his vital signs are within normal limits. During the examination, the sonographer observes unusual patterns in the ultrasound images that do not correspond to the cardiac anatomy. The images show multiple, bright, linear echoes originating from the posterior wall of the left ventricle, and these echoes obscure the visualization of adjacent structures. What is the **MOST LIKELY** explanation for these artifacts in the echocardiogram?

A. Left ventricular thrombus
B. Mitral valve regurgitation
C. Lung tissue interface
D. Reverberation artifact

31.9 A 38-year-old female, who is 35 weeks pregnant, presents to your office for evaluation of a 2-week history of intermittent fatigue and dyspnea. She notes swelling in the ankles over the past few months, which she attributes to "normal pregnancy," but over the past few weeks, she has felt fatigued and increasingly short of breath with minimal exertion, noting occasional "pangs" of chest discomfort. She takes propranolol for a history of migraines and HTN but has no other known medical conditions or drug allergies. She denies any history of similar symptoms with her prior two pregnancies as well. On examination, the patient is tachycardic, with rales and lower extremity and ankle edema, saturating in the upper 90s on ambient air.

Which of the following is the most appropriate imaging modality to investigate this patient's symptoms?

A. TTE
B. CT coronary calcium scoring
C. CT coronary angiogram
D. Cardiac magnetic resonance (MR) angiography

31.10 A 59-year-old male with a past medical history notable for HTN, hyperlipidemia, diabetes mellitus, and tobacco use, presents to the ED with acute-onset severe chest and back pain that began 2 to 3 hours prior, radiating to his shoulders with associated diaphoresis. On examination, he appears flushed and tachycardic with elevated blood pressure of 180s/90s and has a pulse deficit. An ECG performed shows sinus tachycardia, with signs of left ventricular hypertrophy (LVH), and nonspecific ST-T changes. Considering the principles of cardiovascular imaging, which of the following is considered the first-line imaging modality in assessing the likely cause of this patient's symptoms?

A. TTE
B. Transesophageal echocardiogram
C. CT angiography
D. MR angiography

ANSWERS

31.1 The correct answer is B.
Rationale: The statement is false. Anatomically obstructive lesions seen on angiography do not always equate to functionally significant lesions, as assessed by FFR, an index of the physiologic significance of coronary stenosis. Assessing functional significance through FFR is crucial in determining whether a lesion requires revascularization, as not all moderate obstructive lesions lead to reduced blood flow or symptoms. This principle was highlighted in various clinical trials, such as the fractional flow reserve versus angiography for multivessel evaluation (FAME) trial, and underscores the importance of physiologic assessment in guiding treatment decisions for CAD.

31.2 The correct answer is C.
Rationale: In this scenario, cardiac MRI is considered the gold standard for accurate and reproducible measurements of ventricular volumes, myocardial mass, and detection of myocardial scarring due to its superior image quality and tissue characterization capabilities. Cardiac MRI allows for a comprehensive assessment of the patient's cardiac function and myocardial status, making it an excellent choice for this evaluation.

31.3 The correct answer is C.
Rationale: The first-line modality to assess both anatomic and physiologic features of constrictive pericarditis is TTE with respirometric recording. This allows for real-time assessment of pericardial dynamics and can help differentiate constrictive pericarditis from other cardiac conditions. Cardiac MRI and cardiac CT are considered second-line tests and may be utilized if further confirmation or additional information is required.

31.4 The correct answer is D.
Rationale: CAC is a noninvasive imaging technique that quantifies the amount of calcium in the coronary arteries associated with atherosclerosis and increased cardiovascular risk. It is a valuable tool for risk assessment in individuals like the patient in this case scenario. The CAC scoring has emerged as the most predictive single cardiovascular risk marker in asymptomatic subjects and is capable of providing predictive information beyond the traditional cardiovascular risk factors.

31.5 The correct answer is C.
Rationale: The patient's presentation, including skin fibrosis and joint contractures, is highly suggestive of nephrogenic systemic fibrosis (NSF). NSF is a rare disease that predominantly affects individuals with end-stage CKD, particularly those on dialysis. It has been associated with exposure to gadolinium-based contrast agents used in imaging procedures, such as MRI. This condition is characterized by progressive fibrosis of the skin and internal organs. It is a known complication in patients with impaired kidney function who have been exposed to gadolinium-based contrast agents.

31.6 The correct answer is D.
Rationale: In this scenario, the most concerning potential adverse effect is pacing inhibition/dysfunction. MRI can interfere with the normal function of implanted cardiac devices like PPMs. The strong magnetic fields and radiofrequency energy generated during an MRI can disrupt the pacing and sensing functions of the device, leading to asynchronous pacing, pacing inhibition, or even the induction of arrhythmias, such as ventricular tachyarrhythmias. This interference can result in symptoms such as dizziness and palpitations, making pacing inhibition/dysfunction the most concerning potential adverse effect in this context.

31.7 The correct answer is C.
Rationale: The most appropriate initial noninvasive diagnostic test for evaluating CAD in this asymptomatic patient is CCTA. CCTA is a noninvasive imaging technique that provides detailed visualization of the coronary arteries and is valuable for ruling out significant CAD in patients with low to moderate pretest probability. Options such as stress echocardiography, SPECT myocardial perfusion imaging, and coronary angiography are typically reserved for patients with symptoms suggestive of CAD or for further assessment after initial noninvasive testing.

31.8 The correct answer is D.
Rationale: Reverberation artifact is common and occurs when ultrasound waves bounce between two parallel reflectors, creating multiple, bright, linear echoes on the ultrasound image. In this case, the bright, linear echoes originating from the posterior wall of the left ventricle are likely the result of reverberation between the ultrasound beam and a strong reflector, likely the chest wall or lung tissue. This artifact can obscure the visualization of adjacent cardiac structures and create an image that does not correspond to the true cardiac anatomy.

31.9 The correct answer is A.
Rationale: This patient likely has peripartum cardiomyopathy, which can present in the last trimester, most commonly in the first month or so postpregnancy. Few imaging modalities are approved in pregnancy; echocardiography is considered safe for the fetus at all gestational ages. There is approximately a 2.8-fold increase in cancer risk in CT imaging in pregnancy, and while MRI is not associated with radiation exposure, the safety of MRI in pregnancy has not yet been definitively established.

31.10 The correct answer is C.
Rationale: This patient presents with symptoms consistent with aortic dissection. All of the listed imaging modalities are useful diagnostic tools—transthoracic and transesophageal are both helpful in evaluation; however, they are not the most sensitive/specific, and transesophageal echocardiography (TEE) may not be readily available. CT angiography has many advantages, including availability, rapid acquisition of images, value in guiding patient management, and submillimeter special resolution, and is considered the initial imaging modality of choice for aortic dissection. CT angiography is the least operator dependent, provides useful anatomic correlates for surgical and endovascular therapy, and collects information for follow-up analysis and measurement. MR angiography is an alternative to CT angiography, depending on availability. The disadvantages of MRI are inconvenience (patients are required to remain motionless with relatively limited access for >30 minutes) and limited applicability in patients with claustrophobia, pacemakers, or certain types of aneurysm clips or metallic ocular/auricular implants. There are also concerns about patient monitoring and relative patient inaccessibility during prolonged scanning in a critically ill patient. For patients who are hemodynamically unstable, TEE is recommended as an initial study in patients with suspected aortic dissection, wherever available; however, our patient is hemodynamically stable.

SECTION 2 CARDIOVASCULAR IMAGING

CHEST RADIOGRAPHY

Vishal Phogat and Robert L. Carhart

CHAPTER 32

QUESTIONS

32.1 A 78-year-old male with a past medical history of heart failure with reduced ejection fraction, diabetes mellitus, and coronary artery disease, is admitted to the hospital for an elective procedure for placement of a biventricular implantable cardioverter-defibrillator (ICD). Thirty minutes post the procedure, the patient starts complaining of worsening shortness of breath and mild left-sided chest pain that worsens with inspiration. His blood pressure is 120/80 mm Hg, heart rate 96 beats per minute (bpm), respiratory rate of 20/min, temperature of 37.2 °C, and oxygen saturation of 90% on room air. What would be the most appropriate next diagnostic test?

A. Cardiac magnetic resonance imaging (MRI)
B. Chest x-ray
C. Computed tomography (CT) thorax
D. Echocardiogram

32.2 A 55-year-old female with a past medical history of heart failure with reduced ejection fraction, and gall stones, presented to the emergency department (ED) with severe epigastric pain, not relieved by Tylenol. She is hemodynamically stable. Her labs are significant for an elevated lipase level of 500 U/L. CT scan of the abdomen is suggestive of acute pancreatitis. She receives 2 L intravenous (IV) saline. An hour later, the patient starts complaining of difficulty breathing. Her oxygen saturation is now 88% on room air. Bilateral fine crepitations are heard on lung auscultation. What findings would you expect to see on the chest x-ray of this patient?

A. Bilateral moderate-sized pleural effusions
B. Peribronchial cuffing and thickening of the fissures
C. Bilateral centrally distributed patchy fluffy consolidations
D. All of the above

32.3 A 40-year-old male with no significant medical history presented to the ED with a 2-day history of left-sided chest pain, worse with inspiration. He was discharged from the ED 5 days ago, when he presented for flulike symptoms and tested positive for Coxsackievirus infection. His vitals are stable except heart rate (HR) of 99 bpm. Electrocardiogram (ECG) shows sinus tachycardia, low-voltage QRS, and electrical alternans. A bedside echo showed a large-sized pericardial effusion. Which of the following signs seen on this patient's chest x-ray that would correlate to his echo findings?

---

*Questions and Answers are based on Chapter 32: Chest Radiography by Jonathan Alis and Linda B. Haramati in *Cardiovascular Medicine and Surgery*, First Edition.

A. Oreo cookie sign
B. A 1.6 cm increase in the transverse cardiac diameter, compared to a recent x-ray taken 5 days ago
C. Water bottle appearance of the superior mediastinum
D. All of the above

32.4 A 70-year-old female with a past history of coronary artery disease is seen at the primary care office for a 3-day history of a productive cough. Chest x-ray did not show any acute pathology. However, a focal and curvilinear calcification was described at the edge of the left cardiac border. What is the most common cause of the myocardial calcification seen on this patient's chest radiograph?

A. History of MI
B. Metastatic disease
C. Renal failure
D. Cardiac surgery

32.5 An 80-year-old man with no significant past medical history was referred to the cardiology clinic for management of an aortic valve calcification, which was seen incidentally on a recent chest radiograph obtained for flulike illness. He is asymptomatic. Vitals signs are stable and physical examination is unremarkable. What is the most common cause of aortic valve calcification in this patient?

A. Degenerative disease
B. Rheumatic heart disease
C. Syphilis
D. MI

32.6 A 50-year-old man with a past medical history significant for recurrent throat infections was referred to the cardiology clinic for management of an aortic valve calcification, which was seen incidentally on a recent chest radiograph obtained for flulike illness. He is asymptomatic. Vital signs are stable and physical examination is unremarkable. Which of the following should be considered as the **MOST LIKELY** cause of the aortic valve calcifications in this patient?

A. Rheumatic heart disease
B. Bicuspid aortic valve
C. Both A and B
D. Degenerative disease

32.7 A 50-year-old man with a past medical history significant for recurrent throat infections was referred to the cardiology clinic for management of a mitral valve calcification, which was seen incidentally on a recent chest radiograph obtained for productive cough. He is asymptomatic. Vital signs are stable and physical examination is unremarkable. Which of these should be considered as the possible causes of mitral valve calcification in this patient?

A. Syphilis
B. Prior rheumatic heart disease
C. Tuberculosis
D. Degenerative disease

CHAPTER 32 | Chest Radiography

32.8 A 60-year-old man presents to the ED with sudden-onset severe tearing chest pain radiating to the back for 4 hours. His blood pressure (BP) is 190/100 mm Hg on the left arm and 140/90 mm Hg on the right arm, respiratory rate (RR) 19/min, HR 90 bpm, SpO_2 97% on room air. ECG finding is normal. You are concerned about an acute aortic dissection. What is the most common abnormality on chest x-ray in a case of aortic dissection?

A. Widened mediastinum
B. Displacement of intimal aortic calcification from the outer contour of the aortic knob
C. Blurring of the aortic knob
D. Rightward tracheal shift
E. Pleural effusion

32.9 A 55-year-old female came to the primary care office for an annual physical examination. Vital signs are stable and physical examination is unremarkable. She had a chest x-ray to follow up on a positive purified protein derivative (PPD) result, which showed a widened mediastinum. What should be on differentials for the x-ray finding of a widened mediastinum?

A. Aortic dissection
B. Chronic vascular ectasia
C. Enlarged thyroid
D. Mediastinal mass
E. All of the above

32.10 An 80-year-old man with no significant past medical history was referred to the cardiology clinic for management of a curvilinear calcification at the margin of the cardiac silhouette, which was seen incidentally on a recent chest radiograph obtained for flu-like illness. He is asymptomatic. Vitals signs are stable and physical examination is unremarkable. Which of the following from the patient's past history can lead to this pericardial calcification seen on x-ray?

A. Tuberculosis
B. Cardiac surgery
C. Thoracic radiation
D. Uremic pericarditis
E. All of the above

ANSWERS

32.1 The correct answer is B.
Rationale: This patient may have suffered an iatrogenic pneumothorax, a complication of biventricular ICD placement. A chest x-ray would be the most appropriate initial diagnostic test, which is quick and can be easily accessible as a portable test. Although, a CT thorax can diagnose pneumothorax, it is not the first modality of choice due to higher radiation exposure and more time required for the study. Echocardiogram can be considered if there were concerns for cardiac perforation,

or myocardial ischemia, but it is a time-consuming study and not as accessible as an x-ray. Cardiac MRI would be time-consuming and is not indicated in this scenario to rule out any major postoperative complications.

> **KEY POINTS**
>
> ✔ Chest x-ray can be helpful for diagnosing causes of dyspnea and chest pain, such as pneumothorax, pneumonia, pulmonary edema, and so on. It is a quick and easily accessible and widely available test.

32.2 The correct answer is B:
Rationale: This patient with congestive heart failure likely developed pulmonary edema from the volume resuscitation for acute pancreatitis. Interstitial edema is the first phase of pulmonary edema, seen as thickening of the interlobular septa (Kerley B lines). Edema involving other pulmonary interstitial structures such as peribronchovascular and subpleural interstitium results in the x-ray findings of peribronchial cuffing and thickening of the fissures. Pleural effusions are often present. Alveolar edema is seen on x-ray as bilateral patchy fluffy consolidations distributed centrally with sparing of the periphery.

> **KEY POINTS**
>
> ✔ Chest radiographic findings in congestive heart failure vary depending on the acuity and correlate with pulmonary capillary wedge pressures. These findings include Kerley B lines, peribronchial cuffing and thickening of the fissures, bilateral patchy fluffy consolidations distributed centrally with sparing of the periphery (alveolar edema), and pleural effusions. Cardiomegaly can be seen in some chronic cases.

32.3 The correct answer is B:
Rationale: All of the above signs can be seen in cases of pericardial effusion. An increase in transverse cardiac diameter greater than 1.5 cm compared to a recent radiograph taken within 30 days has a reported 80% sensitivity but only 46% specificity. A globular/water bottle appearance of the heart with a normal-sized superior mediastinum can be seen with large pericardial effusions. On the lateral radiographs, the effusion can sometimes be visualized as soft tissue density between the epicardial and pericardial fat, both of which are radiolucent. This is called the pericardial fat stripe, sandwich, or Oreo cookie sign. This is a specific but not sensitive sign. Unilateral left-sided pleural effusions have been seen more commonly in pericardial effusions.

> **KEY POINTS**
>
> ✔ Radiographs are not sensitive to detection of pericardial effusions and can be challenging to differentiate from cardiac chamber enlargement. However, a few signs seen on a chest x-ray that can be suggestive of a pericardial effusion include a rapid increase in cardiac size, globular/water bottle appearance of the heart with a normal-sized superior mediastinum, unilateral left-sided pleural effusions, a pericardial fat stripe, and a sandwich or an Oreo cookie sign.

32.4 The correct answer is A.
Rationale: The myocardial calcification described in this question is a dystrophic calcification. CT is the most sensitive modality to identify these calcifications, but they can also be detected on radiographs. Dystrophic calcifications are a consequence of tissue damage and necrosis, and MI is the most common cause. They are focal and curvilinear calcifications, located at the edge of an infarct of the left ventricular (LV) apex, typically associated with an LV aneurysm.

KEY POINTS
- Dystrophic calcifications are a consequence of tissue damage and necrosis, and MI is the most common cause.

32.5 The correct answer is A.
Rationale: Aortic valve calcifications are the most commonly seen valvular calcifications. Three patterns are described as commissure, complete/partial ring, or plaque-like calcifications. In the majority of patients older than 70 years, aortic valve calcifications are due to degenerative disease.

KEY POINTS
- In the majority of patients older than 70 years, aortic valve calcifications are due to degenerative disease.

32.6 The correct answer is C.
Rationale: Aortic valve calcifications are the most commonly seen valvular calcifications. Three patterns are described as commissure, complete/partial ring, or plaque-like calcifications. In patients younger than 70 years, bicuspid aortic valve or rheumatic heart disease should be considered as the cause of the aortic valve calcification.

KEY POINTS
- In patients younger than 70 years, bicuspid aortic valve or rheumatic heart disease should be considered as the cause of the aortic valve calcification.

32.7 The correct answer is B.
Rationale: Mitral valve calcifications are less commonly seen and are usually secondary to rheumatic heart disease.

KEY POINTS
- Mitral valve calcifications are usually secondary to rheumatic heart disease.

32.8 The correct answer is A.
Rationale: Although all the abovementioned findings can be seen in an acute aortic dissection, widened mediastinum is the most common finding. A greater than 8-cm mediastinal width at the aortic knob on a posteroanterior (PA) radiograph

is defined as a widened mediastinum. It has 64% sensitivity. Care should be taken when interpreting anteroposterior (AP), supine, or rotated radiographs for mediastinal widening because the width can be artificially magnified. If prior radiographs are available, interval progressive widening or change in mediastinal contour has a higher predictive value. Another classically described finding is displacement of intimal aortic calcification from the outer contour of the aortic knob by 6 to 10 mm, which has a poor sensitivity (9%). Additional supportive signs include a pleural cap (apical opacity in a supine radiograph secondary to hemothorax), blurring of the aortic knob, tracheal shift to the right, depression of the left main stem bronchus below 40°, and pleural effusion.

KEY POINTS

✔ A greater than 8-cm mediastinal width at the aortic knob on a PA radiograph is defined as a widened mediastinum and is the most common finding (64% sensitivity) in an acute aortic dissection.

32.9 The correct answer is E.
Rationale: All of the above. A greater than 8-cm mediastinal width at the aortic knob on a PA radiograph is defined as a widened mediastinum. Care should be taken when interpreting AP, supine, or rotated radiographs for mediastinal widening because the width can be artificially magnified. Mediastinal widening can be seen in aortic dissection, chronic vascular ectasia, excessive mediastinal fat, enlarged thyroid, mediastinal mass, or lymphadenopathy.

KEY POINTS

✔ Mediastinal widening can be seen in aortic dissection, chronic vascular ectasia, excessive mediastinal fat, enlarged thyroid, mediastinal mass, or lymphadenopathy.

32.10 The correct answer is E.
Rationale: Pericardial calcifications are caused by end-stage disease from prior injury to the pericardium. There are multiple etiologies including prior infections (tuberculosis, viral), trauma, cardiac surgery, radiation, and uremic pericarditis. Pericardial calcifications appear as curvilinear calcifications at the margin of the cardiac silhouette. Location of the calcifications helps differentiate between pericardial and myocardial calcifications. Pericardial calcifications more often involve the less pulsatile right chambers, along the anterior and diaphragmatic surfaces, and typically involve the atrioventricular grooves. Pericardial calcifications rarely involve the LV apex, and if involvement of the LV apex is noted, this is part of a more diffuse involvement of the entire heart, as opposed to myocardial calcifications that often focally involve the LV apex. In addition, on the lateral radiograph, the extension of calcification above the pulmonic valve involving the pulmonary outflow flow tract is consistent with pericardial calcifications, as opposed to myocardial calcifications that occur inferior to the pulmonic valve. The left atrium is classically spared

from pericardial calcifications. The presence of left atrial pericardial calcification should suggest the diagnosis of constrictive pericarditis, although only present in half of the cases.

KEY POINTS

✔ There are multiple etiologies for pericardial calcifications, including prior infections (tuberculosis, viral), trauma, cardiac surgery, radiation, and uremic pericarditis.

ELECTROCARDIOGRAPHIC EXERCISE TESTING

CHAPTER 33

Meet Patel

QUESTIONS

33.1 A 45-year-old female patient with a history of type 2 diabetes and obesity presents to the clinic for a routine checkup. The physician decides to perform an exercise electrocardiogram (ECG) to evaluate her cardiovascular (CV) function. During the test, ECG showed greater than 1 mm ST elevation in leads V2 to V5 and a drop in systolic blood pressure (SBP) by 15 mm Hg. The patient complains of leg cramps and mild shortness of breath. Her BP drops from 122/82 at rest to 108/84 mm Hg during the test. Which of the following indications alone is an absolute indication to stop the exercise ECG?

A. The patient has achieved their target heart rate (HR).
B. The patient experiences leg cramps or mild shortness of breath.
C. Drop in SBP greater than 10 mm Hg (persistently below baseline) despite an increase in workload, in the absence of other evidence of ischemia.
D. ST-segment elevation (>1.0 mm) in leads without any Q wave changes

33.2 A 65-year-old female with a history of hypertension, hyperlipidemia, and angina presents to the clinic for a routine follow-up appointment. She reports experiencing chest pain and shortness of breath with exertion and her symptoms have been worsening over the past month. A resting ECG reveals normal sinus rhythm without any ST-T wave changes. An exercise ECG is ordered to further evaluate her symptoms.

During the exercise ECG, the patient experiences chest discomfort and shortness of breath at 7 minutes into the test, at which point the ECG reveals the following:

Peaked, tall P waves, 0.8 mm upsloping ST depression in leads V2 to V5, inversion of U waves, and an increase in R-wave amplitude in the precordial leads. Corrected QT (QTc) interval is 380 milliseconds (baseline QTc: 400 milliseconds).

Which of the following is **MORE LIKELY** to be considered as a sign of ischemia?

A. Peaked, tall P waves
B. Inversion of U waves during exercise and an increase in R-wave amplitude in the precordial leads
C. 0.8-mm upsloping ST-segment depression in leads V2 to V5
D. QT interval shortening

33.3 A 65-year-old male with a history of hypertension and hyperlipidemia presents to the clinic with chest discomfort and shortness of breath with exertion for the past week. He reports that the discomfort is central, radiating to the left arm, and lasts for a few minutes, and he has to stop exercising to relieve his symptoms. He denies palpitations or syncope. On physical examination, his blood pressure is 150/95 mm Hg, and his HR is 80 beats per minute (bpm). He has a grade III/VI systolic ejection murmur heard **BEST** at the aortic area, which radiates to the neck.

Questions and Answers are based on Chapter 33: Electrocardiographic Exercise Testing by Zain Ul Abideen Asad and Chittur A. Sivaram in Cardiovascular Medicine and Surgery, First Edition.

An ECG shows sinus rhythm with no ST-segment changes or arrhythmias. A transthoracic echocardiogram is performed, which shows severe aortic stenosis with a peak velocity of 4.5 m/s, mean gradient of 50 mm Hg, and aortic valve area of 0.7 cm². The left ventricular ejection fraction is preserved, and there is no evidence of regional wall motion abnormalities.

While discussing further cardiac testing, the patient reports he was recently admitted to the hospital for stroke with no residual weakness. He also reports a recent deep venous thrombosis in the left lower extremity for which he is on therapeutic anticoagulation. His blood cultures grew *Streptococcus viridians*, and he is receiving intravenous antibiotics for active endocarditis.

Given his clinical history and multiple comorbidities, which of the following is **NOT** an absolute contraindication to exercise stress test?

A. Recent stroke
B. Deep vein thrombosis
C. Severe symptomatic aortic stenosis
D. Active endocarditis

33.4 A 60-year-old female with a history of hypertension, hyperlipidemia, and obesity presents to the clinic with substernal chest discomfort with exertion for the past 3 months. The patient denies any palpitations, shortness of breath, or syncope. On physical examination, her blood pressure is 150/90 mm Hg, and her HR is 72 bpm. The rest of the examination is unremarkable. An ECG shows normal sinus rhythm with no ST-segment changes or arrhythmias. The patient is then scheduled for an exercise stress test, which shows less than 1 mm ST depression at peak exercise. Which of the following is the **BEST** next step in the management of this patient?

A. Repeat the exercise stress test in 1 month.
B. Initiate medical management with beta-blockers and nitroglycerin.
C. Refer the patient for stress echocardiography or myocardial perfusion imaging (MPI).
D. Order a coronary angiogram.

33.5 A 55-year-old male presents to the clinic with chest pain on exertion for the past 2 weeks. He has a history of hypertension and dyslipidemia, but no history of coronary artery disease. On physical examination, his blood pressure is 140/90 mm Hg, and his HR is 80 bpm. An ECG shows normal sinus rhythm with no ST-segment changes or arrhythmias. The patient is then scheduled for an exercise stress test, the patient started to have ST depression during the beginning of exercise but he was unable to complete stage I of the standard Bruce protocol and experienced a drop in SBP. The test was aborted and the patient was noted to have premature ventricular contractions (PVCs) and late resolution of ST depression while the patient was resting. Which of the following is a highly correlated predictor of left main or severe proximal three-vessel coronary artery disease during exercise stress test?

A. Inability to complete stage I of a standard Bruce protocol accompanied by a drop in BP
B. Early appearance of significant ST depression during exercise
C. Slow resolution of ST depression after exercise
D. Development of nonsustained or sustained ventricular ectopy during or immediately after exercise

33.6 A 62-year-old male presents with chest pain on exertion and has a history of hypertension, hyperlipidemia, and a 30-pack-year smoking history. An ECG exercise test is performed, and the results are equivocal. Which of the following diagnostic tests should be considered next to evaluate for suspected ischemic heart disease?

A. Repeated ECG exercise testing
B. MPI with exercise
C. Coronary angiogram
D. Cardiac computed tomography (CT) angiography

33.7 A 62-year-old male patient with a history of hypertension, hyperlipidemia, and smoking presents to his primary care physician with complaints of chest discomfort and shortness of breath during physical activity. The physician suspects coronary artery disease and decides to perform a stress test to establish a diagnosis. The patient is currently taking metoprolol for hypertension. Which of the following would be appropriate recommendations for stress tests in patients taking beta-blockers?

A. Stop taking metoprolol 24 hours before the stress test.
B. Stop taking metoprolol 72 hours before the stress test.
C. No, the patient should continue taking metoprolol before the stress test.
D. Taking beta-blockers won't have any impact on stress test.

33.8 A 58-year-old male with a history of ischemic cardiomyopathy, heart failure with reduced ejection fraction, and implantation of a dual-chamber implantable cardioverter-defibrillator (ICD) presents to the cardiology clinic with complaints of exercise intolerance and occasional chest discomfort. The patient has been on medical management with beta-blockers, angiotensin-converting enzyme (ACE) inhibitors, aspirin, and statins. The patient has been stable on optimal medical therapy for the past year, with no recent hospitalizations for heart failure. The cardiologist plans to perform an exercise ECG stress test to evaluate for myocardial ischemia. Which of the following is **TRUE** regarding stress testing in patients with ICD?

A. ICDs should be turned off for the duration of the stress test.
B. The maximum HR during stress testing should be maintained at 10 to 15 bpm below the device threshold for antitachycardia pacing or defibrillation.
C. Patients with ICDs are not candidates for exercise stress testing.
D. Programming the device to defibrillate at a lower HR during testing

33.9 A 52-year-old male with a history of hypertension and dyslipidemia presents to the cardiology clinic with complaints of chest pain on exertion. He describes the pain as a pressure-like sensation in the center of his chest with exertion, radiating to his left arm and jaw, lasting for a few minutes, and resolving with rest. The patient does **NOT** smoke cigarettes. His physical examination is unremarkable and ECG shows normal sinus rhythm with no ST-T wave abnormalities. Based on his symptoms and history, what is the appropriate pretest probability for ischemic heart disease, and what type of stress test would be most appropriate for this patient?

A. Low-pretest probability, exercise ECG testing
B. Intermediate pretest probability, exercise ECG testing
C. High pretest probability, exercise ECG testing
D. High pretest probability, MPI
E. High pretest probability, cardiac catheterization

33.10 Patient is a 60-year-old male with a past medical history of hypertension and type 2 diabetes mellitus, who presents to the cardiology clinic for a routine follow-up visit. He reports feeling generally well, with no chest pain, shortness of breath, or other CV symptoms. However, he has been struggling to maintain his exercise regimen due to fatigue and decreased stamina. Her current medications include metformin, lisinopril, and hydrochlorothiazide. During his visit, the patient's cardiologist recommends an exercise stress test to assess his CV function and determine her risk for future CV events. The exercise stress test reveals a peak double product (DP) of 25,200, which corresponds to a DP product at rest was 11,050. His maximal HR during exercise is 140 bpm, and his SBP reaches a peak of 180 mm Hg. Which of the following is a strong predictor of CV mortality in patients referred for exercise testing?

A. Maximal HR
B. Maximal SBP
C. Maximal DP reserve
D. Exercise capacity (in metabolic equivalents)

ANSWERS

33.1 The correct answer is D.
Rationale: During an exercise ECG, there are several reasons why the test may need to be stopped early. These include achieving the target HR, leg cramps or mild shortness of breath, and a drop in SBP greater than 10 mm Hg (persistently below baseline) despite an increase in workload, in the absence of other evidence of ischemia. However, these are relative contraindications and should be appropriately evaluated. The absolute indication to stop the exercise ECG test is ST-segment elevation (>1.0 mm) in leads without preexisting Q waves because of prior myocardial infarction (MI; other than aVR, aVL, and V1). Exercise-induced ST elevation in leads without preexisting Q waves indicates the presence of significant proximal coronary stenosis. While less common, exercise-induced ST elevation can also result from coronary vasospasm. Other absolute indications to stop the exercise ECG are drop in SBP greater than 10 mm Hg, despite an increase in workload, when accompanied by any other evidence of ischemia, moderate-to-severe angina, central nervous system symptoms (eg, ataxia, dizziness, near syncope), signs of poor perfusion (cyanosis or pallor), sustained VT or other arrhythmia, including second- or third-degree atrioventricular block, that interferes with normal maintenance of cardiac output during exercise, technical difficulties in monitoring the ECG or SBP or the subject's request to stop. The patient's history of type 2 diabetes and obesity increases the risk of CV disease and may contribute to the development of ischemic symptoms during exercise. Therefore, close monitoring and prompt stopping of the test are essential to ensure patient safety.

33.2 The correct answer is B:
Rationale: This patient's ECG shows 0.8-mm upsloping ST depression. During exercise stress tests, the ST segment can exhibit different types of depression: upsloping, horizontal, and downsloping. While both horizontal and downsloping ST depression indicate myocardial ischemia, upsloping ST depression may be associated with high HRs during exercise. If the ST-segment depression is less than 1 mm, the result is considered equivocal. When evaluating patients with resting ST elevation due to early repolarization changes, it is necessary to measure ST depression relative to the PQ junction. In addition to horizontal and downsloping ST depression more than 1 mm or ST elevation, inversion of U waves during exercise and an increase in R-wave amplitude in the precordial leads resulting from left ventricular cavity dilation are commonly reported as possible signs of myocardial ischemia. However, QT interval shortening does not indicate ischemia, as it is considered normal during exercise ECG testing.

33.3 The correct answer is A:
Rationale: This patient will not be a good candidate for exercise stress test considering the comorbidities he has; however, it is important to note that the decision to perform an exercise stress test should be individualized and based on the clinical scenario and the goals of the test. The presence of a relative contraindication may not necessarily preclude the use of exercise stress testing but rather should be carefully considered in light of the patient's overall condition and the potential risks and benefits of the test. In some cases, an alternative stress modality may be preferred, such as pharmacologic stress testing or imaging modalities like stress echocardiography or MPI. Out of all the risk factors this patient has, the occurrence of a recent stroke is regarded as a relative contraindication to exercise stress testing. In such instances, a thorough evaluation must be conducted on a case-by-case basis, with careful consideration of the associated risks and benefits. Conversely, acute deep vein thrombosis, severe aortic stenosis, and infective endocarditis are all considered absolute contraindications to exercise stress testing. The American Heart Association guidelines provide a comprehensive outline of both absolute and relative contraindications to exercise ECG stress testing.

33.4 The correct answer is C:
Rationale: A nondiagnostic or equivocal exercise stress test, defined as less than 1-mm ST depression at peak exercise, can occur in patients with underlying ischemic heart disease or some normal subjects. Additional stress testing using more expensive modalities such as stress echocardiography or MPI may be necessary for further workup of such patients. In this case, given the patient's risk factors and typical chest discomfort, referral for further evaluation with stress echocardiography or MPI is the most appropriate next step. Repeat exercise stress test in 1 month is not necessary as it is unlikely to yield different results. Coronary angiogram is an invasive procedure that is not indicated as a first-line diagnostic tool in patients with equivocal stress test results. Initiate medical management with beta-blockers and nitroglycerin, which is a possible next step in the management of patients with suspected ischemic heart disease based on current guidelines. Beta-blockers can reduce myocardial oxygen demand, while nitroglycerin can relieve chest discomfort and improve coronary blood flow. However, the optimal management strategy should be individualized based on the patient's clinical presentation, risk factors, and overall CV status.

33.5 The correct answer is A.

Rationale: This patient's inability to complete stage I of a standard Bruce protocol, which equates to a functional capacity of fewer than 5 METs (metabolic equivalent of task), and is accompanied by a drop in SBP is a powerful predictor of adverse prognosis and is highly correlated with left main or severe proximal three-vessel coronary artery disease. A brief exercise duration during a symptom-limited test can also serve as a strong indicator of an unfavorable prognosis. The degree of ST depression, the number of leads showing ST depression, and the early appearance and slow resolution of ST depression after exercise also predict a poor prognosis. Although such features help identify patients in need of early invasive therapy, they are not considered a predictor of left main or severe proximal three-vessel coronary artery disease. The development of nonsustained or sustained ventricular ectopy during or immediately after exercise has been recognized as a sign of an adverse prognosis, but ectopy may also occur in patients with nonischemic conditions, such as arrhythmogenic right ventricular cardiomyopathy and catecholaminergic polymorphic ventricular tachycardia.

33.6 The correct answer is B.

Rationale: In patients with suspected ischemic heart disease, the overall sensitivity of ECG exercise testing has been reported as 45% to 50% and specificity 85% to 90%. Stress echocardiography and MPI have higher sensitivity and specificity, but both are limited by greater cost and lesser availability. Repeated MPIs also expose the patient to significant radiation unlike exercise ECG or stress echocardiography. Equivocal exercise ECG tests are not uncommon, and they result from premature termination of exercise because of fatigue and/or noncardiac comorbid conditions, or when only milder degrees of coronary artery disease are present. MPI with exercise is a reasonable next diagnostic test to evaluate for suspected ischemic heart disease in this patient. It has a reported sensitivity of 73% to 92% for exercise MPI and a specificity of 63% to 87%. This test would be less costly than stress echocardiography or MPI with vasodilator and would expose the patient to less radiation than repeated MPIs.

Coronary angiogram would be the next best step if MPI with exercise is positive.

33.7 The correct answer is A.

Rationale: Beta-blockers such as metoprolol can reduce the HR and blood pressure response during exercise, leading to false-negative results on stress testing. Therefore, the American Heart Association recommends that beta-blockers be stopped **24 hours** before stress testing is performed to establish a diagnosis of coronary artery disease. However, the decision to stop beta-blockers should be individualized based on the patient's underlying condition and the type of stress test being performed. In some cases, it may be appropriate to continue beta-blockers or to perform a pharmacologic stress test instead of an exercise stress test.

33.8 The correct answer is B.

Rationale: Special planning is required before stress testing in patients with implanted cardiac devices such as pacemakers and ICDs. In patients with ICDs, it is important to know the programmed thresholds for defibrillation before exercise testing. Maintaining the maximum HR during the exercise stress test at 10 to 15 bpm below the device threshold for antitachycardia pacing or defibrillation is recommended for the prevention of inappropriate device therapy. Therefore, option B is the correct answer. ICDs should not be turned off for the duration of the stress test because of safety concerns and are not going to provide any benefit. If the device is programmed to defibrillate at a lower HR during testing then it may lead to inappropriate shocks, where the device delivers an unnecessary shock to the heart. This can be uncomfortable and cause anxiety for the patient and may also lead to complications such as damage to the heart muscle or interference with the device's normal functioning. Exercise testing is considered safe for patients with ICDs, as long as appropriate precautions are taken. Furthermore, during exercise, the likelihood of ICD firing remains very low.

33.9 The correct answer is B.

Rationale: This patient has a history of chest pain that occurs with exertion and resolves with rest, which is a typical angina symptom. Based on his age, sex, and other factors, he has an intermediate pretest probability (15%-65%) for ischemic heart disease. The most suitable candidates for exercise ECG testing are patients with intermediate pretest probability (15%-65%) for coronary artery disease and a normal resting ECG. According to current guidelines, the exercise ECG stress test should be the initial diagnostic test for patients with suspected ischemic heart disease and a normal resting ECG, as opposed to other forms of stress testing. It is important to note that stress testing is less useful for the diagnosis of coronary heart disease (CHD) in patients with either a high- or a low-pretest probability. False-positive exercise ECG tests are frequent in those with lower pretest probability, and false-negative tests are of concern in those with higher than 65% pretest probability. Therefore, choosing the appropriate stress test based on pretest probability is crucial for accurate diagnosis and avoiding unnecessary testing.

33.10 The correct answer is C.

Rationale: To accurately measure myocardial oxygen consumption, cardiac catheterization is needed to measure the oxygen content in the coronary arteries and veins. Nonetheless, an estimate of myocardial oxygen consumption during clinical exercise testing can be derived from the product of HR and SBP, known as the DP or rate-pressure product. This measure typically varies from a 10th percentile value of 25,000 to a 90th percentile value of 40,000 at peak exercise. Another critical measure for evaluating mortality and prognostic information is the DP reserve, calculated as the DP at peak exercise minus the DP at rest. A study involving 1,759 male veterans, with an average age of 57 ± 12 years, revealed that DP reserve serves as an effective predictor of CV mortality through both univariable and multivariable Cox survival analyses. The study demonstrated that DP reserve is a more potent indicator of increased mortality risk than traditional risk factors such as smoking, hypertension, diabetes, and other common exercise test parameters like exercise capacity, maximum HR, HR recovery, and ST-segment depression. The findings also highlighted the protective benefit of a higher DP reserve amidst other risk markers. This study highlights that an elevated DP reserve is linked to better survival rates in patients undergoing exercise testing, outperforming other prognostic indicators like METs, maximum HR, SBP, and HR recovery. A diminished DP reserve, defined as 10,000 or less, was identified as an independent prognostic factor.

SUGGESTED READINGS

Fan S, Lyon CE, Savage PD, et al. Outcomes and adverse events among patients with implantable cardiac defibrillators in cardiac rehabilitation: a case-controlled study. *J Cardiopulm Rehabil Prev.* 2009;29:40-43.

Fihn SD, Gardin JM, Abrams J, et al. 2012 ACCF/AHA/ACP/AATS/PCNA/SCAI/STS guideline for the diagnosis and management of patients with stable ischemic heart disease: a report of the American College of Cardiology Foundation/American Heart Association task force on practice guidelines, and the American College of Physicians, American Association for Thoracic Surgery, Preventive Cardiovascular Nurses Association, Society for Cardiovascular Angiography and Interventions, and Society of Thoracic Surgeons. *J Am Coll Cardiol.* 2012;60(24):e44-e164.

Fletcher GF, Ades PA, Kligfield P, et al. Exercise standards for testing and training: a scientific statement from the American Heart Association. *Circulation.* 2013;128(8):873-934.

Montalescot G, Sechtem U, Achenbach S, et al. 2013 ESC guidelines on the management of stable coronary artery disease. *Eur Heart J.* 2013;34:2949-3003.

Sadrzadeh Rafie AH, Sungar GW, Dewey FE, Hadley D, Myers J, Froelicher VF. Prognostic value of double product reserve. *Eur J Cardiovasc Prev Rehabil.* 2008;15:541-547.

ECHOCARDIOGRAPHY

Robert L. Carhart, Atika Azhar, and Subash Nepal

CHAPTER 34

QUESTIONS

34.1 An ultrasound probe emitting ultrasound waves at a frequency of 1 MHz is used for transthoracic echocardiography, while a 12.5-MHz probe is used for transesophageal echocardiography. What are the effects of increasing the frequency of ultrasound waves?

- A. Increase in axial resolution and reduction of depth
- B. Increase in depth and reduction in axial resolution
- C. Increase in temporal resolution and reduction in contrast resolution
- D. Reduction in attenuation and increase in penetrance
- E. Increase in reflection of ultrasound waves from the tissue surface

34.2 A 20-year-old female from Nigeria who immigrated to the United States 1 year ago presented to the clinic with dyspnea on exertion for a year. She also complained of easy fatigability, orthopnea, and paroxysmal nocturnal dyspnea. General physical examination was normal. Vitals showed a pulse rate of 60/min, blood pressure of 120/80 mm Hg, respiratory rate of 29/min, and a temperature of 36.6 °C. Cardiovascular system examination revealed a loud S1 and normal intensity S2 with a mid-diastolic rumble and an opening snap prior to the S2. A right parasternal heave was present on palpation.

Laboratory work showed normal brain-type natriuretic peptide (BMP) and pro B-type natriuretic peptide (proBNP). An electrocardiogram (ECG) showed tall R waves in leads V1 and V2 with an R/S ratio of 2. A broad and notched P wave was seen in lead II. Chest x-ray showed a normal cardiac silhouette with a prominent right descending pulmonary artery. Two-dimensional transthoracic echocardiography showed a normal left ventricular (LV) cavity size, wall thickness, and systolic function. The mitral valve opening was restricted, and the mitral valve area (MVA) was measured to be 0.8 cm^2 by planimetry and the pressure half-time method. Mitral leaflets were moderately calcified from the mid-leaflet to the annulus with restricted mobility, thickened entire leaflets, and chordal shortening and fibrosis extending to the distal third. Moderate mitral regurgitation was present. The left atrium was severely dilated with a volume index of 48 mL/m^2. Pulmonary artery systolic pressure was increased to 50 mm Hg. Which one of the following is the **BEST** next treatment approach?

---

*Questions and Answers are based on Chapter 34: Echocardiography by Edwin Ho and Cynthia Taub in Cardiovascular Medicine and Surgery, First Edition.

A. Percutaneous balloon mitral valvuloplasty
B. Mitral valve replacement
C. Mitral valve repair
D. Start anticoagulation and repeat echocardiography in 6 months.
E. Prescribe diuretics and beta-blockers.

34.3 A 60-year-old male with a past medical history of hypertension, hyperlipidemia, and diabetes mellitus presented with dyspnea on exertion and easy fatigability for 3 months. He denies orthopnea, paroxysmal nocturnal dyspnea, or lower extremity swelling. General physical examination and vitals are within normal limits. Cardiovascular system examination revealed normal S1, an absent A2 component of S2, and a mid-systolic ejection murmur in the aortic area radiating to the common carotid artery and apex of the heart.

BMP and serum proBNP were within normal limits. ECG was remarkable for left ventricular hypertrophy (LVH). Two-dimensional transthoracic echocardiography showed mild, concentric LVH and moderately reduced systolic function with a left ventricular ejection fraction (LVEF) of 35%, with moderate diffuse hypokinesis. The aortic valve was moderately calcified with a calculated aortic valve area (AVA) of 0.8 cm^2 by the continuity equation. The aortic valve peak gradient was 50 mm Hg, the mean gradient was 30, and the dimensionless index (DI) was 0.24. Which of the following is the next **BEST** step?
A. Proceed with aortic valve replacement for severe calcific aortic stenosis.
B. Perform low-dose dobutamine stress echocardiography to assess for low-flow, low-gradient severe aortic stenosis.
C. Consider percutaneous aortic valve valvuloplasty.
D. Evaluate for transcutaneous aortic valve replacement (TAVR).
E. Schedule a repeat echocardiography in 6 months.

34.4 A 56-year-old intravenous (IV) drug abuser presented with fever accompanied by chills and weight loss over the past month. General physical examination revealed splenomegaly. Auscultation revealed normal S1 and S2 heart sounds, along with a systolic murmur heard at the left lower sternal border. The patient is morbidly obese, with a body mass index (BMI) of 45 kg/m^2.

ECG showed a second-degree atrioventricular block. Laboratory work revealed a normal BMP. Complete blood count (CBC) showed leukocytosis with a white blood cell (WBC) count of 21,000, with a neutrophil predominance. Chest x-ray was normal. Blood culture was positive for *Staphylococcus aureus* bacteremia in two samples. Which of the following is the next **BEST** test?
A. Transesophageal echocardiography
B. Transthoracic echocardiography
C. Transthoracic echocardiography with contrast
D. Transthoracic echocardiography followed by transesophageal echocardiography
E. Cardiac computed tomography (CCT) scan

34.5 A 45-year-old male presented with chest pain for a week, described as stabbing, worsened by inspiration and lying down, and relieved by sitting and leaning forward. The chest pain was preceded by cough, fever, and myalgia, which have now subsided.

General physical examination was unremarkable, and vitals were normal. Cardiovascular system examination revealed normal S1 and S2 heart sounds, with scratchy sounds heard in both systole and diastole, best heard in the parasternal area and accentuated in the sitting and leaning forward positions.

ECG showed diffuse concave upward ST-segment elevation, PR depression, and PR elevation in aVR (augmented vector right). CBC and BMP were normal, while troponins were not elevated. Erythrocyte sedimentation rate (ESR) was 75 mm/h, and C-reactive protein (CRP) was 4 mg/dL. Transthoracic echocardiography showed a moderate pericardial effusion with right atrial (RA) diastolic collapse but without right ventricular (RV) diastolic collapse. Transmitral pulse wave Doppler study showed E-wave velocity of 10 cm/s and A-wave velocity of 8 cm/s during inspiration, and 12 and 10 cm/s, respectively, during expiration. The inferior vena cava measured 2 cm in diameter with more than 50% inspiratory collapse. Which of the following is the next **BEST** step in management?

A. Colchicine for 3 months and indomethacin for 2 weeks
B. Pericardiocentesis
C. Steroids
D. Azathioprine
E. Pericardial window

346 A 60-year-old male presented to the emergency room with a 1-month history of progressive dyspnea on exertion, orthopnea, and paroxysmal nocturnal dyspnea. General physical examination is remarkable for jugular venous pressure of 15 cm above the sternal angle and bilateral pitting pedal edema. Cardiovascular system examination was normal, while pulmonary examination revealed normal air entry and bilateral diffuse crackles.

ECG was normal. BMP and CBC were within normal limits, but proBNP was elevated to 1,500 pg/mL. Chest x-ray showed cephalization of pulmonary vessels, interstitial pulmonary infiltrates, and bilateral moderate pleural effusion. Echocardiography showed a dilated LV cavity size with normal wall thickness, reduced systolic function with a calculated ejection fraction of 30%, regional wall motion abnormalities, and grade II diastolic dysfunction. The patient had akinetic basal, mid, and distal anterior and anteroseptal walls, and hypokinetic basal, mid, and distal lateral walls. The inferior and inferolateral walls had normal wall motion.

The patient underwent cardiac catheterization and coronary angiogram, which showed 60% stenosis in the proximal right coronary artery, 90% stenosis in mid-left anterior descending coronary artery with calcification, 70% stenosis in the large first diagonal with calcification, and 70% stenosis in the proximal circumflex artery. A myocardial viability study was considered prior to coronary artery bypass grafting. Which of the following modalities can be used to assess myocardial viability?

A. Low-dose dobutamine stress echocardiography
B. Exercise stress echocardiography
C. Three-dimensional echocardiography
D. Resting two-dimensional echocardiography is a good predictor of myocardial viability.
E. Treadmill stress test

34.7 A 30-year-old female who immigrated from Nigeria presented to the office with complaints of dyspnea on exertion, palpitations, and reduced stamina for about 6 months. Past medical history is unremarkable. General physical examination was normal, and vitals were normal. A cardiovascular system examination revealed normal S1 and S2 heart sounds with a mid-diastolic rumble at the apex.

Chest x-ray showed a dilated right descending pulmonary artery. CBC and BMP were within normal limits, and D-dimer and proBNP were not elevated. ECG showed a normal sinus rhythm with biphasic P waves in V1 and broad and bifid P waves in lead II. Resting two-dimensional transthoracic echocardiography showed a normal LV cavity size and wall thickness, with normal LV systolic and diastolic function. The valvular study was remarkable for moderately thickened mitral valve leaflets without calcification and moderate subvalvular thickening, with a calculated MVA of 1.5 cm^2 by planimetry and pressure half-time method. The mitral valve diastolic gradient was 5 mm Hg. The left atrium was mildly dilated, and the tricuspid, aortic, and pulmonary valves were normal. Pulmonary artery systolic pressure was 30 mm Hg. Which of the following is the next **BEST** step?
A. Perform stress echocardiography and reassess MVA, mean mitral valve diastolic gradient, and pulmonary artery systolic pressure at peak stress.
B. Perform stress echocardiography and assess for diastolic function to evaluate for occult diastolic dysfunction.
C. Consider ventilation-perfusion scan for chronic pulmonary thromboembolic pulmonary hypertension (CTEPH).
D. Proceed with percutaneous valvuloplasty as the patient has symptomatic moderate mitral stenosis.
E. Proceed with mitral valve repair.

34.8 A 50-year-old man with a past medical history of hypertension, hyperlipidemia, and diabetes mellitus is currently undergoing active chemotherapy with a regimen consisting of doxorubicin for Hodgkin lymphoma for the last 3 years. He was referred by his oncologist for the evaluation of his cardiac function. Physical examination was unremarkable. He has received a cumulative doxorubicin dose of 300 mg/m^2 and is being planned for the next cycle. The last transthoracic echocardiography prior to initiation of chemotherapy showed a normal left ventricular systolic function with a calculated LVEF of 60% and a global longitudinal strain of –25%.

ECG was normal. Serum troponin and proBNP were not elevated. Two-dimensional transthoracic echocardiography with strain study was performed. It showed a LVEF of 50%, with normal diastolic function and regional wall motion, and a global longitudinal strain (GLS) of –15%. Which of the following is the next **BEST** step?
A. Initiate carvedilol and enalapril based on echocardiographic findings are suggestive of chemotherapy-induced cardiomyopathy.
B. Consider dexrazoxane for the prevention of doxorubicin-induced cardiomyopathy, as the LVEF is only mildly reduced, suggesting that this may not be chemotherapy-induced cardiomyopathy.
C. Perform cardiac magnetic resonance (CMR) imaging to assess chemotherapy-induced cardiotoxicity, given the echocardiogram shows mildly reduced LV systolic function.
D. Perform a stress echocardiogram to assess for regional wall motion abnormalities.
E. Consider cardiac biopsy for possible cardiotoxicity.

A 30-year-old female with a past medical history of recurrent transient ischemic attacks presented with intermittent chest pain and shortness of breath for 6 months. A review of systems is positive for fever, chronic cough, myalgia, arthralgia, and weight loss. General physical examination is normal. Cardiovascular system examination revealed normal first and second heart sounds with a mid-diastolic murmur at the apex.

CBC and BMP were normal. The chest x-ray was remarkable. A transthoracic echocardiogram followed by a transesophageal echocardiogram was performed (**Figure 34.1**). The patient underwent surgery, and the mass was excised. Gross pathology and histopathology of the specimen are presented (**Figures 34.2 and 34.3**).

Which of the following is the **MOST LIKELY** diagnosis?

A. Thrombus
B. Myxoma
C. Lipoma
D. Leiomyoma
E. Liposarcoma

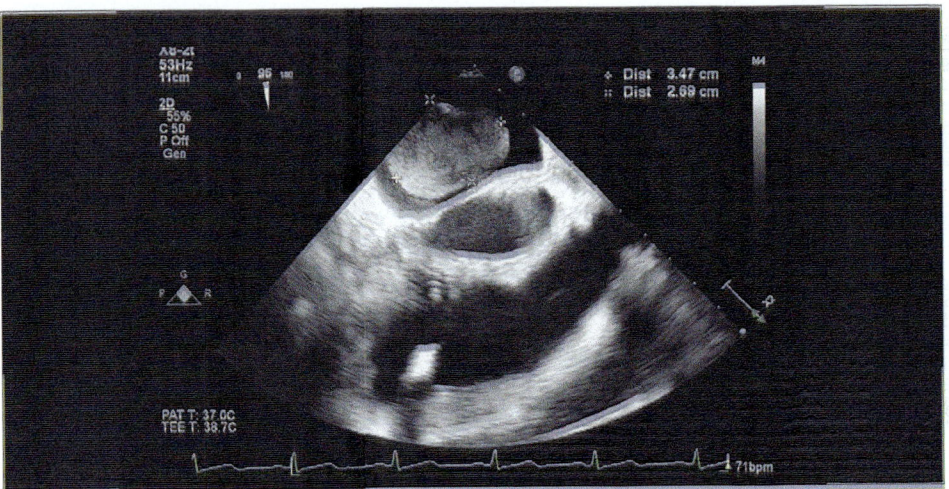

Figure 34.1

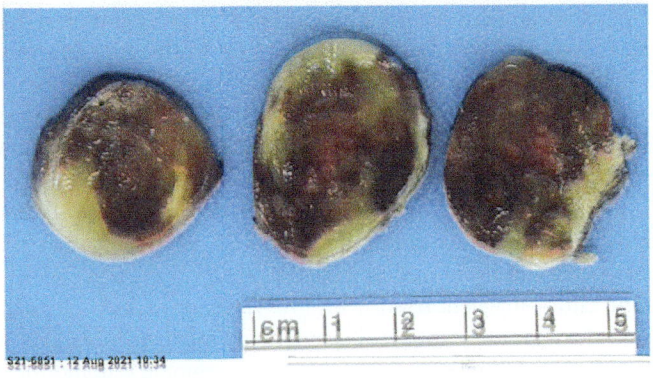

Figure 34.2

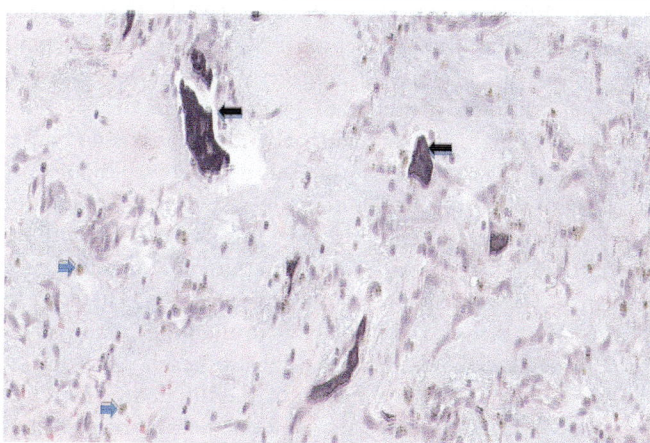

Figure 34.3

34.10 A 60-year-old man with a past medical history of seizure disorder, essential hypertension, paroxysmal atrial fibrillation, diabetes mellitus, and hyperlipidemia presented to the clinic with typical exertional chest pain for 3 months. The patient has cut down his activities due to pain. Vitals were normal. General physical and cardiovascular system examinations were unremarkable.

CBC and BMP were within normal limits. ECG was remarkable for LVH with repolarization abnormalities. The stress test was planned. Which of the following stress test modality is appropriate for this patient?
A. Treadmill stress test
B. Vasodilator nuclear myocardial perfusion imaging using regadenoson and Tc-99m sestamibi
C. Exercise echocardiography
D. Dobutamine stress echocardiography
E. Vasodilator stress echocardiography using dipyridamole

ANSWERS

34.1 The correct answer is A.
Rationale: Increasing the frequency of ultrasound waves enhances axial resolution but reduces depth penetration. Temporal resolution, or frame rate, is the ability to accurately track moving objects over time. It depends on the amount of time needed to complete a scan, which is the function of the ultrasound wave speed, the image depth, and the number of lines of information within the image. Temporal resolution can be increased by narrowing the sector width and imaging at shallower depths.

This is important for structures with high velocity such as valves. It is not dependent on the frequency of the ultrasound probe. M-mode echocardiography has a high temporal resolution of 1,000 to 2,000 images per second. Contrast resolution is the ability to distinguish different shades of gray within the image. This is necessary to differentiate tissue signal from ambient noise, delineate tissue borders, and display texture in the image. Contrast resolution can be improved by pre- and postprocessing of the data as well as the addition of contrast agents. Attenuation is the loss of ultrasound energy by the tissue, leading to a loss in signal strength. Attenuation is a function of ultrasound frequency, with greater attenuation and less penetrance at a higher frequency. The principle of ultrasound imaging is based on the reflection of the transmitted signals from the tissue back to the probe, and images are generated based on the time taken for the reflected signal to reach the probe compared to the incident wave. Reflection is the function of the differences in acoustic impedance between the two tissues as well as the angle of reflection, and not by ultrasound frequency.

KEY POINTS

✔ An increase in the frequency of ultrasound waves enhances axial resolution but at the cost of reduced penetration. Transesophageal echocardiography uses higher frequency ultrasound (12.5-20 MHz), which produces high-resolution images of superficial structures such as the left atrium, left atrial appendage, and mitral valve. However, it may yield lower-resolution images of the apex due to limited penetrance. A lower-frequency transducer for apical views in transthoracic images or larger patients is needed.

34.2 The correct answer is B.
Rationale: This patient is from a tropical region endemic for acute rheumatic fever. She presents with dyspnea on exertion and has a mid-diastolic rumbling murmur at the apex, with calcified leaflets with restricted mobility, thickened leaflets, and chordal fibrosis. The MVA measures 0.8 cm^2, suggestive of severe rheumatic mitral stenosis, with moderate mitral regurgitation and mild pulmonary hypertension, with pulmonary artery systolic pressure of 50 mm Hg. The treatment approach for rheumatic mitral stenosis depends on Wilkin score, the presence of concurrent mitral regurgitation, and the presence of left atrial thrombus. The parameters of Wilkin score are leaflet thickening, mobility, calcification, and subvalvular thickening. With a Wilkin score of 12 and concurrent moderate mitral regurgitation, mitral valve replacement is the preferred option over percutaneous mitral commissurotomy (PTMC). PTMC is reserved for patients with suitable valve anatomy for valvuloplasty (Wilkin score of <8). While mitral valve repair is preferred over replacement whenever feasible, the patient's moderately calcified annulus, along with thickened leaflets with thickened leaflets exhibiting restricted mobility and chordal thickening, suggest poor outcomes with repair. In addition, the patient is not a candidate for anticoagulation therapy, as she does not have left atrial thrombus or atrial fibrillation. Diuretics and beta-blockers are not indicated, as she is neither in congestive heart failure nor atrial fibrillation with tachycardia.

KEY POINTS

- Treatment of severe rheumatic mitral stenosis is guided by the degree of leaflet calcification, mobility, thickening, chordal thickening, concurrent mitral regurgitation, and the presence of left atrial appendage thrombus. Patients with Wilkin score of more than 8 have a better prognosis with mitral valve replacement than PTMC.

34.3 The correct answer is B.

Rationale: This patient has symptoms and signs of severe aortic stenosis, characterized by exertional symptoms and the presence of ejection systolic murmur in the aortic area, along with an absent aortic component of the second heart sound. Assessment reveals severe aortic stenosis with an AVA of 0.8 cm² based on the continuity equation and a DI (LVOT VTI/AV VTI; ratio of the velocity time integral [VTI] of the left ventricular outflow tract [LVOT] to the VTI of the aortic valve [AV]) of 24% (DI <25% qualifies severe aortic stenosis). However, the patient demonstrate moderate aortic stenosis based on peak/mean gradients of 50 mm Hg/30 mm Hg. Given the moderately reduced LVEF of 35%, the possibility of pseudo-severe aortic stenosis (*criteria* for severe aortic stenosis due to incomplete aortic valve opening *related* to reduced myocardial contractility which improves with an augmentation of myocardial contractility) and low-flow, low-gradient severe aortic stenosis is considered. Aortic valve gradients are flow-dependent, and flow is the function of myocardial contractility. To differentiate between these conditions, a low-dose dobutamine stress test is recommended. During low-dose dobutamine stress test echocardiography, in pseudo-severe aortic stenosis, AVA and stroke volume increase without altering mean and peak gradients, whereas in low-flow, low-gradient severe aortic stenosis, stroke volume, peak, and mean gradients increase without changing AVA. This patient indeed has severe calcific aortic stenosis and needs aortic valve replacement, but true aortic valve gradients and the area should be obtained by low-dose dobutamine stress echocardiography by differentiating low-flow, low-gradient aortic stenosis from pseudo-severe aortic stenosis before proceeding to intervention. Percutaneous aortic valve valvuloplasty is inferior to aortic valve replacement in terms of longevity and prognosis. TAVR is considered once severe aortic stenosis is diagnosed. This requires further workup with computed tomography (CT) angiography of the aorta, iliac system, and femoral arteries, as well as cardiac catheterization. Enough data are not available to compare the efficacy and long-term prognosis between surgical aortic valve replacement and TAVR. Severe symptomatic aortic stenosis requires intervention, and expectant management with repeat echocardiography in 6 months is not correct. Severe asymptomatic aortic stenosis can be followed by repeat echocardiography in 6 months.

KEY POINTS

- Aortic valve gradients are flow-dependent, and flow is dependent on LV contractility. In patients with LV systolic dysfunction and severe aortic stenosis, based on a severely reduced AVA calculated by the continuity equation but without gradients within the range of severe aortic stenosis, low-dose dobutamine stress echocardiography can help obtain true aortic valve gradients by improving contractility.

34.4 The correct answer is A.

Rationale: Infective endocarditis is a likely diagnosis in this patient presenting with fever for a month, leukocytosis, *S. aureus* bacteremia, and a new tricuspid regurgitation murmur. This patient has a high pretest probability of infective endocarditis. Transesophageal echocardiography has high sensitivity in diagnosing the complications of infective endocarditis such as abscesses, fistula formation, and perforation. Transthoracic echocardiography has a sensitivity of about 70% for diagnosing infective endocarditis. About 15% of patients with normal transthoracic echocardiography and *S. aureus* bacteremia have vegetations detectable by transesophageal echocardiography. Transthoracic echocardiography with contrast is used to diagnose LV masses, aneurysms, pseudoaneurysms, thrombi, and wall motion abnormalities, particularly when endocardial borders are not clear due to body habitus or position. Cardiac CT is not the first line of investigation for the workup of infective endocarditis due to poor temporal resolution.

KEY POINTS

✔ Transesophageal echocardiography is done when there is a high pretest probability of infective endocarditis, like in patients with *S. aureus* bacteremia, fungemia, or prosthetic valve.

34.5 The correct answer is A.

Rationale: This patient likely presents with acute viral pericarditis, characterized by chest pain worsening by lying down and relieved by sitting or leaning forward, as well as by a friction rub more prominent during sitting or leaning forward. These classical symptoms of acute pericarditis are further supported by classical ECG changes, elevated inflammatory markers, and moderate pericardial effusion observed on transthoracic echocardiography. The treatment for acute pericarditis involves colchicine for 3 months and indomethacin for 2 weeks. This patient does not have cardiac tamponade. Mitral inflow velocity change in inspiration and expiration is 20% (14 − 12/10) × 100% = 20%. Respirophasic mitral inflow variation of 25% or more is consistent with tamponade physiology. Systolic RA collapse more than 1/3 systole has a sensitivity of 94% and specificity of 100% for the diagnosis of tamponade and not diastolic collapse. The presence of RV diastolic collapse is less sensitive (60%-90%) but more specific (85%-90%) for tamponade than brief RA systolic inversion. Normal-sized inferior vena cava has a high negative predictive value for pericardial tamponade. Steroids and azathioprine are not the first-line drugs for pericarditis. Steroids are proven to cause recurrent pericarditis and hence are not the first-line therapy for acute pericarditis. A pericardial window is indicated in malignant pericardial effusion.

KEY POINTS

✔ The treatment for the first episode of idiopathic or viral acute pericarditis or recurrent pericarditis involves indomethacin 50 mg every 8 hours for 15 days along with colchicine. A loading dose of colchicine followed by a maintenance dose for 3 months for the initial episode and 6 months for recurrent pericarditis have proven to have good outcomes. Pericardial effusion due to acute pericarditis but without tamponade physiology should be medically managed with serial monitoring of ESR and CRP, and not with pericardiocentesis.

34.6 The correct answer is A.

Rationale: Low-dose dobutamine stress echocardiography, vasodilator myocardial perfusion imaging with single-photon emission computed tomography (SPECT) Tc-99m sestamibi scan, CMR imaging, thallium-201 stress and redistribution SPECT scan, and ^{18}F-fluorodeoxyglucose positron emission tomography (^{18}F-FDG PET) scan are the modalities used to assess myocardial viability. Viable myocardium, either stunned or hibernating myocardium, has the potential for recovery after revascularization. Distinguishing viable from nonviable myocardium in patients with resting LV dysfunction or chronic total occlusion of the epicardial coronary arteries is important prior to revascularization. The principle behind the low-dose dobutamine stress echocardiography in viability study is that the viable myocardium will have augmentation in contractility with an incremental dose of dobutamine in response to beta-adrenergic stimulation. The classic biphasic response with augmentation in contractility with a low dose followed by worsening at high-dose dobutamine infusion has high predictive value for functional recovery after revascularization. Exercise stress echocardiography helps identify reversible ischemia based on wall motion abnormalities at peak stress and prognosticate coronary artery disease (CAD) based on Duke Treadmill score. Three-dimensional echocardiography is useful in the accurate assessment of chamber volumes as well as the study of valvular anatomy and pathology prior to intervention. It has no use in myocardial viability assessment. Resting echocardiograms have some role in predicting myocardial viability, but with low sensitivity and specificity. Severe wall motion abnormalities, dyskinesia, and thin and scarred myocardium are predictors of nonviable myocardium. A treadmill stress test is used in patients with typical chest pain and a low pretest probability of CAD to assess patients for CAD. It assesses myocardial ischemia based on ST-segment changes (horizontal or downsloping ST depression >2 mm) when the patient is made to exercise to the maximum achievable workload and target heart rate. It is not used for viability assessment.

KEY POINTS

✔ Low-dose dobutamine echocardiography is used for the assessment of myocardial viability in patients with resting LV myocardial dysfunction prior to coronary intervention. Biphasic response with augmentation in contractility with low dose followed by deterioration with high-dose dobutamine infusion is suggestive of viable myocardium and predictive for functional recovery after revascularization.

34.7 The correct answer is A:

Rationale: This patient presents with symptomatic moderate mitral stenosis based on MVA and transmitral gradient, probably due to rheumatic mitral valve disease. The gradient measured at rest is unimpressive. The physiologic impact of mitral stenosis can be studied by measuring the transmitral gradient with exercise. Exercise increases the heart rate, which shortens the diastolic filling time and increases transmitral gradients. Doppler study can be used to study tricuspid regurgitation at exercise and assess exercise-induced pulmonary hypertension. This information obtained at peak exercise can be used to establish the physiologic relation between mitral valve disease and symptoms. This patient has moderate mitral stenosis at rest, and, hence, stress echocardiography is used to measure transmitral gradient and tricuspid regurgitation at stress and assess for exercise-induced pulmonary hypertension and study the physiologic impact of mitral stenosis. The study of exercise-induced diastolic dysfunction is not indicated as the patient has a normal LV systolic and diastolic function at rest. Her symptoms are from rheumatic mitral stenosis and not diastolic dysfunction. Although the finding of dilated right descending pulmonary artery in chest x-ray may suggest pulmonary hypertension, normal serum D-dimer level, and normal resting systolic pulmonary make CTEPH an unlikely diagnosis. Percutaneous valvuloplasty or open mitral valve repair is indicated only after the physiologic relationship between severe mitral stenosis and symptoms is established by stress echocardiography in patients with resting moderate mitral stenosis.

KEY POINTS

- ✓ Exercise echocardiography with the measurement of transmitral gradient and pulmonary artery systolic pressure at peak exercise is indicated when the clinical presentation is disproportionate to the degree of mitral stenosis in resting echocardiography. Exercise increases the heart rate, shortens the diastolic filling time, and increases transmitral gradient, thus establishing the association between mitral valve disease and exertional symptoms.

34.8 The correct answer is A:

Rationale: The 2014 imaging expert consensus statement defines cardiomyopathy related to cancer treatment as a reduction in LVEF by 10% or more from baseline to less than 53%. Subclinical LV dysfunction is defined as a reduction in GLS by more than 15% from baseline. In this patient, chemotherapy-induced cardiomyopathy is evident as there was a decrease in LVEF from 60% to 50% (reduction of 16%) and a decrease in GLS from −25% to −15% (reduction of 40%). For patients in asymptomatic stage B heart failure, the 2013 heart failure guidelines recommend angiotensin-converting enzyme inhibitors (Class 1, level of evidence A) and beta-blockers (Class I, level of evidence C). Dexrazoxane is a cardioprotectant and acts by binding and inhibiting iron-mediated oxygen free radicals, which are responsible for anthracycline-induced cardiomyopathy. It is recommended for the prevention of anthracycline-induced LV dysfunction. CMR imaging is not used for the assessment of chemotherapy-induced cardiomyopathy. A stress echocardiogram to evaluate regional wall motion abnormalities is used for the assessment of CAD in patients with typical chest pain and having a moderate to high pretest probability of CAD. A cardiac biopsy is indicated for the definite diagnosis of cardiac neoplasms, amyloidosis, sarcoidosis, and evaluation of rejection after cardiac transplant, and not chemotherapy-induced cardiomyopathy.

KEY POINTS

✔ Adriamycin and trastuzumab are known to cause cardiotoxicity, and serial echocardiography or a multigated acquisition (MUGA) nuclear scan of the left ventricle is indicated for monitoring chemotherapy-induced cardiomyopathy in patients on these medications. Dexrazoxane is used for the prevention of anthracycline-induced cardiomyopathy. Angiotensin-converting enzyme inhibitor (ACEI) and beta-blockers are indicated for the treatment of chemotherapy-induced cardiomyopathy, as they are cardioprotective and prevent a decline in LV function.

34.9 The correct answer is B.

Rationale: This patient presents with the classical symptom triad of myxoma, with systemic embolic manifestations in the form of transient ischemic attack (TIA), intracardiac obstructive manifestations like dyspnea on exertion, and a mid-diastolic murmur in the apex due to dynamic mitral valve obstruction by the mass. Constitutional symptoms like fever, arthralgia, and weight loss are also present. Myxoma is the most common tumor located in the left atrium and is attached to the interatrial septum by a stalk. The initial transthoracic echocardiogram provides clues to the diagnosis, but a transesophageal echocardiogram has higher sensitivity and helps assess the site of attachment, mobility, and concurrent involvement of the other chambers, as well as study gross pathologic features like hemorrhage and calcification. Multimodality imaging like CMR, cardiac CT, and transcutaneous biopsy are not required for diagnosing typical myxoma. In the transesophageal echocardiogram short-axis view at the aortic valve, a well-circumscribed mass is visible in the left atrium (**Figures 34.1 and 34.4**). Typical gross pathologic features include calcification, necrotic foci, and intratumoral hemorrhage (**Figure 34.2**). High-magnification histopathologic examination reveals Gamna-Gandy bodies and hemosiderin-laden macrophages (**Figure 34.3**, dark and blue arrows, respectively). Although thrombus may also be commonly present in the left atrium, it is less commonly seen in patients in sinus rhythm. Unlike myxoma, a lipoma is well-circumscribed and encapsulated and lacks hemorrhage and necrosis. Liposarcoma is commonly seen in the pericardium, and not the left atrium. Leiomyoma is a tumor of smooth muscle that is not primarily associated with the heart (**Figure 34.4**).

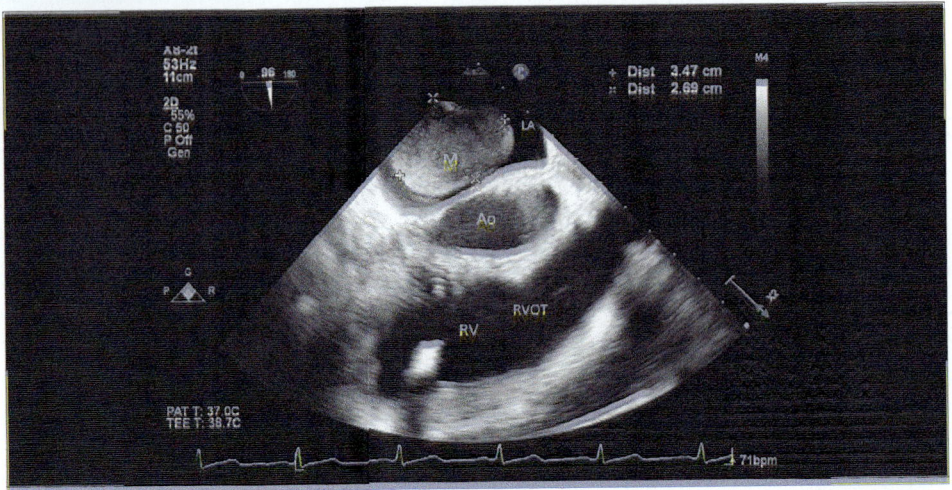

Figure 34.4 Ao, aortic valve; LA, left atrium; M, mass; RV, right ventricle; RVOT, right ventricular outflow tract.

The correct answer is C.

Rationale: This patient presents with a moderate pretest probability of CAD and typical chest pain, indicating the need for a stress test to assess for CAD. Stress echocardiography has a sensitivity of 80% to 85% and a specificity of 80% to 88%. The advantage of exercise echocardiography over the other stress test modalities is the visual determination of wall motion abnormalities and LV cavity dilatation, assessing the functional status, blood pressure, and heart rate response. Hence, stress echocardiography is always preferred over other modalities unless contraindicated (left bundle branch block [LBBB], paced rhythm, patients who cannot run due to joint diseases). During the test, images are obtained at baseline, and the patient is subjected to a treadmill test according to multistage Bruce protocol. Each stage lasts 3 minutes, with assessment of heart rate, blood pressure, and ECG responses. Stress images are obtained at the maximum tolerated stress level and during recovery. For diagnostic purposes, the target heart rate (85% of the maximum age-predicted heart rate) should be achieved prior to obtaining stress images. If the target heart rate is not achieved, or images are obtained below it, the test is labeled as submaximal. A positive test is indicated by the presence of wall motion abnormalities in at least one LV segment and LV dilatation at stress. The treadmill test is suitable for patients with a low pretest probability of CAD. Vasodilator regadenoson Tc-99m sestamibi scan is contraindicated as the patient has a history of seizure disorder. Dobutamine stress echocardiography is also contraindicated due to a history of atrial fibrillation. Functional status assessment and risk stratification with Duke Treadmill score cannot be done with dobutamine stress echocardiography and regadenoson Tc-99m sestamibi scan. Vasodilator stress echocardiography utilizes the coronary steal phenomenon to demonstrate wall motion abnormalities as it lowers the peripheral vascular resistance and venous return to selectively reduce perfusion in the segments supplied by the diseased coronary artery. It has a low sensitivity and high specificity and is not used.

KEY POINTS

✔ Patients with a moderate pretest probability of CAD should undergo an exercise echocardiogram to assess for CAD. Images are obtained at baseline, peak exercise, and during recovery. Images are compared for wall motion abnormalities and LV cavity dilatation. The advantages for exercise echocardiogram include its high sensitivity and specificity for diagnosing CAD, its ability to prognosticate using Duke Treadmill score, its capacity to assess functional status, and its capability to visualize wall motion abnormalities, distinguishing it from other stress test modalities.

NUCLEAR CARDIOLOGY AND MOLECULAR IMAGING

Bilal Talha and Alisha Khan

CHAPTER 35

QUESTIONS

35.1 A 41-year-old male with type 2 diabetes (recently diagnosed), 5-year smoking history, social alcohol use, and right leg amputee after a motor vehicle accident presents for evaluation of chest pain while he was doing some yard work. He describes his chest pain as left sided, usually aggravated by exercise and occasionally occurring at rest as well. There is no family history of premature coronary artery disease (CAD). You are considering myocardial perfusion imaging (MPI) to diagnose underlying CAD rather than a treadmill stress echocardiogram. Which of the following patients would benefit the most from MPI?

A. A patient with high pretest probability
B. A patient with intermediate pretest probability
C. A patient with low pretest probability
D. A patient with very low pretest probability

35.2 A 63-year-old male with obesity, poorly controlled type 2 diabetes, 50-pack-year smoking history, and rheumatoid arthritis presents for evaluation of chest pain that has been ongoing for 1 month. Chest pain is described as typical, worse with exertion, and resolves with rest and nitroglycerin. You have ordered a pharmacologic stress test on this patient with regadenoson as opposed to dipyridamole or adenosine. What receptor does regadenoson work on primarily as opposed to the other two agents?

A. A_1
B. A_{2A}
C. A_{2B}
D. A_3

35.3 A 30-year-old African American female is undergoing testing after she presented with fatigue and weight loss. Her chest x-ray revealed bilateral hilar lymphadenopathy. She underwent lymph node biopsy and was diagnosed with sarcoidosis. Subsequently, she was started on steroids and her symptoms improved significantly. Today, she presents to the emergency department with syncope. The electrocardiogram (ECG) shows second-degree atrioventricular (AV) block and concern for cardiac sarcoidosis is raised. Patient is hesitant to undergo another biopsy but is agreeable with pursuing imaging. Which of the following nuclear imaging studies would you choose?

Questions and Answers are based on Chapter 35: Nuclear Cardiology and Molecular Imaging by Sean R. McMahon, Josiah Bote, and William Lane Duvall in Cardiovascular Medicine and Surgery, First Edition.

A. ^{18}F-fluorodeoxyglucose positron emission tomography (^{18}F-FDG PET)
B. Technetium pyrophosphate (^{99m}Tc-PYP)
C. I-metaiodobenzylguanidine (^{123}I-*m*IBG) D. Single-photon emission computed tomography (SPECT) scan

35.4 A 33-year-old female with sarcoidosis has had a complicated disease course. She was initially asymptomatic and diagnosed incidentally; however, she developed ventricular arrhythmia and had a syncopal event. She then underwent extensive workup including lymph node biopsy, cardiac magnetic resonance imaging (MRI), and endomyocardial biopsy and was diagnosed with cardiac sarcoidosis. She was started on steroids and her symptoms have resolved. Which of the following tests can be used to monitor response to immunosuppressive therapy?

A. ^{18}F-FDG PET
B. ^{99m}Tc-PYP
C. ^{123}I-*m*IBG
D. SPECT scan

35.5 A 52-year-old male with past medical history significant for intravenous drug use (IVDU) complicated by mitral valve (MV) endocarditis requiring prosthetic MV placement presents to the emergency department with persistent fever for the past 3 days. His symptoms initially started with night sweats, shivers, and shakes accompanied by fevers. On further questioning, he admits to spending time with a new girl who has been pressuring him to experiment with a new drug on the market. Vital signs on presentation include a temperature of 38.1 °C, BP 90/62 mm Hg, pulse 112, and respiratory rate (RR) of 20. Physical examination is significant for diffuse sweating with warm skin. Blood cultures are positive for *Staphylococcus aureus*. He was started on vancomycin; however, his repeat culture results continue to stay positive 8 days into his admission. He undergoes transthoracic echocardiogram (TTE), which is negative for endocarditis, followed by transesophageal echocardiogram (TEE), which is not able to isolate a lesion. MRI of his entire spine is also negative for abscess or source of infection. Which of the following nuclear imaging choices would benefit in isolating the infectious source in this patient?

A. ^{18}F-FDG PET
B. ^{99m}Tc-PYP
C. ^{123}I-*m*IBG
D. SPECT scan

35.6 Which of the following is not an indication of ^{123}I-*m*IBG imaging?

A. Monitoring for cardiac toxicity in a patient receiving doxorubicin for breast cancer
B. A patient with long-standing diabetes mellitus complaining of jumping heart rates and orthostatic hypotension
C. Further evaluation of a patient noted to have Brugada sign on ECG
D. Predicting survival in a patient with congestive heart failure (CHF) with shortness of breath and palpitations at rest

35.7 A 60-year-old woman with breast cancer receiving trastuzumab as a part of her treatment regimen complains of increasing fatigue and dyspnea on exertion. She is referred for equilibrium radionuclide angiography (ERNA) to reassess her cardiac function. Which of the following methods results in the highest labeling efficiency?

A. The in vitro method
B. The in vivo method
C. The modified in vivo method
D. Direct intravenous injection of ^{99m}Tc

35.8 A 65-year-old African American male with a past medical history of heart failure with preserved ejection fraction, left ventricular (LV) hypertrophy and bilateral carpal tunnel syndrome is being evaluated for suspected amyloidosis. The patient arrives in the nuclear medicine department for a ^{99m}Tc-PYP scan. Which of the following statements is correct?

A. The patient cannot undergo the test at this time as he is not in a fasting state.
B. Due to the 100% specificity of the scan in identifying transthyretin amyloidosis (ATTR), a heart-to-contralateral ratio of 2 confirms the diagnosis of ATTR.
C. The patient will need to undergo imaging at 1 and 3 hours.
D. SPECT imaging must be performed if there is radiotracer uptake on planar images.

35.9 Which of the following statements pertaining to the metabolism of cells is **INCORRECT**?

A. Diseased myocardium is adapted to predominantly utilizing glucose as its energy source.
B. Healthy myocardium can shift between utilizing fatty acids or glucose.
C. In PET sarcoid studies, a special diet is used to enhance healthy myocyte metabolism of carbohydrates while suppressing uptake of fatty acids, thus favoring ^{18}F-FDG uptake to active inflammatory cells.
D. In PET viability studies, myocyte metabolism of glucose over fatty acids is preferred to maximize ^{18}F-FDG uptake in the myocardium.

35.10 In which patient would stress myocardial perfusion **NOT** be contraindicated?

A. A pregnant woman who presents with epigastric pain
B. A man who presented with chest pain, ST depressions on ECG and an elevated troponin value 4 days ago
C. A patient with diffuse wheezing and tachypnea on physical examination
D. A patient who was recently found to have second-degree Mobitz type 2 on recent ECG and is awaiting pacemaker placement

ANSWERS

35.1 The correct answer is B.
Rationale: A pretest probability of greater than 90% is defined as high, 10% to 90% as intermediate, less than 10% as low, and less than 5% as very low. Anyone with low pretest probability (<10%) likely does not have CAD, whereas anyone with high (>90%) very likely has CAD and perfusion imaging will likely not alter posttest

probability, with the downside of exposing the individual to unneeded radiation. Patients with high pretest probability will likely require intervention but their clinical picture can dictate whether this is done acutely or electively. MPI is reserved for patients with intermediate pretest probability (10%-90%) as the yield of the test and its effect on patient management will be highest in this group.

KEY POINTS

- ✔ MPI is most useful in patients with intermediate pretest probability (10%-90%) to evaluate for symptoms of CAD.

35.2 The correct answer is B.

Rationale: Options for pharmacologic stress testing include adenosine, dipyridamole, and regadenoson. These are coronary vasodilators that can be used for pharmacologic stress testing in patients who are unable to undergo exercise stress testing. Adenosine and dipyridamole are nonselective adenosine agonists that activate A_1, A_{2A}, A_{2B}, and A_3 receptors, whereas regadenoson primarily works on the A_{2A} receptor, resulting in fewer side effects of vasodilation such as flushing and hypotension. Dobutamine can also be used to increase myocardial work by stimulating beta-1 and beta-2 receptors. The result is similar to exercise stress with increased myocardial blood flow in the coronary arteries.

KEY POINTS

- ✔ Adenosine and dipyridamole are nonselective adenosine agonists that activate A_1, A_{2A}, A_{2B}, and A_3 receptors, whereas regadenoson primarily works on the A_{2A} receptor, resulting in fewer side effects of vasodilation such as flushing and hypotension.

35.3 The correct answer is A.

Rationale: FDG PET can be used to image inflammation in sarcoidosis because glucose metabolism is increased in inflammatory cells such as the macrophages in sarcoid granulomas. However, in order to diagnose cardiac sarcoidosis, diagnostic lab work is also needed.

^{99m}Tc-PYP scan is usually reserved for workup of amyloidosis, specifically wild-type transthyretin amyloidosis (wtATTR) and hereditary transthyretin amyloidosis (mATTR). *m*IBG can isolate sympathetic innervation and when directed toward cardiac causes, can identify cardiac neuropathies, diabetes with autonomic neuropathies, and many more. One- and two-day SPECT scans are mostly employed in the setting of evaluating for CAD.

KEY POINTS

- ✔ FDG PET can be used to image the inflammation in sarcoidosis because glucose metabolism is increased in inflammatory cells such as the macrophages in sarcoid granulomas.

35.4 The correct answer is A:

Rationale: Cardiac PET metabolic imaging with ^{18}F-FDG is used for imaging the initial steps of glucose metabolism in cardiac tissue. It works by taking advantage of glucose analogue (deoxyglucose), which becomes trapped intracellularly after undergoing initial phosphorylation and allows for identification of metabolically active or hyperactive cells. It is a great modality of choice in someone who has been diagnosed with cardiac sarcoidosis and is on immunosuppressive therapy to monitor clinical response. In serial assessments by FDG PET, a reduction in ^{18}F-FDG uptake in patients on immunosuppression is associated with improvement in LV systolic function and reduction in ventricular arrhythmia.

^{99m}Tc-PYP is used in the diagnosis of cardiac amyloid. ^{123}I-*m*IBG is indicated for the assessment of sympathetic innervation and can be used for innervation studies including cardiac toxicities secondary to chemotherapy, cardiac neuropathies, diabetes with autonomic neuropathies, and many more. SPECT is most frequently employed in a single-day, rest-stress study.

KEY POINTS

✔ FDG PET imaging may be clinically useful for the investigation of suspected cardiac sarcoidosis or as a method of monitoring response to therapy in patients with known cardiac sarcoidosis and on immunosuppressive therapy.

35.5 The correct answer is A:

Rationale: FDG PET can be used for imaging infection because both activated immune cells and bacteria at the site of infection utilize large quantities of glucose, allowing for localization. FDG PET has shown the greatest promise in the diagnosis of prosthetic valve endocarditis, with sensitivities between 73% and 100% and specificity of 71% to 100% per some literature.

KEY POINTS

✔ PET infection studies are assessed visually with regions of abnormal FDG uptake. Once increased uptake is noted, CT scan acquired as part of the PET/CT study can then be used to anatomically localize the areas of increased tracer uptake. Prosthetic valves, pacemaker wires and generators, and left ventricular anterior descending (LVAD) components can all be identified on the CT images as a site of infection or extracardiac locations of injection or embolization can be seen.

35.6 The correct answer is D:

Rationale: Monitoring cardiac toxicity from chemotherapy, investigating patients with diabetes for autonomic dysfunction and identifying patients with increased risk of cardiac arrhythmias are some of the common indications for performing ^{123}I-*m*IBG imaging.

In addition, ^{123}I-mIBG imaging is used to evaluate primary cardioneuropathies, assess pre- and postcardiac transplant patients and assess the risk of ischemic heart disease.

^{123}I-mIBG imaging has been studied to predict survival (ie, 1- and 2-year mortality risk) in patients with New York Heart Association (NYHA) class II and III heart failure with an ejection fraction of less than 35% using the heart-to-mediastinum ratio (HMR). An HMR of less than 1.6 was shown to be associated with increased likelihood of worsening NYHA class, life-threatening arrhythmias, and cardiac death.

KEY POINTS

✓ ^{123}I-mIBG is indicated for the assessment of cardiac neuronal dysfunction even in the absence of structural abnormalities.

35.7 The correct answer is A.

Rationale: Red blood cells need to be labeled with ^{99m}Tc when performing ERNA. For radioactive labeling, the red blood cells must first be combined with stannous pyrophosphate in order to facilitate binding of ^{99m}Tc to the red cells. The stannous pyrophosphate acts as a reducing agent. The ^{99m}Tc can then be labeled onto the red blood cells using the in vitro, in vivo, or modified in vivo methods.

Direct intravenous injection of ^{99m}Tc is not a valid method of labeling red blood cells as stannous pyrophosphate must be used as a reducing agent for the labeling to be effective.

KEY POINTS

✓ The in vitro method has the highest labeling efficiency, followed by the modified in vivo method, and lastly by the in vivo method.

35.8 The correct answer is D.

Rationale: No specific patient preparation is required for a ^{99m}Tc-pyrophosphate scan when assessing for amyloidosis. Following a special or restricted diet or presenting in a fasting state is not required.

In order to confirm the diagnosis of ATTRs, light chain amyloidosis (AL) must be excluded using serum and urine immunofixation and a serum free light chain assay in all patients referred for a ^{99m}Tc-PYP scan irrespective of the scan results.

After injection of 10 to 20 mCi of ^{99m}Tc-PYP at rest, imaging should be performed 1 hour later. Additional imaging at 3 hours is only required if excess blood pool activity is noted on the 1-hour images.

If planar images suggest myocardial uptake, SPECT images must be reviewed to confirm myocardial uptake as they provide better spatial resolution. The diagnostic standard is diffuse uptake on SPECT.

KEY POINTS

✔ Reviewing SPECT images is required when interpreting images with radiotracer uptake. No specific patient preparation is required for a ^{99m}Tc-PYP scan. AL must always be ruled out when evaluating a patient for ATTR. Repeat imaging at 3 hours is not required if there was no blood pool radiotracer uptake on the 1-hour images.

35.9 The correct answer is C.

Rationale: Statements A, B, and D are correct. Statement C should read as, "In PET sarcoid studies, a special diet is used to enhance healthy myocyte metabolism of fatty acids while suppressing uptake of carbohydrates, thus favoring ^{18}F-FDG uptake to active inflammatory cells."

In other words, PET sarcoid studies and PET viability studies differ in their patient preparation protocols in order to achieve different imaging results. In PET sarcoid imaging, the patient is asked to consume a high-fat, high-protein diet for 24 hours while avoiding carbohydrates and followed by a fast. This technique favors uptake of ^{18}F-FDG to cells with active sarcoidosis. On the other hand, in PET viability studies, patients are asked to fast and are then administered an oral glucose load. This technique favors uptake of ^{18}F-FDG to viable myocardium while sparing nonviable myocardium.

KEY POINTS

✔ In PET sarcoid studies, a high-fat, high-protein diet, followed by a fast, is used to enhance healthy myocyte metabolism of fatty acids while suppressing uptake of carbohydrates, thus favoring ^{18}F-FDG uptake to the active inflammatory cells of sarcoidosis.

35.10 The correct answer is B.

Rationale: In pregnant women, alternative imaging modalities should be pursued in order to avoid exposure to radiation and radioactive isotopes. Active bronchospasm as indicated by diffuse wheezing and tachypnea is an absolute contraindication to performing a pharmacologic nuclear stress test. Advanced conduction disease (ie, high-grade AV block or sick sinus syndrome) without an artificial pacemaker is also contraindicated.

The patient in answer choice B presented with a non–ST-elevation myocardial infarction (NSTEMI) 4 days ago. Vasodilator stress testing has been shown to be safe in patients who are greater than 48 hours post a myocardial infarction.

KEY POINTS

✔ Vasodilator stress testing has been shown to be safe in patients who are greater than 48 hours post a myocardial infarction.

CARDIAC COMPUTED TOMOGRAPHY

Alisha Khan and Vishal Phogat

CHAPTER 36

QUESTIONS

36.1 In which of these patients is coronary artery calcium (CAC) testing **NOT** indicated?

   A. A 41-year-old male presents to your clinic for evaluation of sharp chest pain that occurred while he was lifting weights at the gym. His BP in the office is 140/90 mm Hg. Lipid panel reveals a total cholesterol of 260 mg/dL, high-density lipoprotein (HDL) cholesterol of 35 mg/dL, and low-density lipoprotein (LDL) cholesterol of 110 mg/dL. He has a 10 pack-year smoking history but quit smoking 15 years ago. He forgot to take his amlodipine-benazepril this morning. Upon further questioning, he reveals he often does not take his medications as he is worried about the possible side effects, even though he has not experienced anything so far. Based on this information, his current 10-year atherosclerotic cardiovascular disease (ASCVD) risk is 14.5%.

   B. A 53-year-old African American male with a past medical history of hypertension, hyperlipidemia, and depression presents to your clinic as a new patient. His BP is 119/75 mm Hg and pulse is 70 bpm. He is currently taking hydrochlorothiazide and amlodipine for his hypertension. He states he was previously on atorvastatin but it had to be discontinued due to a significant rise in his liver enzymes associated with myalgias. Lipid panel reveals a total cholesterol of 295 mg/dL, HDL cholesterol of 30 mg/dL, LDL cholesterol of 145 mg/dL, and a triglyceride level of 160 mg/dL.

   C. A 40-year-old South Asian female with a recent diagnosis of Crohn disease presents for risk factor management. She is worried about her cardiovascular health as her father had bypass surgery at the age of 56. Her lipid panel is within normal limits.

   D. A 70-year-old female with a past medical history of hypertension, hyperlipidemia, peripheral vascular disease, and type 2 diabetes mellitus presents for follow-up. She is taking telmisartan, amlodipine, aspirin, rosuvastatin, and metformin.

36.2 A 55-year-old male presents to the emergency department (ED) with atypical chest pain of 4-hour duration. His initial troponin, chest x-ray, and electrocardiogram (ECG) are unremarkable. He has had two other ED visits in the past 3 months with similar complaints. A coronary computed tomographic angiography (CCTA) is performed. The CCTA reveals a small amount of noncalcified plaque in the mid-right coronary artery (RCA), resulting in a 40% stenosis. What is the Coronary Artery Disease-Reporting and Data System (CAD-RADS) classification of his lesion?

*Questions and Answers are based on Chapter 36: Cardiac Computed Tomography by Ron Blankstein and Vasvi Singh in Cardiovascular Medicine and Surgery, First Edition.

A. CAD-RADS 0
B. CAD-RADS 2
C. CAD-RADS 4
D. CAD-RADS 5

36.3 A 68-year-old woman presents to the ED with complaints of chest pressure that started 1 hour ago with radiation down the left arm and to the jaw. She has a past medical history of CAD status post placement of a stent in the mid-left anterior descending (LAD), uncontrolled hypertension, and hyperlipidemia. BP is 160/90 mm Hg with a pulse of 90 bpm. Initial troponin results at 12 ng/L (normal <14 ng/L). ECG does not show any ischemic changes. A CCTA is performed in order to evaluate her coronary anatomy. CCTA reveals a 50% lesion in the proximal LAD. CT-FFR (fractional flow reserve) value of 0.72 is obtained. What is the next **BEST** step?

A. Reassurance and no additional cardiac testing
B. Recommend invasive coronary angiography.
C. Recommend nuclear stress test to assess for reversibility.
D. Only offer medical therapy

36.4 Which of the following scenarios would have the highest quality CCTA images?

A. A patient with rate-controlled atrial fibrillation who has overlapping stents in multiple coronary territories presenting with chest pain
B. A patient with a body mass index (BMI) of 53 kg/m² who is in atrial flutter with rapid ventricular response despite receiving beta-blockers in whom a left atrial appendage thrombus needs to be ruled out
C. An older patient with dementia and a BMI of 22 kg/m² who is unable to follow instructions and has an elevated troponin value
D. A patient with a glomerular filtration rate (GFR) of 40 mL/min/1.73 m² who has sinus bradycardia with a heart rate of 55 bpm in whom a cardiac mass is suspected

36.5 A 75-year-old man with a prior history of coronary artery bypass graft (CABG) presents with more frequent episodes of chest pressure over the past 2 weeks. His current medications include aspirin, rosuvastatin, lisinopril, spironolactone, and carvedilol. His ECG, chest x-ray, and high-sensitivity troponin levels are all unremarkable. A CT-FFR is performed to assess his coronary anatomy. A CT-FFR value of 0.9 is noted for a 60% lesion in the distal LAD after the attachment point of the left internal mammary artery (LIMA) graft. What should be done about this new finding?

A. Coronary angiography with revascularization
B. Medical management for CAD and angina
C. Reassurance only
D. Redo CABG

36.6 A 60-year-old male presents to the ED with complaints of substernal chest pressure and dyspnea on exertion for the past 3 days. His symptoms are relieved with rest. An ECG, chest x-ray, and troponin levels are unremarkable. He has no prior history of CAD, but his past medical history includes tobacco use disorder. CCTA is performed shortly thereafter. His CCTA report indicates that he has a CAD-RADS 4 lesion in the RCA. Which of the following options should **NOT** be pursued?

A. Coronary angiography with percutaneous coronary intervention (PCI)
B. Medical management of CAD
C. Symptomatic treatment of angina
D. Reassurance and investigation of alternative causes of chest pressure and dyspnea on exertion

36.7 A 40-year-old female with a past medical history of obesity, hypertension, and gastroesophageal reflux disease (GERD) presents with a substernal burning sensation. She reports longstanding dyspnea on exertion as well as heartburn after eating certain foods. Due to the atypical nature of her symptoms, CCTA was performed. She was found to have a CAC score of 90 and a lesion in the left circumflex artery with a CAD-RADS of 1. What can you recommend on the basis of these results?

A. Statin therapy
B. Aspirin
C. Lifestyle modifications
D. All of the above

36.8 A 32-year-old man with a past medical history of intravenous drug use and esophageal ulcers presents with fevers, night sweats, malaise, and chest discomfort. He is found to be hypotensive and febrile. Blood culture results reveal gram-positive cocci in clusters. A cine-cardiac CT is performed for further evaluation. The finding is shown in **Figure 36.1**.

What pathology can be seen in the cine-cardiac computed tomography (cine-CCT) image (**Figure 36.1**)?

A. Aortic valve calcification
B. Mitral valve endocarditis
C. Aortic valve endocarditis
D. Aortic stenosis

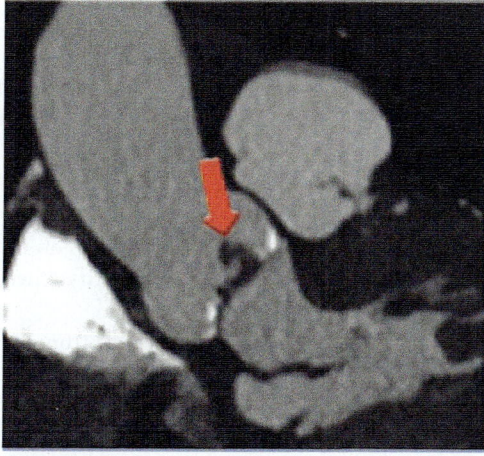

Figure 36.1

36.9 A 38-year-old female with no significant past medical history is coming to establish care. She reports a significant family history of her father passing away from myocardial infarction at the age of 70 years. She is anxious about her risk of sustaining a myocardial infarction herself. She denies any symptoms. Vitals are stable. Physical examination is unremarkable. She requests for a coronary CT to assess her cardiac risk. What would be the most appropriate next step?

A. Order the coronary CT per patient's request.
B. Explain to the patient that CT is not indicated.
C. Order cardiac magnetic resonance (CMR) imaging as there is no risk of radiation.
D. Refer for a diagnostic angiography as it is a more accurate test to assess coronaries.

36.10 A 55-year-old male with a past medical history of CAD, congestive heart failure, atrial fibrillation, and multiple myeloma presents to the clinic for a follow-up. He reports mild intermittent dyspnea upon exertion and chest pain. He heard about a cardiac CT scan from his friend and wants to discuss the role of a cardiac CT scan for his symptoms. CCT can be recommended for evaluation of all of the following **EXCEPT**:

A. Cardiac amyloidosis
B. Severity of aortic stenosis
C. Evaluation of coronary arteries
D. Left atrial appendage thrombus

ANSWERS

36.1 The correct answer is B.
Rationale: The patient in answer choice A would benefit from CAC testing as he is between the age of 40 and 75 with an intermediate 10-year ASCVD risk (ie, a risk of 7.5%-20%). He is also averse to taking certain medications due to fear of side effects; therefore, calculating his CAC score will help counsel the patient.

The patient in answer choice B would benefit from CAC testing as he is statin intolerant given his history of transaminitis after starting a statin in the past. An elevated CAC score will help make the case to start alternative lipid-lowering therapies.

The patient in answer choice C would benefit from CAC testing as she falls in the appropriate age range (ie, between the age of 40 and 75). Although her 10-year ASCVD risk is low based on the ASCVD risk calculator, due to her South Asian ancestry, borderline elevated familial risk, and diagnosis of an inflammatory condition such as Crohn disease, she should be screened to clarify whether statin therapy will be beneficial.

The patient in answer choice D would not benefit from CAC testing as she is an elevated risk patient who is already on a statin for her diabetes mellitus, peripheral arterial disease, and hyperlipidemia. Regardless of the results of the CAC score, she will need to be on a statin for her diabetes and peripheral arterial disease as long as she can tolerate it.

KEY POINTS

✔ CAC testing is indicated in statin-averse and statin-intolerant patients, as well as for screening of lower risk patients with additional traditional and nontraditional risk factors. Using CAC testing in patients younger than 40, high-risk patients, or patients who are on a statin for another diagnosis has limited benefits.

36.2 The correct answer is B.

Rationale: CCTA is indicated in the evaluation of acute chest pain in the ED. CCTA can assist the providers in obtaining a diagnosis and reducing the length of stay in the ED. Not only will CCTA define the coronary anatomy but it will also evaluate for alternative diagnoses such as aortic pathologies, pericardial disease, lung diseases, and musculoskeletal pathologies.

Table 36.1 summarizes the grading scale for stenosis severity according to the recent CAD-RADS 2.0—2022 Coronary Artery Disease-Reporting and Data System.

The updated CAD-RADS classification also introduces P1 to P4 descriptors to indicate increasing severity of plaque burden (**Table 36.2**).

In addition, the updated CAD-RADS classification also includes the modifier "I" to provide an assessment of lesion-specific ischemia using CT-FFR or myocardial CT perfusion (CTP) when these tests are performed (**Table 36.3**).

TABLE 36.1 Coronary Artery Disease-Reporting and Data System Summary

CAD-RADS Classification	Degree of Luminal Diameter Stenosis (%)	Terminology
CAD-RADS 0	0	No visible stenosis
CAD-RADS 1	1-24	Minimal stenosis
CAD-RADS 2	25-49	Mild stenosis
CAD-RADS 3	50-69	Moderate stenosis
CAD-RADS 4	70-99	Severe stenosis
CAD-RADS 5	100	Occluded

TABLE 36.2 P1 to P4 Descriptors

Terminology	Overall Plaque Burden	CAC
P1	Mild amount of plaque	1-100
P2	Moderate amount of plaque	101-300
P3	Severe amount of plaque	301-999
P4	Extensive amount of plaque	>1,000

CAC, coronary artery calcium.

TABLE 36.3 CT-FFR or Myocardial CTP Classification

Terminology	Meaning
I+	CT-FFR or CTP shows lesion-specific ischemia or reversible perfusion defect.
I−	CT-FFR or CTP is negative for lesion-specific ischemia or reversible ischemia.
I±	CT-FFR or CTP is borderline.

CT-FFR, computed tomography fractional flow reserve; CTP, computed tomography perfusion.

KEY POINTS

- Increasing degrees of luminal stenosis correspond to a higher CAD-RADS classification number. The plaque burden in the arteries is denoted with the P1 to P4 modifiers. The "I" modifier indicates the presence or absence of ischemia and reversibility.

36.3 The correct answer is B.
Rationale: This woman with known CAD and history of PCI presents with chest pain concerning for angina. CCTA revealed an intermediate lesion in the proximal LAD, which should be further investigated with CT-FFR. A CT-FFR value of 0.72 is considered hemodynamically significant and has been shown to correlate with findings obtained on an invasive FFR.

KEY POINTS

- A CT-FFR value of greater than 0.8 corresponds to a hemodynamically insignificant lesion in which it is safe to defer coronary revascularization. A CT-FFR value of 0.76 to 0.80 is considered borderline. A CT-FFR value less than 0.75 is considered hemodynamically significant in which coronary angiography should be considered.

36.4 The correct answer is D.
Rationale: CCTA image quality is reduced in patients with an irregular heart rhythm, even if the heart rate is controlled as it can lead to misalignment artifacts. Evaluation of the coronary artery is also limited when high-attenuation objects such as overlapping stents create beam hardening artifacts and scatter.

Patients who are obese with a BMI greater than 40 kg/m^2 have a higher likelihood of nondiagnostic scans, missed diagnoses, and receiving increased radiation doses. Excess adiposity leads to increased noise and beam hardening artifacts. If heart rate cannot be adequately controlled by beta-blockers, motion artifacts and inappropriate gating will negatively affect image quality.

Following instructions is an important factor when undergoing CCT imaging, as being able to perform breath holds and holding still are needed for high-quality images. With improvement in technology, however, the duration of the scan time is getting progressively shorter and easier to perform.

Although CCT is relatively contraindicated in patients with GFR below 30 mL/min/ 1.73 m² due to the risk of contrast-associated nephropathy, image quality is not reduced by this factor alone. A patient with sinus bradycardia already has an ideal heart rate for this test and will not require any further rate-controlling medications prior to the test.

KEY POINTS

- ✔ Image quality is reduced in patients with an irregular rhythm, patients with tachycardia, patients who are obese, and patients who are unable to follow instructions. Image quality is also limited by high-attenuation objects in the field of view.

36.5 The correct answer is B.

Rationale: A CT-FFR value of greater than 0.8 corresponds to a hemodynamically insignificant lesion in which it is safe to defer coronary revascularization with PCI or bypass grafting. Therefore, it would be reasonable to medically manage this patient's CAD and prescribe antianginal medications. However, if symptoms remain uncontrolled on optimized medical therapy, it would be reasonable to pursue coronary angiography.

Reassurance alone would not be sufficient as this patient is not on antianginal medications such as isosorbide mononitrate, ranolazine, or amlodipine, or even a short-acting sublingual nitroglycerin tablet.

KEY POINTS

- ✔ This patient with a CT-FFR value of 0.9 (ie, >0.8) has a hemodynamically insignificant lesion in which it is safe to defer coronary revascularization. A CT-FFR value of less than 0.75 is considered hemodynamically significant in which coronary angiography should be considered, whereas a CT-FFR value of 0.76 to 0.80 is considered borderline.

36.6 The correct answer is D.

Rationale: A CAD-RADS 4 lesion corresponds to an area with severe stenosis, occupying 70% to 99% of the luminal diameter. Obstructive lesions such as these require further intervention. Answer choices A, B, and C are all options that can be pursued.

The ISCHEMIA trial showed that in stable patients with symptomatic CAD, the use of coronary revascularization was not associated with a reduction in the risk of cardiovascular events when compared to optimal medical therapy. Therefore, both coronary angiography and optimal medical management are options.

In addition to medical treatment for CAD, symptomatic treatment of angina using medications such as isosorbide mononitrate, ranolazine, sublingual nitroglycerin, and amlodipine can be implemented. Treatment of angina alone, without medical management of CAD, would not be appropriate.

Reassurance would be inappropriate in this case as significant obstructive pathology has been identified on CCTA. In addition, unless further information is provided, looking for an alternative diagnosis would not be required given this patient's cardiac chest pain and supporting imaging findings.

> **KEY POINTS**
>
> ✓ CAD-RADS 4 corresponds to a severely stenotic lesion occupying 70% to 99% of the luminal diameter. Such lesions in a stable patient can be managed conservatively, with medications, or with invasive coronary angiography and revascularization.

36.7 The correct answer is D.

Rationale: This patient's CAC and CAD-RADS scores are sufficient to diagnose her with nonobstructive CAD. Therefore, she warrants treatment with a statin and aspirin. Both of these will prevent progression of her atherosclerosis, provide plaque stabilization, and even cause plaque regression in some cases.

All patients with CAD also benefit from lifestyle modifications that include diet, exercise, weight reduction, and controlling risk factors such as hypertension, hyperlipidemia, diabetes mellitus, and stress.

> **KEY POINTS**
>
> ✓ The diagnosis of CAD can be established with a CCTA and CAC score. Treatment of CAD warrants treatment with an aspirin, statin, and lifestyle modifications.

36.8 The correct answer is C.

Rationale: The red arrow in **Figure 36.1** points to an aortic valve vegetation. Aortic valve calcification would appear as an area of high attenuation. The area indicated by the red arrow is, however, an area of low attenuation.

The valve represented in the image is the aortic valve and not the mitral valve. This view represents the left ventricular outflow tract and the long axis of the aortic root and ascending aorta.

Aortic stenosis is most commonly accompanied with aortic calcification. Although minimal calcification is seen in this image, the patient's presentation is most consistent with an infective pathology.

Cine-CCT can be useful in evaluating patients with known or suspected endocarditis, especially when an initial evaluation using transthoracic echocardiography is inconclusive, or when transesophageal echocardiography is not feasible, such as in this patient with esophageal ulcers. The cine-CCT has a diagnostic accuracy similar to that of transesophageal echocardiography for detecting vegetations. A unique advantage of cine-CCT over other imaging techniques is the ability to evaluate mechanical valves.

In addition, cine-CCT is well suited for detecting perivalvular involvement, including pseudoaneurysm or fistulas. Accordingly, the current European Society of Cardiology guidelines support the modified Duke Criteria, where the identification of paravalvular involvement by CCT is considered a major criterion toward the diagnosis of infective endocarditis.

KEY POINTS

✔ Cine-cardiac CT can be used to evaluate valvular heart diseases, including evaluation of patients with known or suspected endocarditis. The diagnostic accuracy of cine-CCT is similar to that of transesophageal echocardiography.

36.9 The correct answer is B.

Rationale: Similar to any diagnostic imaging test, CCT should be obtained only in cases where the test results can impact patient management. CAC testing is only useful in patients without known CAD and is of limited value in most individuals younger than 40 years of age. CCTA is most useful in symptomatic individuals who do not have known CAD. CCTA in asymptomatic individuals is generally not recommended, although there are current trials assessing the efficacy of such testing. A particular concern is that testing asymptomatic individuals could lead to unnecessary downstream testing and procedures such as invasive angiography and coronary revascularization.

KEY POINTS

✔ CCTA in asymptomatic individuals is generally not recommended, and could lead to unnecessary testing and procedures such as invasive angiography.

36.10 The correct answer is A.

Rationale: Cardiac CT is not the diagnostic test of choice for infiltrative diseases, such as cardiac amyloidosis. A ^{99m}Tc-pyrophosphate scan and CMR imaging with late gadolinium enhancement imaging would be better imaging studies for the diagnosis of cardiac amyloidosis.

CCT still enables detailed visualization of all cardiac structures, including pericardium, pericardial and epicardial fat, myocardium, coronary arteries and veins, and valves. The strength of CCT is the ability to obtain high spatial resolution images. Accordingly, CCT can provide detailed visualization of coronary artery plaque and stenosis. In addition to evaluation of the coronary arteries, a cine-CCT can be used to obtain information on valvular function, and cardiac morphology, structure, and function.

KEY POINTS

✔ CCT has lower contrast resolution than do other techniques such as CMR imaging. Thus, CCT is not suited for evaluating infiltrative disease of the myocardium.

CARDIAC MAGNETIC RESONANCE IMAGING

Rohan Desai, Bhavi Trivedi, Rakhee Makhija, and Debabrata Mukherjee

CHAPTER 37

QUESTIONS

37.1 A 47-year-old female with no prior medical history presents with pressure-like substernal chest pain persisting for 3 hours. A 12-lead electrocardiogram (ECG) showed ST-segment elevation in inferior leads along with elevated troponin levels. The patient undergoes emergent coronary angiography, which reveals only nonobstructive coronary artery disease (stenosis <50%). Patient's echocardiogram shows normal left ventricular function, and other laboratory results remain unremarkable. Which of the following is the next **BEST** step in management?

  A. Obtain cardiac magnetic resonance (CMR) imaging within 2 weeks.
  B. Discharge with aspirin, $P2Y_{12}$ receptor inhibitor, and statin.
  C. Monitor the intensive cardiac unit and repeat angiography.
  D. Pursue intravascular imaging and assessment of coronary physiology.

37.2 A 40-year-old female with no significant medical history presents with progressive dyspnea on exertion, fatigue, and chest pain persisting for 3 months. She reports no medication use. Physical examination is unremarkable, and laboratory investigations are within normal limits. A 12-lead ECG shows normal sinus rhythm, second-degree heart block, and right bundle branch block. The patient undergoes CMR imaging for further evaluation, which shows patchy areas of subepicardial late gadolinium enhancement (LGE) in the basal septal in noncoronary distribution. Which of the following is the **MOST LIKELY** diagnosis?

  A. Hypertrophic cardiomyopathy (HCM)
  B. Dilated cardiomyopathy
  C. Ischemic heart disease
  D. Sarcoidosis

37.3 A 65-year-old male patient with a recent ST-elevation myocardial infarction (STEMI) 2 weeks ago, treated with percutaneous coronary intervention (PCI) and stent placement, presents with left-sided weakness, difficulty speaking, and confusion. A noncontrast computed tomography (CT) of the head is unremarkable, but a brain magnetic resonance imaging (MRI) indicates concern for an embolic stroke. Contrast-enhanced transthoracic echocardiogram (TTE) showed antero-apical akinesis, though it is inconclusive for excluding a left ventricular apical thrombus due to apex not well seen in the available acoustic windows. What is the **MOST** appropriate next step in the management of this patient?

Questions and Answers are based on Chapter 37: Cardiac Magnetic Resonance Imaging by Louis-Philippe David, Panagiotis Antiochos, and Raymond Y. Kwong in Cardiovascular Medicine and Surgery, First Edition.

A. Repeat TTE in 2 weeks.
B. Obtain transesophageal echocardiogram (TEE).
C. Initiate empiric treatment with anticoagulation.
D. Obtain CMR imaging.

374 A 65-year-old male patient presents with exertional dyspnea and bilateral lower extremity edema. Echocardiogram shows a thickened interventricular septum, while an ECG shows low-voltage QRS complexes. CMR imaging reveals diffuse subendocardial LGE with preserved apical contractility. What is the **MOST LIKELY** diagnosis?

A. HCM
B. Fabry disease
C. Sarcoidosis
D. Amyloidosis

375 A 50-year-old male with uncontrolled hypertension, experiencing paresthesia in hands and feet, decreased hearing, tinnitus, heat intolerance, and small dark red spots on skin, presents with recent-onset dyspnea on exertion. His family history is notable for heart failure in his grandfather. A 12-lead ECG shows a short PR interval. Echocardiography reveals moderate left ventricular hypertrophy, mild diastolic dysfunction, and mild aortic root dilation. CMR imaging reveals concentric increase in left ventricular thickness, mid-myocardial LGE in the basal to mid-inferolateral wall, and shortening of T1 values. What is the **MOST LIKELY** diagnosis?

A. HCM
B. Chagas disease
C. Anderson-Fabry disease (AFD)
D. Sarcoidosis

376 A 35-year-old male with a history of thalassemia major receiving frequent blood transfusion presents with shortness of breath and fatigue. CMR imaging shows evidence of myocardial iron overload with a T2* value of 9 minutes. He is started on chelation therapy. After 6 months of therapy, a follow-up CMR imaging is performed, which shows a T2* value of 15 minutes. Which of the following statements is **MOST ACCURATE** regarding the role of CMR imaging in chelation therapy for siderotic cardiomyopathy?

A. CMR imaging is not useful in monitoring response to chelation therapy.
B. An increase in myocardial T2* relaxation value indicates an improvement in cardiac siderosis.
C. CMR imaging should only be performed before initiating chelation therapy.
D. T1 relaxation time is a more accurate measure of cardiac siderosis after starting chelation therapy.

377 A 25-year-old male, professional cyclist, presents with occasional episodes of palpitations but is otherwise asymptomatic. Physical examination and ECG reveal sinus bradycardia. Echocardiography and CMR imaging show left ventricular wall thickness of 15 mm. The patient is recommended to stop all endurance exercises by his primary care physician until further workup can be obtained. A repeat CMR imaging performed 3 months later shows left ventricular thickness of 15 mm and patchy multifocal mid-wall LGE. What is the **MOST LIKELY** diagnosis?

A. HCM
B. Athlete's heart
C. Arrhythmogenic right ventricular cardiomyopathy (ARVC)
D. Dilated cardiomyopathy

37.8 A 38-year-old male with a history of palpitations presents with syncope while running on a treadmill. His 12-lead ECG shows T-wave inversions in leads V1 to V3 and a small deflection at the end of the QRS complex. Echocardiography shows normal left ventricular size and function, along with mild right ventricular dilatation and dysfunction. CMR imaging shows severe global dilatation of the right ventricle (RV) with severe systolic dysfunction and fatty infiltration. What is the **MOST LIKELY** diagnosis?

A. Dilated cardiomyopathy
B. Hypertrophic cardiomyopathy
C. ARVC
D. Right ventricular outflow tract ventricular tachycardia

37.9 A 35-year-old male patient with no significant medical history presents with sudden left-sided weakness. Brain imaging shows an acute infarct of the right middle cerebral artery territory. An echocardiogram reveals a left ventricular ejection fraction of 30% to 35% with prominent trabeculations and deep recesses suggestive of left ventricular noncompaction cardiomyopathy (LVNC). CMR imaging is ordered to confirm the diagnosis. Which of the following MRI findings **CANNOT** be used to diagnose LVNC?

A. Ratio between noncompacted and compacted myocardium
B. Mass ratio between total and trabeculae mass
C. Quantitative measure of myocardial trabeculae complexity
D. Septal mid-wall LGE

37.10 A 65-year-old male with a history of mitral valve replacement surgery, coronary artery bypass grafting, and right hip replacement presents for a CMR imaging to evaluate myocardial function. Which of the following is a limiting factor that could prevent the patient from undergoing a CMR imaging at a field strength of 2.0 T?

A. Prosthetic heart valve
B. Prosthetic joint
C. Sternal wires
D. No contraindication for CMR imaging

37.11 A 65-year-old male patient with a history of hypertension and dyslipidemia presents to the emergency department with severe chest pain and shortness of breath. He is diagnosed with STEMI and undergoes thrombolytic therapy within 3 hours of symptom onset before being transferred to a tertiary care center. A CMR imaging is performed the following day to assess myocardial salvage. The MRI reveals an area of hypoenhancement on T2-weighted images and hyperenhancement on LGE images. The myocardial salvage index (MSI) is calculated. What is the significance of the MSI in this scenario?

A. It quantifies the proportion of myocardium that can be salvaged after acute myocardial infarction (AMI).
B. It reflects the severity of the AMI.
C. It predicts the likelihood of reperfusion injury.
D. It correlates with the degree of collateral circulation to the infarcted area.

37.12 A 50-year-old male with a history of hypertension and hyperlipidemia presents with chest pain and ST-segment elevation on ECG. He is taken emergently to the cardiac catheterization laboratory where he undergoes successful PCI of the culprit lesion in the left anterior descending artery. CMR imaging is performed 3 days later to assess for myocardial injury, revealing an area of hypoenhancement within the infarcted region. Which of the following **BEST** describes this finding?

A. Myocardial edema
B. Microvascular obstruction
C. Intramyocardial hemorrhage
D. Myocardial scar

ANSWERS

37.1 The correct answer is A.

Rationale: Despite the patient's lack of notable risk factors, the presenting symptoms, ECG changes, and elevated troponin levels raise concern for acute coronary syndrome. However, coronary angiography did not reveal significant stenosis (<50% stenosis). In the setting of normal echocardiography, this raises suspicion for MINOCA (myocardial infarction with nonobstructive coronary arteries). A CMR imaging is recommended for patients with suspected MINOCA to evaluate for coronary microvascular obstruction and noncoronary etiologies such as myocarditis, takotsubo cardiomyopathy, and other cardiomyopathies, preferably within 2 weeks. Reviewing the angiography for missed subtle findings such as plaque, emboli, or dissection is important, and intravascular imaging may be considered to evaluate for spontaneous coronary artery dissection; however, coronary physiologic assessment is not recommended in cases with less than 50% stenotic disease.

KEY POINTS

✓ MINOCA should be suspected in patients meeting AMI criteria, with less than 50% coronary obstruction and no other causes. All patients with suspected MINOCA should ideally undergo CMR imaging for further investigation, preferably within 2 weeks.

37.2 The correct answer is D.

Rationale: CMR imaging or positron emission tomography with fluorodeoxyglucose (PET-FDG) are recommended in cases of suggestive symptoms and ECG findings concerning for sarcoidosis. Although no LGE pattern is specific for sarcoidosis, typically subepicardial and mid-myocardial patchy areas of LGE at the basal septum following a noncoronary distribution are noted. Other common findings include septal thinning or aneurysm development in the left ventricle (LV). Furthermore, on T2-weighted images, hyperintense signal suggests active inflammation and myocardial edema. In contrast, hypertrophic cardiomyopathy is characterized by diffuse hypertrophy of the LV, typically involving the interventricular septum, with or without areas of LGE. Dilated cardiomyopathy is characterized by left ventricular dilatation and reduced ejection fraction, with or without areas of LGE. While coronary artery disease–type LGE can be seen in nearly 50% of patients with sarcoidosis, the pattern described is typical of sarcoidosis rather than ischemic heart disease.

> **KEY POINTS**
>
> ✔ CMR imaging should be obtained in patients with symptoms, ECG, or echocardiography findings suspicious for sarcoidosis. Patchy LGE in a noncoronary distribution is typical; however, it is not specific to cardiac sarcoidosis.

37.3 The correct answer is B.

Rationale: This patient, with ischemic cardiomyopathy with wall motion abnormality, is at an increased risk of developing a left ventricular thrombus, likely resulting in the cardioembolic stroke. TTE is the standard imaging technique for detecting left ventricular thrombus, and the use of contrast enhances its sensitivity. CMR imaging is a validated technique for thrombus detection and is the imaging of choice if an echo with contrast is not diagnostic and there is a high clinical suspicion. The left ventricular apex is typically not well visualized by TEE and is not considered to evaluating apical thrombus. Current guidelines do not recommend empiric treatment without adequate imaging confirmation of left ventricular thrombus.

> **KEY POINTS**
>
> ✔ Left ventricular thrombus should be suspected in patients with AMI with antero-apical akinesis or cardioembolic stroke. Contrast-enhanced TTE has significantly higher sensitivity than noncontrast-enhanced echo. CMR imaging should be pursued if noncontrast-enhanced echo is nondiagnostic but if there is clinical concern.

See also **Table 37.1**

37.4 The correct answer is B.

Rationale: The clinical presentation of exertional dyspnea and lower extremity edema, along with the thickened interventricular septum and low-voltage QRS complexes on the ECG, suggests amyloid cardiomyopathy. Concentric increase in wall thickness with small ventricles and biatrial enlargement are classic CMR imaging findings of cardiac amyloidosis, as seen on echocardiogram. Amyloid proteins infiltrate basal segments, and hence preserved apical contractility is noted in both CMR imaging and strain imaging on TTE ("cherry-on-top" pattern). Since cardiac amyloid infiltrates the interstitium, diffuse subendocardial LGE is noted on CMR imaging, along with abnormal gadolinium kinetics (ie, nulling of myocardium before or at

TABLE 37.1 Clinical Indications for Cardiac Magnetic Resonance (CMR) Imaging

ISCHEMIC HEART DISEASE
Assessment of ventricular volumes, function, and mass
Assessment of myocardial ischemia
Assessment of myocardial infarction
Assessment of myocardial viability
Assessment of ventricular thrombus
Assessment of microvascular obstruction

CARDIOMYOPATHIES
Nonischemic cardiomyopathy
Hypertrophic cardiomyopathy: apical/nonapical
Arrhythmogenic right ventricular cardiomyopathy (dysplasia)
Restrictive cardiomyopathy
Siderotic cardiomyopathy
Left ventricular noncompaction
Cardiac involvement in Anderson-Fabry disease and amyloidosis
Cardiac sarcoidosis
Postcardiac transplantation rejection

MYOCARDITIS

Pericardial Disease
Acute pericarditis
Pericardial effusion
Constrictive pericarditis

ARRHYTHMIAS AND PREVENTION OF SUDDEN CARDIAC DEATH
Pulmonary vein anatomy for management of atrial fibrillation
Atrial function evaluation
Evaluation of patients with ventricular arrhythmias

VALVULAR HEART DISEASE
Quantification of aortic regurgitation
Quantification of mitral regurgitation

CONGENITAL HEART DISEASE
Assessment of shunt size (Q_p/Q_s)
Anomalies of the atria and venous return
Anomalies of the valves
Anomalies of the atria, ventricles, and coronary arteries

ACQUIRED DISEASES OF THE VESSELS
Assessment of acute aortic syndromes
Assessment and follow-up of chronic aortic syndromes
Management of aortic root dilation in patients with bicuspid aortic valve
Follow-up after aortic surgery and evaluation of CMR-compatible stent grafts
Diagnosis and follow-up of thoracic aortic aneurysm in Marfan disease

CHARACTERIZATION OF CARDIAC MASSES

Future Clinical Developments
Atherosclerosis detection
Interventional CMR
Novel contrast agents
Hardware developments (high-field systems)

the same inversion time as the blood pool, and extensive extracellular volume expansion detected by newer T1 mapping techniques). In hypertrophic cardiomyopathy, LGE is patchy and involves the mid-myocardium or epicardium, sparing the sub-endocardium, whereas in Fabry disease, mid-myocardial LGE in the basal to mid-inferolateral wall is typical. Sarcoidosis is characterized by patchy LGE in non-coronary distribution.

KEY POINTS

- ✓ While CMR imaging is neither necessary nor sufficient for establishing the diagnosis of cardiac amyloidosis, it can help differentiate amyloidosis from other cardiomyopathies. Diffuse LGE, abnormal gadolinium contrast kinetics, and expansion of extracellular volume noted on CMR imaging should prompt further workup for cardiac amyloidosis. See also **Figure 37.1**.

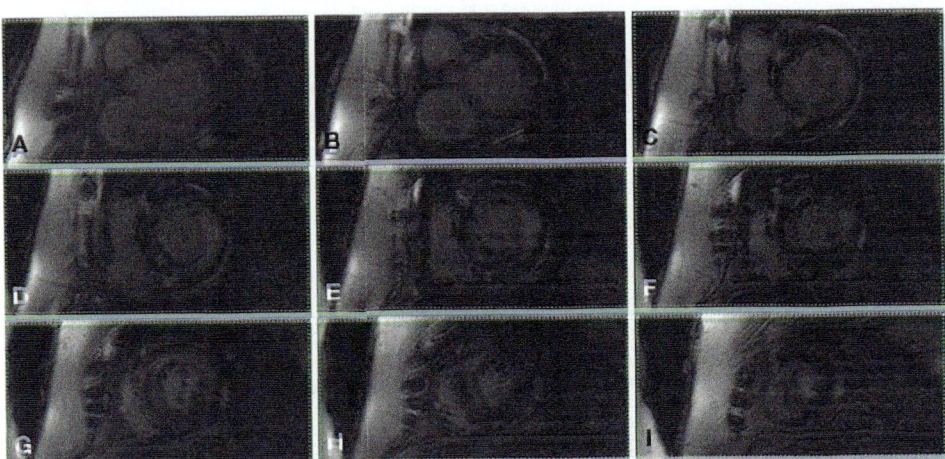

Figure 37.1 Cardiac amyloidosis. Late gadolinium enhancement images of the basal (**A-D**), mid (**E-G**), and apical (**H, I**) left ventricle and right ventricle reveal extensive concentric early and late gadolinium enhancement in a subendocardial pattern, with relatively spared epicardium, in a pattern classic for cardiac amyloidosis. (Reprinted with permission from Morgan RB, Kwong RY. Assessment of cardiomyopathies and cardiac transplantation. In: Kwong R, Jerosch-Herold M, Heydari B, eds. *Cardiovascular Magnetic Resonance Imaging. Contemporary Cardiology*. Springer; 2019:249-272. Copyright © 2019 Springer Science+Business Media, LLC.)

The correct answer is C:

Rationale: AFD is an X-linked lysosomal storage disorder caused by deficient alpha-galactosidase-A activity, leading to the accumulation of glycosphingolipids in various organs including the heart. Classic symptoms include acroparesthesia, hypohidrosis, angiokeratoma, hearing loss, psychomotor instability, pain during physical activity, and gastrointestinal problems. Late complications involve heart and kidney failure, stroke, and neuropathy. LGE in the inferolateral wall of LV is the most common pattern in patients with concentric LV wall hypertrophy. Shortening of native

T1 (longitudinal relaxation) values is due to intracellular glycosphingolipid accumulation and provides additional evidence. Similar LGE pattern can also be seen in Chagas disease, HCM, and sarcoidosis, but shortened T1 time would not be present. Presence of LGE in AFD is a poor prognostic factor and has been associated with a higher risk of ventricular arrhythmias and sudden cardiac death.

KEY POINTS

- ✔ LGE of the inferolateral wall is the most common pattern noted in AFD, often with shortened native T1 values.

376. The correct answer is B.

Rationale: CMR imaging is a useful tool in the assessment of cardiac siderosis, which is a common complication in patients with thalassemia major and other forms of transfusional iron overload. The T2* relaxation time on CMR imaging is a sensitive and specific measure of cardiac iron deposition, with an inverse relationship between T2* values and iron overload. T2* values, ideally assessed in the septal wall, less than 20 minutes are considered the threshold for cardiac siderosis, while less than 10 minutes indicate severe iron overload requiring chelation therapy, which is associated with a poor prognosis. Shortened T1 values can be seen in Fabry disease but are not useful in monitoring cardiac siderosis.

KEY POINTS

- ✔ CMR imaging plays a crucial role in the management of siderotic cardiomyopathy. T2* value falls linearly with increasing iron overload. A T2* value less than 20 minutes is diagnostic of cardiac siderosis, and a value less than 10 minutes should prompt chelation therapy initiation.

377. The correct answer is A.

Rationale: In trained athletes, LV wall thickness of 13 to 15 mm falls in the gray zone between pathologic and physiologic LV hypertrophy. Regression of more than 2 mm in LV thickness following forced deconditioning over a short time, approximately 3 months, is consistent with athlete's heart. In this case, since the patient's LV thickness did not regress, it meets the criteria for HCM. LGE on CMR imaging is suggestive of heterogeneous fibrosis and myocardial disarray, with patchy LGE in affected segments of the wall being most common. Other CMR findings supporting HCM include aberrant LV muscle bundles, basal crypts, apical pouching, and anomalous papillary muscle insertion. ARVC, a genetic disease characterized by fibrofatty replacement of the right ventricular free wall, typically presents with RV dilatation. Dilated cardiomyopathy presents with LV dilatation. Mild phenotypes of both pathologies can overlap with RV and LV remodeling in athletes and need to be differentiated. CMR imaging plays an important role by providing accurate measurements of chamber volumes and function.

KEY POINTS

- ✔ Forced deconditioning for a short duration is a useful strategy to differentiate between HCM and athlete's heart. Regression of more than 2 mm in LV thickness is consistent with athlete's heart.

37.8 The correct answer is C:

Rationale: ARVC is an inherited disease that causes normal myocardium to be replaced by fibrofatty tissue, predisposing to ventricular arrhythmias. Patients typically present with palpitation, syncope, especially after exercise, or sudden cardiac death, with arrhythmias ranging from premature ventricular contractions (PVCs) and sustained ventricular tachycardia to ventricular fibrillation. ECG findings in this patient are concerning for ARVC. CMR imaging is a useful tool in the diagnosis and evaluation of patients with suspected ARVC. It typically shows functional abnormalities such as right ventricular dilatation and systolic dysfunction. Patients with hypertrophic cardiomyopathy may present similarly, but on CMR imaging, diffuse hypertrophy of the LV with or without areas of LGE is typically seen. Dilated cardiomyopathy typically involves left ventricular dilatation.

KEY POINTS

✔ CMR imaging is of great use in patients with suspected ARVC. Morphologic abnormalities such as RV dilatation and RV systolic dysfunction are major criteria for diagnosis, while fat deposition in the myocardium is least specific and should not be a focus in ARVC diagnosis. See also **Figure 37.2**.

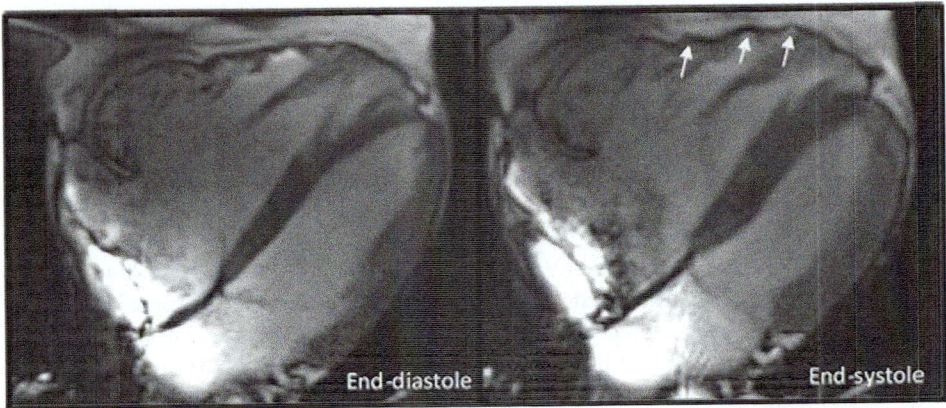

Figure 37.2 End-diastolic and end-systolic cine images in a 34-year-old male patient with a family history of sudden cardiac death and dilated right ventricle on echocardiogram. Both images show severe right ventricular (RV) dilatation (RV end-diastolic volume: 150 mL/m^2) and RV systolic dysfunction (RV ejection fraction: 38%). There are significant wall motion abnormalities of the RV free wall (white arrows) consistent with RV microaneurysms. Imaging features fulfilled one major task force criterion for arrhythmogenic RV cardiomyopathy.

37.9 The correct answer is D:

Rationale: LVNC is characterized by prominent trabeculation and deep recesses in the LV. While such trabeculations have been reported in pregnant women and athletes, they are typically pathologic and increase the risk for heart failure, thromboembolism, arrhythmias, and so on. CMR imaging provides highly accurate visualization of the myocardial tissue, and various criteria have been proposed to confirm LVNC. While septal mid-wall LGE is the most common pattern, LGE is only seen in up to 55% of cases and is not definitive of LVNC. Of the other options, a ratio of noncompacted to compacted myocardium greater than 2.3:1 in end-diastole is the most widely used criterion.

KEY POINTS

- CMR imaging plays an important role in LVNC diagnosis as it allows accurate visualization of the myocardium. Various criteria comparing trabeculated and nontrabeculated myocardium are utilized to diagnose LVNC, but LGE is not specific enough for this diagnosis.

37.10 The correct answer is D.

Rationale: Metallic implants and implanted cardiac devices are increasingly common in today's population, and a large number of these patients require CMR imaging over their lifetime. Devices are categorized into three groups: CMR-safe, CMR-conditional, and CMR-unsafe. Ferromagnetic material–containing devices known to pose hazards in all CMR environments are labeled CMR-unsafe, while those that are safe under specified conditions are considered CMR-conditional. The above implants are categorized as CMR-conditional and are considered safe for CMR imaging at strengths of 1.5 to 3 T.

KEY POINTS

- CMR-conditional devices or metallic implants contain ferromagnetic material and can be safely imaged under specific conditions. It is recommended to check the manufacturer's specifications and follow those to safely obtain a CMR.

37.11 The correct answer is A.

Rationale: The myocardium supplied by an acutely occluded artery defines the area at risk (AAR) for infarction if reperfusion is not established. The AAR contains both the infarcted and salvaged myocardium once reperfusion in achieved. Myocardial salvage is calculated by subtracting the infarct size from AAR, and MSI is the ratio of myocardial salvage to AAR. MSI acts as an assessment tool to compare the effectiveness of novel cardioprotective therapies. T2-based CMR sequences, reflecting the myocardial edema extent, can identify the AAR, while LGE reflects the infarct size. Overall, MSI reflects the effectiveness of reperfusion therapy rather than the severity of AMI or collateral circulation. CMR imaging is typically performed 5 ± 2 days after reperfusion, and it does not have a role in predicting reperfusion injury after PCI.

KEY POINTS

- MSI is defined as the proportion of myocardium that remains viable and is calculated as (area at risk − final infarct size)/area at risk.

37.12 The correct answer is B.

Rationale: Microvascular obstruction is a common complication of AMI and is characterized by incomplete microvascular perfusion within the infarcted myocardium, despite successful revascularization. This results in an area of hypoenhancement on CMR imaging, typically located within the infarcted region. On delayed postcontrast sequences, which are T1-weighted inversion recovery sequences, MVO appears as a dark core surrounded by a zone of hyperenhancement on LGE images,. Myocardial edema is a common finding in the acute phase of myocardial infarction but would present as an area of hyperintense signal on T2-weighted images. Intramyocardial hemorrhage is typically seen as an area of hypointensity on T2-weighted MRI sequences. Myocardial scar appears as a region of hyperenhancement on LGE imaging and would be unlikely to develop within 3 days of AMI.

> **KEY POINTS**
>
> ✔ Microvascular obstruction is defined as an inability to reestablish coronary microcirculation in the ischemic region despite achieving good flow in epicardial artery. On CMR imaging, MVO is visualized as a dark core within areas of hyperenhancement.

HYBRID AND MULTIMODALITY IMAGING CORRELATION*

Karan Sarode and Debabrata Mukherjee

CHAPTER 38

QUESTIONS

38.1 Which of the following statements is **FALSE** regarding the benefit of hybrid imaging technology compared with single-modality imaging?

   A. Hybrid imaging provides the ability to combine functional assessment with anatomic localization, resulting in improved diagnostic accuracy compared to single-modality imaging.
   B. Integrated hybrid imaging technology provides synergistic information compared to aggregating the information obtained from the individual modalities.
   C. Because of its increased diagnostic capability compared to single-modality imaging, it is recommended to use hybrid imaging, when available, as the first-line diagnostic tool for any clinical scenario.
   D. When cardiac positron emission tomography (PET) is required, it is the standard of care to perform hybrid cardiac PET/computed tomography (CT) rather than single-modality cardiac PET.

38.2 Hybrid single-photon emission computed tomography (SPECT)/CT imaging would be **MOST** appropriate for the diagnosis of which of the following clinical entities?

   A. Anomalous origin of a coronary artery in a teenage male with typical angina
   B. Hypertrophic obstructive cardiomyopathy (HOCM) in a teenage male with unexplained syncope while exercising
   C. Restrictive cardiomyopathy in an older female admitted for shortness of breath and leg swelling
   D. Diagnosis of a culprit coronary artery lesion in a patient presenting with typical angina and elevated troponin levels without ischemic changes seen on the electrocardiogram (ECG)

38.3 A 77-year-old male with a history of obesity, hypertension, and hyperlipidemia presents with an 8-week history of progressive shortness of breath on exertion and bilateral lower extremity swelling. He also complains of light-headedness on exertion and easy fatigability. On admission, the ECG showed normal sinus rhythm with 2:1 AV block and low-voltage QRS. Echocardiogram showed left ventricular hypertrophy, ejection fraction of 50% to 55%, and grade 3 diastolic dysfunction. The global longitudinal strain pattern showed an apical-sparing pattern consistent with cardiac amyloidosis. In attempting to diagnose this patient for transthyretin (ATTR)

---

*Questions and Answers are based on Chapter 38: Hybrid and Multimodality Imaging by Albert J. Sinusas in *Cardiovascular Medicine and Surgery*, First Edition.

cardiac amyloidosis, multimodality imaging is planned. Which of the following multimodality combinations would be **MOST** useful in the diagnosis of ATTR cardiac amyloidosis?
   A. Hybrid pyrophosphate (PYP) SPECT/CT
   B. Myocardial perfusion SPECT with subsequent coronary angiography
   C. Transesophageal echocardiography with subsequent combined left and right heart catheterization
   D. None of the above

38.4 A 65-year-old male with hypertension and hyperlipidemia presents with a 1-week history of chest pain. The pain is localized to the left sternal region, occurs on exertion but also at times while at rest, and is described as a sharp sensation. He is normotensive, nontachycardic, and saturating well on room air. His troponin-I levels are negative on three successive tests. An ECG performed while the patient was without chest pain shows normal sinus rhythm with nonspecific ST-segment changes in the anterolateral leads. Transthoracic echocardiogram shows a 60% to 65% left ventricular ejection fraction without regional wall motion abnormality. The patient is anxious regarding his chest pain, and the primary team has decided to order coronary CT angiography (CCTA) to evaluate for coronary artery disease. Which of the following is **FALSE** regarding the use of CCTA?
   A. CCTA tends to overestimate the severity of stenosis when compared with angiography.
   B. CCTA has a very high positive predictive value for diagnosing coronary artery disease.
   C. CCTA hybridized with fractional flow reserve (FFR) improves the specificity for the diagnosis of significant coronary artery disease.
   D. CCTA hybridized with PET can reduce the amount of unnecessary invasive angiographies if used in appropriate patients.

38.5 Which of the following scenarios would the use of hybrid PET/CT imaging be **MOST** helpful?
   A. Patient with complex congenital coronary disease presenting with exertional chest pain and ECG changes suggestive of ischemia
   B. Patient with critical limb ischemia of the right lower extremity, with gangrenous ulcers on the first toe and severe rest pain of the foot
   C. Patient with severe aortic stenosis undergoing preoperative evaluation prior to planned transcatheter aortic valve implantation
   D. Patient with a history of coronary artery bypass graft presenting with non–ST-elevation myocardial infarction

38.6 Hybrid PET/cardiac magnetic resonance (CMR) is **BEST** used for evaluating which of the following diseases?
   A. Cardiac sarcoidosis
   B. Cardiac amyloidosis
   C. Comprehensive evaluation of coronary arteries
   D. All of the above

38.7 What is one potential benefit of hybrid x-ray fluoroscopy with CT technology?

A. This approach helps lower the amount of contrast used and radiation exposure by reducing fluoroscopy time and improving procedural efficiency.
B. It can be easily gated with the ECG to provide real-time coupling with the cardiac cycle.
C. Hybrid x-ray fluoroscopy and CT technology have very short acquisition times (1-2 seconds) that facilitate its ease of use in a variety of cardiac applications.
D. All of the above

38.8 In which of the following scenarios would hybrid x-ray fluoroscopy with echocardiography be used?
A. Watchman device implantation
B. Transcatheter edge-to-edge repair of the mitral valve
C. Transcatheter closure of an atrial septal defect
D. Transcatheter aortic valve replacement
E. All of the above

38.9 The advancement of multimodality imaging has led to the development of hybrid multimodality imaging probes. What is one potential advantage of these multimodality imaging probes?
A. The use of multimodality imaging probes in combination with hybrid imaging technology has led to the development of "theranostics," which integrates diagnostic and therapeutic capabilities.
B. Multimodality imaging probes are preferred over single-modality imaging due to the improved diagnostic accuracy offered by multimodality studies.
C. Multimodality imaging probes are typically more cost-effective than single-modality imaging methods due to improved diagnostic accuracy and less need for downstream testing.
D. All of the above

38.10 What are some possible limitations of hybrid imaging technology?
A. Combining two technologies in a single device may reduce the efficacy of either technology.
B. There may be delays in developing the appropriate knowledge and skills to optimally implement hybrid technology.
C. There may be inefficient use of hybrid technology as the health care environment adapts to these new developments.
D. All of the above

ANSWERS

38.1 **The correct answer is C.**

Rationale: Although hybrid imaging has improved diagnostic, prognostic, and therapeutic capabilities compared to single-modality imaging, it is more costly. There are many clinical scenarios where data acquired from single-modality imaging are sufficient. Therefore, the use of hybrid imaging should be restricted to clinical scenarios where single-modality imaging has limited benefits. A—This choice is true. One of the main benefits of hybrid imaging is to improve the traditionally poor anatomic resolution of functional imaging such as SPECT or PET by integrating these data with high-resolution anatomic imaging such as magnetic resonance imaging (MRI) and CT. B—This choice is true. Hybrid imaging is particularly useful when integrated technology co-registers both sets of imaging data, thereby minimizing patient positional changes compared to separate analysis of each individual imaging modality. D—This choice is true. Hybridization of cardiac PET with CT is the standard of care because of the very poor anatomic resolution of cardiac PET as a single-modality imaging.

KEY POINTS

- Hybrid imaging improves the diagnostic, prognostic, and therapeutic capabilities compared to single-modality imaging; however, it is significantly more expensive. Therefore, hybrid imaging should be used only in scenarios where the benefits of single-modality imaging are limited. Hybrid imaging provides synergistic information compared to analyzing each imaging component individually because co-registering the data minimizes patient positional changes and attenuation artifacts.

38.2 The correct answer is A.

Rationale: Hybrid SPECT/CT allows for the assessment of perfusion deficits mapped to a particular segment of an epicardial coronary artery due to the capability to visualize the origin and course of each coronary artery. In a young male with typical angina, the list of possible diagnoses is limited and may include congenital defects such as anomalous coronary artery origin. B—This choice is incorrect. HOCM is best diagnosed using echocardiography. Echocardiography provides a cost-effective structural and functional assessment of septal thickness and left ventricular outflow tract (LVOT) gradients, which are essential in the diagnosis of HOCM. Syncope in HOCM is less likely due to ischemia, especially in a teenage male. Although CT may help assess septal thickness, perfusion assessment using SPECT is not likely to provide much benefit. C—This choice is incorrect. Restrictive cardiomyopathy is best diagnosed via cardiac catheterization due to the ability to quantify chamber pressures and measure respirophasic pressure variations. Neither the anatomic nor functional component of SPECT/CT would be helpful in measuring intracardiac chamber pressures. D—This choice is incorrect. This patient is presenting with non–ST-segment myocardial infarction. Although SPECT/CT would be useful in localizing the culprit lesion, the patient would preferably be taken for coronary angiography in the setting of an acute coronary syndrome.

KEY POINTS

- Hybrid SPECT/CT provides the ability to localize perfusion defects to a specific anatomic distribution. Because of its high-resolution anatomic capabilities, it is particularly useful in diagnosing congenital anatomic anomalies while also evaluating whether such anomalies result in an ischemic burden.

See also **Figure 38.1**.

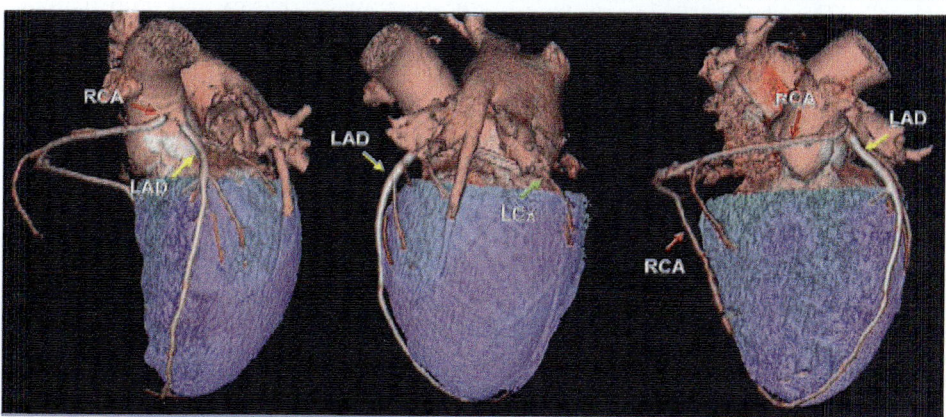

Figure 38.1 Hybrid exercise single-photon emission computed tomography/computed tomography (SPECT/CT) imaging. Images from a 10-year-old male who presented with chest pain and dyspnea with exertion and was found to have an anomalous right coronary artery (RCA) from the left main without an intramural course. Hybrid exercise SPECT/CT imaging was performed after injection of 99mTc-tetrofosmin (4.2 mCi) at peak exercise using a high-sensitivity cadmium-zinc-telluride (CZT) SPECT 64-slice CT scanner, demonstrating normal myocardial perfusion. Multidetector 64-slice CT angiography did not demonstrate any significant stenosis. LAD, left anterior descending; LCx, left circumflex coronary artery; RCA, right coronary artery.

38.3 The correct answer is A.

Rationale: Choice A is the correct answer. The use of Technetium-99m-PYP SPECT scintigraphy hybridized with CT imaging has been shown to be an effective method for diagnosing ATTR cardiac amyloidosis. This hybridization allows for reliable differentiation of the myocardium from the left ventricular cavity, which improves the accuracy of heart-to-mediastinal uptake ratios that are used to diagnose ATTR cardiac amyloidosis. B—This choice is incorrect. Coronary perfusion testing is not specific to ATTR cardiac amyloidosis; thus, pursuing perfusion testing is not necessary for diagnosis. C—This choice is incorrect. Although cardiac amyloidosis can result in restrictive cardiomyopathy that can be demonstrated by invasive hemodynamics, a more specific test is required for diagnosis.

> **KEY POINTS**
>
> ✓ Technetium-99m-PYP SPECT hybridized with CT imaging is an effective method for diagnosing ATTR cardiac amyloidosis. It improves the ability to differentiate the myocardium from the left ventricular cavity and offers higher diagnostic accuracy compared to standalone PYP SPECT.

38.4 The correct answer is B.

Rationale: CCTA has a very high negative predictive value for ruling out coronary artery disease. However, because CCTA tends to overestimate the severity of stenosis, its positive predictive value may be limited. A—This choice is incorrect. It is true that CCTA overestimates the severity of stenosis when compared with angiography.

C—This choice is incorrect. It is true that hybridizing CCTA with FFR improves the specificity for the diagnosis of coronary artery disease. FFR provides functional analysis of anatomically severe-appearing lesions. D—This choice is incorrect. It is true that CCTA hybridized with PET reduces the number of unnecessary angiographies. PET adds a functional component to the anatomic data provided by CCTA; however, this increased diagnostic accuracy comes at a higher cost and increased radiation exposure.

KEY POINTS

- The most recent American College of Cardiology and the American Heart Association (ACC/AHA) guidelines assign CCTA a Class 1 indication for the diagnosis of coronary artery disease in intermediate-risk patients presenting with stable chest pain, such as the patient in this vignette. CCTA is a highly sensitive test for ruling out coronary artery disease; however, a limitation is its tendency to overestimate the degree of stenosis. Therefore, hybridizing CCTA with FFR can improve the diagnostic accuracy of this noninvasive test.

38.5 The correct answer is A.

Rationale: Hybrid PET/CT allows for simultaneous anatomic and functional assessment, which is most useful in scenarios where patients present with functional limitations with an unclear underlying coronary anatomy, such as in patients with a history of congenital heart disease. B—This choice is incorrect. This patient would benefit from invasive angiography of the right lower extremity as it provides the ability to simultaneously treat culprit lesions. C—This choice is incorrect. This patient would not benefit from functional assessment, as the decision to perform transcatheter aortic valve implantation has already been made. Anatomic assessment with CT may be useful in sizing the prosthetic valve. D—This choice is incorrect. This patient would benefit from invasive angiography, which is the standard of care in treating acute coronary syndrome.

KEY POINTS

- Hybrid PET/CT provides the ability to assess functional significance in patients with complex coronary anatomy.

38.6 The correct answer is B.

Rationale: PET/CMR is preferable to PET/CT in evaluating myopathies, as late gadolinium enhancement can detect scar tissue in the myocardium. Cardiac sarcoidosis, amyloidosis, and coronary atherosclerosis all cause scars that are detectable via CMR. Hybridization with PET provides additional data regarding metabolic activity, which is useful in determining disease activity. See also **Figure 38.2**.

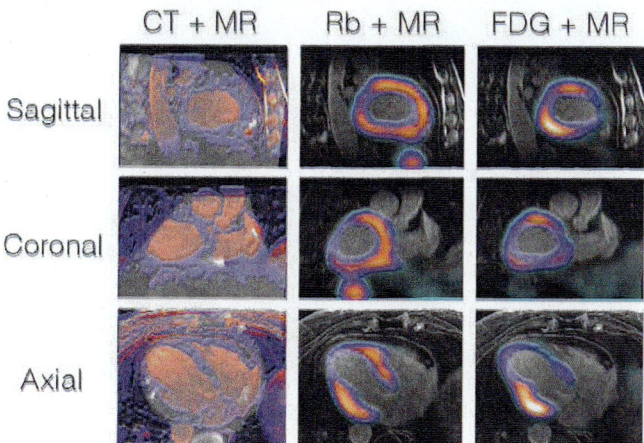

Figure 38.2 Positron emission tomography/computed tomography (PET/CT) and magnetic resonance (MR) image fusion. Separately acquired cardiac PET/CT and MR images were fused in a patient with cardiac sarcoidosis. CT images from a hybrid PET-CT scanner were used to fuse the PET images (color) with MR images (black and white). Shown are fused CT and cardiac magnetic resonance (CMR) images (left), fused 82-rubidium (Rb) perfusion PET and MR (middle), and fused cardiac 18-fluorodeoxyglucose (FDG) PET and MR (right) studies. (From Quail MA, Sinusas AJ. PET-CMR in heart failure: synergistic or redundant imaging? *Heart Fail Rev.* 2017;22(4):477-489. Image fusion and figure provided courtesy of Mary Germino. http://creativecommons.org/licenses/by/4.0/.)

38.7 The correct answer is A.

Rationale: Hybridizing CT with x-ray fluoroscopy can contribute to shorter procedural durations because of the 3D anatomic data provided by CT, compared to the 2D fluoroscopic data. This, in turn, reduces fluoroscopy time and contrast used. B—This choice is incorrect. X-ray fluoroscopy and CT are usually not gated to the ECG or to respirations. C—This choice is incorrect. X-ray fluoroscopy and CT have relatively short acquisition times (5-10 seconds), which limits their use in many cardiac applications. See also **Figure 38.3**.

> **KEY POINTS**
>
> ✓ Hybrid x-ray fluoroscopy with CT is used to improve procedural efficiency in patients with complex anatomy or where anatomic precision is needed. Benefits include decreased radiation and contrast exposure. Limitations include long acquisition times, which restricts its use to select cardiac procedures, and the inability to gate the images to time it with either the cardiac or respiratory cycle.

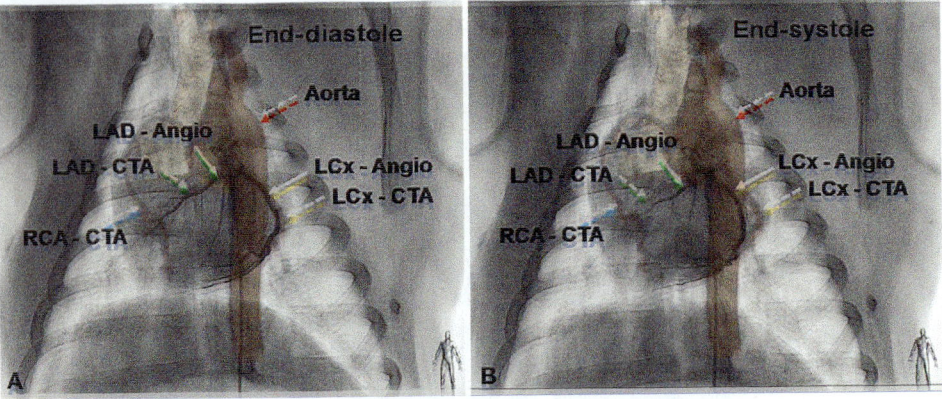

Figure 38.3 Fusion of contrast fluoroscopic angiography with multislice contrast coronary computed tomography angiography (CCTA). A prospective contrast CCTA was obtained using a 64-slice computed tomography (CT) scanner with the coronary anatomy frozen at end-diastole. The coronary anatomy and aorta were rendered in three-dimensions (3D) and color-coded (orange), and the multislice CT was registered with a cone-beam CT image acquired on a digital C-arm. This allowed registration of the real-time contrast angiography with the 3D CT. Images are shown at end-diastole (left, A) and end-systole (right, B). Notice that at end-diastole, the coronary angiogram is superimposed on the outline of the coronary anatomy from the CT angiography. At end-systole, this registration is lost because of cardiac motion over the cardiac cycle. LAD, left anterior descending; LCx, left circumflex coronary artery; RCA, right coronary artery.

38.8 The correct answer is E:
Rationale: Hybrid x-ray fluoroscopy with echocardiography has long been used to guide complex endovascular procedures. The development of 3D echocardiography has improved the ability of echocardiography to assist in procedures.

38.9 The correct answer is A:
Rationale: Multimodality imaging probes can track complex biologic processes, which may lead to the development of novel therapeutics. This ability to simultaneously diagnose and treat disease processes is represented by the term "theranostics." B—This answer is incorrect. While multimodality imaging probes are relatively novel, guidelines have not yet recommended their routine use in practice. C—This answer is incorrect. Appropriate testing should always be guided by pretest probability. Many single-modality imaging methods have very high sensitivity and specificity when used in appropriate patients and clinical scenarios. Furthermore, multimodality imaging is significantly more expensive and may not be necessary for most patients.

38.10 The correct answer is D:
Rationale: All of the choices listed are potential limitations of hybrid imaging technology.

PERIPROCEDURAL IMAGING

Shweta Paulraj

CHAPTER 39

QUESTIONS

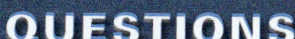

39.1 A 70-year-old female undergoes successful transcatheter left atrial appendage occlusion (LAAO). No pericardial effusion or device leak is noted at the end of the procedure. What is the ideal time post-LAAO to assess for leaks and device thrombosis?

  A. 1 week
  B. 2 months
  C. 6 months
  D. 1 year

39.2 In which of the following scenarios would it **NOT** be suitable to use intraprocedural intracardiac echocardiography (ICE)?

  A. A 57-year-old male with a cryptogenic stroke undergoing patent foramen ovale (PFO) closure
  B. A 66-year-old female undergoing atrial fibrillation (Afib) ablation
  C. A 28-year-old female undergoing atrial septal defect (ASD) closure
  D. A 24-year-old male undergoing alcohol septal ablation for hypertrophic obstructive cardiomyopathy (HOCM)

39.3 An 85-year-old male presents with dyspnea on exertion and fatigue. On further evaluation with a transthoracic echocardiogram (TTE), he is found to have severe aortic stenosis with a mean gradient of 48 mm Hg. He is scheduled to undergo transcatheter aortic valve replacement (TAVR) for symptomatic severe aortic stenosis. Prior to the procedure, which of the following imaging modalities are suitable to perform aortic annular sizing?

  A. Two-dimensional (2D) TTE with multiple views of the aortic valve
  B. Computed tomography angiography (CTA) for aortic annular sizing
  C. Three-dimensional (3D) transesophageal echocardiogram (TEE)
  D. Both B and C are appropriate.

39.4 What are the limitations of ICE?

  A. Inadequate to identify pericardial effusions
  B. Limited visualization of proximal structures
  C. Lack of color Doppler acquisition in all ICE catheters
  D. Poor spatial resolution

Questions and Answers are based on Chapter 39: Periprocedural Imaging by Federico Asch in Cardiovascular Medicine and Surgery, First Edition.

39.5 Which of the following statements are **NOT TRUE** regarding the limitations of cardiac magnetic resonance (CMR) compared to ultrasound?
   A. Limited temporal resolution
   B. Limited spatial resolution
   C. Superior spatial resolution
   D. Superior contrast resolution

39.6 What is the **BEST** imaging technique to visualize highly mobile structures?
   A. TEE
   B. CMR
   C. Cardiac CT
   D. Both A and B

39.7 What is the **BEST** imaging modality to routinely assess valve hemodynamics post-TAVR?
   A. Cardiac CT
   B. TEE
   C. TTE
   D. CMR

39.8 Which of the following studies should serve as the "baseline" for future assessment of valvular hemodynamics after structural heart interventions?
   A. The earliest available images postprocedure (at discharge or 30 days postprocedure)
   B. The echocardiogram performed just prior to the procedure
   C. The intraoperative/interventional echocardiogram measurement of gradients and leaks
   D. Images obtained 6 to 12 months postprocedure

39.9 Which among the following is the **BEST** imaging modality for further evaluation of a suspected immobile prosthetic disk?
   A. TTE
   B. Gated 4D cardiac CT
   C. TEE
   D. Either B or C

39.10 A 73-year-old male with dyspnea undergoes further evaluation to determine the etiology. His TTE demonstrates excellent views of severe mitral regurgitation, and he is interested in possible mitral valve transcatheter edge to edge repair (TEER). He has no evidence of coronary artery disease on a coronary angiogram. Which of the following tests is routinely indicated prior to consideration for the same?
   A. CMR
   B. TEE
   C. Cardiac CT
   D. No further testing is indicated given excellent windows on TTE.

ANSWERS

39.1 The correct answer is B.
Rationale: The ideal follow-up window after left atrial appendage closure devices is 1 to 3 months to assess device position, leaks, and thrombosis.

39.2 The correct answer is D.
Rationale: A 24-year-old male undergoing alcohol septal ablation for HOCM does not require an ICE-guided procedure. However, in options A, B, and C, ICE can aid in visualizing the interatrial septum and facilitate transeptal access.

39.3 The correct answer is D.
Rationale: Both CTA and 3D TEE are reasonable options to measure annular size.

39.4 The correct answer is B.
Rationale: Limited visualization of proximal structures.

39.5 The correct answer is C.
Rationale: CMR has limited spatial resolution but superior contrast resolution.

39.6 The correct answer is A.
Rationale: Highly mobile structures require high temporal resolution, and therefore ultrasound techniques are best suited. Examples include evaluation of the integrity of leaflets that have normal mobility, evaluation for endocarditis, and so on.

39.7 The correct answer is C.
Rationale: Routine postprocedure evaluation after a TAVR includes assessment for paravalvular leak, new or worsening left ventricular (LV) wall motion and MR, pericardial effusion or tamponade, and long-term follow-up to evaluate device function and cardiac response (predischarge, 30 days, and yearly by TTE). Worsening gradients, leaks, or regurgitation may warrant a more detailed evaluation with additional imaging modalities (CT, TEE, or CMR).

39.8 The correct answer is A.
Rationale: The earliest follow-up available (at discharge or 30 days) should serve as the reference or "device baseline" to be compared to in subsequent examinations.

39.9 The correct answer is D.
Rationale: Evaluation of structures that lack high mobility is best achieved by gated 4D cardiac CT or by TEE. Examples include integrity and detailed position of hardware (stents or clips), immobile prosthetic disks, and thickened leaflets due to thrombosis or pannus.

39.10 The correct answer is B.
Rationale: In patients with severe MR being planned for TEER, current guidelines recommend TEE as a class I recommendation to identify if the valve morphology is amenable to TEER.

SECTION 3 CARDIAC CATHETERIZATION

CARDIAC CATHETERIZATION AND HEMODYNAMIC ASSESSMENT

Joseph Cade Owens and Mohamed Khalid Munshi[*]

CHAPTER 40

QUESTIONS

40.1 In which of the following would you **NOT** see an elevated or prominent v-wave?

   A. Mitral regurgitation
   B. Cardiac tamponade
   C. Left ventricular (LV) failure
   D. Reduced left atrial compliance

40.2 When obtaining a pulmonary artery wedge pressure (PAWP), how can an appropriate "wedge" position be confirmed?

   A. If done under fluoroscopy, visualization of the PAWP balloon in the pulmonary artery (PA) confirms appropriate position.
   B. It is confirmed if the measured PAWP is higher than the PA diastolic pressure.
   C. It is confirmed when the O_2 saturation obtained from the end-hole catheter while in "wedge" position is more than 95%.
   D. A PAWP waveform with the appropriate "waves and descents" indicates appropriate placement.

40.3 When converting Wood units to dynes.s/cm^5, what conversion factor is used?

   A. 80
   B. 60
   C. 40
   D. 225

40.4 In a left-to-right shunt, what shunt fraction (Q_p/Q_s) is considered significant?

   A. Greater than 1
   B. Greater than 1.5
   C. Less than 1
   D. Less than 1.5

40.5 A 48-year-old woman presents to her primary care physician complaining of progressively worsening shortness of breath for the past 1 year. A transthoracic echo is obtained, which shows a dilated right atrium and ventricle as well as an atrial septal defect with color flow indicating a left-to-right shunt. The patient is referred for right heart catheterization with a shunt run to evaluate the significance of the atrial septal defect. The results of the shunt run are listed in the following table. Using those results and assuming a systemic arterial saturation of 100%, calculate the shunt fraction (Q_p/Q_s).

[*]Questions and Answers are based on Chapter 40: Cardiac Catheterization and Hemodynamic Assessment by Punag Divanji and Joseph Yang in Cardiovascular Medicine and Surgery, First Edition.

Chamber	O₂ Saturation (%)
Superior vena cava	70
Right atrium	85
Right ventricle	85
Pulmonary artery	85

A. 1.2
B. 1.7
C. 2.0
D. 2.3

40.6 An 18-year-old female who recently immigrated from sub-Saharan Africa presents to her primary care physician with progressively worsening dyspnea on exertion. She has a history of rheumatic fever as well as tuberculosis as a child. Transthoracic echo shows moderate mitral stenosis and significantly elevated pulmonary pressure. She is referred for invasive hemodynamic assessment to further elucidate the underlying cause of her dyspnea. The patient is anxious throughout the procedure, causing her heart rate to range between 110 and 120 beats per minute and her blood pressure to increase to more than 160 systolic. When calculating her valve area, why is the Gorlin equation superior to the Hakki equation in this patient?

A. The patient's age and relative increase in vascular compliance make the Hakki equation unreliable.
B. At heart rates more than 100 bpm, the Hakki equation is inaccurate.
C. Either the Gorlin or the Hakki equation can be used to obtain accurate measurements.
D. At systolic blood pressures greater than 150 mm Hg, the Hakki equation will overestimate mitral valve area.

40.7 When evaluating jugular venous distention as a surrogate for right atrial pressure (RAP), which of the following would **NOT** cause "cannon a-waves"?

A. Third-degree atrioventricular (AV) block
B. Ventricular tachycardia
C. Ventricular pacemaker
D. Atrial fibrillation

40.8 A 55-year-old male is brought by ambulance to the hospital after the sudden onset of chest pain while shoveling snow in his driveway. Electrocardiogram (ECG) by emergency medical service (EMS) shows 3-mm ST elevations in leads V2 to V6 with reciprocal ST depressions in leads II, III, and aVF. On arrival at the hospital, the patient is somnolent with an initial blood pressure of 81/43 (mean arterial pressure [MAP] 56 mm Hg). O₂ saturation is 84%. The patient is emergently intubated, with an improvement in his O₂ saturation, and taken to the cath lab where right heart catheterization is performed, revealing the following information—Svo₂: 61%; mean RAP: 7 mm Hg; right ventricle pressure (RVP): 25/7 mm Hg; pulmonary artery pressure

(PAP): 26/14 mm Hg; pulmonary capillary wedge pressure (PCWP): 22 mm Hg at end-inspiration; and cardiac output (CO): 3.2. Norepinephrine is started. Based on the cardiac power output (CPO) and pulmonary artery pulsatility index (PAPi), what is the **MOST** appropriate next step according to the National Cardiogenic Shock Initiative?

A. Immediate placement of invasive right ventricular mechanical support (Impella RP)
B. Proceed with coronary angiography and percutaneous coronary intervention as indicated.
C. Placement of invasive LV mechanical support (Impella) followed by coronary angiography and percutaneous coronary intervention as indicated
D. Extracorporeal membrane oxygenation (ECMO)

40.9 A patient has been referred for a right heart catheterization. What ECG finding would necessitate the placement of transcutaneous pacing pads prior to starting the procedure?

A. Left bundle branch block (LBBB)
B. First-degree AV block
C. Mobitz type-I block
D. Atrial fibrillation

40.10 In patients undergoing right heart catheterization, why is the brachial approach preferred if the patient has a coagulopathy or blood dyscrasia?

A. It is a lower pressure system compared to other arterial sites.
B. It is a larger caliber vessel compared to other sites and allows for more rapid transfusion of blood if a bleeding complication occurs.
C. The brachial site is the preferred access point in all patients given the anatomic pathway to the PA and is easier to navigate.
D. This site allows for easier compressibility if bleeding occurs.

ANSWERS

40.1 The correct answer is B.

Rationale: Interpretation of PAWP waveforms is a vital part of invasive hemodynamics. Recall that the "v-wave" represents passive atrial filling that occurs during ventricular systole and is related to atrial compliance. Of the available answer choices, only cardiac tamponade would not give you an elevated "v-wave." In tamponade, central venous pressure (CVP) will be elevated, and the notable findings on PAWP waveforms are a rapid "x-descent" and an absent "y-descent" (**Table 40.1**).

TABLE 40.1 Right Atrial Pressure Waveform and Common Abnormalities

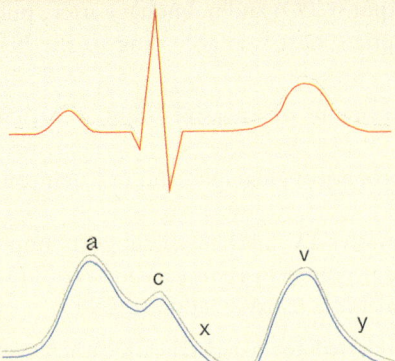

Elevated a-wave	**Equal a- and v-waves**
• Tricuspid stenosis	• Tamponade
• Decreased RV compliance	• Constrictive pericarditis
Cannon a-wave	**Prominent x-descent**
• Third-degree AV block	• Tamponade
• Ventricular tachycardia	• RV ischemia
• Ventricular pacemaker	**Prominent y-descent**
Absent a-wave	• Tricuspid regurgitation
• Atrial fibrillation	• Constrictive pericarditis
• Junctional rhythm	• Restrictive myopathy
Elevated v-wave	**Blunted x-descent**
• Tricuspid regurgitation	• Atrial fibrillation
• RV failure	• RA ischemia
• Reduced RA compliance	**Blunted y-descent**
• Left-to-right shunting	• Tricuspid stenosis
	• RV ischemia
	• Tamponade

Of note, left-to-right shunting produces a prominent v-wave in the RA if shunting occurs at the atrial level.
AV, atrioventricular; RA, right atrium; RV, right ventricle.

40.2 The correct answer is C:

Rationale: An O_2 saturation of more than 95% indicates the PAWP balloon is likely "underwedged," indicating incomplete occlusion, and therefore does not represent a true PAWP. "Overwedging" can also occur and typically shows a dampened waveform and PAWP higher than the PA diastolic pressure. Fluoroscopy, while helpful during right heart catheterization, cannot be used to confirm appropriate wedge position.

40.3 The correct answer is A:

Rationale: When converting from Wood units to dynes.s/cm^5, multiplying by 80 will convert to metric dynes.s/cm^5.

40.4 The correct answer is B.
Rationale: A calculated shunt fraction greater than 1.5 is considered significant. A shunt fraction of 1 is considered normal, indicating equal systemic and pulmonary flow.

40.5 The correct answer is C.
Rationale: Based on the shunt run, the shunt fraction is 2. The step-up in saturation occurring in the right atrium is consistent with an atrial septal defect, as seen on echo. This indicates a significant shunt and may warrant closure. The equation for calculating the shunt fraction is as follows:

$$Q_p/Q_s = \frac{(Sao_2 - Svo_2)}{(Pvo_2 - Pao_2)} = \frac{(100 - 70)}{(100 - 85)} = 2$$

40.6 The correct answer is B.
Rationale: The Hakki can be inaccurate at extremes of heart rate (<60 or >100). It is useful for a quick assessment of valve area as it only requires the CO and peak-to-peak gradient to calculate. However, due to the limitations mentioned, the Hakki equation may not be appropriate for use in all patients. In this patient, the Gorlin equation would be more appropriate.

40.7 The correct answer is D.
Rationale: The "a-waves" are the result of atrial contraction in late diastole. Answers A-C can all result in atrial contraction against a closed tricuspid valve that will cause an exaggerated (cannon) "a-wave." However, in atrial fibrillation, the loss of atrial contraction results in the absence of "a-waves" (see **Table 40.1**).

40.8 The correct answer is C.
Rationale: This patient is experiencing cardiogenic shock following an acute myocardial infarction (MI) (anterior ST-segment elevation myocardial infarction [STEMI]). Right heart catheterization was performed, revealing a low CO but normal functioning RV based on PAPi. The National Cariogenic Shock Initiative (NCSI) recommends right heart catheterization prior to coronary angiography to guide advanced therapies. In this case, the CPO is 0.4. According to the NCSI, a CPO of less than 0.6 indicates the use of LV support devices such as the Impella (2.5/CP/5.0/5.5). The patient's PAPi is 1.7, indicating no component of RV failure. A PAPi of less than 0.9 supports the use of RV support devices and, depending on the CPO, may indicate escalation to ECMO. For this patient currently in cardiogenic shock secondary to an acute MI, already receiving norepinephrine, and with intact RV function but low CO and CPO, using an LV mechanical support device is appropriate, making Impella the correct answer. See calculations that follow.

CPO = (3.2 × 56)/451 = 0.4

PAPi = (26 − 14)/7 = 1.7

As a side note, since the patient is intubated, measuring PCWP at end-inspiration is appropriate. In contrast, for a nonintubated patient, end-expiration is the preferred timing for this measurement (**Table 40.2**).

TABLE 40.2 Measure of Right Ventricular Function

Parameter	Calculation	Normal Value
RAP/PAWP		<0.63
Stroke volume index	CI/HR × 1000	33-47 mL/m^2/beat
RV stroke work index	(MAP − RAP) × SVI	300-900 mm Hg·mL/m^2
PA pulsatility index	(PASP − PADP)/RAP	>1.0
Pulmonary vascular resistance	(MPAP − PAWP)/CO	<3 Wood Units

CI, cardiac index; CO, cardiac output; HR, heart rate; MAP, mean arterial pressure; MPAP, mean pulmonary artery pressure; PA, pulmonary artery; PADP, pulmonary artery diastolic pressure; PASP, pulmonary artery systolic pressure; PAWP, pulmonary artery wedge pressure; RAP, right atrial pressure; RV, right ventricle; SVI, stroke volume index.

40.9 The correct answer is A.
Rationale: While performing a right heart catheterization, there is a possibility of irritating the right ventricular septal myocardium, which can transiently induce a right bundle branch block (RBBB). In patients with an underlying LBBB, the introduction of an RBBB can completely disrupt the native electrical conduction to the ventricles, causing complete heart block. Hence, in patients undergoing a right heart catheterization with an LBBB, it is advisable to place transcutaneous pacing pads prior to the procedure. Choices B to D do not require any artificial pacing precautions.

40.10 The correct answer is B.
Rationale: Other sites such the internal jugular, subclavian, and femoral veins are less easily compressed if bleeding occurs.

DIAGNOSTIC CORONARY AND PULMONARY ANGIOGRAPHY AND LEFT VENTRICULOGRAPHY*

Joseph Cade Owens and Mohamed Khalid Munshi

CHAPTER 41

QUESTIONS

41.1 In which of the following cases is diagnostic coronary angiography **NOT** indicated?
A. In a patient with severe symptomatic aortic stenosis who is planning to undergo aortic valve replacement
B. In a patient presenting to the emergency department with chest pain and a high sensitivity troponin of 500 ng/L
C. In a patient admitted to the hospital with acute decompensated heart failure with a newly discovered reduced left ventricular (LV) ejection fraction
D. In a patient presenting to the emergency department with new-onset atrial fibrillation with rapid ventricular response requiring electrical cardioversion due to hemodynamic instability

41.2 Which of the following anatomic locations describes the ideal location for femoral artery access in coronary angiography?
A. In the femoral artery, in an area that overlies the femoral head and is above the bifurcation of the common femoral artery (into the profunda femoris and superficial femoral artery) but below the takeoff of the inferior epigastric artery
B. In the external iliac artery just above the inguinal ligament where the artery crosses over the pelvic girdle
C. In the superficial femoral artery in an area that overlies the femoral shaft but is below the bifurcation of the deep femoral artery
D. Any location below the bifurcation of the aorta into the common iliac artery but above the bifurcation of the common femoral artery into the deep and superficial femoral artery

41.3 Which of the following is **NOT** a factor that would indicate a left radial approach over a right radial approach during a coronary angiogram?
A. Age above 70
B. Height more than 64 in
C. Female
D. Hypertension

41.4 Which of the following will **NOT** reduce radiation exposure?
A. Minimize the use of cine.
B. Decrease magnification.
C. Reduce the frame rate.
D. Minimize the distance from the image receptor to the patient.

*Questions and Answers are based on Chapter 41: Diagnostic Coronary and Pulmonary Angiography and Left Ventriculography by Jennifer A. Rymer, Sunil V. Rao, Richard A. Krasuski, and Rajesh V. Swaminathan in Cardiovascular Medicine and Surgery, First Edition.

Section 3: Cardiac Catheterization

415 What are the four standard views for quick visualization of the left coronary system during coronary angiography? Known as the "4 corners."
   A. Anteroposterior (AP) cranial, AP caudal, right anterior oblique (RAO) caudal, left anterior oblique (LAO) caudal
   B. LAO caudal, straight AP, RAO cranial, LAO cranial
   C. RAO caudal, RAO cranial, LAO cranial, LAO caudal
   D. LAO caudal, AP caudal, AP cranial, RAO cranial

416 What percentage of the population will have a right dominant coronary anatomy?
   A. 5% to 10%
   B. 10% to 20%
   C. 50% to 60%
   D. 70% to 80%

417 A 55-year-old-female presents to the emergency department with an acute myocardial infarction (MI). She is taken emergently to the catheterization lab where coronary angiogram reveals complete occlusion of the mid-left anterior descending artery with no flow beyond the lesion. Following percutaneous coronary intervention (PCI), flow is restored and contrast completely opacifies the distal artery, but the flow is sluggish compared to the other coronary arteries. How would the thrombolysis in myocardial infarction (TIMI) flow in the patient be described before PCI and following PCI?
   A. TIMI 0 to TIMI 3
   B. TIMI 1 to TIMI 2
   C. TIMI 0 to TIMI 2
   D. TIMI 0 to TIMI 1

418 A 50-year-old male presents to the emergency department with a 4 day history of constant substernal chest pain. Initial vitals show mild tachycardia and a blood pressure of 100/55 mm Hg. Electrocardiogram (ECG) shows ST elevations with associated deep Q waves in the inferior leads, and the patient is taken to the catheterization lab where coronary angiography shows complete occlusion of his mid-right coronary artery (RCA). Successful PCI is performed on the RCA with resultant TIMI 3 flow. His left coronary system shows nonobstructive coronary artery disease (CAD). Throughout the procedure, the patient's blood pressure continues to drop and is now requiring pressor support. Telemetry shows normal sinus rhythm without evidence of heart block. What is the next **BEST** step in the assessment of this patient's hemodynamic collapse?
   A. Repeat diagnostic coronary angiography on the left coronary system to evaluate for the possible development of a new lesion.
   B. Perform LV angiography to evaluate for a possible mechanical complication of the patient's acute MI.
   C. Place a transvenous pacemaker.
   D. Place an Impella 5.0 to offload the LV.

419 A 77-year-old male with type 2 diabetes, chronic kidney disease stage 3, and hypertension presents to the emergency department with a non–ST-elevation MI. His labs show his creatinine and glomerular filtration rate (GFR) are at his baseline. After discussion with the patient, the patient would like to proceed with a coronary

catheterization. With his chronic kidney disease in mind, what is the most appropriate way to assess this patient's coronary anatomy?
- A. Perform coronary CTA to avoid the contrast load used when performing a coronary angiogram.
- B. Place a dialysis catheter and contact nephrology to dialyze the patient after he undergoes a coronary angiogram.
- C. Medical management of non–ST-elevation myocardial infarction (NSTEMI)
- D. The patient should receive preprocedural hydration with normal saline and post-procedural hydration based on his left ventricular end diastolic pressure (LVEDP). During the coronary angiogram, biplane imaging, if available, should be used to minimize contrast exposure.

41.10 Anomalous coronary arteries are rare and generally benign. What feature of coronary artery anomalies is associated with an increased risk of sudden cardiac death?
- A. Interarterial course between the aorta and the pulmonary artery
- B. Separate ostia for the left anterior descending and left circumflex (LCx) arteries
- C. Myocardial bridging
- D. Origin of the LCx coronary artery from the RCA

41.11 Indications for performing diagnostic pulmonary angiography include:
- A. Assessment for suspected pulmonary embolism
- B. Determining the extent of disease and chronic thromboembolic pulmonary hypertension before planning pulmonary endarterectomy or balloon pulmonary angioplasty
- C. Evaluate for pulmonary arteriovenous malformations
- D. B and C
- E. All of the above

ANSWERS

41.1 The correct answer is D.
Rationale: New-onset atrial fibrillation, regardless of hemodynamic status, is not an indication for diagnostic coronary angiography. Answer options A to C all include an indication for diagnostic coronary angiography.

41.2 The correct answer is A.
Rationale: This location which overlies the femoral head allows for adequate compression to the puncture site if a bleeding complication occurs. A puncture site above the inferior epigastric artery leads to a greater risk of a retroperitoneal bleed. A puncture site below the bifurcation of the common femoral artery into the superficial and deep femoral artery leads to a greater risk of pseudoaneurysm, dissection, and arteriovenous fistulae (**Figure 41.1**).

41.3 The correct answer is B.
Rationale: If three or more of the following criteria are met (age > 70 years, female sex, height less than or equal to 64 in and hypertension), left radial approach is

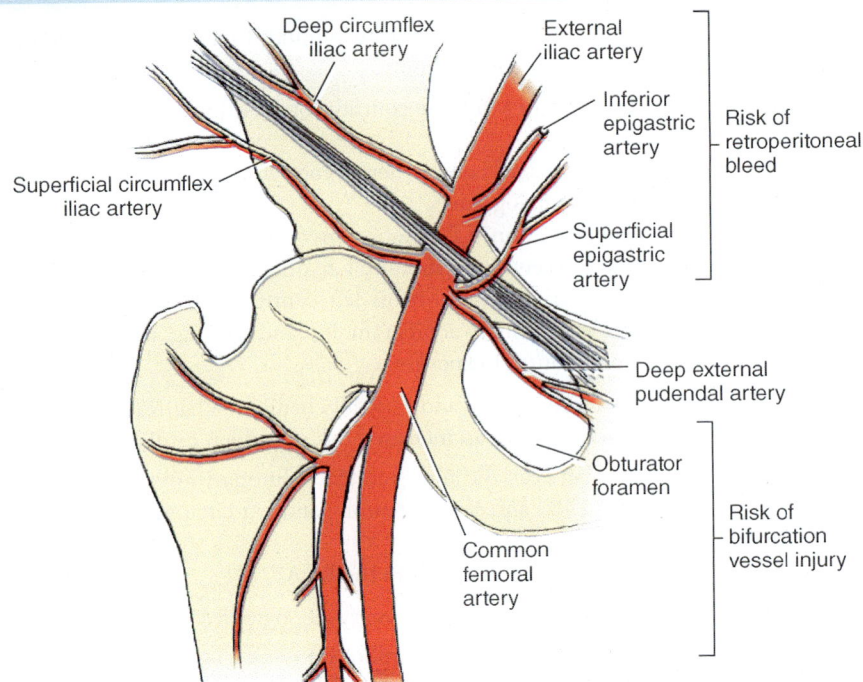

Figure 41.1 Femoral artery anatomy for cardiac catheterization access. Bony landmarks are useful for identifying the level of the common femoral artery. The inguinal ligament runs between the pubic tubercle and the anterior superior iliac spine, marking the top of the common femoral artery. High puncture or laceration of the inferior epigastric artery can lead to serious retroperitoneal bleeding. Puncture at or below the femoral bifurcation is also to be avoided. (Reprinted with permission from Rasmussen TE, Clouse WD, Tonnessen BH. *Handbook of Patient Care in Vascular Diseases*. 6th ed. Wolters Kluwer; 2018. Figure 9.1.)

preferred over a right radial approach due to less subclavian artery tortuosity. In patients with prior coronary artery bypass grafting (CABG), left radial access may also be beneficial due to the ease of access to the left internal mammary artery as well as vein grafts. However, an individual approach should be taken in patients with prior CABG and graft anatomy known, as a left radial approach will not be appropriate in all CABG patients.

41.4 The correct answer is B:
Rationale: Minimizing the use of cine, minimizing the use of steep angles, increasing magnification, reducing the frame rate, minimizing the distance from the image receptor to the patient, and use of collimation will all aid in reducing radiation exposure.

41.5 The correct answer is C:
Rationale: The "four corners" or "around the world" approach includes the RAO caudal and cranial views, as well as the LAO caudal and cranial views. Other projections including the AP projections are beneficial, as not all coronary anatomy is identical, but are not typically included in the "standard" views (**Figure 41.2**).

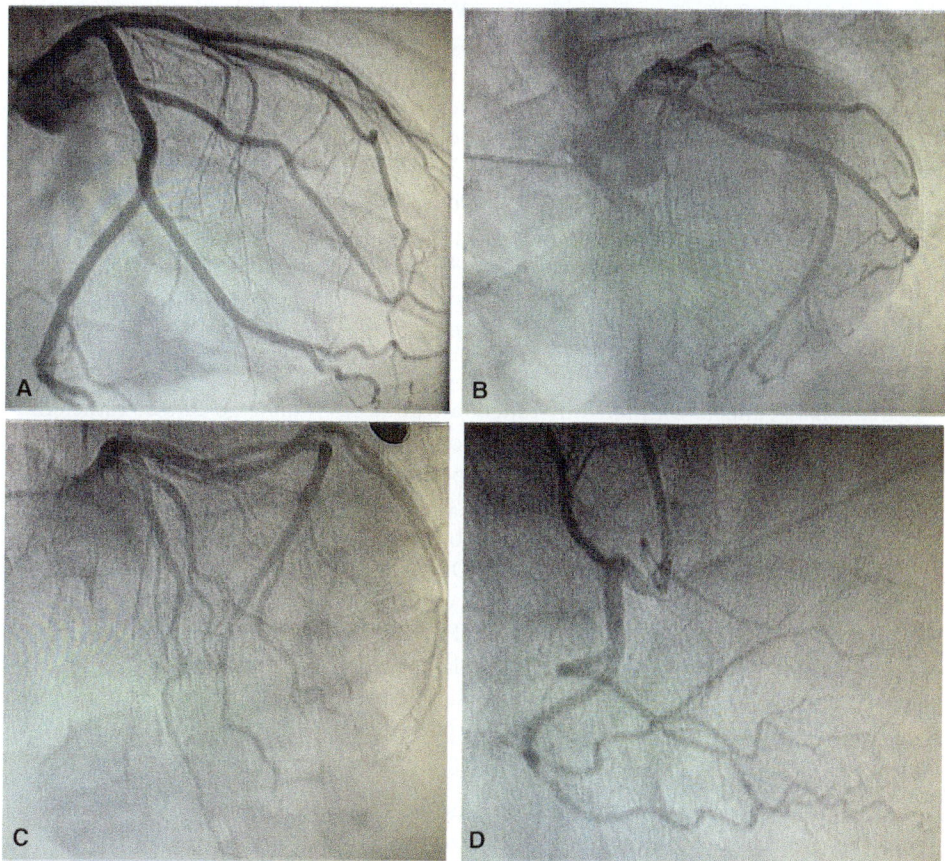

Figure 41.2 Standard coronary angiogram views. **A:** Right anterior oblique caudal view. **B:** Left anterior oblique caudal view. **C:** Left anterior oblique cranial view. **D:** Anterior-posterior cranial view.

41.6 The correct answer is D.

Rationale: Coronary dominance is determined by where the posterior descending artery (PDA) originates. 70% to 80% of the population is right dominant (the PDA arises from the distal RCA), 5% to 10% will be left dominant (PDA arises from the LCx), and 10% to 20% will be codominant (PDA is supplied by both the RCA and LCx).

41.7 The correct answer is C.

Rationale: Complete occlusion with no antegrade flow indicates TIMI 0. TIMI 1 indicates faint flow beyond the lesion but incompletely opacifies the distal coronary bed. TIMI 2 indicates flow beyond with lesion with complete opacification of the distal coronary bed but with sluggish/slow flow. TIMI 3 flow indicates normal flow with complete filling of the distal coronary bed within three cardiac cycles.

41.8 The correct answer is B.

Rationale: In the patient, with several days of chest pain, Q waves on ECG indicative of MI, and hemodynamic compromise that is not explained by a RCA lesion, further investigation is warranted. In this case, LV angiography can help identify mechanical complication of MI including acute mitral regurgitation, ventricular septal rupture, or ventricular free wall rupture. A "v-gram" will also give a quantitative assessment of the ejection fraction. A right heart catheterization would also be appropriate to determine if mechanical circulatory support is needed and what type would be most appropriate (see Chapter 40 section on Cardiac Catheterization and Hemodynamic Assessment). Answer option A is inappropriate as the left coronary system was already evaluated. Answer option C is inappropriate as telemetry shows no evidence of bradycardia or high-degree heart block. Answer option D is inappropriate because, while an Impella may eventually be placed, it is premature as the underlying cause of this patient's shock has yet to be elucidated.

41.9 The correct answer is B:
Rationale: Patients with renal dysfunction who need to undergo cardiac catheterization present a challenge as contrast-induced nephropathy can occur. In this patient, it is most appropriate to use a pre- and post-hydration protocol to mitigate the risk to his kidney function. Biplane imaging should be used to minimize contrast exposure, which allows two separate views to be obtained with a single contrast injection. Post-hydration protocols based on LVEDP have proven to be most successful at reducing contrast-induced nephropathy. A coronary CTA would give some diagnostic information but uses contrast and would expose the patient to the risk of contrast-induced nephropathy without the potential for coronary intervention. Placing a dialysis catheter and planning for hemodialysis would be premature. Treating this patient medically would be a viable option if the patient preferred a noninvasive approach.

41.10 The correct answer is A:
Rationale: While coronary artery anomalies are generally benign and often incidentally discovered, some features are considered high risk. Of the available answers, only an interarterial course is associated with an increased risk of sudden cardiac death. The pathophysiology of this is attributed to compression between the major arteries during exercise or to compression of an intramural segment within the aortic wall that is compressed with the aortic stretch that occurs with systole. Other features, such as anomalous pulmonary artery origin, slit-like ostia, and acute angle takeoff, are also considered high-risk features. Myocardial bridging is when a portion of a coronary artery takes an intramuscular course and has an overlying muscular "bridge." This tunneled section is compressed during systole and can appear as a transient narrowing during coronary angiography. This condition is generally clinically silent. The anomalous origin of a coronary artery alone is generally not considered a high-risk feature in isolation.

41.11 The correct answer is E:
Rationale: Choices A, B, and C are all indications for performing pulmonary angiography. To perform pulmonary angiography, access is obtained in the femoral, internal jugular, antecubital, or forearm vein with a 6 or 7 Fr sheath. The operator often performs a right heart catheterization first to assess hemodynamics and cardiac output. When acquiring images, the patient should be instructed to take a full breath, and then hold it for several seconds and avoid any movement. A standard pulmonary angiogram should include both AP and lateral projections to avoid missing any lesions that could be overlapped (**Figure 41.3**).

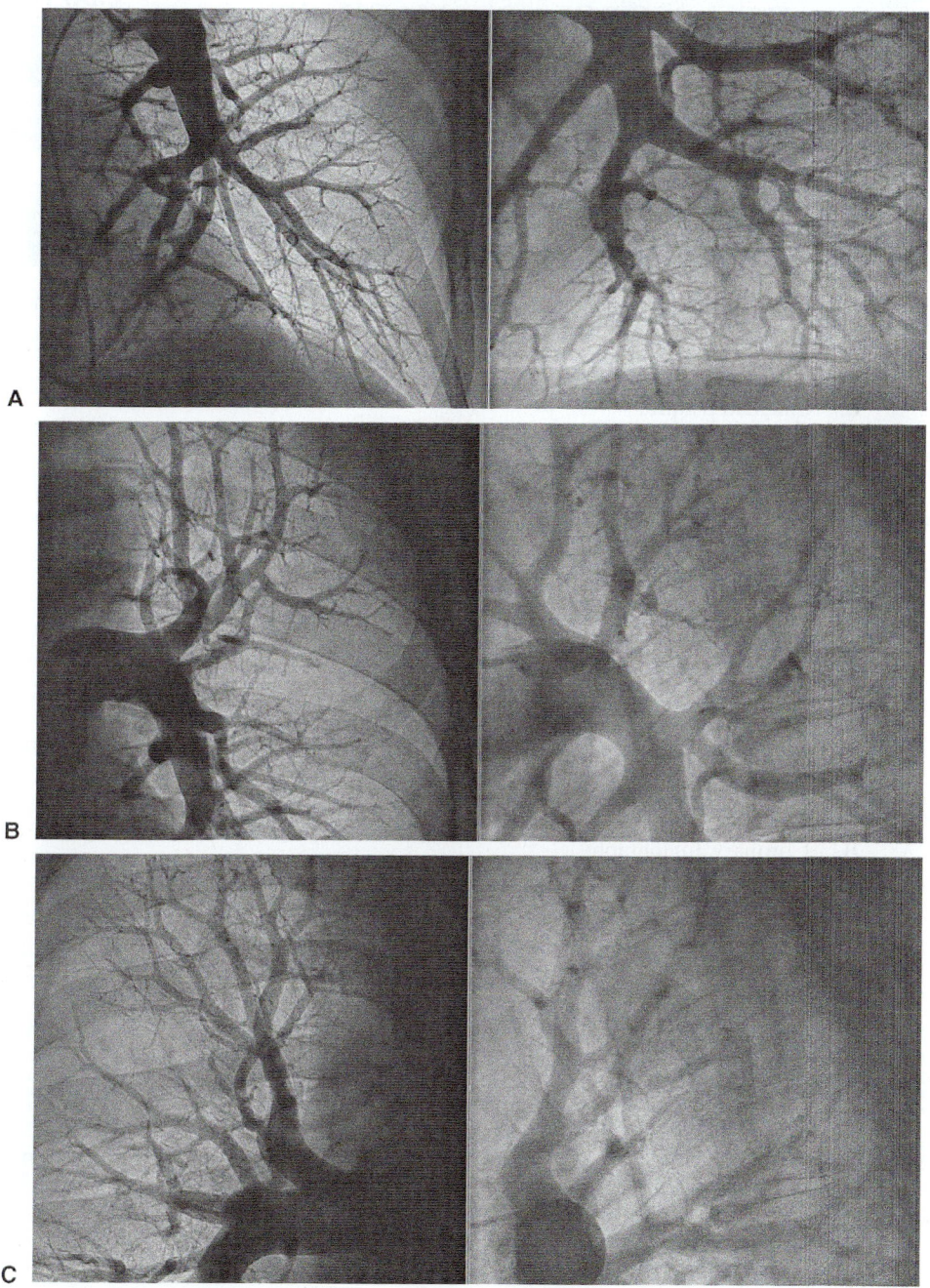

Figure 41.3 Pulmonary angiography standard views. **A:** Left lower lobe anteroposterior (AP) and lateral. **B:** Left upper lobe AP and lateral. **C:** Right upper lobe AP and lateral.

INTRACORONARY IMAGING*

CHAPTER 42

Neil Yager and Joseph Cade Owens

QUESTIONS

42.1 Which of the following does intravascular ultrasound (IVUS) have a significantly higher sensitivity than angiography in detecting?
   A. Soft, noncalcified plaques
   B. Calcified plaques
   C. Coronary lesion length
   D. The hemodynamic significance of a coronary lesion

42.2 Optical coherence tomography (OCT) uses infrared light as opposed to IVUS, which uses sound waves. This difference allows for OCT to have better _____ resolution but at the cost of _____.
   A. spatial, tissue penetration
   B. temporal, image quality
   C. spectral, acquisition time
   D. radiometric, increased artifact

42.3 Which of the following modalities is superior in identifying early-stage and progression of transplant vasculopathy in donor hearts?
   A. IVUS
   B. Coronary angiography
   C. OCT
   D. Fractional flow reserve (FFR)

42.4 What is the minimum luminal area of the left main coronary artery, as measured by IVUS, that indicates a hemodynamically significant stenosis?
   A. Less than 7.5 mm^2
   B. Less than 6.2 mm^2
   C. Less than 6.8 mm^2
   D. Less than 4.8 mm^2

42.5 Which imaging modality (OCT or IVUS) would be more appropriate to use in a patient at high risk of developing contrast-induced nephropathy?

---

*Questions and Answers are based on Chapter 42: Intracoronary Imaging by Catalin Toma and Jeff Fowler in *Cardiovascular Medicine and Surgery*, First Edition.

A. IVUS because it allows for stent sizing (both diameter and length) and can assess post-stent expansion without the use of contrast
B. OCT since its relative ease of use leads to less required contrast and shorter procedure times
C. IVUS given that saline required during IVUS deployment helps prevent contrast-induced nephropathy
D. OCT since contrast is not needed during image acquisition

42.6 OCT is superior to IVUS in all of the following areas **EXCEPT**:
A. Vessel size measurements
B. Thickness of calcified plaque
C. Detection of thrombus
D. Procedural guidance in patients undergoing PCI

42.7 What is the maximal tissue penetration with intracardiac echocardiography (ICE)?
A. 5 to 10 cm
B. 10 to 20 cm
C. 20 to 30 cm
D. 30 to 40 cm

42.8 Intracardiac echo (ICE) is becoming more commonly used in structural heart disease interventions. There are two types of ICE transducer systems: mechanical/rotational and phased-array. Phased-array ICE systems are preferred in structural heart disease interventions over mechanical/rotational ICE systems for all of the following reasons **EXCEPT**:
A. Ability to steer the probe
B. Doppler capability
C. Allow for both near- and far-field imaging
D. Reduced fluoroscopy exposure

42.9 When using IVUS, an arc of calcium more than _____ indicates potential benefit of rotational or orbital atherectomy for adequate lesion preparation prior to stenting.
A. 180°
B. 270°
C. 90°
D. 225°

42.10 Intracardiac echo (ICE) is superior to transesophageal echo (TEE) in all the following ways **EXCEPT**:
A. Visualizing the inferior-posterior border of the intra-atrial septum
B. Minimal sedation required
C. Being maneuvered into the coronary sinus
D. Hemodynamic assessment following transcatheter aortic valve replacement

ANSWERS

42.1 The correct answer is B.

Rationale: Sound waves emitted from the IVUS catheter bounce off calcified surfaces, creating a distinct image that allows it to be more sensitive compared to angiography. However, IVUS is less optimal for softer plaque characterization. While IVUS can measure the minimal luminal area, which correlates with functional significance, it does not consider the length of the lesion.

42.2 The correct answer is A.

Rationale: Due to OCT's increased spatial resolution, luminal area measurements are closure to the true values than IVUS (**Figure 42.1**).

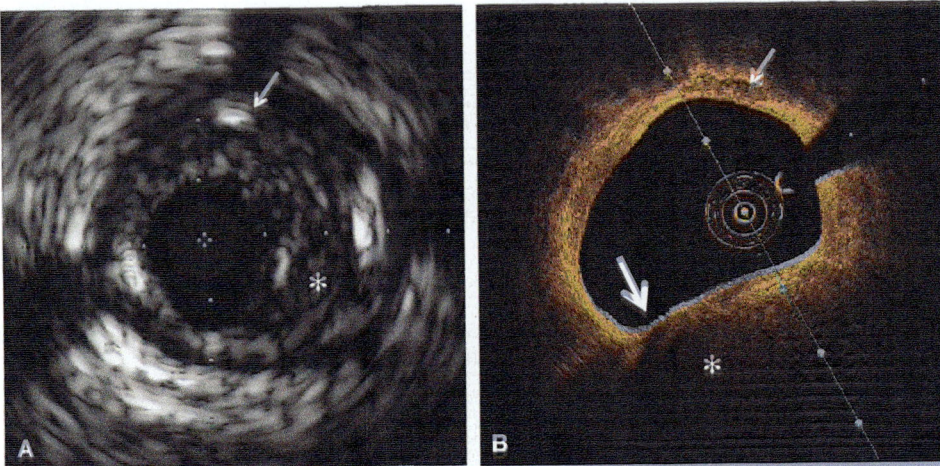

Figure 42.1 Lesion characterization by intravascular imaging. **A:** Heterogeneous lesion detected by intravascular ultrasound (IVUS), showing calcifications with characteristic signal dropout (arrow) and mixed intensity signal plaque suggestive of a large necrotic core (asterisk). **B:** Optical coherence tomography's (OCT's) higher spatial definition allows for greater detail. Calcium nodules are well-delineated (arrow), whereas lipid-rich atherosclerotic plaques have marked signal attenuation (asterisk). Thin-cap atheroma, considered the precursor to plaque rupture, can be identified by OCT at the plaque edges (arrowhead).

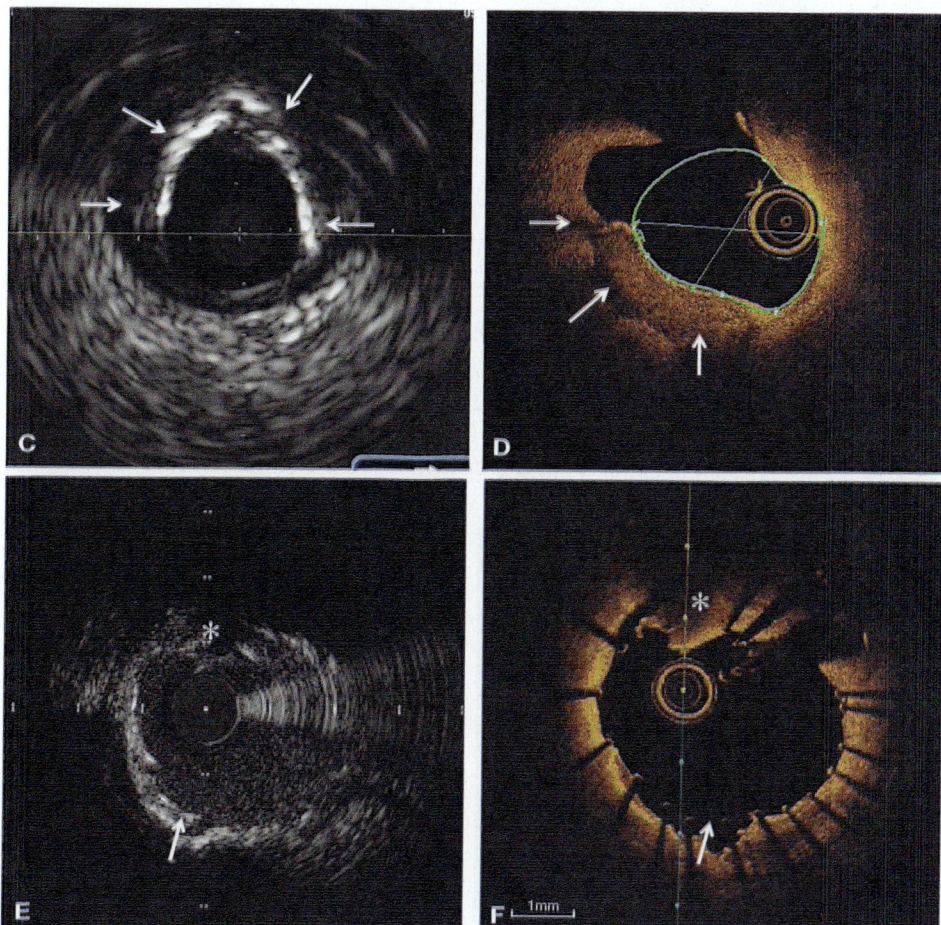

Figure 42.1 (*continued*) **C:** The circumferential extent of the plaque calcification can be easily identified by IVUS (arrows, about 180° in this case); circumferential calcium is an important predictor of the need for atherectomy to ensure optimal stent implantation. **D:** Similarly, OCT readily detects calcified plaque (arrows) and allows for an assessment of the thickness of plaque calcium, with thicker calcium more likely to require atherectomy. **E:** Although stent expansion can be readily assessed by IVUS, stent malapposition (arrow) and the presence of thrombus (asterisk) can be challenging. **F:** OCT is an excellent tool for detecting vascular thrombus, which has a particular lobulated appearance with signal scatter (asterisk), as well as accurately assesses strut malapposition (arrow).

42.3 The correct answer is C.

Rationale: Angiography has traditionally been used to screen for the development of transplant vasculopathy but only detects changes at later stages of the disease. Although IVUS can also be used to detect transplant vasculopathy, OCT is superior, specifically in identifying early stages of the disease process.

42.4 The correct answer is D.

Rationale: A left main minimal luminal area of less than 4.8 mm^2 has shown to be hemodynamically significant. Findings from the LITRO study proposed a cutoff of less than 6 mm² for left main minimal luminal area. Cutoffs for minimal area in non–left main coronary arteries, below which stenoses are considered hemodynamically significant, vary more widely.

42.5 The correct answer is A:
Rationale: IVUS would be preferred over OCT in patients at risk for developing contrast-induced nephropathy, because IVUS enables vessel and lesion assessment without the need for contrast. OCT requires contrast boluses during each image acquisition.

42.6 The correct answer is D:
Rationale: OCT and IVUS are equivalent regarding procedural guidance in patients undergoing PCI.

42.7 The correct answer is B:
Rationale: The maximal tissues penetration of ICE is 10 to 20 cm, allowing for both near- and far-field imaging (**Figure 42.2**).

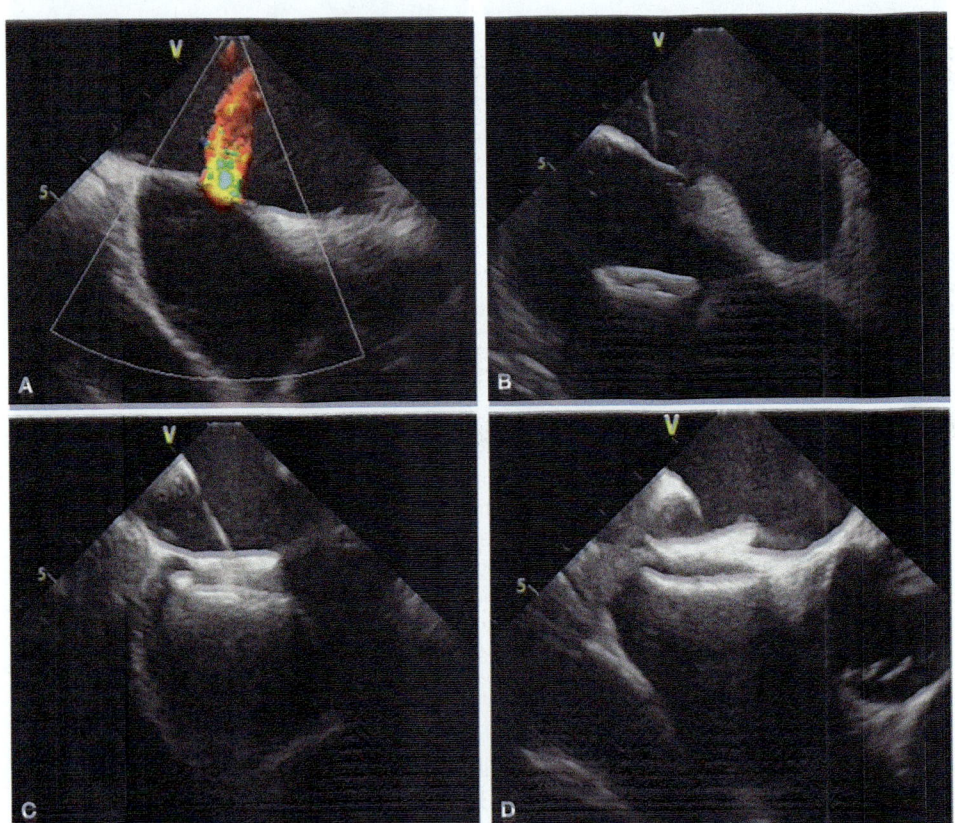

Figure 42.2 Guidance for percutaneous atrial septal occlusion. **A:** Intracardiac echocardiography septal view with color Doppler clearly identifies an atrial septal defect (ASD). **B:** Left atrial disc of the ASD occlusion device is deployed in the left atrium. **C:** After pulling the disc against the intra-atrial septum, the right atrial disc is deployed. **D:** Aortic valve short-axis view demonstrates additional inspection of rims prior to release.

42.8 The correct answer is D.
Rationale: A phased-array ICE system is preferred over a mechanical/rotational ICE system due to its ability to steer the probe, Doppler capabilities, and presence of both near- and far-field imaging capabilities. Also, reduced fluoroscopy exposure is an advantage that ICE systems have over TEE during structural heart disease interventions.

42.9 The correct answer is B.
Rationale: Calcium arc of 270° or greater by IVUS identifies calcified lesions that are at risk for stent under expansion and may benefit from atherectomy (Doan et al., 2023).

42.10 The correct answer is D.
Rationale: ICE and TEE are equivalent in providing hemodynamic assessments following transcatheter aortic valve replacement.

SUGGESTED READINGS

de la Torre Hernandez J, Hernández Hernandez F, Alfonso F, et al. Prospective application of pre-defined intravascular ultrasound criteria for assessment of intermediate left main coronary artery lesions: results from the multicenter LITRO study. *J Am Coll Cardiol.* 2011;58(4):351-358.

Doan KH, Liu TL, Yun WS, et al. Intravascular ultrasound guided intervention in calcified coronary lesions showed good clinical outcomes during one year follow-up. *J Clin Med.* 2023;12(12):4073.

PERCUTANEOUS CORONARY INTERVENTION

Joseph Cade Owens and Mohammad El-Hajjar

CHAPTER 43

QUESTIONS

43.1 Both rotational and orbital atherectomy improve deliverability of balloons or stents in calcific or densely packed coronary lesions but have yet to show improvement in restenosis rates or clinical outcomes. However, the use of rotational or orbital atherectomy both increases the risk of what complication?
   A. Stent strut malapposition
   B. Significant tachyarrhythmia due to release of adenosine
   C. Under-sizing of the stent
   D. No-reflow phenomenon

43.2 A 65-year-old male presents to the emergency department with an acute inferior myocardial infarction (MI). He is taken emergently to the catheterization lab where a coronary angiogram shows 100% occlusion of his mid-right coronary artery (RCA). The patient undergoes successful percutaneous intervention (PCI) with resultant thrombolysis in myocardial infarction (TIMI) III flow. Angiogram of his left coronary system reveals a 60% to 70% mid-left anterior descending (LAD) artery lesion by visual estimation. Fractional flow reserve (FFR) is performed which shows the ratio of distal coronary pressure to proximal coronary pressure across the lesion to be 0.85. Based on the FFR, how should the nonculprit lesion in the mid-LAD be treated?
   A. PCI of the mid-LAD in 2 to 3 days
   B. Immediate PCI
   C. No intervention
   D. Reassess the lesion with repeat coronary angiogram in 3 months.

43.3 What is the most commonly used agent to induce hyperemia when performing FFR?
   A. Adenosine
   B. Atropine
   C. Nitroprusside
   D. Dobutamine

43.4 Which of the following statements comparing FFR and instantaneous wave-free ratio (iFR) is **FALSE**?
   A. FFR is performed under hyperemic conditions and iFR is performed under resting conditions.
   B. The hemodynamically significant value for FFR is less than 0.8 and for iFR is less than 0.89.
   C. iFR uses a different pressure wire that significantly increases cost as compared to FFR.
   D. Multiple trials have demonstrated no significant difference between FFR and iFR when evaluating the hemodynamic significance of coronary lesions.

*Questions and Answers are based on Chapter 43: Percutaneous Coronary Intervention by Olabisi Akanbi and David Lee in Cardiovascular Medicine and Surgery, First Edition

43.5 A 57-year-old female with a past medical history of chronic obstructive pulmonary disease (COPD), type 2 diabetes, and hypertension is admitted to her local hospital with acute decompensated heart failure. Her initial transthoracic echocardiogram shows a reduced ejection fraction (EF <25%) with segmental wall motion abnormalities. After the patient was stabilized and diuresed, she undergoes a coronary angiogram which reveals the following: 80% mid- RCA stenosis, 70% proximal LAD artery stenosis (FFR 0.78), and 90% proximal left circumflex (LCx) and stenosis. Which of the following is the most appropriate next step in her management?

A. Immediate PCI to her LAD with a planned staged PCI to her LCx and RCA at a later date
B. Medical management
C. Cardiothoracic surgery evaluation for possible coronary artery bypass grafting (CABG)
D. Place an Impella and consult advanced heart failure to evaluate for possible heart transplant.

43.6 A 75-year-old male with known coronary artery disease and prior CABG × 4 in the distant past presents to the emergency department one evening with chest pain. He is vitally stable but his high-sensitivity troponin results at 1,500 ng/mL and trends to 3,000 ng/mL over the next 8 hours. His electrocardiogram reveals subtle ST-segment depressions. His home aspirin and Plavix are continued, and he is placed on a heparin drip with plans for a coronary angiogram in the morning. The coronary angiogram shows a 90% occlusion in the proximal segment of a saphenous vein graft (SVG) to his LCx artery. PCI is planned for the SVG lesion. What additional intervention will help prevent complications from his PCI?

A. Use of an embolic protection device
B. Rotational atherectomy before PCI
C. FFR assessment before PCI
D. Retrograde approach through the native LCx artery to ensure patency of the native artery throughout the procedure

43.7 A 67-year-old female with a past medical history of mechanical aortic valve replacement (AVR), currently on warfarin, and hypertension presents to the hospital with an acute MI. She undergoes PCI to her RCA. What is a reasonable antiplatelet and anticoagulation regimen in this patient?

A. Lifelong aspirin, Plavix, and warfarin
B. Hold warfarin while the patient is on dual antiplatelet therapy.
C. Treat with aspirin, Plavix, and warfarin (triple therapy) for a short time while the patient is hospitalized but discharged on Plavix and warfarin only.
D. Treat with aspirin, Plavix, and warfarin for a short time while the patient is hospitalized but discharged on warfarin monotherapy.

43.8 A 65-year-old male presents to the emergency department with an acute inferior MI. He is taken emergently to the catheterization lab where coronary angiogram shows 100% occlusion of his mid- RCA. He undergoes successful PCI with resultant TIMI III flow. On visualization of this left coronary system, there is a 60% to 70% mid-left anterior (LAD) lesion. FFR is performed which shows the ratio of distal coronary pressure to proximal coronary pressure across the lesion to be 0.75. Based on this information, which of the following treatments would be inappropriate?

A. PCI of the mid-LAD in 2 to 3 days
B. Immediate PCI of the mid-LAD
C. PCI of the mid-LAD following hospital discharge
D. Perform a myocardial perfusion imaging (MPI) following discharge.

43.9 In patients with stable ischemic heart disease, what is the role does PCI?

A. Coronary angiography should be performed routinely to investigate for progression of known ischemic heart disease and PCI performed based on the findings.
B. PCI can be beneficial in relieving angina.
C. PCI has no role in stable ischemic heart disease.
D. Optimal medical therapy is superior to PCI in stable ischemic heart disease.

43.10 A 57-year-old female with a past medical history of COPD, type 2 diabetes, and hypertension presents to the hospital with chest pain. Initial high-sensitivity troponin is 6,500 ng/mL with an electrocardiogram showing ST depressions. She is taken urgently to the catheterization lab where her coronary angiogram shows a 60% stenosis of her distal left main coronary artery with the remainder of her coronary arteries having no notable disease. Intravascular ultrasound (IVUS) is performed on the left main lesion showing a minimal luminal area of 4.5 mm². Which of the following is the appropriate next step in her management?

A. Immediate PCI to the left main coronary artery
B. Medical management
C. Multidisciplinary meeting between cardiothoracic surgery and interventional cardiology regarding the most appropriate revascularization approach for this patient
D. Orbital atherectomy followed by PCI`

ANSWERS

43.1 The correct answer is D.
Rationale: Rotational and orbital atherectomy can increase the risk of no-reflow phenomenon due to distal embolization of small plaque particles. Other risks include coronary dissection and perforation, and tamponade. Adenosine can be released from calcified as well as thrombotic lesions but typically causes bradyarrhythmias and can be mitigated with the use of aminophylline. Malapposition and under-sizing of the stent are not associated with rotational or orbital atherectomy.

43.2 The correct answer is C.
Rationale: A FFR of less than 0.8 is considered hemodynamically significant and warrants intervention. In this patient, the FFR of 0.85 indicates this lesion is not hemodynamically significant and needs no further intervention. The patient will be treated medically for his acute MI. Medical therapy and not PCI will aid in preventing the progression of his coronary artery disease. For this particular patient, there is currently no indication to repeat a coronary angiogram in 3 months.

43.3 The correct answer is A.

Rationale: Adenosine, nitroprusside, and dobutamine are all used to induce hyperemia during FFR, but adenosine is the most commonly used. Atropine is not used (**Table 43.1**).

TABLE 43.1 Hyperemic Agents Used in Coronary Fractional Flow Reserve Measurements

Drug	Dose	Plateau	$T_{1/2}$	Side Effect	Pitfall
Papaverine IC	15 mg LCA 10 mg RCA	30-60 s	2 min	Transient QT prolongation and T-wave abnormalities: very rarely, ventricular tachycardia/torsade de pointes	Do not use with heparin or heparinized saline, as it forms a precipitate.
Adenosine IC	40-60 μg LCA 24-36 μg RCA	5-10 s	30-60 s	Occasional transient AV block after injection in RCA	Submaximum stimulus in some patients; interruption of aortic pressure. Must repeat with escalating doses to ensure that maximal hyperemia is reached. No pullback curve possible
Adenosine IV	140 mg/kg/min	≤1-2 min	1-2 min	Decrease in blood pressure by 10%-15%. Burning or angina-like chest pain during infusion (harmless, not ischemia). Not to be used in patients with severe obstructive lung disease (potential for bronchospasm).	
Dobutamine IV	10-40 μg/kg/min	1-2 min	3-5 min	Tachycardia, mild increase in blood pressure	
Nitroprusside IC	0.3-0.9 μg/kg	20 s	1 min	20% decrease in blood pressure	

AV, atrioventricular; IC, intracoronary; IV, intravenous; LCA, left coronary artery; min, minutes; RCA, right coronary artery; s, seconds; $T_{1/2}$, half-life.
Modified from Pijls NH, Kern MJ, Yock PG, De Bruyne. Practice and potential pitfalls of coronary pressure measurement. *Catheter Cardiovasc Interv.* 2000;49(1):1-16. Copyright © 2000 Wiley-Liss, Inc. Reprinted by permission of John Wiley & Sons, Inc.

43.4 The correct answer is C.

Rationale: FFR and iFR can use the same pressure wire to perform measurements. Otherwise, all listed statements are true (**Table 43.2**).

TABLE 43.2 Invasive Physiologic Indices to Assess the Functional Significance of Coronary Artery Stenosis

Index	Conditions of Measurement	Interrogation Level	Advantages	Disadvantages
FFR	Hyperemia	Epicardial level	• Established cutoff	• Need for hyperemic agents • High interpatient variability in microvascular resistance during vasodilatation induced by adenosine • Affected by hemodynamic variables
iFR	Baseline	Epicardial level	• No need for hyperemic agents • Established cutoff • Assessment of tandem and/or diffuse coronary lesions	• Requires proprietary software • Longer term outcome results warranted • Outcome data in higher-risk patient subgroups needed
Resting P_d/P_a	Baseline	Epicardial level	• No need for hyperemic agents	• Not validated in randomized controlled trials
Contrast FFR	Hyperemia	Epicardial level	• Resting index correlating best with FFR	• No contrast dose established in randomized controlled trials • Contrast induces short-lived hyperemia.
CFR	Hyperemia	Epicardial level and microcirculation	• Prognostic marker	• Inability to differentiate the effects of microvascular dysfunction from effects of the epicardial lesion • Need for hyperemic agents • Affected by hemodynamic variables

(continued)

TABLE 43.2 Invasive Physiologic Indices to Assess the Functional Significance of Coronary Artery Stenosis (*continued*)

Index	Conditions of Measurement	Interrogation Level	Advantages	Disadvantages
HSR	Hyperemia	Epicardial level	• Combination of flow and pressure measurement • Established cutoff	• Need for hyperemic agents • Largely confined to research setting owing to difficulty of measurement technique
BSR	Baseline	Epicardial level	• Combination of flow and pressure measurement • No need for hyperemic agents	• No established cutoff • Less accurate than HSR • Largely confined to research setting owing to difficulty of measurement technique

BSR, basal stenosis resistance; CFR, coronary flow reserve; FFR, fractional flow reserve; HSR, hyperemic stenosis resistance; iFR, instantaneous wave-free ratio; P_d/P_a, ratio of the mean distal coronary pressure to the mean proximal coronary pressure.

43.5 The correct answer is C.

Rationale: The patient has triple vessel disease (LAD FFR <0.8) and should be evaluated by cardiothoracic surgery for possible CABG. In patients with severe multivessel disease, CABG remains the preferred revascularization strategy over PCI. This patient may eventually undergo PCI if she refused CABG or was deemed too high risk to undergo surgery, but it would be premature to perform PCI on this patient before cardiothoracic surgery evaluation. Medical management could also be a potential treatment strategy, but CABG should be offered to the patient followed by PCI, with both CABG and PCI refused by the patient, before pursuing a less invasive approach. The question mentions the patient is stable and therefore she does not need any mechanical circulatory support at this time and evaluation for heart transplant would be premature.

43.6 The correct answer is A.

Rationale: Compared to native coronary intervention, SVG interventions have been associated with poorer outcomes due to distal embolization of small plaque particles and contribute to higher rates of no-reflow phenomenon. Given this, embolic protection devices are often employed before PCI of select SVG lesions. The question stem makes no mention of a calcific plaque or difficulty passing the wire or balloon beyond the lesion making rotational atherectomy of no benefit. FFR is used to determine hemodynamic significance in borderline lesions where visual estimation based on angiography alone is uncertain. This patient has a 90% lesion and therefore FFR is not appropriate. Retrograde approach through the native artery would add to the complexity of the intervention and increase its risk but may be useful in select cases.

43.7 The correct answer is C.
Rationale: The optimal treatment strategy for patients undergoing PCI who also have an indication for anticoagulation is not certain. What is known is that triple therapy significantly increases the risk of bleeding. Therefore, long-term triple therapy is avoided and instead, a single antiplatelet agent in conjunction with anticoagulation is used. It would not be appropriate to discontinue warfarin in a patient with a mechanical valve.

43.8 The correct answer is D.
Rationale: An FFR of less than 0.8 is considered hemodynamically significant and warrants intervention. In this patient, the FFR of 0.75 indicates this lesion is hemodynamically significant and warrants intervention. Depending on patient characteristics and operator discretion, answer options A, B, and C would all be appropriate based on The Complete vs Culprit-only Revascularization to Treat Multivessel Disease After Early PCI for STEMI (COMPLETE) Trial which states that complete revascularization is superior to culprit-only revascularization in a patient presenting with ST-elevation myocardial infarction (STEMI). The significance of the mid-LAD lesion has already been established and there is no need for further investigation.

43.9 The correct answer is B.
Rationale: Based on the current guidelines, in patients with stable ischemic heart disease, PCI should be reserved for patients with medically refractory angina or with large areas of ischemia on stress testing. Routine coronary angiography is not appropriate and optimal medical therapy is equivocal to PCI in patients with stable ischemic heart disease who do not fall into the category of those with medically refractory angina or who have a large area of ischemia on stress testing.

43.10 The correct answer is C.
Rationale: The patient has a left main lesion that is significant based on IVUS criteria (<4.8 mm^2 is significant, see Diagnostic Utility: Intravascular Ultrasound in Chapter 42: Intracoronary Imaging for further information) and should be evaluated by cardiothoracic surgery to decide the optimal revascularization strategy. Immediate PCI would be inappropriate. Medical management could be pursued based on the patient's preference, but some form of revascularization should be advised.

PERCUTANEOUS VALVULAR INTERVENTION*

Joseph Cade Owens and Mohammad El-Hajjar

CHAPTER 44

QUESTIONS

44.1 In which of the following patients would transcatheter aortic valve replacement (TAVR) be **MOST** appropriate?

- A. 55-year-old male with severe symptomatic aortic insufficiency due to infective endocarditis who has no contraindication to warfarin
- B. 75-year-old female with moderate asymptomatic aortic stenosis
- C. 81-year-old male with severe symptomatic aortic stenosis at a prohibitively high risk to surgical aortic valve replacement (SAVR)
- D. 92-year-old male with severe symptomatic aortic stenosis and pancreatic cancer, with a life expectancy of less than 1 year

44.2 Which of the following is an explanation why TAVR is **NOT** considered mainstream for the treatment of aortic insufficiency (AI)?

- A. The typically noncalcified and dilated aortic annulus found in patients with AI makes anchoring the valve difficult.
- B. The compensatory hemodynamic changes that occur due to long-standing AI make TAVR less viable in patients with AI compared to aortic stenosis.
- C. Redundant leaflet tissue, often seen in regurgitant valves, makes appropriate sizing of the valve difficult, leading to increased complications.
- D. AI typically occurs in a much younger population than aortic stenosis, making SAVR the more appropriate choice.

44.3 Which of the following is **NOT** a limitation of TAVR?

- A. The life of the bioprosthetic valve is shorter compared to a mechanical valve.
- B. The procedure is taxing on the patient and requires prolonged recovery time.
- C. Manipulation of catheters within the aorta can lead to embolic debris causing TIA/stroke.
- D. Leakage around the prosthetic valve following TAVR is higher when compared to SAVR.

44.4 Following the success of TAVR, much interest has been generated regarding possible transcatheter interventions for the tricuspid valve. However, many challenges exist, and transcatheter interventions for the treatment of tricuspid regurgitation remain

---

*Questions and Answers are based on Chapter 44: Percutaneous Valvular Intervention by Gurion Lantz and Firas Zahr in Cardiovascular Medicine and Surgery, First Edition.

investigational. Which of the following is **NOT** a challenge facing transcatheter tricuspid valve interventions?

- **A.** Difficulty in positioning the valve prosthesis due to angulation between the superior and inferior vena cava in relation to the tricuspid annular plane
- **B.** Patients often have preexisting device leads (permanent pacemaker [PPM]/implantable cardioverter-defibrillator [ICD]) in the right atrium and ventricle.
- **C.** The low pressures experienced on the right side of the heart increase the risk of valve thrombosis.
- **D.** The vascular complications of transcatheter interventions are significantly increased when approaching through the venous system.

44.5 MitraClip was developed to mimic which surgical intervention?

- **A.** Lariat procedure
- **B.** Alfieri stitch
- **C.** Maze procedure
- **D.** Mitral annuloplasty

44.6 A 78-year-old female with severe secondary mitral regurgitation presents to the hospital with acute decompensated heart failure. She has multiple prior admissions under similar circumstances. She is compliant with her medications and follows a salt-restricted diet. She responds well to diuresis and is now stable. Cardiothoracic surgery is consulted for possible surgical mitral valve repair, but the patient is deemed too high risk. The patient opts to have a MitraClip placed. She undergoes the procedure without complication, and her mitral regurgitation is significantly improved without the introduction of iatrogenic mitral stenosis. She is feeling much better and is discharged home. One month later, she again presents with symptoms of dyspnea on exertion and lower extremity edema. A transthoracic echo is ordered. Besides evaluating the mitral valve, what other abnormalities should this patient be evaluated for?

- **A.** Left ventricular outflow tract (LVOT) obstruction
- **B.** Pulmonic stenosis
- **C.** Atrial septal defect (ASD) with left-to-right shunting
- **D.** Left ventricular (LV) thrombus

44.7 Which of the following clinical trial(s) was the landmark clinical trial in comparing TAVR to SAVR in patients with severe, symptomatic aortic stenosis?

- **A.** Placement of Aortic Transcatheter Valves (PARTNER)
- **B.** Surgical Replacement and Transcatheter Aortic Valve Implantation (SURTAVI)
- **C.** Management of Moderate Aortic Stenosis by Clinical Surveillance or TAVR (PROGRESS)
- **D.** Transcatheter Aortic Valve Replacement System a U.S. Pivotal Trial (SALUS)

44.8 A 75-year-old male with a distant history of mitral valve annuloplasty ring, subsequent development of severe mitral stenosis, presents to the hospital with acute decompensated heart failure. He has multiple prior admissions under similar circumstances. He is compliant with his medications and follows a salt-restricted diet. He responds well to diuresis and is now stable. Cardiothoracic surgery is consulted for possible surgical mitral valve replacement, but the patient is deemed too high risk. The patient opts to have a transcatheter mitral valve replacement (TMVR). Following the procedure, the patient goes into cardiogenic shock and requires an emergent alcohol septal ablation, which resolves the patient's shock. What complication developed as a result of the TMVR?

A. LVOT obstruction
B. Retroperitoneal hemorrhage
C. ASD with left-to-right shunting
D. Cardiac tamponade

44.9 A bicuspid aortic valve can present many unique challenges or complications when undergoing TAVR. Which of the following is **NOT** a challenge or complication associated with a patient undergoing TAVR with a bicuspid aortic valve?

A. Difficult valve sizing due to the more elliptical annulus
B. Increased risk of paravalvular regurgitation
C. Increased risk of conduction abnormalities requiring pacemaker implantation
D. Increased risk of embolic stroke

44.10 As technology progresses, TAVR costs are coming down. What is the largest component of TAVR costs?

A. The length of hospital stay
B. The incurred cost of complications from TAVR
C. The cost of the TAVR valve
D. The complex delivery system

ANSWERS

44.1 The correct answer is C.
Rationale: This patient fits the "classic" profile for which TAVR is indicated. Option A is more appropriate for SAVR. Option B is not indicated for either SAVR or TAVR. Option D is not appropriate for TAVR due to the patient's limited life expectancy.

44.2 The correct answer is A.
Rationale: The underlying cause of AI, compared to AS, makes TAVR a less viable option in patients with AI. The aortic annulus in patients with AS is typically calcified, providing a more stable background for TAVR. Hemodynamic changes occur in patients with aortic stenosis, resulting in LV hypertrophy and greater forces to overcome the stenotic aortic valve. Resolving this fixed obstruction following TAVR can sometimes lead to a hyperdynamic left ventricle, causing complete obliteration of the LV cavity and leading to shock. A hypertrophic left ventricle is not seen in AI, where the ventricle is dilated. Statements C and D are false.

44.3 The correct answer is B.
Rationale: TAVR is generally a well-tolerated procedure that requires minimal recovery times, with patients often discharged the day after the procedure barring any significant complications. Otherwise, options A, C, and D are all limitations of TAVR.

44.4 The correct answer is D.

Rationale: Transcatheter interventions that require venous access have a lower rate of complications rather than higher. Options A to C are all challenges to developing transcatheter interventions for the treatment of tricuspid regurgitation (**Figure 44.1**).

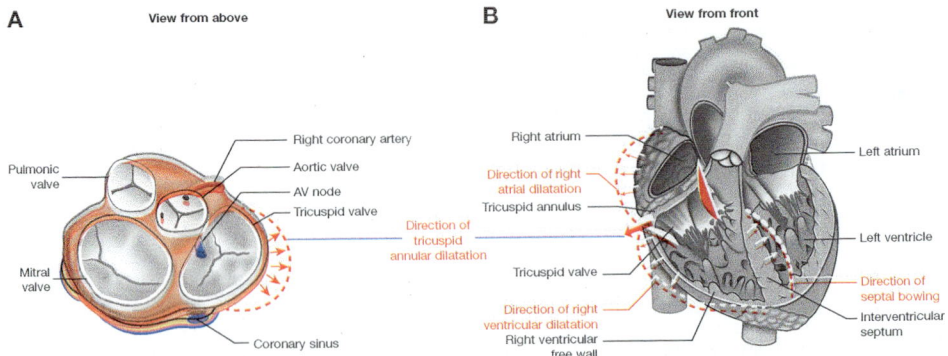

Figure 44.1 Complex tricuspid valve anatomy and pathophysiology of tricuspid regurgitation. **A:** Dilation of the tricuspid annulus occurs in the portion corresponding to the right ventricular free wall, sparing the septal portion of the annulus. **B:** Right atrial and ventricular distention and dilatation occur predominantly away from the septae and drive tricuspid annular dilatation. AV, atrioventricular.

44.5 The correct answer is B.

Rationale: The Alfieri stitch is a surgical technique used to treat severe mitral regurgitation, in which a stitch is placed between the A2 and P2 segments of the mitral valve. The MitraClip attempts to mimic this, but through a transcatheter approach (**Figure 44.2**).

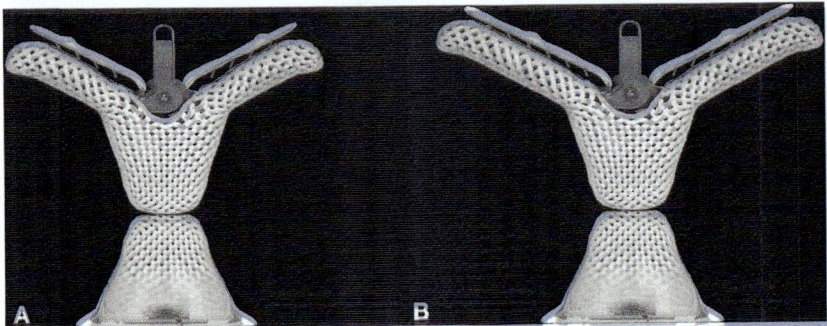

Figure 44.2 The latest generation of currently available devices for transcatheter edge-to-edge mitral repair include the Abbott Vascular MitraClip G4 Clip Delivery System, NT **(A)** and XTR **(B)**. (MitraClip is a trademark of Abbott or its related companies. Reproduced with permission of Abbott, © 2024. All rights reserved.)

44.6 The correct answer is C.

Rationale: Placement of the MitraClip necessitates crossing the interatrial septum and creation of an iatrogenic ASD. These ASDs typically do not cause complications but should be considered in a patient with recent mitral valve intervention (or any procedure requiring transseptal puncture) who is presenting with symptoms concerning for heart failure. LVOT obstruction can be seen following TMVR. There would be no reason to suspect pulmonic stenosis or LV thrombus after MitraClip.

44.7 The correct answer is A.

Rationale: The PARTNER trial was the first prospective, randomized controlled trial to investigate transcatheter heart valve replacement in patients with severe, symptomatic aortic stenosis. It consisted of two individually powered cohorts: Partner 1A and 1B. Cohort A compared TAVR to surgery among patients at high surgical risk for operative mortality, while cohort B compared TAVR to best medical management in patients with a prohibitive risk for surgery. PARTNER 1B revealed that at 1 and 5 years, all-cause mortality was significantly lower in the TAVR arm compared with the conservative arm. Subsequently, PARTNER 1A demonstrated TAVR outcomes (all-cause mortality at 30 days, 1 year, and 5 years) were noninferior to SAVR in patients at high risk for cardiac mortality.

44.8 The correct answer is A.

Rationale: LVOT obstruction is a known complication of TMVR. Patients at risk of developing LVOT obstruction often undergo septal reduction therapy prior to intervention. Options B to D all describe complications of TMVR but would not be resolved by an alcohol septal ablation.

44.9 The correct answer is D.

Rationale: A bicuspid aortic valve presents many additional challenges to TAVR. Options A to C all describe challenges or complications associated with bicuspid aortic valves, in addition to aortic injury. However, the risk of embolic stroke is not increased in patients with a bicuspid aortic valve.

44.10 The correct answer is C.

Rationale: While the cost of TAVR is coming down, the valve itself remains the largest contributor to the overall cost and is several times that of surgical aortic valves. Current manufacturers use either bovine or porcine pericardium mounted on a stent. In intermediate-risk patients in the PARTNER 2 trial, the cost of TAVR was approximately $20,000 higher than SAVR but $4,155 lower for the third-generation S3 valve, owing to a reduction in length of stay. Total hospitalization costs were $2,888 higher for the second-generation SAPIEN XT valve versus SAVR. Follow-up costs were significantly lower with both types of TAVR compared with SAVR. TAVR cost continue to decline; however, the largest component of the cost of TAVR remains the valve itself, which is several times more expensive than SAVR valves.

CATHETER INTERVENTIONS IN CONGENITAL HEART DISEASE

CHAPTER 45

Robert L. Carhart

QUESTIONS

45.1 You are seeing a healthy 18-year-old male for the first time. He is being considered for a scholarship to play collegiate lacrosse. He is known to have a bicuspid aortic valve. He is active and totally asymptomatic. He has been periodically monitored during his childhood. He has had no symptoms related to his valve. He underwent an echocardiogram as part of his evaluation. His bicuspid valve was confirmed. He has an otherwise benign echocardiogram. His Doppler reveals a peak gradient of 45 mm Hg across the aortic valve. His examination reveals an appropriate systolic murmur. His blood pressure is 116/74 in his right arm and 132 systolic in his right leg. He and his parents are very anxious about his ability to play collegiate lacrosse. At this point, what would your recommendation include?

A. Clearance to play lacrosse with annual echocardiogram follow-up
B. Referral for a computed tomography angiography (CTA) of the thorax
C. Referral for balloon valvuloplasty of the aortic valve
D. Referral for aortic valve replacement surgery
E. Recommend that he never participates in competitive sports because of his underlying congenital heart problems.

45.2 A 28-year-old woman presents to our office for evaluation of exertional dyspnea while climbing stairs and mild lower extremity edema. She states being informed about a "murmur" on previous examinations. She has no recent illnesses and no significant past medical history. On examination, she has a III/VI mid-systolic high-pitched crescendo murmur heard in the left upper sternal border. Her lungs examination is clear she has some mild pitting edema in her lower shins. Based on her examination, an echocardiogram is ordered. The study reveals turbulent flow through the pulmonic valve with a peak gradient of 34 mm Hg. The right ventricle appears enlarged. The tricuspid annular plane systolic excursion (TAPSE) is 12 mm, and the S′ velocity is 7 mm/s. What would be the **MOST** appropriate intervention at this point?

A. Right heart catheterization with probable pulmonary valvuloplasty
B. Cardiac magnetic resonance imaging (MRI)
C. CTA of the thorax
D. Initiation of sildenafil
E. Prescription for a diuretic with reassurance

Questions and Answers are based on Chapter 45: Catheter Interventions in Congenital Heart Disease by Thomas M. Zellers, Carrie Herbert, Surendranath Veeram Reddy, and V. Vivian Dimas in Cardiovascular Medicine and Surgery, First Edition.

45.3 You are asked to see a 32-year-old man with a known history of a bicuspid aortic valve. He is relatively healthy and has been undergoing periodic echocardiograms to monitor the status of his aortic valve. He remains asymptomatic and states that he is not exercising regularly due to his work schedule. His most recent study reveals normal left ventricular systolic function. The peak gradient across to his aortic valve is 64 mm Hg, and there is also aortic regurgitation, with a measured pressure half-time of 250 milliseconds. He seeks your advice as he wishes to avoid an aortic valve replacement. What would be the **MOST** appropriate intervention?

A. A transesophageal echocardiogram
B. Cardiac MRI
C. Initiation of a vasodilator and scheduling for repeat echocardiogram within 1 year
D. Referral for aortic balloon valvuloplasty
E. Referral for aortic valve replacement

45.4 You are seeing a 26-year-old patient for the first time. Five years ago, he underwent a balloon angioplasty of his pulmonary valve for stenosis. However, he was lost to follow-up, even though the procedure was successful. Understanding the importance of periodic monitoring, he has now made this appointment. He is asymptomatic and exercises several times a week without limitation. During his visit, an echocardiogram reveals mild pulmonary regurgitation. At the end of the visit, he asks about the next step. What would be the **MOST** appropriate next step?

A. Reassure him that the valve is stable after 5 years, so he can make another appointment in 3 to 5 years.
B. Schedule a follow-up echocardiogram in 1 year.
C. Schedule a follow-up echocardiogram in 6 months.
D. Refer him for a right heart catheterization.
E. Reassure him that the valve is stable, but advise him to call if symptoms arise.

45.5 Your patient had previously undergone a pulmonary artery stent placement when she was much younger. It is now determined that the stent placed is too small as the patient has grown into adulthood, resulting in relative stenosis of the pulmonary artery. What would be the **MOST** appropriate intervention?

A. Attempting to dilate the stent further while avoiding high pressures to prevent stent fracture
B. Referring to surgery for resection of the stented section
C. Referring to surgery for a bypass around the stented section
D. Attempting dilation of the existing stent. If the stent fractures, then placing a larger stent
E. Prescribing a pulmonary vasodilator to allow for collateral development

45.6 You have been asked to see a 35-year-old patient who had previously undergone a Ross-Konno procedure as a child. She is complaining of increasing shortness of breath while climbing stairs, making daily activities more difficult. An echocardiogram reveals a peak gradient across the right ventricular outflow tract (RVOT) of 4.1 m/s, and her TAPSE is noted at 12 mm. Under which condition would she **NOT** be considered a candidate for percutaneous pulmonic valve implantation?

A. The presence of severe tricuspid regurgitation
B. A right ventricular (RV) end-systolic volume of 125 mL/m^2
C. A body mass index (BMI) more than 36
D. The presence of RV dysfunction
E. The presence of a previous conduit

45.7 A 42-year-old man presents to you because of hypertension. He reports a history of a heart murmur since childhood. He is noted to have a blood pressure of 158/88 mm Hg in his left arm. He has a blood pressure of 126 mm Hg systolic in his left leg. He admits to experiencing leg cramping when walking long distances. A systolic murmur is appreciated in the left interscapular area. Further testing would involve all of the following, **EXCEPT**:

A. Magnetic resonance angiography (MRA) of the brain
B. CTA of the chest
C. Lower extremity Doppler study
D. Transthoracic echocardiogram
E. Left heart catheterization

45.8 A 25-year-old woman is considering pregnancy and was evaluated by her gynecologist. A murmur was noted on examination, and the patient was referred to you for further evaluation. She reports being previously told about a murmur but did not undergo further evaluation. On examination, she indeed has a continuous murmur with a somewhat shortened diastolic component. You order an echocardiogram, which suggests the presence of a patent ductus arteriosus (PDA). In preparation for potential next steps, you refer the patient for a left and right heart catheterization. These studies are important to measure pulmonary artery pressures, shunt flow, and pulmonary vascular resistance. At what pulmonary vascular resistance is closure of the PDA contraindicated?

A. 3 Wood units/m^2
B. 2 Wood units/m^2
C. 5 Wood units/m^2
D. 8 Wood units/m^2
E. The pulmonary vascular resistance is not used to determine eligibility for PDA closure.

45.9 Stenting of a coarctation can be done with a bare metal stent. What is the primary indication to use a covered stent for stenting of a coarctation?

A. Decreasing the risk of aneurysm formation
B. Allows use of a low-pressure balloon
C. Bare metal stents are never used.
D. Covered stents are never used.
E. There is no difference in the type of stent used.

45.10 What is the 10-year rate for freedom from reintervention in patients with aortic stenosis who undergo balloon valvuloplasty?

A. 10%
B. 25%
C. 46%
D. 76%
E. 33%

ANSWERS

45.1 The correct answer is C.
Rationale: Balloon valvuloplasty would still be considered first-line treatment based on the patient's young age and lack of other cardiac issues. The blood pressures would suggest the absence of coarctation. Typically, intervention would not be necessary unless the peak gradient was above 50 mm Hg, but in this case, despite the patient's lack of symptoms, the appropriate cutoff for intervention is 40 mm Hg because of his desire to play competitive sports.

45.2 The correct answer is A.
Rationale: Right heart catheterization with probable pulmonary valvuloplasty is recommended. While a peak-to-peak gradient of greater than 40 mm Hg is the typical indication for pulmonary valvuloplasty, this patient also presents evidence of RV dysfunction. Despite the lower peak-to-peak gradient, the RV dysfunction indicates a clinically significant obstruction and should prompt intervention. Further evaluation of the valvular structures or treatment for elevated pulmonary pressures are not appropriate at this time.

45.3 The correct answer is E.
Rationale: The peak gradient suggests the presence of severe aortic stenosis. While his young age might allow consideration for an aortic valvuloplasty, the Doppler study indicates a minimum moderate aortic insufficiency, making him ineligible for a balloon procedure. The peak gradient would imply severe aortic stenosis and thus warrants a referral for potential valve replacement. Further evaluation of the structure of the valve is unnecessary at this point. The presence of severe aortic stenosis makes the use of vasodilators problematic.

45.4 The correct answer is B.
Rationale: The recommended follow-up would be yearly because of the potential for increasing regurgitation. Typically, follow-up consists of an echocardiogram at 1 month, 6 months, and then yearly going forward.

45.5 The correct answer is D.
Rationale: Intentional fracturing of a small stent is typically well tolerated and allows for placement of a larger stent. There is no indication for surgery or the use of vasodilating medication in this scenario.

45.6 The correct answer is A.
Rationale: The elevated gradient across the RVOT suggests the existence of severe stenosis in the RVOT conduit. This, in addition to symptoms, indicates the need for intervention on the preexisting conduit. Ideally a percutaneous approach would be favored in a young patient. However, the presence of severe tricuspid regurgitation would likely necessitate repair of the tricuspid valve, which at present would require a surgical approach. While not an absolute contraindication, an RV end-systolic volume of more than 140 mL/m^2 is associated with a lack of RV recovery. The patient must have large enough femoral vessels to accommodate the catheter. The presence of RV dysfunction is another indication to intervention. Finally, while the presence of a previous conduit is not a contraindication, appropriate precautions need to be in place for the possibility of conduit rupture.

45.7 The correct answer is C.
Rationale: The patient likely has a coarctation of the aorta based on the blood pressure deficit in the lower extremities. The presence of claudication symptoms suggests vascular insufficiency and warrants. Because coarctation can be associated with a bicuspid aortic valve and cerebral aneurysms, further evaluation is appropriate. Identifying the location of the lesion is helpful for planning the appropriate intervention and documenting aortic pressures. Given the unlikely association with peripheral vascular disease, a lower extremity Doppler is not indicated.

45.8 The correct answer is D.
Rationale: Pulmonary vascular resistance greater than 8 Wood units/m^2 is considered a contraindication to closure of a PDA.

45.9 The correct answer is A.
Rationale: Use of a covered stent decreases the risk of aneurysm formation. It also allows for the use of higher pressure balloons to maximize the dilation of the stent.

45.10 The correct answer is C.
Rationale: At 10 years, the freedom from reintervention rate is 46%, while the freedom from aortic valve replacement is 76%. Both of these rates support the choice of surgical approach as opposed to a transcatheter approach for aortic valve interventions.

PERCUTANEOUS CLOSURE OF PATENT FORAMEN OVALE AND ATRIAL SEPTAL DEFECT*

Jacqueline Kenitz and Neil Yager

CHAPTER 46

QUESTIONS

46.1 All of the following are modalities for possible diagnosis of patent foramen ovale (PFO), **EXCEPT**?

- A. Transthoracic echocardiography with agitated saline
- B. Transcranial Doppler (TCD)
- C. Transesophageal echocardiography
- D. Cardiac computed tomography (CT) scan
- E. Intracardiac echocardiography (ICE)

46.2 A 75 year-old male with significant past medical history of hypertension and type 2 diabetes mellitus presents to the emergency room with right-sided neurologic deficits that started about 1 hour ago. He was diagnosed with an acute cerebrovascular event and admitted to the hospital. Inpatient workup included a transesophageal echocardiogram (TEE) with a bubble study, which revealed a small PFO with no interatrial septal aneurysm. What is the next step in his treatment?

- A. Start aspirin 81 mg daily.
- B. Start systemic anticoagulation for presumed atrial fibrillation.
- C. Perform percutaneous closure of the PFO.
- D. Conduct a TEE.
- E. Discharge home with cardiology follow-up.

46.3 Based on the 2018 American Heart Association and American College of Cardiology (AHA/ACC) guidelines for the management of adults with congenital heart disease, for which of the following reasons would you recommend closure of an atrial septal defect (ASD)?

- A. Normal right atrium (RA) size
- B. Unchanged exercise capacity
- C. Pulmonary hypertension with pulmonary vascular resistance (PVR) more than 1/3 of systemic vascular resistance
- D. Normal right ventricular (RV) size
- E. Left-to-right shunting with a shunt magnitude of greater than or equal to 1.5:1

46.4 How common is a PFO in the general adult population?

- A. 50%
- B. 90%
- C. 1%
- D. 25%
- E. 10%

*Questions and Answers are based on Chapter 46: Percutaneous Closure of Patent Foramen Ovale and Atrial Septal Defect by Ricardo Cigarroa and Ignacio Inglessis in Cardiovascular Medicine and Surgery, First Edition.

46.5 After the placement of an atrial septal occluder device, which of the following is **NOT** appropriate in the postoperative management?
- A. Follow-up transthoracic echocardiography (TTE) at 1 day, 1 month, 6 months, and 12 months
- B. Dual-antiplatelet therapy indefinitely
- C. Antibiotic prophylaxis for dental procedures for up to 6 months after procedure
- D. Observation for development of atrial fibrillation
- E. 81 mg aspirin indefinitely

46.6 Which of the following findings is an absolute contraindication to closing PFO/ASD?
- A. Mild atherosclerosis
- B. Intracardiac thrombus in the apex of left ventricle
- C. Migraine headaches
- D. Nickel allergy
- E. Documented inferior vena cava thrombus

46.7 What additional feature found on echocardiogram would indicate a patient is likely to benefit more from PFO closure after cryptogenic stroke?
- A. Less than six bubbles in LA after three cardiac cycles
- B. Atrial septal aneurysm
- C. Normal RA volume
- D. Late appearance of bubbles in LA
- E. Left ventricular ejection fraction 50% to 55%

46.8 What is the purpose of the PFO in fetal development?
- A. Allows blood from the systemic circulation to be oxygenated by the pulmonary circuit
- B. Equalizes oxygen content between the left atrium and the RA
- C. Allows blood from the venous system to bypass the lungs and directly enter the systemic circulation
- D. Carries blood away from the lungs and sends it directly to systemic circulation
- E. To shunt oxygenated blood from the placenta to the RA via the umbilical veins and then to the inferior vena cava

46.9 Which of the following are thought to be associated with a PFO?
- A. Decompression sickness
- B. Migraine with aura
- C. Cryptogenic stroke
- D. Platypnea-orthodeoxia
- E. All of the above

46.10 Which noninvasive imaging modality is able to detect an ASD and calculate shunt fraction?
- A. Magnetic resonance imaging (MRI)
- B. Cardiac CT scan
- C. Transthoracic echocardiogram
- D. ICE

CHAPTER 46 | Percutaneous Closure of Patent Foramen Ovale and Atrial Septal Defect

ANSWERS

46.1 The correct answer is D.
Rationale: The most inclusive criteria for a "positive" bubble study include bubbles appearing in the LA within the first seven cardiac cycles with provocative maneuvers. TEE can diagnose PFO using both Doppler ultrasound and bubble study. ICE can directly visualize the atrial septal flat and may be even more sensitive that TTE for the detection of PFO. TCD is another noninvasive method useful for screening for PFO, measuring cerebral blood flow, and identifying microbubbles passing though intracranial arteries to detect the presence of a right-to-left shunt.

46.2 The correct answer is A.
Rationale: Recently, three large randomized controlled trials found a significant reduction in recurrent stroke in patients who underwent transcatheter PFO closure (**Table 46.2**). However, older patients, greater than age 60, and those with uncontrolled risk factors were excluded from these studies. Given this patient's age and chronic comorbidities, routine medical therapy for a first-time stroke is the best option. However, to rule out other cryptogenic causes of stroke, it would be appropriate to monitor for atrial fibrillation, check for hypercoagulable state, and obtain carotid ultrasound to rule out significant stenosis. Recurrent cryptogenic stroke has been associated with factors such as age less than 60, moderate or large size PFO, and the presence of an interatrial septal aneurysm.

46.3 The correct answer is E.
Rationale: Indications for closure of ASD include enlarged RA or RV, impaired exercise tolerance, pulmonary hypertension as long as the systolic pulmonary artery pressure is less than 50% of systemic pressure and PVR is less than one-third of the systemic vascular resistance, or if there is left-to-right shunting large enough to cause physiologic effects, corresponding to a shunt magnitude (ratio of pulmonary to systemic blood flow) of greater than or equal to 1:5:1.

46.4 The correct answer is D.
Rationale: Approximately 25% of the adult general population has a PFO. The condition of having a PFO by itself has not been shown to increase the risk of ischemic stroke.

46.5 The correct answer is B.
Rationale: Follow-up transthoracic echocardiography should be completed at day 1, 1 month, 6 months, and 12 months to monitor the placement and continued occlusion of the septal occluder. Patients with a septal occluder should receive prophylactic antibiotics for all dental procedures for 6 months. Approximately, 4% to 6% of patients develop atrial fibrillation in the postoperative period. Appropriate medical therapy postprocedure includes dual-antiplatelet therapy for 3 to 6 months, followed by continued aspirin 81 mg indefinitely.

46.6 The correct answer is E.
Rationale: Contraindications to closing a PFO/ASD include the presence of intracardiac masses such as vegetation or thrombus, particularly if located near the PFO/ASD, as this could make the intervention technically challenging. Inadequate vasculature

to support the devices, such as severe atherosclerosis, and documented thrombus along the venous pathway to the RA are also contraindications. For patients with a documented nickel allergy, certain devices like the GORE CARDIOFORM Septal Occluder device can be used. Also, migraine headaches are currently under study as another potential indication for closing a PFO.

46.7 The correct answer is B:
Rationale: The randomized evaluation of recurrent stroke comparing PFO closure to established current standard of care treatment (RESPECT) trial found that PFO closure in patients with an atrial septal aneurysm (ASA) significantly protected against recurrent stroke when compared to medical therapy alone. ASA are present in 2% to 3% of the general population, are associated with intracardiac shunts, and are believed to act as a nidus for thrombus formation (**Figure 46.1**).

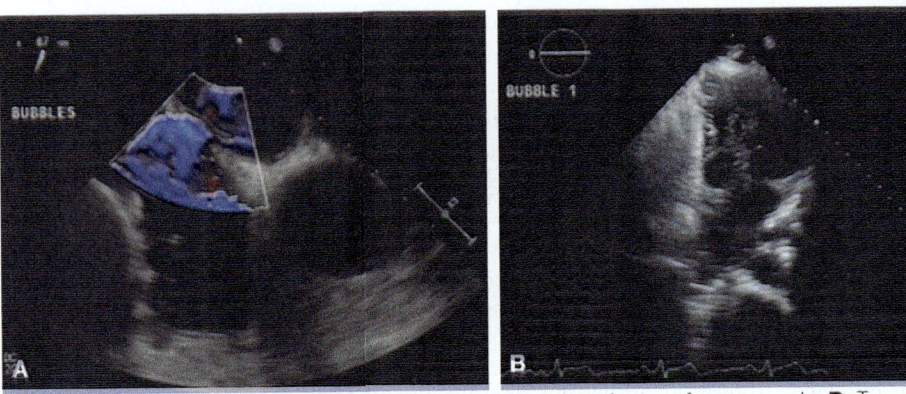

Figure 46.1 **A:** Transesophageal echocardiographic imaging of patent foramen ovale. **B:** Transthoracic echocardiography with positive agitated saline/bubble study.

46.8 The correct answer is C:
Rationale: The function of the PFO in fetal circulation allows highly oxygenated placental blood to flow directly from the RA to the LA, bypassing the lungs. Patent ductus arteriosus is described in option D, and ductus venosus is described in option E. Options A and B do not describe any components of fetal circulation.

46.9 The correct answer is E:
Rationale: PFOs are implicated in all of the choices listed. Decompression sickness occurs when nitrogen dissolved in the blood and tissues under high pressure forms bubbles as pressure decreases. These bubbles may cross into the arterial system via PFO and cause a constellation of symptoms. Other pathologic disease processes associated with PFO include migraine, cryptogenic stroke, and platypnea-orthodeoxia (dyspnea and hypoxia that occurs when transitioning from a supine to upright position due to increased right-to-left shunting).

46.10 The correct answer is A:
Rationale: MRI has emerged as a noninvasive option for evaluating ASD anatomy and providing high-quality imaging, as well as the ability to calculate shunt fraction. Routine diagnostic cardiac catheterization, which carries some risk, prior to ASD closure is no longer necessary.

ETHANOL SEPTAL ABLATION*

Ciril Khorolsky and Mohammad El-Hajjar

CHAPTER 47

QUESTIONS

47.1 A 39-year-old female with hypertrophic cardiomyopathy (HCM) and type-2 diabetes mellitus presents to the cardiology clinic for evaluation of 1 month of exertional dyspnea. Her current medications are metformin 500 mg twice daily and metoprolol succinate 25 mg daily. Physical examination is notable for a blood pressure of 145/85 mm Hg, heart rate of 89 bpm (beats per min), and a harsh crescendo-decrescendo systolic murmur at the left lower sternal border. There is no jugular venous distension, and the lungs are clear. A transthoracic echocardiogram performed in the office demonstrates a left ventricular ejection fraction (LVEF) more than 55%, septal thickness of 14 mm, and a resting left ventricular outflow tract (LVOT) gradient of 70 mm Hg. What is the **MOST** appropriate next step in her management?

   A. Refer the patient for septal myectomy.
   B. Refer the patient for alcohol septal ablation (ASA).
   C. Uptitrate beta-blocker to maximally tolerated dose.
   D. Repeat echocardiogram with provocative maneuver.

47.2 Which of the following statements regarding ASA and septal myectomy is **TRUE**?

   A. ASA is considered the gold standard therapy for LVOT obstruction reduction.
   B. Mortality for surgical myectomy and ASA are both less than 1%.
   C. The rate of pacemaker implantation is higher with surgical myectomy than with ASA.
   D. ASA and surgical myectomy have similar clinical efficacy in terms of reduction in NYHA (New York Heart Association) class, syncope, and angina.
   E. Both B and D are true.

47.3 Which of the following is **NOT** a contraindication to ASA?

   A. Age less than 21 years
   B. Apical phenotype
   C. Patients with well-controlled symptoms on optimal medical therapy
   D. Septal thickness greater than or equal to 15 mm at point of systolic anterior motion (SAM)-septal contact
   E. All of the above

47.4 You are evaluating a patient with HCM and severe LVOT obstruction for potential septal reduction therapy. The presence of which of the following factors would favor

---

*Questions and Answers are based on Chapter 47: Ethanol Septal Ablation by Srikanth Yandrapalli, Risheek Kaul, and Srihari S. Naidu in Cardiovascular Medicine and Surgery, First Edition.

the selection of ASA over septal myectomy as the treatment of choice for LVOT reduction?

A. Preexisting left bundle branch block (LBBB)
B. Septal thickness more than 15 mm
C. Midventricular obstruction
D. Young age (<40 years old)
E. All of the above

475 Which of the following statements regarding the ASA procedure is **CORRECT**?

A. The correct septal artery that targets the septum is always the first septal branch of the left anterior descending (LAD) artery.
B. For optimal result, 6 to 8 mL of 98% ethanol should be injected rapidly.
C. It is recommended to use 4 mL of ethanol for every 1 cm of septal thickness.
D. Intraprocedural echocardiography is performed during ethanol infusion to evaluate LVOT gradient changes.
E. All of the above

476 A 62-year-old male with HCM and severe LVOT obstruction presents for an elective ASA. He tolerates the procedure well without complications and is transferred to the coronary care unit (CCU) for postprocedural care. His vital signs are stable, and physical examination is unremarkable. The patient is placed on continuous telemetry monitoring, and electrocardiogram (ECG) is ordered. Which of the following would be the **MOST LIKELY** finding on the ECG?

A. New right bundle branch block (RBBB)
B. New LBBB
C. First-degree atrioventricular (AV) block
D. Complete heart block

477 Each of the following statements about transvenous pacing during ASA is correct **EXCEPT**:

A. A temporary transvenous pacemaker (TVP) is only required in patients with an underlying RBBB.
B. TVP must be placed in all patients undergoing ASA who do not have a permanent pacemaker.
C. There is no way to predict the development of complete heart block that would necessitate permanent pacing.
D. The use of balloon-tip pacemaker wire is preferred over a flexible screw-in pacemaker electrode.
E. None of the above

478 A 74-year-old male with long-standing HCM and severe LVOT obstruction presents to the cardiology clinic for follow-up. He reports having recurrent exertional syncope despite being on maximally tolerated medical therapy. His most recent transthoracic echocardiogram demonstrated an LVEF greater than 55%, a septal thickness of 19 mm, and a resting LVOT gradient of 77 mm Hg. The patient expresses interest in septal reduction therapy with ASA and inquiries about the potential benefits of this procedure. All of the following statements regarding outcomes of ASA are true **EXCEPT**:

A. Diastolic function improvement and regression of left ventricular hypertrophy (LVH) may continue for up to 2 years postprocedure.
B. Approximately 25% patients will require repeat septal reduction therapy following ASA.
C. Improvement in NYHA functional class by at least one class and a reduction of greater than 50% in the peak resting or provoked LVOT gradient, with a final resting gradient of less than 20 mm Hg is required for procedural success.
D. Procedural success is attained in approximately 80% to 90% of ASA procedures.

47.9 A 68-year-old male with HCM and recurrent symptomatic LVOT obstruction after a prior septal myectomy in the distant past is being evaluated for repeat septal reduction therapy with ASA. Left heart catheterization with coronary angiography reveals a significant stenosis in the proximal LAD, just around the origin of target septal perforator artery. What would be the next **BEST** step in the management of this patient?

A. Proceed with percutaneous coronary intervention (PCI) of the LAD.
B. Refer the patient for repeat septal myectomy.
C. Proceed with ASA.
D. Refer the patient for percutaneous intramyocardial septal radiofrequency ablation.

47.10 A 57-year-old female with history of HCM and severe LVOT obstruction arrives to the CCU following an uncomplicated ASA. Her vitals are stable, and physical examination is unremarkable. Postprocedural myocardial enzymes are ordered. Which of the following statements regarding postprocedural creatine phosphokinase (CPK) and ASA is **TRUE**?

A. CPK levels are not useful for assessing ASA procedural success.
B. High level of CPK more than or equal to 5,000 is expected following a successful ASA procedure.
C. CPK level of 800 to 1,200 is suggestive of a successful ASA.
D. None of the above

ANSWERS

47.1 The correct answer is C.
Rationale: Both the American College of Cardiology/American Heart Association (ACC/AHA) and the European Society of Cardiology (ESC) guidelines recommend that septal reduction therapy be offered to patients with HCM and significant symptoms despite being on maximally tolerated drug therapy. This patient, although symptomatic with an elevated LVOT gradient, is on suboptimal medical therapy as evident by the low-dose beta-blocker and inadequately reduced heart rate of 91. Therefore, uptitration of beta-blockers to maximally tolerated dose should first be attempted prior to undergoing septal reduction therapy such as ASA or septal myectomy. Repeating the echocardiogram with a provocative maneuver is unlikely to

change management since the patient's resting LVOT gradient of 70 mm Hg already fulfills one of the ASA indication criteria of having a resting or provoked LVOT gradient of more than 50 mm Hg.

472. The correct answer is E.
Rationale: Surgical myectomy is considered the gold standard therapy for LVOT obstruction reduction; however, no randomized controlled trials have compared surgical myectomy with ASA. In observational experience, while surgical myectomy resulted in greater improvements in LVOT gradients than ASA, clinical efficacy was similar between strategies in terms of reduction in NYHA class, syncope, and angina. The difference in outcomes lies primarily in the development of conduction system abnormalities with a 2% to 3% pacemaker implantation rate after surgical myectomy and approximately 7% to 10% pacemaker implantation rate after ASA. The mortality for surgical myectomy and ASA are both less than 1%.

473. The correct answer is D.
Rationale: Contraindications to ASA include patients who are asymptomatic or with well-controlled symptoms on maximally tolerated optimal medical therapy, apical and midcavitary phenotypes, age less than 21 years, and septal thickness less than 15 mm at point of SAM-septal contact (**Table 47.1**).

TABLE 47.1 Indications and Contraindications for Alcohol Septal Ablation

INDICATIONS FOR ALCOHOL SEPTAL ABLATION
- Symptoms that interfere substantially with lifestyle despite optimal medical therapy (New York Heart Association [NYHA] class II, III, or IV; CCS [Canadian Cardiovascular] class 2, 3, or 4 angina or recurrent gradient-related lightheadedness or syncope)
- Resting or provoked left ventricular outflow tract gradient of >50 mm Hg
- Adequately sized and accessible septal branches supplying the target myocardial segment
- Absence of important intrinsic abnormality of mitral valve and of other conditions for which cardiac surgery is independently indicated

CONTRAINDICATIONS TO ALCOHOL SEPTAL ABLATION
- Asymptomatic disease or minimal symptoms
- Septal thickness <15 mm at point of systolic anterior motion contact
- Patients with well-controlled symptoms on optimal medical therapy
- Children and adults aged <21 y
- Apical and midcavitary phenotypes are absolute and contraindications, respectively.

474. The correct answer is B.
Rationale: One of the multiple factors favoring ASA over septal myectomy is having an adequately hypertrophied septum of at least 15 mm in thickness. This is strongly recommended since performing an ASA in patients with septal thickness less than 15 mm is associated with higher risk of iatrogenic ventricular septal defect. Additional factors that favor ASA include older patients over 60 years, preexisting RBBB, resting or provoked gradient more than 50 mm Hg, presence of preexisting

permanent pacemaker (PPM) or implantable cardioverter-defibrillator (ICD), favorable coronary anatomy, patients at high or prohibitive cardiac risk, and prior failed myectomy. Surgical myectomy, on the other hand, is preferred in patients who have surgically correctable cardiac comorbidities, presence of midventricular obstruction, severe LVOT gradients of more than 100 mm Hg resting and more than 200 mm Hg provoked, preexisting LBBB, unfavorable coronary anatomy, septal thickness less than 15 mm, and younger patients below 40 years (in patients <21 years, ASA is contraindicated with a class III recommendation) (**Table 47.2**).

TABLE 47.2 Factors Favoring Alcohol Septal Ablation and Septal Myomectomy in Hypertrophic Obstructive Cardiomyopathy

	Factors Favoring Septal Ablation	Factors Favoring Septal Myectomy
Patient and Clinical Factors	• Patient's age: >60 y • Adults of any age with particularly favorable anatomy • Patients at high or prohibitive cardiac risk • Patients with preexisting RBBB • Patients with preexisting PPM/ICD • Prior failed myectomy	• Younger patients, especially those <21 y • Patients with surgically correctable cardiac comorbidities • Preexisting left bundle branch block • Prior failed alcohol septal ablation
Anatomic and Hemodynamic Factors	• Septal thickness >15 mm • Resting or provoked gradient >50 mm Hg • Accessible septal branches supplying the target myocardium • Presence of a focal septal bulge • Obstructive LVOT gradients localized to the proximal basal ventricular septum	• Septal thickness <15 mm • Lack of accessible septal branches • Massive diffuse LVH with septal thickness >25-30 mm • Presence of midventricular obstruction • Presence of subvalvular membranes • Presence of anomalous papillary muscles • Severe LVOT gradients of >100 mm Hg resting and >200 mm Hg provoked

ICD, implantable cardioverter-defibrillator; LVH, left ventricular hypertrophy; LVOT, left ventricular outflow tract; PPM, permanent pacemaker; RBBB, right bundle branch block.

475 The correct answer is D.

Rationale: Intraprocedural echocardiography is performed to localize the area of myocardial infarction during alcohol injection and determine improvements in LVOT gradient and SAM in real time. The target septal branch usually originates from the proximal segment of the LAD artery; however, it is not always the first septal. It may be the second or third septal, or it may originate from diagonal or ramus intermediate branches of the left coronary artery. In general, no more than 1 mL for every 1-cm maximal wall thickness at the point of SAM contact or at the point of maximal flow acceleration should be used, with average alcohol doses of approximately 1 to 2 mL.

476. The correct answer is A:
Rationale: Damage to the AV conduction system is a frequent complication of ASA, with RBBB being the most common. Approximately 40% to 60% of patients will develop a RBBB, and 20% of them will have an associated left anterior fascicular block. Around 10% to 15% develop a new LBBB, and first-degree AV block complicates 7% to 17% of procedures. Approximately 25% to 50% of patients will develop transient complete AV block during the ASA procedure. In most cases, the conduction system recovers by day 3 or day 4 post-ASA; however, 10% to 20% of patients will have persistent AV block.

477. The correct answer is B:
Rationale: In all patients without an implanted cardiac electronic device with ventricular sensing and pacing feature, a TVP is required prior to ASA, regardless of their underlying conduction disease. This is due to the high rate of injury to the AV conduction system during or after the procedure (up to 55% of patients may develop transient complete heart block during the procedure). The use of a flexible screw-in pacemaker electrode is the preferred pacing wire because it may lower the incidence of pericardial tamponade resulting from cardiac perforation, improve lead stability and threshold, and promote earlier ambulation and more prolonged monitoring when compared to the balloon-tip pacemaker wire. The following electrophysiologic features predict the development of complete heart block necessitating permanent pacing: complete heart block during the ASA, preexisting or new bundle branch conduction disturbances, post-ASA prolonged PR duration/first-degree AV block, and absence of retrograde AV-nodal conduction after ASA.

478. The correct answer is B:
Rationale: Approximately 80% to 90% of ASA procedure achieve procedural success, which is defined by postprocedural improvement in NYHA functional class by at least one class and a reduction of greater than 50% in the peak resting or provoked LVOT gradient, with a final resting gradient of less than 20 mm Hg. Diastolic function improvement and regression of LVH may continue up to 2 years later. Roughly 10% of patients require repeat septal reduction therapy because of procedural failure or recurrent symptoms with dynamic obstruction despite optimal medical therapy.

479. The correct answer is C:
Rationale: In patients with obstructive coronary artery disease (CAD) in the LAD located around the origin of a target septal perforator artery, it is preferred to proceed with ASA first, prior to performing PCI of the obstructive LAD lesion, in order to avoid difficulties in accessing the septal artery for the ASA. In this particular case, given the history of a prior failed myectomy, ASA would be the preferred nonpharmacologic treatment option. Referring the patient for percutaneous intramyocardial septal radiofrequency ablation would not be appropriate since the use of radiofrequency catheter ablation (RFCA) for the treatment of HCM is still under investigation and development.

47.10 The correct answer is C.

Rationale: The mechanism of ASA involves the creation of a localized myocardial infarction in the septal artery territory, and, therefore, elevation of cardiac enzymes postprocedure is expected. Peak myocardial enzyme levels (usually CPK level obtained at 6-hour intervals) correlate well with the infarct size, procedural success, and long-term efficacy. Optimal CPK level is usually in the range of 800 to 1,200 units. Lower levels of CPK suggest potentially too small a septal myocardial ablation, whereas higher CPK levels indicate potential spillage of ethanol to other regions of the myocardium.

LEFT ATRIAL APPENDAGE CLOSURE*

Ravi Kiran Vutheeri and Mohammad El-Hajjar

CHAPTER 48

QUESTIONS

48.1 All of the following factors increase the propensity of thrombus formation in the left atrial appendage (LAA) in patients with atrial fibrillation **EXCEPT**:
- A. Decrease in appendage blood flow velocity
- B. Inflammation
- C. Increase in appendage velocity
- D. Endothelial dysfunction

48.2 The rationale for LAA closure is based on the thought that most thrombi originate in the LAA. What percentage of thrombi occur in the LAA?
- A. 55%
- B. 80%
- C. 90%
- D. 75%

48.3 **CORRECTLY** match the following anatomic patterns of the LAA to one of the choices listed:

Anatomic Patterns
- A. Cactus
- B. Windsock
- C. Chicken wing
- D. Cauliflower

Description
- Dominant lobe in its proximal or middle portion
- Multiple branches arising from the dominant lobe
- Complex branching of multiple lobes without a dominant lobe
- Relatively straight dominant lobe

- A. Dominant lobe in its proximal or middle portion: C; Multiple branches arising from the dominant lobe: A; Complex branching of multiple lobes without a dominant lobe: D; Relatively straight dominant lobe: B
- B. Dominant lobe in its proximal or middle portion: A; Multiple branches arising from the dominant lobe: B; Complex branching of multiple lobes without a dominant lobe: C; Relatively straight dominant lobe: D

---

*Questions and Answers are based on Chapter 48: Left Atrial Appendage Closure by Thomas A. Dewland and Randall J. Lee in Cardiovascular Medicine and Surgery, First Edition.

C. Dominant lobe in its proximal or middle portion: B; Multiple branches arising from the dominant lobe: C; Complex branching of multiple lobes without a dominant lobe: D; Relatively straight dominant lobe: A

D. Dominant lobe in its proximal or middle portion: D; Multiple branches arising from the dominant lobe: C; Complex branching of multiple lobes without a dominant lobe: B; Relatively straight dominant lobe: A

48.4 A 74-year-old female with a history of atrial fibrillation presents to the hospital for elective Watchman implantation. Her other history includes hypertension, diabetes, and previous stroke. After her procedure, she becomes tachycardic and hypotensive. Which of the following is the **MOST LIKELY** complication the patient is experiencing?

A. Pulmonary embolism
B. Cardiac tamponade
C. Hemorrhagic stroke
D. Nephritis

48.5 John is a 67-year-old male with a history of atrial fibrillation, hypertension, and previous stroke. He is unable to take long-term anticoagulation due to gastrointestinal bleeding issues. The patient is interested in a Watchman implant but wants to know more about the recovery process and medication requirements after the procedure. Which of the following statements is **CORRECT**?

A. Patients are discharged on daily anticoagulation and aspirin 81 mg daily. After a repeat transesophageal echocardiogram (TEE) is performed at 45 days and shows an adequate seal, anticoagulation is stopped and the patient starts aspirin 325 mg and clopidogrel 75 mg daily. After 6 months, the patient continues on aspirin 325 mg indefinitely.

B. Patients are discharged on clopidogrel 75 mg and aspirin 81 mg. After a repeat TEE is performed at 45 days and shows an adequate seal, anticoagulation is started and aspirin is increased to 325 mg daily. After 6 months, the patient continues on aspirin 325 mg indefinitely.

C. Patients are discharged on daily anticoagulation and aspirin 81 mg daily. After a repeat TEE is performed at 60 days and shows an adequate seal, anticoagulation is stopped and the patient starts aspirin 325 mg and clopidogrel 75 mg daily. After 6 months, the patient continues on aspirin 325 mg indefinitely.

D. Patients are discharged on daily anticoagulation and aspirin 325 mg. After a repeat TEE is performed at 45 days and shows an adequate seal, anticoagulation is stopped and the patient starts aspirin 81 mg and clopidogrel 75 mg daily. After 6 months, the patient continues on aspirin 81 mg indefinitely.

48.6 The **BEST** transeptal puncture location to facilitate efficient device delivery is inferior.

A. True
B. False
C. There is not enough data to answer this question.

48.7 Which of the following is **INCORRECT** in the PASS (Pull, Aim, Squeeze, and Sweep) criteria prior to release of the device?
   A. Position—Proximal aspect of the device should sit at the appendage ostium and cover all lobes.
   B. Anchor—Documenting stability of the device after the tug test
   C. Size—Device should be between 80% and 92% of the nominal diameter (8%-20% compressed) and should be confirmed by multiple TEE views.
   D. Seal—Defined as absence or minimal flow (<10 mm) around the device

48.8 A 74-year-old man is evaluated for LAA occlusion with the Watchman device in your clinic. His imaging with TEE preprocedure shows a maximum LAA ostium of 25 mm. A 27-mm device was chosen and deployed in the appendage with no complications. Imaging shows that the device is 12% compressed. Before the device is released, imaging shows that there is a leak around the device 7 mm in width. Which of the following statements is **TRUE**?
   A. Although there is a 7-mm leak, this is within normal limits and demonstrates an adequate seal.
   B. A computed tomography (CT) scan should have been used to assess size and characteristics of the LAA.
   C. The device is too small and does not adequately occlude the appendage.
   D. Since the device is within the normal compression range, this means the device is correctly sized and occluding the appendage.

48.9 Which one of the following patients with atrial fibrillation is **NOT** a good candidate for the Watchman LAA closure procedure?
   A. A 65-year-old female with diabetes, hypertension, and prior gastrointestinal bleed
   B. A 91-year-old male with hypertension, congestive heart failure, Parkinson disease, and recurrent falls
   C. A 58-year-old female with prior cryptogenic stroke and deep vein thrombosis (DVT)
   D. A 55-year-old male roofer with history of diabetes, peripheral vascular disease, and hypertension

ANSWERS

48.1 The correct answer is C.
Rationale: Due to reduction of mechanical atrial function and LAA contractility with atrial fibrillation, there is a *decrease* and not an increase in appendage velocity. In addition, inflammation and endothelial dysfunction contribute to the formation of thrombi in approximately 90% of the time in the LAA due to atrial fibrillation.

48.2 The correct answer is C.
Rationale: It is thought that approximately 90% of thrombi that develop secondary to atrial fibrillation originate in the LAA.

48.3 Correct matching: A-C; B-D; C-A; D-B

48.4 The correct answer is B.
Rationale: Patient has two signs consistent with tamponade. Pericardial effusion is a known complication during LAA closure procedures. In the PROTECT-AF trial, pericardial effusion requiring intervention was reported to be 4.3%. In more recent pooled data from registries and studies, this incidence was shown to be lower, around 1.3%. Other complications include vascular complications, periprocedural stroke, device embolization, device erosion, death, and cardiac arrest.

48.5 The correct answer is A.
Rationale: Patients continue their oral anticoagulation with aspirin 81 mg for 45 days postprocedure. A repeat TEE is performed at that time, and if there is an adequate seal without thrombus, the patient can be transitioned to aspirin 325 mg and clopidogrel 75 mg daily for 6 months. Thereafter, they will be continued on aspirin 325 mg daily. Option B is incorrect as they are not started on dual antiplatelet therapy after the procedure. Option C is incorrect as the repeat TEE is at 45 days, not 60 days. Option D is incorrect as the patient is started on aspirin 81 mg and not 325 mg postprocedure.

48.6 The correct answer is True.
Rationale: This is the best puncture location as the dominant lobe in most appendages is anterior and superior. This allows for coaxial orientation of the delivery sheath and appendage.

48.7 The correct answer is D.
Rationale: This is incorrect as minimal flow around the device should be less than 5 mm using TEE color Doppler and fluoroscopic contrast.

48.8 The correct answer is C.
Rationale: A leak greater than 5 mm exceeds the acceptable range, indicating inadequate occlusion of the appendage by the device. TEE sizing was used in the landmark trials, providing accurate sizing for the device. Since there is a large leak, the current device should be removed, and a larger size Watchman device should be chosen (**Figures 48.1 and 48.2**).

48.9 The correct answer is C.
Rationale: This patient does not have a contraindication for long-term anticoagulation, and her DVT history alone indicates anticoagulation. The other patients are better candidates for the Watchman procedure since they are poor candidates for long-term anticoagulation due to prior gastrointestinal bleeding, recurrent falls, and a profession with exposure to such risks.

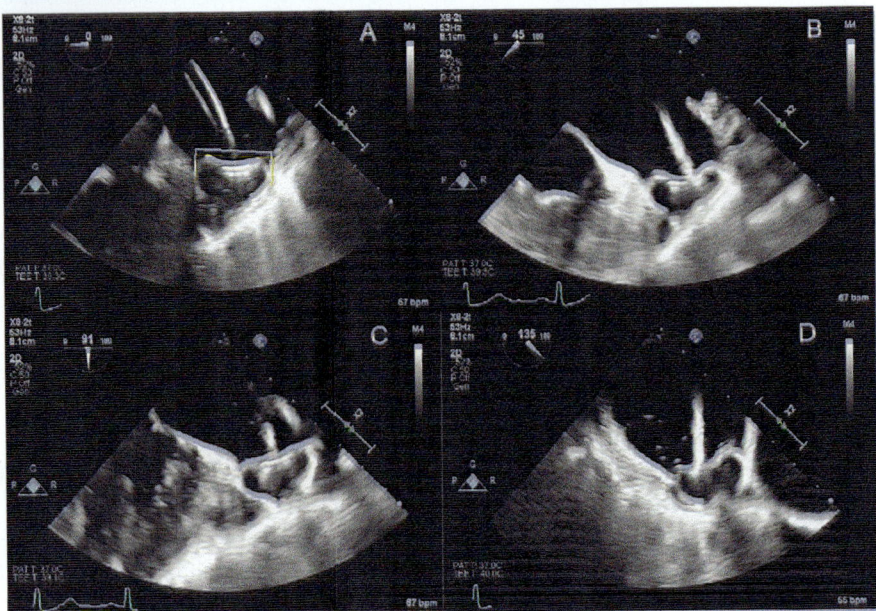

Figure 48.1 Post-deployment Watchman transesophageal echocardiographic evaluation. After device delivery, assessment for compression, appropriate positioning, and adequate seal is performed using transesophageal echocardiography in the 0° (**A**), 45° (**B**), 90° (**C**), and 135° (**D**) views. To ensure accurate assessment of maximal compression, diameter measurements (**A**, yellow line) should be obtained in a plane that also images the central threaded insert.

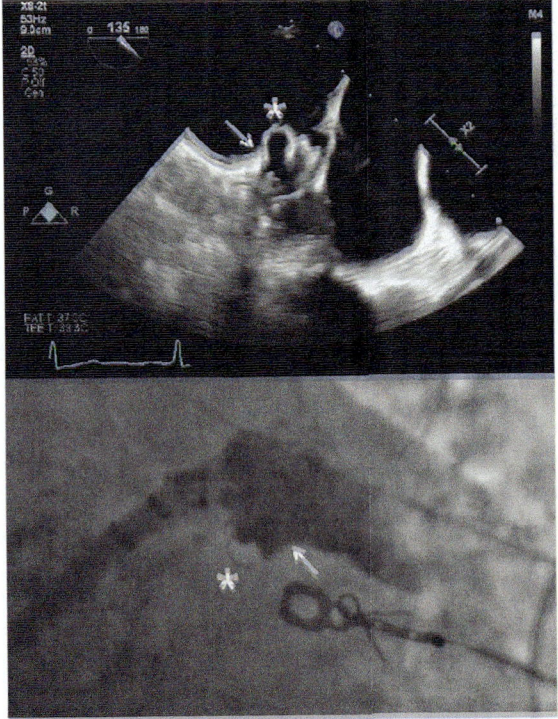

Figure 48.2 Unacceptable Watchman device shoulder. An example of a Watchman device placed too proximally, resulting in a large inferior shoulder (*) that extends far beyond the appendage ostium (arrow). This particular device was recaptured and repositioned.

ELECTROCARDIOGRAM*

Robert L. Carhart, Shweta Paulraj, and Sean Byrnes

CHAPTER 49

QUESTIONS

49.1 A 34-year-old male comes into the office with complaints of chest pain. He recently got over a viral illness. His electrocardiogram (ECG) shows diffuse ST elevations and PR (**Figure 49.1**).

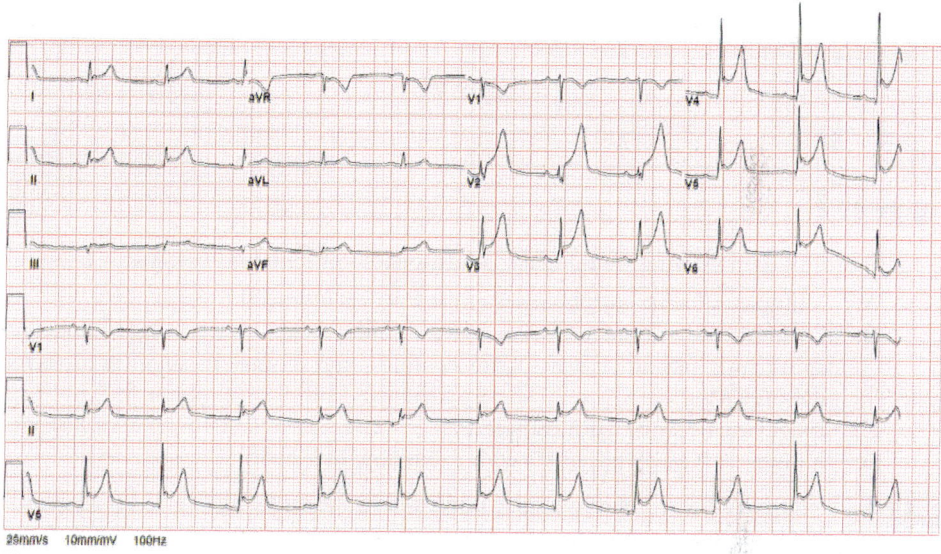

Figure 49.1

What is the likely chest pain characteristic in this patient?
- **A.** Chest pain that is worse when supine
- **B.** Chest pain that radiates down his arm and is worsened with exercise
- **C.** Chest pain that is worse with palpation
- **D.** Chest pain that does not have any exacerbating or alleviating factors

49.2 All of the following are causes of poor R wave progression **EXCEPT** for what?
- **A.** Obesity
- **B.** Anterior myocardial infarction (MI)
- **C.** Poor lead placement
- **D.** Wolff-Parkinson-White

*Questions and Answers are based on Chapter 49: Electrocardiogram by Duc H. Do and Noel G. Boyle in Cardiovascular Medicine and Surgery, First Edition.

49.3 A 56-year-old male presents to the clinic for follow-up of hypertension. His ECG is presented to you for review (**Figure 49.2**).

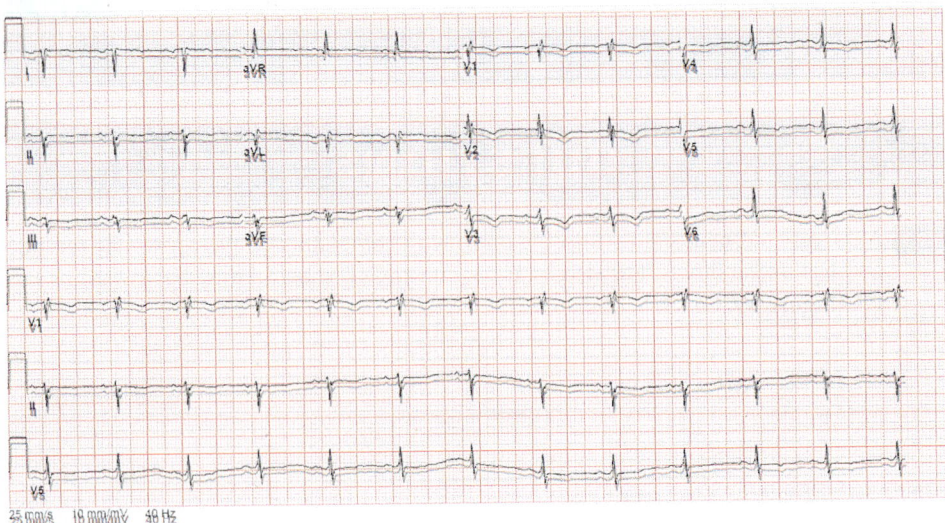
Figure 49.2

Which of the following would make you suspicious of limb lead reversal?
A. Multiple different morphologies of the P waves in lead II
B. Predominantly negative P wave, QRS complex, and T wave in lead I and predominantly upward P wave, QRS complex, and T wave in augmented vector right (aVR)
C. Irregularly irregular QRS complexes
D. A biphasic P wave in lead V1 with a notching in lead II

49.4 A 25-year-old African American male is referred to the cardiology clinic for an abnormal ECG. He saw his primary care physician (PCP) for a regular checkup and was without complaints. ECG obtained by the PCP showed ST elevation in the anterior leads. Today the ECG again shows ST elevations in the anterior leads at the J point with a notched pattern. He remains asymptomatic. What is the likely diagnosis?
A. Left ventricular (LV) apical aneurysm
B. Brugada syndrome
C. Benign early repolarization
D. Hyperkalemia

49.5 A 56-year-old male with a past medical history of hypertension, hyperlipidemia, and a drug-eluting stent to his right coronary artery 4 years ago is admitted to the hospital with a hemorrhagic stroke. His ECG on presentation shows deep T-wave inversions diffusely. His high-sensitivity troponin is normal, and he does not endorse any chest pain. What is the likely cause of these ECG abnormalities?
A. Stent thrombosis
B. Hemorrhagic stroke
C. Pericarditis
D. Lead misplacement

49.6 Which of the following statements is **TRUE**?
- A. The normal axis of the heart is more vertical in older adults (90°-100°), with a gradual shift rightward throughout life.
- B. The normal axis of the heart is more vertical in young individuals (90°-100°), with a gradual shift leftward throughout life.
- C. The axis of the heart remains fixed between −30° and 90° and does not change with age in the absence of underlying cardiac conditions.
- D. The normal axis of the heart is more vertical in women irrespective of age.

49.7 What is the **CORRECT** method to measure the QT interval?
- A. The QT is measured in lead V2 or V3 as this is the most accurate lead for measurement.
- B. Average the QT measurement over the one precordial QT and the one limb lead QT measurement.
- C. The QT is measured in the lead with the longest QT interval.
- D. The QT can be measured in any lead and will give the same value when corrected for heart rate.

49.8 All of the following are causes of right axis deviation **EXCEPT**:
- A. Inferior MI
- B. Ostium secundum atrial septal defect
- C. Normal variant in young individuals
- D. Wolf-Parkinson-White syndrome

49.9 A 54-year-old male comes in with chest pain that he describes as a burning sensation at the center of his chest for the past 1 week. His ECG shows sinus rhythm with Q waves in lead III and aVR. No significant abnormalities were noted on other leads, and ST segments are normal. What are your differentials?
- A. Old inferior/right-sided MI, given Q waves in lead III and aVR
- B. Based on the information provided, this is likely a normal ECG.
- C. Suspect left posterior fascicular block, given Q waves in lead III.
- D. Early manifestation of an acute right ventricular MI

49.10 What is the sensitivity and specificity of the stress ECG for diagnosing ischemia?
- A. 97% sensitivity and specificity
- B. Approximately 30% sensitivity and specificity
- C. It is sensitive but not specific.
- D. Approximately 70% sensitivity and specificity

ANSWERS

49.1 The correct answer is A.
Rationale: Pericarditis presents with diffuse ST elevations and PR depressions. The pain is usually described as pleuritic and worse when supine. It commonly is preceded by a viral illness or MI.

49.2 The correct answer is B.
Rationale: While there are many causes for poor R wave progression, the most common include obesity, lead misplacement, anterior MI, and LV hypertrophy.

49.3 The correct answer is B.
Rationale: In limb lead reversal, the normally upright P wave in sinus rhythm in lead I becomes negative, and leads II and III and aVR and augmented vector left (aVL) appear switched. In limb lead reversal, there is normal R wave progression across the precordium, unlike in dextrocardia.

49.4 The correct answer is C.
Rationale: LV apical aneurysm can present with persistent ST elevations; however, this is in the setting of a recent MI. Brugada syndrome is a specific ECG pattern of coved ST segment elevation in V1 and V2 with T-wave inversions in a symptomatic patient (such as ventricular arrhythmias, syncope, and family history of sudden cardiac death). Benign early repolarization is described as being in a young asymptomatic patient, usually of African American descent, with ST-segment elevations with J waves. Hyperkalemia classically presents peaked T waves, loss of P waves, and eventually sinusoidal QRS morphology.

49.5 The correct answer is B.
Rationale: Any acute neurologic event, especially hemorrhage in nature, has been reported to cause diffuse symmetric T-wave inversions, along with QT prolongation. Stent thrombosis would present with acute coronary syndrome such as chest pain, ST-segment changes, and elevated troponin, depending on the acuity. Pericarditis presents with diffuse ST elevations and PR depressions along with chest pain worse when supine. Lead misplacement does not cause diffuse T-wave inversions.

49.6 The correct answer is B.
Rationale: The normal axis of the heart is more vertical in young individuals (90°-100°) with a gradual shift leftward throughout life.

49.7 The correct answer is C.
Rationale: The QT interval is measured from the beginning of the QRS complex to the end of the T wave (using a tangent line along the steepest downslope of the T wave, the end of the T wave is marked where this crosses the isoelectric line). The QT interval should be measured in the lead with the longest such interval.

49.8 The correct answer is A.
Rationale: Inferior MI causes left axis deviation. Note that ostium secundum atrial septal defects (ASDs) cause right axis deviation, but ostium primum ASDs can cause left axis deviation.

49.9 The correct answer is B.
Rationale: Q waves can appear normally in leads III and aVR, although they should not also be present in contiguous leads if normal (ie, leads III and augmented vector foot [aVF]).

49.10 The correct answer is D.
Rationale: Stress ECG has approximately 70% sensitivity and specificity for diagnosing ischemia. In patients where a strong clinical suspicion exists, additional imaging modalities such as stress echocardiogram or myocardial perfusion scan should be considered, or proceeding with anatomic evaluation by computed tomography angiography or coronary angiography.

SECTION 4 ELECTROPHYSIOLOGY

CHAPTER 50

MECHANISMS OF CARDIAC ARRHYTHMIAS*

Casey White and Amole Ojo

QUESTIONS

50.1 A 72-year-old woman with past medical history significant for hypertension, hyperlipidemia, and extensive tobacco smoking dependence presents to the hospital with ongoing chest pain. She rules in for an acute inferior ST-segment elevation myocardial infarction (STEMI). She subsequently undergoes successful percutaneous intervention with a single drug-eluting stent placed to the distal right coronary artery. Afterward, she is observed to have sustained, asymptomatic sinus bradycardia on the cardiac telemetry floor. What is the **MOST LIKELY** physiologic explanation for the observed bradycardia?

A. Decreased vagal stimulation leading to phosphorylation-regulated calcium cycling proteins
B. Augmentation of I_f via sympathetic nervous system upregulation
C. Parasympathetic nervous system activation and increase in I_f
D. Activation of muscarinic potassium channels and decrease in I_f activity

50.2 A genetic mutation resulting in an acquired channelopathy may be expected to prolong phase 3 repolarization under which of the following circumstances?

A. Gain of function in either or both I_{Kr} (rapid) and I_{Ks} (slow) delayed rectifier potassium currents
B. Loss of function in either or both I_{Kr} (rapid) and I_{Ks} (slow) delayed rectifier potassium currents
C. Gain of function in only I_{Ks} (slow) delayed rectifier potassium currents
D. Loss of function in only I_{Kr} (rapid) delayed rectifier potassium currents

50.3 Which of the following is **CORRECT** regarding triggered activity?

A. Early afterdepolarizations typically occur during the rapid upstroke of the action potential, correlating with sodium channel activation.
B. Class III antiarrhythmics may induce early afterdepolarizations at faster heart rates due to use-dependence properties.
C. Delayed afterdepolarizations (DADs) may occur secondary to a calcium-induced, calcium-release mechanism.
D. Digitalis leads to direct inhibition of potassium efflux channels, resulting in increased cytoplasmic intracellular potassium concentrations.

*Questions and Answers are based on Chapter 50: Mechanisms of Cardiac Arrhythmias by Peter Hanna, Kalyanam Shivkumar, and James N. Weiss in Cardiovascular Medicine and Surgery, First Edition.

50.4 Propagation of a reentrant tachycardia around a fixed anatomic obstacle typically requires all the following **EXCEPT**:
- A. Anatomic circuit length less than the tachycardia wavelength
- B. Time between the recovery of tissue in the reentrant circuit trailing the waveback and leading the wavefront
- C. Unidirectional block
- D. An inciting premature stimulus

50.5 Which of the following is **INACCURATE** regarding reentry?
- A. Functional reentry entails a functionally refractory core with a depolarizing spiral or scroll wave rotor.
- B. The regional properties leading to heterogeneity in dispersion of excitability and refractoriness contribute to functional reentry.
- C. Monomorphic tachycardias often entail a scroll wave rotor with a stationary refractory core.
- D. A rotator arm with 1:1 conduction, closest to the refractory core, is most likely to degrade to fibrillatory waves.

50.6 An otherwise healthy 30-year-old patient experiencing paroxysmal episodes of palpitations undergoes an electrophysiology (EP) study. Diagnostic catheters are placed in the coronary sinus, at the level of the His bundle, and the right ventricular apical septum. With successive burst pacing down to 200 milliseconds (300 bpm [beats per minute]), atrial fibrillation briefly develops before spontaneously terminating with sinus rhythm restored. What would be the **MOST LIKELY** interpretation?
- A. Paroxysmal atrial fibrillation is confirmed, likely accounting for symptoms.
- B. Rapid pacing likely results in a repolarization core with subsequent unstable rotator arm degrading into fibrillatory waves.
- C. Pacing-induced reentry through dispersion in a region with a short action potential duration (APD) results in unidirectional block and propagation to an adjacent region with long APD.
- D. Triggered activity leads to unidirectional block, conduction slowing, and reentry at the level of the tricuspid valve/inferior vena cava isthmus.

50.7 The intrinsic automaticity of ventricular cardiomyocytes typically remains latent secondary which of the following?
- A. Refractoriness
- B. Autonomic regulation of funny current activity in ventricular cardiomyocytes
- C. Overdrive suppression
- D. Reflection

50.8 A 75-year-old patient with a known history of nonischemic cardiomyopathy, ventricular tachycardia, and subsequent implantable cardioverter-defibrillator is brought to the local emergency department following several delivered shocks from the defibrillator. Interrogation of the device confirms appropriate shocks for recurrent sustained ventricular tachycardia episodes. Over the subsequent hospital course, antiarrhythmic therapy is initiated, in addition to up-titration of beta-blocker therapy. What is one mechanism by which beta-blocker therapies mitigate subsequent reentrant tachycardia?

A. Decreased L-type Ca^{2+} activity
B. Augmentation of inward I_{NCX}
C. Direct decrease in outward repolarizing potassium
D. Inhibition of sodium channels with decreased phase 0 slope

50.9 Which of the following statements is **CORRECT**?
A. Early afterdepolarizations typically occur only under conditions of abbreviated action potential.
B. DADs are mechanistically culprit in catecholaminergic polymorphic ventricular tachycardia (CPVT).
C. States of hyperkalemia and hypocalcemia increase the likelihood of DADs reaching threshold.
D. The ryanodine receptor or calsequestrin promote potassium sarcolemma release.

50.10 Which of the following is characteristic of phase 2 reentry?
A. Regional areas of highly concentrated transient outward potassium current can result in dispersion of refractoriness, allowing propagation of current from areas of heterogeneous APD.
B. Most commonly occurs in regional areas with low-density transient outward potassium activity (I_{to}).
C. Thought to be an important mechanism in focal atrial tachycardias.
D. Regions and conditions of low repolarization reserve favor reentry through an all-or-none action potential mechanism.

ANSWERS

50.1 The correct answer is D.
Rationale: Following an inferior myocardial infarction, increased vagal activity is frequently observed, accounting for observed sinus bradycardia. In more severe cases, activation of muscarinic potassium channels can decrease nodal I_f activity, resulting in decreased sinus rates or even escape rhythms. While enhanced automaticity and sympathetic nervous system upregulation can lead to increased atrioventricular (AV) junctional activity, the observation of sinus bradycardia in this scenario is likely consistent with increased vagal activity; moreover, the identified distal right coronary artery lesion makes involvement of a nodal branch clinically less likely.

50.2 The correct answer is B.
Rationale: The basis of several notable clinical conditions, such as LQTS1 and LQTS2, involve ion channelopathies. In particular, loss of function in repolarizing outward potassium currents prolongs phase 3 repolarization, which clinically can manifest as prolongation of the QT interval. Prolongation of repolarization can potentially allow for triggered activity and reentry.

50.3 The correct answer is C.
Rationale: Triggered activity includes early afterdepolarizations and DADs. Early depolarizations tend to occur during phase 2 and phase 3 of the action potential

correlating with calcium and potassium channel activation. Class III antiarrhythmics, by modulation of phase 3 potassium channels, may induce early afterdepolarizations at slower heart rates secondary to reverse-use dependence. Under conditions promoting increased cytosolic calcium concentrations, excess calcium may result in calcium-induced, calcium-release via the sarcoplasmic reticulum, typically during phase 4 of the action potential. Whereas digitalis has its inhibiting effect on the sodium-potassium ATPase, pronounced in toxicity, leading to an increase in intracellular sodium concentration and subsequent reduction in the sodium driving gradient, thereby decreasing cytoplasmic calcium exchange via the sodium-calcium exchanger.

50.4 The correct answer is A.
Rationale: Reentry requires the anatomic circuit to exceed the wavelength, allowing for an excitable gap between the waveback and wavefront. The excitable gap is the time between the recovery of tissue in the reentrant circuit trailing the waveback and leading the wavefront. Initiation under these circumstances is dependent on a premature stimulus with unidirectional conduction.

50.5 The correct answer is D.
Rationale: Options A, B, and C describe functional reentry and conditions for reentry. A rotator arm may become unstable, degrading further into multiple fibrillatory waves, clinically resulting in fibrillation. A rotator arm is likely to degrade further into fibrillatory waves if distant from the core, thus unable to maintain 1:1 conduction, or by unstable dynamic oscillations.

50.6 The correct answer is C.
Rationale: The clinical scenario describes a common mechanism by which rapid pacing can induce atrial fibrillation in otherwise normal cardiac substrate. Option C describes a reentrant mechanism by spatially discordant APD alterans. Option B describes functional reentry, which is less likely in this clinical context. Likewise, option D describes an anatomic reentrant mechanism, specific to typical atrial flutter.

50.7 The correct answer is C.
Rationale: Automaticity of cardiomyocytes and pacemaker cells remain hierarchically latent secondary to overdrive suppression; that is, the intrinsic rate of the higher pacemaker cells exceeds that of lower sites. As an example, the intrinsic rates of the sinus node exceed that of the lower ventricular intrinsic rates. This may translate clinically in cases of AV nodal disease states, whereby the normally latent activity of lower sites becomes the predominant unopposed pacemaker (ie, ventricular escape rhythm in third-degree AV block).

50.8 The correct answer is A.
Rationale: One of the many effects of beta-blockers is reduction of Ca^{2+} influx via decreased activity of L-type Ca^{2+} channels. Beta-blockers decrease autonomic catecholaminergic activity and cyclic adenosine monophosphate (cAMP), an important part of management in recurrent ventricular tachycardias.

50.9 The correct answer is B.
Rationale: CPVT onset is thought to mechanistically occur with DADs. Mutations in the ryanodine receptor or calsequestrin ultimately result in spontaneous calcium

release from the sarcoplasmic reticulum, triggering a calcium-release, calcium-induced mechanism. Early afterdepolarizations generally occur under conditions of prolonged action potential, but have also been associated with APD shortening. Electrolyte conditions of hypokalemia and hypercalcemia increase DAD likelihood of reaching threshold.

50.10 The correct answer is A.
Rationale: Phase-2 functional reentry entails regional areas of excessive repolarization reserve, occurring in regions with high density of transient outward potassium current activity, such as the right ventricular epicardium. These areas of excessive repolarization reserve can set up for regional APD heterogeneity, resulting in marked dispersion of refractoriness. Through these regional variations, current flow from areas of prominent dome in plateau to short plateau-less action potential areas, that have already undergone repolarization, can set up for premature extrasystole. This is thought to be an important mechanism in congenital short QT syndrome and Brugada syndrome.

GENETICS OF ARRHYTHMIAS*

Casey White and Amele Oje

CHAPTER 51

QUESTIONS

51.1 Which of the following regarding Long QT syndrome (LQTS) is **MOST ACCURATE**?
   A. All subtypes of LQTS entail a loss-of-function potassium channelopathy.
   B. In LQTS type 3, loss-of-function mutations in SCN5A result in action potential prolongation.
   C. Loss-of-function mutations in potassium channels KCNQ1 and KCNH2 correspond to subsequent prolongation of the action potential duration due to aberrant slowly and rapidly activated delayed rectifying potassium current activity.
   D. Calcium channelopathies and calcium-binding protein mutations do not contribute to LQTSs.

51.2 Which of the following genotype-phenotype relationships is **CORRECT**?
   A. LQTS1: auditory-triggered events
   B. LQTS3: sudden cardiac death at rest or sleep state
   C. LQTS2: prominent electrocardiogram (ECG) with long isoelectric segment followed by narrow-based T-wave
   D. LQTS3: greatest response to beta-blocker therapy

51.3 A patient with suspected LQTS2 is observed during monitored exercise testing to have QT prolongation at intermediate heart rates on continuous ECG, while at higher exertional states there is observed appropriate QT shortening. Which of the following is a likely explanation for this observation?
   A. Increased recruitment of I_{Na} at higher exertional levels
   B. Decreased I_{Kr} activity at moderate exertion; recruitment of I_{Ks} at higher exertion
   C. Increased I_{Kr} recruitment at moderate exertion; decreased activity of I_{Ks} at higher exertion
   D. Increased recruitment of I_{Na} at rest state

51.4 Which of the following regarding LQTS diagnosis and treatment is **MOST ACCURATE**?
   A. With a confirmed diagnosis of LQTS, all patients should be referred for implantable cardioverter-defibrillator (ICD) for primary prevention of sudden cardiac death irrespective of symptoms, prior treatments, or genotype.
   B. Despite a high probability Schwartz score (≥ 3.5), genetic testing carries a low likelihood of yielding a known genetic mutation.
   C. Left cardiac sympathetic denervation should be considered a first-line therapy in LQTS.
   D. Initiation of beta-blocker therapy should be considered first-line therapy for all patients unless contraindicated.

*Questions and Answers are based on Chapter 51: Genetics of Arrhythmias by Aadhavi Sridharan, Jason S. Bradfield, and James N. Weiss in Cardiovascular Medicine and Surgery, First Edition.

51.5 A 20-year-old patient with short QT syndrome type 1 (SQTS1), with a confirmed *KCNH2*, mutation, presents after recurrent ICD shocks. ECG reveals sinus rhythm with QTc 340 milliseconds and symmetric peaked T-waves in the precordial leads. Interrogation of the ICD reveals several episodes of non-sustained ventricular tachycardia, as well as recurrent episodes of sustained ventricular tachycardia over the past 48 hours, treated appropriately with anti-tachycardia pacing and ICD shocks. Which of the following is the **BEST** treatment recommendation?

A. Reprogram the ICD with decreased T-wave sensitivity.
B. Initiate amiodarone.
C. Initiate a non-dihydropyridine calcium channel blocker.
D. Initiate quinidine.

51.6 A 30-year-old patient is undergoing a new office evaluation. A 12-lead ECG reveals coved-type ST-segment elevations of 2.5 mm with a negative T-wave in precordial leads V1 and V2. Echocardiogram is without structural abnormalities. The patient has no history of syncope or near-syncopal episodes. There is no established family history of sudden cardiac death. Which of the following is the **BEST** next step?

A. Obtain a repeat ECG with higher repositioning of the precordial V1 and V2 leads at the level of the second intercostal space.
B. Proceed with provocation pharmacologic testing with a sodium channel blocker for the diagnosis of Brugada syndrome (BrS).
C. Referral for cardiac magnetic resonance imaging (MRI)
D. Referral for ICD implantation

51.7 Which of the following regarding catecholaminergic polymorphic ventricular tachycardia (CPVT) is **CORRECT**?

A. The underlying mechanism entails potassium-induced, calcium-release activation of a mutated RyR_2-encoded ryanodine receptor.
B. Arrhythmogenesis is most commonly secondary to outward Na-Ca exchange current triggering early afterdepolarizations.
C. Compared to mutations in the calsequestrin-encoding gene *CASQ2*, mutations in *RyR2* result in a clinically more severe phenotype characterized by higher penetrance, younger age of onset, and younger age at death.
D. Maximally tolerated beta-blocker is considered first-line therapy.

51.8 An 18-year-old patient with CPVT with known *RyR2* mutation presents to the hospital after recurrent syncopal episodes. ICD interrogation confirms recurrent, sustained ventricular tachycardia. To this point, the patient has been maintained on a maximally tolerated beta-blocker dose, as well as flecainide. What is the next appropriate step in therapy?

A. Referral for left cardiac sympathetic denervation
B. Stop flecainide, start a Class III antiarrhythmic.
C. Repeat exercise stress test on current medical therapies.
D. Addition of a non-dihydropyridine calcium channel blocker

51.9 Which of the following is **TRUE** regarding BrS?
  A. Arrhythmogenesis occurs via phase 3 reentry by regional variations in outward potassium current density with predisposition to early repolarization and conduction slowing.
  B. Type 2 ECG pattern (*saddleback*) is strongly correlated with *SCN5A* mutation.
  C. ICD implantation is recommended in patients with type 1 pattern and a history of syncope.
  D. Asymptomatic patients with spontaneous type 1 patterns should be initiated on quinidine for the prevention of ventricular arrhythmias.

51.10 Pair the diagnosis with the **CORRECT** statement:

Statements

i. Age-related fibrosis of native His-Purkinje conduction system that is most frequently inherited in an autosomal dominant pattern. Can present with bundle branch blocks, intraventricular conduction delay, syncope, or sudden cardiac death
ii. Fetal bradycardia, pronounced QT prolongation, T-wave alternans, and 2:1 atrioventricular block due to a gene mutation-encoding cardiac L-type calcium channels
iii. Mutations in sodium and potassium ion channels and non-ion channel variants connexin 40, renin-angiotensin system, and atrial natriuretic peptide
iv. Loss-of-function mutation in *KCNJ2* encoding the inward rectifier potassium channel. Prominent U-waves, QTU prolongation, polymorphic ventricular tachycardia, and bidirectional ventricular tachycardia

Diagnosis

- A Atrial fibrillation
- B. Timothy syndrome
- C. Lev-Lenegre disease
- D. SQTS
- E. BrS
- F. CPVT
- G. Andersen-Tawil syndrome

  A. 1-C, 2-B, 3-A, 4-G
  B. 1-D, 2-A, 3-B, 4-G
  C. 1-G, 2-A, 3-B, 4-C
  D. 1-B, 2-G, 3-C, 4-D

ANSWERS

51.1 The correct answer is C.
Rationale: There are several recognized subtypes of LQTS to date; while many recognized gene mutations affect potassium currents, other chromosomal loci and gene mutations are known to affect sodium and calcium trafficking. In LQT3, gain-of-function mutation in SCN5A increases late Na$^+$ activity resulting in increased action potential duration. In LQTS1 and LQTS2, loss-of-function mutations, commonly encoding potassium channel activity, lead to action potential prolongation.

51.2 The correct answer is B.

Rationale: Events in LQTS1 are associated with higher exertional states, such as swimming. Due to increased events at higher exertional states, beta-blocker response is greatest in the LQTS1 subtype, compared to LQTS2 and LQTS3. Auditory-triggered events have been classically described in LQTS2, whereas events occurring at rest/sleep state have been well-described in LQTS3. ECG morphology in LQTS1 is classically characterized by a broad-based T-wave, LQTS2 a low-amplitude or biphasic T-wave, and LQTS3 a long isoelectric ST segment followed by a narrow-based T-wave.

51.3 The correct answer is B.

Rationale: QT hysteresis may offer clinical insight into LQTS phenotype. In LQTS2, loss-of-function mutations in *KCNH2* result in decreased recruitment activity of I_{Kr}, which is active at moderate exertional levels. At higher levels of exertion, there is greater recruitment of I_{Ks}. LQTS2, therefore, may demonstrate an exaggerated QT-prolonging response to a moderate exertional state but exhibit normal QT shortening at high exertional and rest states due to normal I_{Ks} and I_{Na} activity.

51.4 The correct answer is D.

Rationale: All patients diagnosed with LQTS should be initiated on beta-blocker therapy, unless contraindicated. A nonselective beta-blocker, such as nadolol or propranolol, is preferable. Other therapies, such as left cardiac sympathetic denervation, generally should be reserved for patients with symptoms or arrhythmias refractory to beta-blocker therapy or for those who cannot tolerate beta-blocker therapy. A high probability Schwartz score carries an 80% likelihood of a positive LQTS genetic test. ICD for primary prevention should be considered in patients with refractory symptoms despite beta-blocker therapy and in high-risk asymptomatic patients (QTc >500 milliseconds, LQTS2 and LQTS3 genotypes, history of recurrent syncope, onset of symptoms <10 years of age, age <40).

51.5 The correct answer is D.

Rationale: In this case, the patient has confirmed SQTS1 with a *KCNH2* mutation and presents with recurrent ventricular tachycardic episodes, both sustained and nonsustained in duration. This patient already has a previously implanted ICD; given sustained ventricular arrhythmia, an ICD should otherwise be recommended in such a high-risk patient. As defined in the vignette, the ICD appropriately delivers therapy via anti-tachycardia pacing and shocks. In SQTS, due to prominent T-waves, oversensing can be potentially problematic with *inappropriate* delivery of therapy. However, there is no indication to reprogram the ICD here given that these are appropriate device therapies. Amiodarone could be considered for ventricular tachycardia; however, due to potential long-term side effects such as pulmonary fibrosis, this is a less ideal therapy in a 20-year-old patient. Patients with *KCNH2* mutations have a shorter QT interval and observed greater response to quinidine. In this patient, initiation of the QT-prolonging drug, quinidine, is the next best step in therapy. A non-dihydropyridine calcium channel blocker may be of benefit in supraventricular tachycardias but is not considered first-line therapy for ventricular tachycardias.

51.6 The correct answer is C.

Rationale: The 12-lead ECG describes a spontaneous type 1 Brugada pattern. Repositioning the precordial leads higher to the second intercostal space can be helpful in increasing the sensitivity of the ECG for diagnosing Brugada. This is a particularly helpful adjustment when the presenting ECG reveals a type 2 or 3 pattern; in this case, there is no indication for repositioning given presenting type 1 pattern. Likewise, proceeding with pharmacologic provocation testing is useful in further assessing type 2 or 3 patterns, or when BrS is suspected without a spontaneous type 1 pattern. Patients with asymptomatic spontaneous type 1 pattern should undergo cardiac imaging, including echocardiogram and cardiac MRI. Right ventricular outflow tract (RVOT) localization determined by using cardiac MRI correlates highly with the type I Brugada pattern. In asymptomatic patients with type 1 patterns, an electrophysiology (EP) study could be considered for further risk stratification. The presence of an ECG type 1 pattern in isolation does not reflexively warrant ICD implantation.

51.7 The correct answer is D.

Rationale: CPVT is a hereditary arrhythmia with a hallmark presentation of exercise-induced syncope or sudden cardiac death. ECG commonly demonstrates bidirectional ventricular tachycardia. Beta-blocker therapy initiation is recommended with diagnosis. The underlying mechanism entails a calcium-induced, calcium-release mechanism (choice A) secondary to a mutation in the ryanodine receptor protein/associated ryanodine receptor protein or calcium-binding sarcoplasmic reticulum protein, resulting in inward Na-Ca exchange current activity, which can trigger delayed afterdepolarizations (choice B). The autosomal recessive calsequestrin form, secondary to *CASQ2* mutation, results in a more severe phenotype as described earlier (choice C). Therapeutic management for patients with CPVT includes maximally tolerated beta-blockers without intrinsic sympathomimetic activity. Nadolol is the beta-blocker of choice in a high dosage, 1–2 mg/kg (correct choice D).

51.8 The correct answer is A.

Rationale: This young patient with established CPVT is on a maximally tolerated beta-blocker, as well as a Class IC antiarrhythmic, namely flecainide. The patient also previously underwent ICD implantation. Given recurrent ventricular arrhythmias on maximal medical therapies, the next reasonable step in therapy is a referral for left cardiac sympathetic denervation.

51.9 The correct answer is C.

Rationale: Arrhythmogenesis in BrS occurs as a result of regional variations in repolarization and conduction slowing, most notably due to a loss-of-function sodium channelopathy. In areas with high *Ito* density, regional conduction and repolarization differences set up for potential phase 2 functional reentry, not phase 3. *SCN5A* mutations do not phenotypically correlate with ECG patterns. Asymptomatic patients with spontaneous type 1 ECG pattern should undergo further workup and testing including structural evaluation via echocardiogram and/or cardiac MRI. ICD implantation is recommended in patients with type 1 pattern presenting with syncope.

51.10 The correct answer is A.

Rationale: A pairs the condition descriptions with the clinical conditions correctly. Statement i: Describes choice (C) Lev-Lenegre disease; Statement ii: Describes choice (B) Timothy syndrome; Statement iii: Describes choice (A) atrial fibrillation; and Statement iv: Describes choice (G) Andersen-Tawil syndrome.

AMBULATORY RHYTHM MONITORING*

Casey White and Amole Ojo

CHAPTER 52

QUESTIONS

52.1 A 26-year-old patient presents to the outpatient office with ongoing symptoms of intermittent palpitations experienced 1 to 2 times per week over the past week. The episodes are distressing to the patient, often requiring cessation of activity until palpitations resolve after several minutes to an hour. It seems that the palpitations can stop with vagal maneuvers but not always. Physical examination is unrevealing. 12-lead electrocardiogram (ECG) reveals sinus rhythm with nonspecific T-wave abnormalities. Laboratory testing, including thyroid function and assessment of electrolytes, is unremarkable. What is the next **BEST** step in management?

A. Start empiric beta-blocker therapy.
B. Order a 24-hour Holter monitor to assess for underlying arrhythmia.
C. Order a 30-day event monitor to assess for underlying arrhythmia.
D. Proceed with implantation of an implantable loop recorder.

52.2 Which of the following regarding Holter monitoring is **MOST** accurate?

A. Holter monitoring offers high diagnostic sensitivity, comparable to implantable loop recorders.
B. Offers event-only (auto or patient triggered) intermittent monitoring
C. Ideal monitoring system to assess atrial arrhythmia burden over a several months period
D. Requires wearable leads and external device

52.3 A 56-year-old patient has a known history of nonischemic cardiomyopathy. The patient is admitted to the hospital following a syncopal episode while driving, resulting in a motor vehicle accident sustaining a right humeral fracture. There are no reports of preceding prodrome before the syncope. Telemetry monitoring during the hospital course reveals sinus rhythm with occasional premature ventricular ectopy. An echocardiogram reveals global hypokinesis, moderate mitral regurgitation, and a left ventricular ejection fraction (LVEF) of 40%. An electrophysiology (EP) study is recommended. EP study was non-inducible for ventricular tachycardia (VT), as well as supra-VTs. Conduction study was normal. Which of the following is the most reasonable next step?

A. Implantable cardioverter-defibrillator (ICD) implantation for probable ventricular arrhythmia
B. Event monitor for 30 days
C. Extended Holter monitor for 2 weeks
D. Implantable loop recorder

*Questions and Answers are based on Chapter 52: Ambulatory Rhythm Monitoring by Kevin Sung, Justin Hayase, and Jason S. Bradfield in Cardiovascular Medicine and Surgery, First Edition.

52.4 A 70-year-old female with a history of hypertension maintained on amlodipine presents to the office for evaluation after experiencing recent, intermittent symptoms of overt fatigue, pre-syncope, and a decline in exertional status. A resting 12-lead ECG is obtained, which is notable for a PR interval of 260 milliseconds, sinus bradycardia with a ventricular rate of 58 beats per minute (bpm), and an incomplete right bundle branch block. While walking in the hallway, telemetry monitoring demonstrates peak heart rate into the 90 bpm range. She is asymptomatic at this time and cannot reproduce the symptoms previously experienced. Which of the following management strategies is recommended?

A. Event monitor
B. 24- to 48-hour Holter monitor
C. Implantable loop recorder
D. Coronary angiogram

52.5 A 45-year-old patient with intermittent palpitations undergoes placement of an event monitor for continuous, real-time monitoring. The monitoring service calls for an auto-triggered event noting a 4.1-second pause and bradycardic nadir to 35 bpm occurring at 3:00 AM. The patient was asymptomatic during this episode and reports sleeping during this time. What is the next **BEST** step in management?

A. Continued monitoring
B. Exercise treadmill test
C. Permanent pacemaker implantation
D. EP study

52.6 A 78-year-old female with a history of hypertension and paroxysmal atrial fibrillation is wearing an event monitor for recurrent symptoms of lightheadedness and palpitations. She is maintained on metoprolol succinate 100 mg daily and a direct oral anticoagulant. Auto-triggered and patient-triggered events are notable for daytime pauses up to 6 seconds, average heart rate of 55 bpm, and lowest heart rate of 38 bpm. Pauses occur in sinus rhythm and with conversion from atrial fibrillation to sinus rhythm. Symptomatic tachycardic episodes occurring 18% of the time correspond to atrial fibrillation with rapid ventricle rates, with a maximal heart rate of 140 bpm. What is the next **BEST** step in management?

A. Increase metoprolol for prevention of tachycardic episodes.
B. Start flecainide for rhythm control.
C. Dual-chamber permanent pacemaker implant
D. Observation

52.7 A 72-year-old patient was recently admitted for decompensated heart failure in the setting of newly diagnosed cardiomyopathy. He was found to be in atrial fibrillation with rapid ventricular rate at the time. The patient was not aware of the atrial fibrillation as he never felt any palpitations. Coronary angiogram showed nonobstructive coronary artery disease. His cardiomyopathy was considered to be tachycardia mediated. He later underwent radiofrequency ablation of all his pulmonary veins. Entrance and exit blocks were confirmed at the conclusion of the case. Which of the following monitoring strategies is the **BEST** to evaluate for atrial fibrillation recurrence following ablation?

A. Implantable loop recorder
B. Extended Holter monitor
C. Event monitor
D. Wearable watch monitor

52.8 Which of the following clinical scenarios is ambulatory monitoring **MOST** indicated?

A. 20-year-old-college student with some palpitations occurring with caffeine consumption
B. 56-year-old patient with incidental left bundle branch on 12-lead ECG during employment health assessment
C. 72-year-old patient with baseline right bundle branch block presenting with syncope following transcatheter aortic valve replacement
D. 48-year-old patient with recently diagnosed hypertrophic cardiomyopathy (HCM)

52.9 Which of the following statements regarding direct-to-consumer monitors is **MOST** accurate?

A. The REHEARSE-AF trial demonstrated efficacy in detecting asymptomatic atrial fibrillation in patients with elevated CHA2DS2-VASc score using aggressive monitoring.
B. Head-to-head comparisons between 12-lead ECGs and direct-to-consumer monitors were found to be dissimilar.
C. Assessment of arrhythmias on direct-to-consumer monitors has shown superior detection compared to conventional ambulatory monitors.
D. Direct-to-consumer monitors are contraindicated in patients with implantable loop recorders.

52.10 A 67-year-old female with a history of diabetes mellitus type 2 and hypertension develops transient left-sided weakness prompting hospital evaluation. She recently experienced an episode of dysarthria just 1 week prior. Now, symptoms resolved shortly after reaching the hospital emergency department. Laboratory tests were normal. Neuroimaging did not demonstrate overt large vessel vascular occlusion. Evaluation and assessment were consistent with a transient ischemic attack (TIA). Carotid artery duplex ultrasonography revealed nonobstructive atherosclerotic disease. Transthoracic echocardiogram revealed normal left ventricular size and function, normal valvular structure and function, and mildly increased left atrial size by volume. Continuous telemetry monitoring during the hospital course demonstrated predominantly sinus rhythm with occasional atrial premature complexes. A 30-day event monitor did not show any atrial fibrillation. Which of the following monitoring is recommended for further atrial fibrillation surveillance?

A. Another event monitor
B. Extended Holter monitor
C. Implantable loop recorder
D. Observation only

ANSWERS

52.1 The correct answer is C.
Rationale: In this 26-year-old patient, who is experiencing ongoing distressing symptoms, monitoring for underlying arrhythmia should be offered. Presentation and historical details are suggestive of a possible supra-VT. Therefore, diagnosis is largely dependent on the appropriate monitoring period. As symptoms have been occurring 1 to 2 times per week for the past week, a 24-hour Holter monitor may or may not capture the event. Hence, a 30-day symptomatic event monitor is recommended given the less-than-daily frequency. Starting empiric beta-blocker therapy could curb symptoms but not ideal without first confirming the diagnosis. Likewise, proceeding with a more invasive monitoring strategy first is not recommended.

52.2 The correct answer is D.
Rationale: Holter monitoring offers continuous monitoring over a 24- to 48-hour period. The diagnostic sensitivity can be low due to this monitoring period, especially if clinical events occur on an infrequent basis. It is important to note that Holter monitoring requires wearable leads connected to an external device. This can be cumbersome, at times, for patients making this less of an ideal long-term monitoring solution.

52.3 The correct answer is D.
Rationale: This patient presents after a syncopal episode resulting in a significant mechanism of injury, concerning for a cardiogenic etiology. As noted on the transthoracic echocardiogram, LVEF is reduced but in the absence of documented VT, does not meet the criteria for ICD implantation (for primary or secondary prevention). Clinical suspicion for VT prompted inducibility study, and VT was non-inducible at the time of the study. An arrhythmogenic etiology has not been ruled out, as there is still potential for supraventricular and ventricular tachyarrhythmias; thus, prospective, long-term monitoring in this situation is recommended. Implantable loop recorder offers long-term monitoring over the course of at least 3 years. An event, patient-triggered monitor is not ideal for non-prodromal syncope.

52.4 The correct answer is A.
Rationale: The best answer in this clinical scenario is the placement of an event monitor. The patient has features of baseline conduction disease as evidenced by the presence of a first-degree atrioventricular (AV) block and right bundle branch block. There is evidence of chronotropic competency in the office; however, clinical suspicion for intermittent bradyarrhythmia or high-degree symptomatic AV block is high. An event monitor is recommended, which offers both continuous real-time monitoring and patient-triggered event monitoring. A 24 to 48 Holter monitor does not offer real-time monitoring, important in monitoring symptomatic patients with syncope and baseline conduction disease. Pending data acquisition from the event monitor, implantation of a loop recorder may be premature. Coronary angiography is unlikely to offer an etiologic explanation for symptoms in this case.

52.5 The correct answer is A.
Rationale: In the absence of symptoms and nocturnal onset of the pause/bradycardia during sleep, there is no indication for permanent pacemaker implantation. Modifiable risk factors and conditions, such as obstructive sleep apnea, should be considered. EP study for nocturnal bradycardia during sleep is not indicated, nor is an exercise treadmill test.

52.6 The correct answer is C.
Rationale: This is a patient with evidence of sinoatrial nodal dysfunction and clinical tachy-brady syndrome. She is symptomatic from pauses, occurring in both sinus rhythm and with conversion from atrial fibrillation. Baseline low heart rate and sinus pauses preclude further up-titration of beta-blocker therapy at this time without anti-bradycardia pacing. As atrial fibrillation burden is paroxysmal and not permanent, a dual-chamber pacemaker is recommended. Anti-bradycardia pacing will allow for further management of atrial fibrillation with rapid ventricular rate as clinically indicated.

52.7 The correct answer is A.
Rationale: An implantable loop recorder is most ideal in this setting. Given that the patient is not aware of when he is in atrial fibrillation and longer period of monitoring is needed, an event monitor is unlikely to be beneficial. Wearable watch monitors are particularly helpful in monitoring but do not necessarily offer continuous, real-time data acquisition that is readily accessible by providers. An implantable loop recorder is recommended as it provides continuous monitoring and data transmissions, whether scheduled or unscheduled, are readily available for review.

52.8 The correct answer is D.
Rationale: Nearly a quarter of patients with diagnosed HCM have non-sustained VT, which is associated with an increased risk of sudden cardiac death. Ambulatory monitoring is recommended as an initial evaluation in patients diagnosed with HCM. The patient in choice C should be referred for prompt inpatient evaluation as there is likely development of high-degree heart block meeting clinical indication for permanent pacemaker implantation. Ambulatory monitoring for incidental left bundle branch block is not empirically indicated, as in choice B. If symptoms develop, there may be an indication at that time. In choice A, modifiable intake of caffeine should be addressed first. Without further information, the patient is otherwise low risk. If overtly symptomatic or requested by the patient, ambulatory monitoring could be considered.

52.9 The correct answer is A.
Rationale: The REHEARSE-AF trial demonstrated efficacy in detecting asymptomatic atrial fibrillation in patients with elevated CHA2DS2-VASc score using aggressive monitoring. Direct-to-consumer monitors are evolving and becoming prevalent in rhythm and health monitoring. Comparisons with 12-lead ECG were found to be similar but not necessarily superior to conventional ambulatory monitors. Studies are ongoing and data are emerging. At this time, there are no overt contraindications to direct-to-consumer monitor use with concurrent implantable loop recorder.

52.10 The correct answer is C:

Rationale: This patient is suspected of having a cryptogenic stroke/TIA. Subtle features on examination and workup suggest a possible recurrent cardioembolic etiology, namely bi-hemispheric neurologic symptoms and paucity of evidence for primary neurovascular phenomenon. Echocardiogram further reveals left atrial enlargement. While there is no formal diagnosis of atrial fibrillation, an arrhythmogenic etiology cannot be excluded at this time. The patient has risk factors for developing atrial fibrillation (age, hypertension), which if confirmed, places the patient at high risk for stroke. Long-term arrhythmia monitoring is recommended. In this case, implantable loop recorder is recommended for further prospective monitoring and workup of cryptogenic stroke.

ELECTROPHYSIOLOGY TESTING*

Casey White and Amole Ojo

CHAPTER 53

QUESTIONS

53.1 Which of the following findings during an electrophysiology (EP) study would strongly indicate the need for a permanent pacemaker in a patient with a history of syncope?

   A. Atrial to His (AH) interval 70 millisecond
   B. His to ventricular (HV) interval 100 millisecond
   C. Sinus node recovery time (SNRT) 1,000 millisecond
   D. Corrected sinus node recovery time (cSNRT) 450 millisecond

53.2 A 26-year-old female with a history of supraventricular tachycardia (VT) presents for an elective EP study after evaluation by a cardiologist. Intracardiac catheters are positioned at the high right atrium, His bundle, coronary sinus, and right ventricular apex. During programmed stimulation from the ventricular apex, with progressively shorter coupling intervals, VA conduction was observed to be nondecremental, with the earliest atrial activation on CS1,2 on the coronary sinus catheter. Which of the following is **MOST LIKELY** suggested by these findings?

   A. Concentric atrial activation
   B. Presence of a left-sided accessory pathway (AP)
   C. His-Purkinje disease
   D. Focal atrial tachycardia near the coronary sinus

53.3 A 50-year-old female is noted to have recurrent episodes of supraventricular tachycardia on outpatient Holter monitoring. Due to significant symptoms during the clinical tachycardia, an EP study is recommended for both definitive diagnosis and possible treatment with ablation. Standard intracardiac catheters are used during the study and positioned at the high right atrium, coronary sinus, His bundle, and ventricular apex. A focal atrial tachycardia along the lateral aspect of the mid-right atrial wall is confirmed with pacing maneuvers and activation, propagation, and voltage mapping. The focus is successfully ablated. Postprocedural electrocardiogram (ECG) in the recovery area reveals sinus tachycardia at 116 bpm. Blood pressure is 88/60 mm Hg. She complains of vague chest discomfort that worsens on inspiration and is marginally improved with positional change. What is the next **BEST** step?

   A. Echocardiogram
   B. Anteroposterior (AP) chest radiograph
   C. Start colchicine for pericarditis.
   D. Continue monitoring.

---

*Questions and Answers are based on Chapter 53: Electrophysiology Testing by Duc H. Do and Noel G. Boyle in *Cardiovascular Medicine and Surgery*, First Edition.

53.4 During an EP study, the AH interval is observed to prolong gradually during programmed atrial extrastimuli. At 600 millisecond (S1), with a coupled extrastimulus (S2) at 290 millisecond, there is a sudden increase of more than 50 millisecond in the AH interval. Which of the following is **MOST LIKELY** reflected by this observation?

A. Transition from the atrioventricular (AV) nodal slow pathway to the fast pathway
B. Slow pathway refractory period
C. Typical atrioventricular nodal reentrant tachycardia (AVNRT)
D. Transition from the AV nodal fast pathway to the slow pathway

53.5 Which of the following is **TRUE** regarding invasive EP study?

A. SNRT of 1,100 millisecond is an indication for a pacemaker.
B. Short AV Wenckebach cycle lengths generally reflect nodal dysfunction.
C. The shortest interval at which an electrical input is conducted to tissue is the effective refractory period (ERP).
D. The measured difference in cycle length variability in sinus rhythm represents the SNRT.

53.6 Which of the following cases pertaining to asymptomatic Wolff-Parkinson-White pattern represents a potentially high-risk pathway?

A. Loss of manifest preexcitation pattern during exercise testing
B. Atrial fibrillation induction during EP study with shortest preexcited RR interval (SPERRI) less than 240 millisecond
C. Atrial fibrillation induction during EP study with SPERRI more than 240 millisecond
D. Absence of inducible supraventricular tachycardia (SVT)

53.7 Isoproterenol can be used during EP studies to increase the likelihood of inducing arrhythmia. Which statement **BEST** explains its use in the EP laboratory?

A. Physiologic decreased dromotropy of pacemaker cells
B. Beta-1 adrenergic antagonism
C. Increase in adenylyl cyclase activity
D. Parasympathetic stimulation

53.8 Which of the following statements regarding VT/ventricular fibrillation (VF) inducibility testing is **MOST** accurate?

A. Patients with confirmed cardiac channelopathies should undergo programmed ventricular stimulation for risk stratification.
B. Patients with nonischemic cardiomyopathy and inducible VT/VF during EP study have higher rates of implantable cardioverter-defibrillator (ICD) therapy delivery.
C. Patients with ischemic heart disease and reduced left ventricular ejection fraction (LVEF) less than 30% should undergo ventricular arrhythmia inducibility testing prior to consideration for ICD implantation.
D. Patients with cardiac sarcoidosis should never undergo inducibility testing for risk stratification.

53.9 Which of the following statements regarding electroanatomic mapping (EAM) is **MOST** accurate?

A. Spatial EAM is dependent on fluoroscopy.
B. Areas of high voltage collected during voltage mapping correlate with cardiac scar and are often associated with reentrant VT.
C. Activation mapping is independent of local electrograms (EGMs).
D. Electroanatomic substrate mapping can identify areas of slow conduction useful during VT ablation procedure.

53.10 Which of the following clinical scenarios is **MOST** appropriate for EP testing?
A. Patient with ischemic heart disease and LVEF 35% to 40% with nonsustained VT
B. Patient with ischemic heart disease and longstanding LVEF less than 30%
C. Patient with cardiac sarcoidosis, reduced LVEF less than 35%, and sustained VT
D. Asymptomatic patient with progressive PR-interval prolongation and nonconducted P waves

ANSWERS

53.1 The correct answer is B.
Rationale: The HV interval is the measured time between the His-bundle depolarization and the earliest ventricular depolarization measured on surface ECG or EGM. A normal HV interval is 35 to 55 millisecond. Prolongation in this interval generally indicates Purkinje fiber disease, which, in a patient with a history of syncope, warrants consideration for placement of a permanent pacemaker. All other listed choices are within normal limits.

53.2 The correct answer is B.
Rationale: Retrograde conduction through the AV node depolarizes the atrium in a midline (or concentric) manner, where atrial EGMs propagate from CS9,10, which is the most midline electrode pair in the CS catheter, toward CS1,2, which is the most lateral electrode pair. In this case, eccentric atrial activation was observed, with the earliest atrial activation in CS1,2 (the most lateral electrode pair). This eccentric activation pattern is suggestive of the presence of a left lateral AP.

53.3 The correct answer is A.
Rationale: A rare but known complication of intracardiac EP studies and ablations is cardiac perforation, which can lead to pericardial effusion. While there are several possible sites of perforation in this example, the most likely place of perforation is along the anatomically thin right atrial free wall, which probably happened during radiofrequency ablation. Another common site of perforation is the right ventricular true apex; thus, caution must be utilized especially when placing diagnostic catheters at this location. In the described scenario, clinical signs suggestive of tamponade are evident from the patient's vital signs. The next best step here is to assess for pericardial effusion with tamponade physiology, which should start with a thorough clinical examination, including bedside assessment for pulsus paradoxus. An echocardiogram will be particularly useful in assessing for the presence of pericardial effusion.

If pericardial effusion is present, with clinical features of tamponade, pericardiocentesis should be performed.

53.4 The correct answer is D:
Rationale: Assessment of refractoriness is often conducted during an EP study. Delivery of an atrial programmed drive train with a coupled extrastimulus helps define the refractoriness of the fast and slow pathways, if present. Progressive prolongation of the AH interval, followed by a sudden prolongation exceeding 50 millisecond (AH jump), reflects the fast pathway refractory period and a subsequent "jump" to the slow pathway. AH jump signifies antegrade conduction down the slow pathway with retrograde activation to the atrium via the fast pathway. While dual nodal physiology is necessary for typical AVNRT, the presence of a slow pathway does not equate with typical AVNRT.

53.5 The correct answer is C:
Rationale: The shortest interval at which an electrical input is conducted to tissue is the ERP. All myocardial tissues have an ERP. SNRT during an EP study represents the interval from the last paced beat to the first spontaneous sinus activity. With sinoatrial node dysfunction, the recovery time may be longer. A normal SNRT is considered to be less than 1,500 millisecond. Short AV Wenckebach cycle length is common in young healthy patients. AV Wenckebach cycle length can increase with age, disease, or with vagal stimulation.

53.6 The correct answer is B:
Rationale: The conduction properties of an AP determine the potential high-risk nature of the pathway. Loss of the manifest preexcitation pattern during exercise testing suggests refractoriness of the AP (loss of preexcitation on ECG) with antegrade AV nodal conduction. Atrial fibrillation in the presence of a high-risk AP is a potentially serious condition. Atrial fibrillation with rapid conduction via the AP is considered high-risk if the shorten preexcited RR interval is less than 240 millisecond. The absence of inducible SVT is not overtly specific in assessing high-risk AP features.

53.7 The correct answer is C:
Rationale: Isoproterenol is a beta-agonist with affinity for beta-1 and -2 receptors, resulting in both chronotropic effects (beta-1) and vasodilatory smooth muscle effects (beta-2) through adenylyl cyclase activity stimulation, leading to downstream effects on calcium channels via cyclic adenosine monophosphate (cAMP). In the heart, this results in increased intracellular cAMP, which binds to HCN4 channels to augment I_f, as well as modulation of the phosphorylation of calcium cycling proteins.

53.8 The correct answer is B:
Rationale: Inducibility testing for ventricular arrhythmias is an important risk stratification approach in several patients with underlying cardiac conditions. Patients with confirmed cardiac channelopathies are stratified according to the specific genetic mutation and phenotypic manifestation, as well as with other risk stratifying assessment such as treadmill and/or pharmacologic provocative testing. Ventricular arrhythmia inducibility testing in these patients is not broadly or prognostically used. In patients with ischemic heart disease and LVEF less than 30%, inducibility testing is typically foregone in favor of implantation of an ICD for primary prevention. This guideline-based practice is strongly supported by several landmark clinical

trials. For patients with evidence of cardiac sarcoidosis, inducibility testing can be a helpful tool for risk stratification in those who have not displayed evidence of ventricular arrhythmia prior to EP testing. In patients with nonischemic cardiomyopathy, inducible ventricular arrhythmia during EP testing is associated with higher rates of ICD therapy delivery.

53.9 The correct answer is D.

Rationale: Electroanatomic spatial mapping does not necessarily require the use of fluoroscopy and in many cases can eliminate or significantly reduce the amount of fluoroscopy needed in a case. Areas of low voltage are often associated with scar substrate. Substrate mapping can also identify areas of slow conduction, particularly useful in VT mapping. Whereas the premise of activation mapping is dependent on timing from local EGMs.

53.10 The correct answer is A.

Rationale: Patients with ischemic heart disease and a reduced LVEF 35% to 40% with nonsustained ventricular tachycardia (NSVT) should be considered for EP testing, specifically ventricular arrhythmia inducibility testing. Patients with persistent LVEF less than 30% from an ischemic etiology should be considered for primary prevention ICD implantation. Patients with cardiac sarcoidosis presenting with reduced LVEF and sustained VT should be considered for secondary prevention ICD implantation, among other therapeutic considerations. A patient with second-degree AV block Mobitz I may not necessarily require an EP study.

BRADYCARDIAS: SINUS NODE DYSFUNCTION AND ATRIOVENTRICULAR CONDUCTION DISTURBANCES*

Casey White and Amole Ojo

CHAPTER 54

QUESTIONS

54.1 Which of the following statements regarding sinus node dysfunction is **CORRECT**?
   A. Sinus node dysfunction always presents with bradycardia first.
   B. Sinus node dysfunction is a life-threatening condition, which should always be treated with prompt placement of a permanent pacemaker.
   C. Sinus node dysfunction is considered significant when sinus pause is greater than 3 seconds and sinus rate is less than 40 beats per minute (bpm) irrespective of sleep/wake status.
   D. A sinus node recovery time greater than 3,000 millisecond, especially if associated with symptoms, is diagnostic of sick sinus syndrome.

54.2 Which of the following is **NOT** an indication for permanent pacemaker in sinoatrial nodal dysfunction?
   A. Patient with symptomatic chronotropic incompetency
   B. Patient with nocturnal bradycardia and sinus pauses of 4 seconds while sleeping
   C. Patient with tachy-brady syndrome and symptomatic bradycardia
   D. Patient with symptomatic bradycardia requiring further uptitration in guideline therapies

54.3 Which of the following statements regarding atrioventricular (AV) nodal disease etiology is **MOST** accurate?
   A. Most cases of acquired AV nodal disease are related to decreased perfusion to the node.
   B. Acquired AV nodal disease is more common in coronary artery bypass and mitral valve surgeries than in aortic valve surgeries.
   C. Most cases of complete heart block caused by *Borrelia burgdorferi* infection are reversible when appropriately treated with antibiotics.
   D. Infiltrative disease secondary to cardiac sarcoidosis can affect the His-Purkinje system.

54.4 Which of the following findings **MOST LIKELY** reflects block at the level of the AV node?
   A. Exercise-induced 2:1 block
   B. Wide QRS escape rhythm in a patient with narrow complex QRS at baseline
   C. Presence of left bundle branch block at baseline
   D. AV block improved with isoproterenol

Questions and Answers are based on Chapter 54: Bradycardias: Sinus Node Dysfunction and Atrioventricular Conduction Disturbances by Osamu Fujimura and Houman Khakpour in Cardiovascular Medicine and Surgery, First Edition.

54.5 Which of the following clinical scenarios may depict complete AV block?
  A. A 72-year-old patient with 12-lead electrocardiogram (ECG) revealing sinus rhythm, PR duration of 260 millisecond, and QRS duration of 100 millisecond
  B. An 18-year-old patient with palpitations and 12-lead ECG revealing sinus bradycardia with rate of 54 bpm, QRS duration of 106 millisecond, and nonspecific ST changes consistent with early repolarization abnormality
  C. A 78-year-old patient with permanent atrial fibrillation with 12-lead ECG demonstrating atrial fibrillation, QRS duration of 128 millisecond, and regular R-R interval of 1,000 millisecond
  D. A 64-year-old patient with 12-lead ECG demonstrating sinus rhythm, nonspecific QRS duration of 122 millisecond, and nonspecific T-wave abnormalities

54.6 Which of the following preoperative examination findings for aortic valve replacement indicates the highest risk for needing a permanent pacemaker postoperatively?
  A. PR interval of 260 millisecond
  B. Left bundle branch block with QRS duration of 130 millisecond
  C. Right bundle branch block with QRS duration of 128 millisecond
  D. Atrial fibrillation with average ventricular rates of 80 bpm

54.7 All of the following favor second-degree AV block or higher, **EXCEPT** for which of the following?
  A. Junctional premature beat blocking in both antegrade and retrograde directions
  B. Sinus rate faster than the ventricular rate without evidence of AV conduction
  C. Ventricular rate faster than the sinus rate without evidence of AV conduction
  D. Constant PP intervals and similar P-wave morphology with "dropped" QRS complexes

54.8 In which of the following scenarios is permanent pacemaker implantation **NOT** recommended?
  A. Second-degree AV block Mobitz II without identifiable reversible cause
  B. Symptomatic AV block secondary to indicated guideline-directed medical therapies
  C. Infiltrative cardiomyopathy with acquired high-grade AV block
  D. Acute anterior wall myocardial infarction with new left bundle branch block

54.9 In which of the following situations is bradycardia management with a transvenous permanent pacemaker recommended for patients with adult congenital heart disease?
  A. Asymptomatic patients with first-degree AV block and chronotropically competent
  B. Asymptomatic patients with congenital second-degree AV block Mobitz I and venous-to-systemic intracardiac shunt
  C. Congenital complete AV block with QRS duration of 150 millisecond and daytime heart rate of 48 bpm
  D. Transient intermittent Mobitz I activity in the first 24 hours following cardiac surgery

54.10

CORRECTLY match the pharmacologic agent with the appropriate physiologic effect in heart block:

Physiologic Effect

i. Limited effect on the His-Purkinje system; improves sinus rate and AV nodal conduction
ii. Nonselective adenosine receptor and phosphodiesterase inhibitor
iii. Treatment in beta-blocker overdose
iv. Beta-adrenergic agonist leading to increased nodal rates and conduction

Pharmacologic Agent

- **A.** Glucagon
- **B.** Isoproterenol
- **C.** Atropine
- **D.** Aminophylline

A. i—C; ii—D; iii—A; iv—B
B. i—A; ii—B; iii—C; iv—D
C. i—D; ii—B; iii—C; iv—A
D. i—D; ii—C; iii—B; iv—A

ANSWERS

54.1 The correct answer is B.

Rationale: A sinus node recovery time greater than 1,500 millisecond is considered abnormal, with a value exceeding 3,000 millisecond being diagnostic of sick sinus syndrome, especially when accompanied by symptoms. Sinus node dysfunction may present with persisting bradycardia, sinus pauses, sinus arrest, or chronotropic incompetence. In all cases of sinus node dysfunction, reversible causes should be explored. Sinus node dysfunction is considered significant when the sinus pause exceeds 3 seconds and the sinus rate falls below 40 bpm while awake.

54.2 The correct answer is B.

Rationale: All options except choice B are class I and class IIa indications for permanent pacemaker implantation. Nocturnal bradycardia and pauses during sleep states are not considered indications for permanent pacemaker implantation.

54.3 The correct answer is C.

Rationale: Most cases of acquired AV nodal disease result from degenerative sclerosis of the conduction system. Aortic valve surgeries are more likely to cause direct trauma leading to AV nodal dysfunction compared to coronary artery bypass and mitral valve cardiac surgeries. Complete heart block secondary to Lyme disease, when appropriately diagnosed and treated, is often reversible and rarely requires placement of a permanent pacemaker. Infiltrative disease secondary to cardiac sarcoidosis can affect the entire conduction system; thus, a dual-chamber permanent pacemaker is often implanted at the time of placement for acquired AV block to both preserve AV synchrony and to address the possibility of progression of infiltrative disease affecting the sinoatrial node.

54.4 The correct answer is D.
Rationale: When the site of AV block is at the level of the AV node, it usually improves with exercise, atropine, and isoproterenol, while carotid sinus pressure usually worsens the AV block. Administration of isoproterenol mitigates vagal activity and improves the block. The remaining options all describe block at or below the His-Purkinje system.

54.5 The correct answer is C.
Rationale: Of the clinical scenarios, choice C is most indicative of complete AV block. The regularization of the R-R interval in permanent atrial fibrillation burden should always raise clinical suspicion for complete AV block. Choice A describes an ECG with first-degree AV block, which is above the level of the AV node. Choice B describes an ECG with common findings in younger patients, such as elevation of the J-point consistent with early repolarization. Choice D describes an ECG with nonspecific intraventricular conduction delay (IVCD), indicating a degree of infra-Hisian disease, but in isolation, it is not indicative of AV block.

54.6 The correct answer is C.
Rationale: The presence of a chronic right bundle branch block increases the perioperative risk of high-degree or complete heart block due to the possibility of injury to the left bundle during aortic valve replacement. Injury and inflammatory changes to the left bundle branch and interventricular septum can result in branch block, high-degree AV block, and complete heart block.

54.7 The correct answer is C.
Rationale: All choices describe second-degree AV block, with the exception of choice C, which is most consistent with ventricular tachycardia.

54.8 The correct answer is D.
Rationale: Choices A and B describe class I indications for permanent pacemaker implantation, while choice C describes a class IIa indication. As in choice D, in the absence of second- or third-degree AV block, permanent pacemaker implantation is not indicated following an acute myocardial infarction with new bundle branch block or isolated fascicular block.

54.9 The correct answer is C.
Rationale: Permanent pacing is recommended for patients with congenital complete AV block exhibiting a wide QRS rhythm and daytime bradycardia with rates less than 50 bpm. Permanent pacing is not recommended in the remaining scenarios.

54.10 The correct answer is A.
Rationale: i—Atropine (choice C) has a limited effect on the His-Purkinje system, but improves sinus rates and AV nodal conduction. ii—Aminophylline (choice D) is a non-selective adenosine receptor and phosphodiesterase inhibitor. iii—Glucagon (choice A) is considered a treatment in beta blocker overdose. iv—Isoproterenol is a beta-adrenergic agonist leading to increased nodal rates and conduction.

SUPRAVENTRICULAR TACHYCARDIAS

Jeanwoo Yoo, Evan C. Adelstein, and Alfred M. Loka

CHAPTER 55

QUESTIONS

55.1 A 32-year-old male with a history of hypertension, treated with diet and lifestyle modifications, presents to the cardiology clinic with intermittent palpitations lasting a few minutes each time. He denies any loss of consciousness and cannot recall if his palpitations occur with exertion or at rest. On physical examination, his blood pressure (BP) is 134/78 mm Hg, pulse rate is 108 beats per minute (bpm), S1 and S2 heart sounds are normal, there is no S3 gallop, and no lower extremity edema is noted. An electrocardiogram (ECG) is obtained, as shown in **Figure 55.1**.

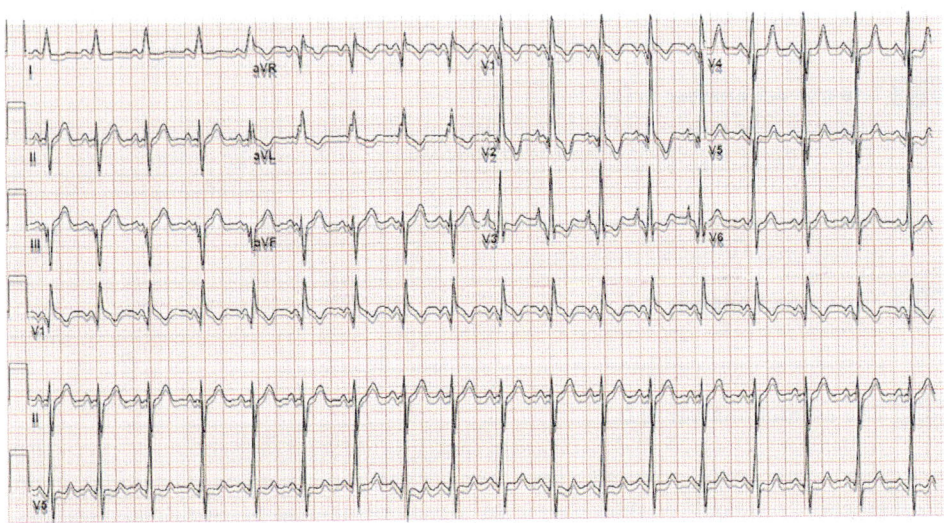

Figure 55.1

Which of the following findings would indicate a low risk of sudden cardiac death?

A. Loss of preexcitation at fast heart rates
B. Increase in the degree of preexcitation at fast heart rates
C. Paroxysmal atrial fibrillation (AF) seen on event monitoring
D. History of seizures as an adolescent

55.2 A 17-year-old girl presents with a week of intermittent palpitations associated with dizziness. An ECG is obtained, as shown in **Figure 55.2**.

Questions and Answers are based on Chapter 55: Supraventricular Tachycardias by Roberto G. Gallotti, Kevin M. Shannon, and Jeremy P. Moore in Cardiovascular Medicine and Surgery, First Edition.

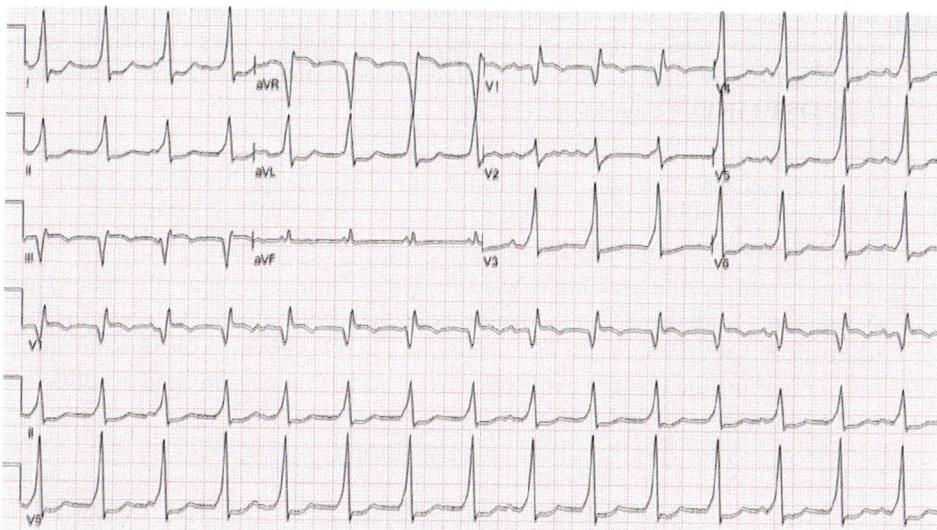

Figure 55.2

Her physical examination reveals a regular heart rhythm, normal S1 and S2 heart sounds, no murmurs, and no lower extremity edema. She denies syncope or falls. What is the **MOST LIKELY** mechanism of her tachyarrhythmia?

A. Macro-reentrant circuit between the atrium and ventricle utilizing an accessory pathway (AP)
B. Macro-reentrant circuit between the atrium and ventricle with reentry within the atrioventricular (AV) node
C. Focal tachycardia resulting from enhanced automaticity within the atrium
D. Micro-reentrant circuit within the atrium

55.3 Which of the following is **NOT TRUE** regarding the tachyarrhythmia for the patient described in **Question 55.2**?

A. The arrhythmia is always associated with a delta wave.
B. The arrhythmia may overlap with other atrial arrhythmias.
C. The arrhythmia may travel down a pathway that has decremental conduction.
D. The arrhythmia may be initiated with a premature atrial contraction (PAC) or a premature ventricular contraction (PVC).

55.4 A 46-year-old man presents to the cardiology clinic with palpitations associated with dizziness and shortness of breath. His symptoms occur a few times a week, approximately every 2 to 3 days. On examination, his heart rate and rhythm are regular, and he has normal S1 and S2 heart sounds. There are no murmurs, jugular venous distention (JVD), or lower extremity edema noted. He denies chest pain, paroxysmal nocturnal dyspnea, orthopnea, or syncope. What is the next appropriate step?

A. A 24- or 48-hour Holter monitor
B. A 7-day cardiac event monitor
C. A 30-day patch monitor
D. Inpatient telemetry monitoring

55.5 The same patient described in **Question 55.4** has his tachyarrhythmia captured with the appropriate monitoring approach. The recorded rhythm shows a regular tachycardia with a narrow QRS complex and visible P waves with a long RP interval. What is the **MOST LIKELY** diagnosis?

A. AF
B. Atypical atrioventricular nodal reentrant tachycardia (AVNRT)
C. Typical AVNRT
D. Multifocal atrial tachycardia

55.6 A 26-year-old woman presents to the emergency department with palpitations and shortness of breath that began suddenly 8 hours ago. Her examination reveals a regular heart rhythm at 165 bpm, BP of 110/60 mm Hg, O$_2$ saturation of 99%, no appreciable murmurs, no lower extremity edema, and clear lung fields upon auscultation. An ECG is shown in **Figure 55.3**.

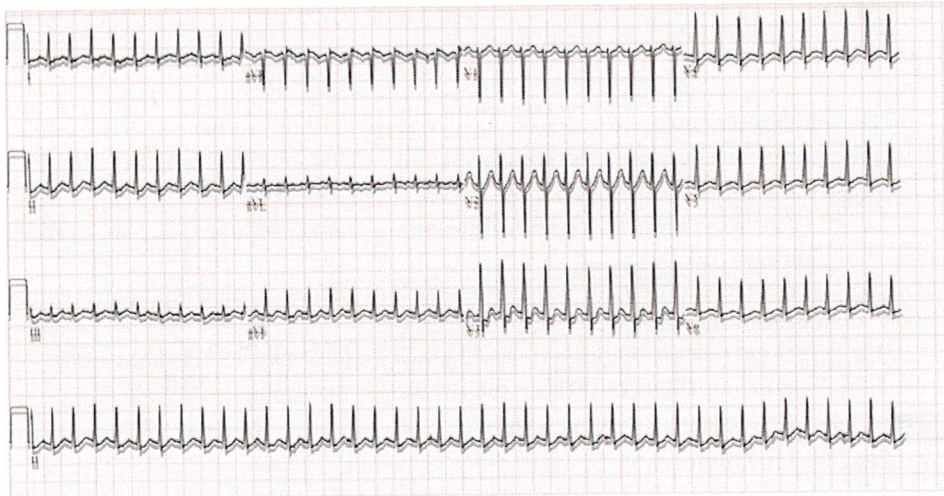

Figure 55.3

What is the next appropriate step in management?

A. Vagal maneuvers
B. Intravenous amiodarone
C. Synchronized cardioversion
D. Intravenous metoprolol

55.7 For the patient described in **Question 55.6**, appropriate therapy converts the patient to sinus rhythm, and she is discharged with outpatient follow-up. Given the profound nature of her symptoms, the patient expresses her wish to eliminate the tachycardia, if possible. Consequently, she undergoes electrophysiology (EP) study. Which of the following findings is **MOST** suggestive of orthodromic AV reentrant tachycardia?

CHAPTER 55 | Supraventricular Tachycardias

A. Ventriculoatrial conduction with eccentric activation in the coronary sinus recordings and late His catheter activation
B. Ventriculoatrial conduction with concentric atrial activation and earliest atrial signal in the His catheter
C. Dual AV node physiology
D. Simultaneous activation of the atrium and ventricle

55.8 The patient described in **Question 55.7** undergoes successful ablation for the supraventricular tachycardia (SVT). Which of the following aspects of follow-up care is **NOT** appropriate?
A. Follow-up in ambulatory clinic within 1 to 2 weeks to check venipuncture sites
B. Periodic assessment within the first 12 months to assess for recurrence
C. Same day discharge after ablation
D. No follow-up is needed given the high success rate of SVT ablation 90% to 98%.

55.9 A 72-year-old woman with a history of hypertension, hyperlipidemia, and coronary artery disease with a three-vessel coronary artery bypass grafting (CABG) 10 years prior, presents to the hospital with palpitations and shortness of breath. She also has a history of paroxysmal AF. A list of her home medications reveals apixaban, furosemide, metoprolol, and atorvastatin, none of which she has been taking for the past 2 weeks while on a cruise vacation.

Vital signs: BP 110/55 mm Hg, heart rate 125 bpm, 18 breaths per minute

General: She is diaphoretic

Cardiac: Irregular heart rhythm

Extremities: Bilateral pitting edema extends above her ankles

Her ECG is concerning for AF. Which of the following is **MOST LIKELY TRUE** regarding her tachyarrhythmia?
A. She should undergo immediate cardioversion without further testing.
B. She is at high risk of developing syncope with her tachyarrhythmia.
C. Acute heart failure is the cause for her tachyarrhythmia, not the result.
D. Cardioversion to sinus may not be successful in the setting of acute heart failure.

55.10 A 40-year-old man with a history of hypertension and diabetes presents to the cardiology clinic after a recent hospital admission for palpitations. He reports several hours of palpitations and feeling short of breath with mild exertion for several days before going to the hospital, where he was found to have tachycardia at 135 bpm. His ECG shows a regular tachycardia (**Figure 55.4**).

His echocardiogram noted mild left ventricular hypertrophy, a left ventricular ejection fraction of 65%, and a left atrial volume indexed to 37 mL/m^2. He was then placed on metoprolol and diltiazem, with improvement in his heart rate. He was also started on apixaban and discharged to follow-up with cardiology. He states that he feels well at rest but still has dyspnea on exertion. Select the following that applies to the management of his arrhythmia.

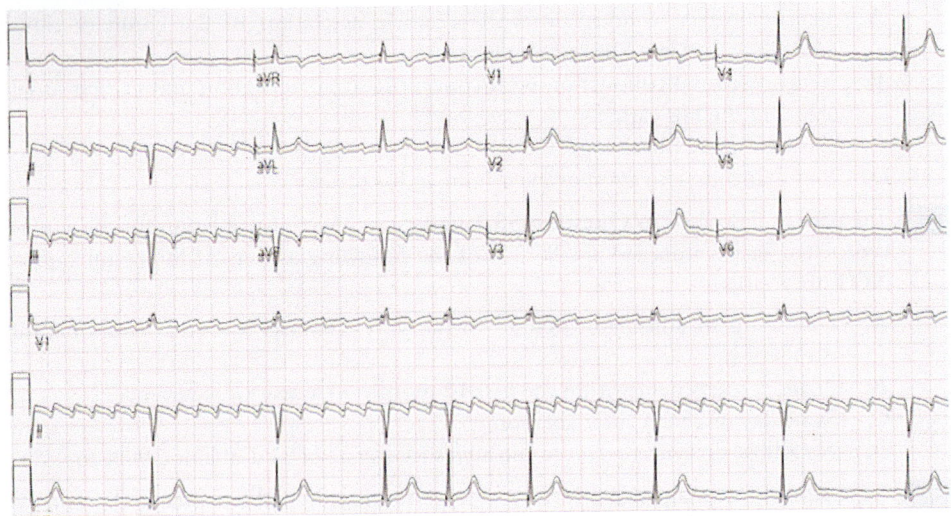

Figure 55.4

A. He has atypical atrial flutter and is unlikely to have a successful electrical cardioversion.
B. His atrial flutter circuit is clockwise and so cannot be dependent on the cavo-tricuspid isthmus.
C. He would likely benefit from cavo-tricuspid isthmus ablation.
D. He would not need anticoagulation unless he undergoes ablation or cardioversion.

55.11 A 21-year-old woman presents with palpitations while in the hospital after delivering her first child. The episodes of palpitations are brief, lasting several minutes. On telemetry, they are noted to be narrow complex with rates of 140 to 150 bpm and regular. Which of the following is **NOT** necessary for the development of a reentrant mechanism as part of the etiology of her tachycardia?

A. Two functionally or anatomically distinct conduction pathways
B. Unidirectional conduction block must occur in a potential pathway
C. Conduction slowing in one pathway or long anatomic distance to allow for recovery of conduction
D. Enhanced automaticity or triggered activity

ANSWERS

55.1 The correct answer is A.
Rationale: Sudden loss of preexcitation at fast sinus rates indicates that antegrade conduction down the AP has reached refractoriness. This indicates that antegrade conduction down the pathway ceases, and conduction instead occurs only down the AV node as the sinus rate increases. Otherwise, AF or atrial flutter may conduct

down the AP at a rapid rate and degenerate into ventricular fibrillation, possibly causing sudden cardiac death. An increase in the degree of preexcitation at fast heart rates would indicate a higher risk of sudden cardiac death, as this suggests that antegrade pathway conduction is rapid. AF in the presence of rapid conduction down the AP increases the risk of degenerating into ventricular fibrillation. A history of seizures may suggest prior episodes of ventricular fibrillation that self-terminated.

55.2 The correct answer is A.
Rationale: Accessory AV pathways with antegrade conduction will display a classic delta wave on the surface ECG with a prolonged, slurred QRS complex. The presence of these findings, along with symptoms compatible with SVT, characterizes Wolff-Parkinson-White (WPW) syndrome. Patients with WPW are at risk for SVT, which can occur via orthodromic reentry (down AV node, up AP) or antidromic reentry (down AP, up AV node). AVNRT is a reentrant tachycardia involving two functional limbs of the AV node, typically a slow and fast pathway, in the setting of dual AV nodal physiology. Focal atrial tachycardias (AT) were historically associated with enhanced automaticity; however, in recent decades, the definition has been expanded to include ATs of automatic, triggered, and micro-reentrant etiologies. Patients with WPW may have other arrhythmias and may have bystander APs, but pathway-medicated orthodromic reentrant tachycardia is the most likely cause of their symptoms.

55.3 The correct answer is A.
Rationale: This patient has WPW syndrome, characterized by the presence of an AP that allows conduction between the atrium and ventricle by means other than the AV node. Concealed APs are those that only allow retrograde conduction (from the ventricle to the atrium) and do not manifest a delta wave, whereas manifest APs have a visible delta wave. Orthodromic AV reentry commonly occurs in patients with APs, in which the circuit comprises antegrade conduction down the AV node and retrograde conduction up the AP. WPW may occur in the setting of other atrial arrhythmias, including AF, atrial flutter, atrial tachycardia, or AVNRT. Mahaim fibers are an uncommon type of AP that have antegrade decremental conduction between the right atrium and ventricle, but unlike the AV node, have not been shown to exhibit retrograde conduction. Reentry occurs when a PAC blocks in the AP but conducts down the AV node and the His-Purkinje system. Reentry can also initiate when a PVC occurs and blocks in the His-Purkinje system but conducts to the atrium by the AP.

55.4 The correct answer is B.
Rationale: The key to diagnosing arrhythmias causing symptoms is to capture the event on an ECG. This may be challenging, especially in patients with paroxysmal SVT or AF, in which episodes are sporadic and brief. Historically, Holter monitoring has been used for 24-hour ambulatory ECG recording; however, in recent years, this technology has expanded, with patch monitors now lasting up to 4 weeks and wearable single-lead electrode monitoring being commercially available. This patient has events every 2 to 3 days, so 7-day cardiac event monitoring would suffice in capturing an arrhythmic event.

55.5 The correct answer is B.
Rationale: AF does not display visible P waves. Typical AVNRT has a short RP interval, often with P waves obscured in the latter part of the QRS complex. Atypical AVNRT usually has a long RP interval. Multifocal atrial tachycardia has various P-wave morphologies and does not have a regular ventricular rate.

55.6 The correct answer is A.
Rationale: This patient has SVT for which the mainstay of initial treatment involves slowing or temporarily blocking AV nodal conduction. Vagal maneuvers are first line and are quickly performed or taught to patients. For adults, these maneuvers include Valsalva and carotid massage. If vagal maneuvers do not work, intravenous bolus adenosine is recommended for the patient with regular SVT. Synchronized cardioversion should only be performed in the setting of hemodynamically unstable SVT, which is rather unusual. Other acute therapies include intravenous metoprolol or diltiazem. However, these medications should only be used after adenosine.

55.7 The correct answer is A.
Rationale: In patients in whom VA conduction occurs through the AV node, the pattern of atrial activation is concentric (earliest in the His catheter and proximal coronary sinus) and decremental. If the pattern of activation is eccentric, this is suggestive of an AP connecting the left atrium and left ventricle and therefore AVNRT. When dual AV node physiology occurs, the AV node has properties of both fast and slow pathways and has the substrate necessary for AVNRT. Typical (slow/fast) AVNRT has near-simultaneous activation of the atrium and ventricle.

55.8 The correct answer is B.
Rationale: Patients choosing to undergo catheter ablation for SVT will be routinely seen in the ambulatory setting within 1 to 2 weeks of their procedure to check the venipuncture sites. They will then have periodic assessments in the first 12 months, following ablation to assess for recurrence. Despite the high success rate of SVT ablation, patients will need appropriate follow-up care and monitoring post ablation. Most patients who undergo SVT ablation may be safely discharged several hours after their procedure is completed.

55.9 The correct answer is B.
Rationale: There are multiple potential triggers for AF, including infection, thyrotoxicosis, pulmonary embolism, cardiac surgery, electrolyte abnormalities, and acute heart failure. If the underlying cause triggering AF is not addressed, electrical cardioversion is less likely to be successful. Patients with AF are at no greater risk for syncope except for conversion pauses when there is concomitant sick sinus syndrome. AF may cause tachycardia-induced cardiomyopathy. This patient will need to undergo transesophageal echocardiography prior to cardioversion if performed during this hospitalization, as she has not been taking apixaban for some time. However, she likely has been retaining fluid from excessive salt intake on vacation combined with not taking furosemide, triggering her AF that has only exacerbated her heart failure.

55.10 The correct answer is C.

Rationale: The patient has typical atrial flutter based on the ECG. Although he now is asymptomatic at rest, he may still have significant tachycardia with activity. Negative saw-tooth waves in leads II, III, and aVF and positive P waves in V1 are indicative of typical, counterclockwise atrial flutter. Typical flutter is dependent on the cavo-tricuspid isthmus for reentry and may be either counterclockwise or clockwise, more commonly the former. Although the CHA_2DS_2-VASc is validated for AF, guidelines suggest that patients with atrial flutter should be treated in the same manner as patients with AF for preventing ischemic stroke. This patient has an elevated CHA_2DS_2-VASc score of 2 (hypertension and diabetes), indicating an indication for stroke prevention with anticoagulation. CHA2DS2-VASc refers to risk factors for stroke related to atrial fibrillation and flutter and includes Congestive heart failure, Hypertension, Age 75 or older, Diabetes, Stroke or Systemic embolism, Vascular disease, Age 65–74, and Sex category.

55.11 The correct answer is D.

Rationale: A reentrant tachycardia occurs when there is continuous wavefront propagation over an anatomic or functional circuit loop. For this to occur, three distinct criteria must be met. First, there must be two distinct pathways present forming a closed loop, thus allowing continuous circular movement of the tachycardia wavefront. Second, unidirectional conduction block must occur in one of the two pathways. Third, an area of this loop must have slow conduction, or the loop must be adequately large enough anatomically to allow recovery of conduction before the next electrical wavefront returns. The other mechanisms of SVT occur when there is abnormal impulse formation from either enhanced automaticity or triggered activity. These are focal tachycardias.

ATRIAL FIBRILLATION AND ATRIAL FLUTTER*

Jeanwoo Yoo, Evan C. Adelstein, and Alfred M. Loka

CHAPTER 56

QUESTIONS

56.1 A 54-year-old man with a past medical history of atrial fibrillation, sleep apnea, obesity, and chronic obstructive pulmonary disease (COPD) presents with recurrent palpitations. His examination reveals a heart rate of 135 beats per minute (bpm), an irregular rhythm, cannon a waves on jugular venous inspection, lower extremity edema, and bilateral rales. He is found to have the following electrocardiogram (ECG) shown in **Figure 56.1**.

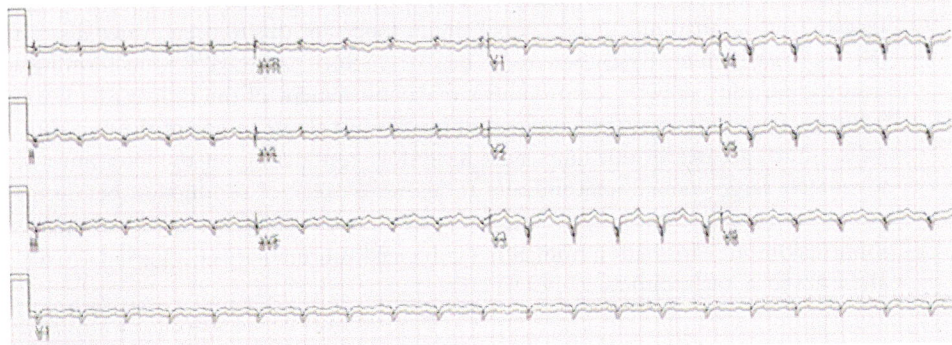

Figure 56.1

Which of the following is **MOSTLY LIKELY** to predispose him to developing this arrhythmia?

A. Sleep apnea
B. Atrial fibrillation
C. Prior atrial surgery or ablation
D. Obesity

56.2 A 45-year-old woman with a history of hypertension, diabetes, obesity, and sleep apnea presents to the cardiology clinic with shortness of breath and palpitations. A 28-day-event monitor reveals episodes of atrial fibrillation lasting from minutes to hours, and her heart rate in atrial fibrillation ranges from 65 to 145 bpm. An echocardiogram shows preserved left and right ventricular function and no significant valvular disease. Metoprolol succinate 50 mg daily is started, but her symptoms persist. In addition to lifestyle modification, which of the following would be the **BEST** initial management strategy for her atrial fibrillation?

*Questions and Answers are based on Chapter 56: Atrial Fibrillation and Atrial Flutter by Aron Bender, Joseph Hadaya, Peyman Benharash, Eric Buch, and Richard J. Shemin in Cardiovascular Medicine and Surgery, First Edition.

A. Digoxin and anticoagulation with dabigatran
B. Amiodarone and anticoagulation with apixaban
C. Catheter ablation and anticoagulation with apixaban
D. Diltiazem without anticoagulation

56.3 A 30-year-old woman presents with shortness of breath and lower extremity edema that had not improved since she underwent vaginal delivery at home 2 weeks prior with the help of a midwife. She was born in Haiti and moved to the United States when she was 12 years old. Her examination reveals an irregular rhythm, a loud opening snap at the apex with radiation to the axilla, and jugular venous distension (JVD) to the angle of her mandible. The abdomen is soft with no fluid shift. Bilateral pitting edema is noted to the knees. An ECG reveals atrial fibrillation with a heart rate of 112 bpm. What of the following is the **BEST** next step for prevention of thromboembolism?

A. Start aspirin 325 mg daily.
B. Start warfarin and monitor international normalized ratio (INR).
C. Start apixaban 5 mg BID.
D. Anticoagulation is not indicated.

56.4 A 45-year-old gastroenterologist with a past medical history of sleep apnea presents to the hospital with 1 day of palpitations. He denies prior episodes of palpitations, dizziness, or syncope. His ECG reveals atrial fibrillation. His examination reveals an irregularly irregular rhythm and no appreciable murmurs. What is the **BEST** management for his atrial fibrillation?

A. Transesophageal echocardiogram, perform electrical cardioversion, and initiate anticoagulation for at least 1 month
B. Transesophageal echocardiogram, perform electrical cardioversion, no anticoagulation
C. No transesophageal echocardiogram, perform electrical cardioversion, and initiate anticoagulation for at least 1 month
D. No transesophageal echocardiogram, perform electrical cardioversion, no anticoagulation

56.5 A 43-year-old man with history of hypertension, hyperlipidemia, diabetes, obesity, and hyperlipidemia is noted to have atrial fibrillation on a routine ECG by his primary care provider. He drinks 2 cups of coffee daily and drinks 12 cans of beer weekly. His primary care physician initiates metoprolol succinate and apixaban. Which of the following will have the **MOST** benefit in reducing his atrial fibrillation burden?

A. Lowering hemoglobin A1c from 7.5 to 7.0
B. Start atorvastatin therapy.
C. Eliminate caffeine from his diet.
D. Reduce or eliminate alcohol use.

56.6 A 68-year-old woman with history of asthma, hypertension, chronic kidney disease, and paroxysmal atrial fibrillation presents to cardiology clinic with palpitations. Her physical examination notes a blood pressure of 134/92 mm Hg, a heart rate of 115 bpm with an irregular rhythm, a respiratory rate of 14 breaths per minute, no appreciable JVD or lower extremity edema, and no wheezing or rhonchi. Her medications include albuterol inhaler, apixaban, chlorthalidone, and lisinopril. Her most recent echocardiogram noted preserved left ventricular (LV) systolic function and no significant valvular abnormalities. She had been on amiodarone after a recent cardioversion, but she would prefer to switch to an alternative regimen, as she has read about the potential for long-term side effects of amiodarone. What is the next **BEST** step after stopping amiodarone?

A. Start dofetilide.
B. Start sotalol.
C. Monitor off amiodarone.
D. Refer for pulmonary vein isolation.

56.7 A 61-year-old woman with a history of hypertension presents to the cardiology clinic after a Holter monitor had revealed paroxysmal atrial fibrillation. She is currently taking amlodipine and apixaban. She undergoes a stress echocardiogram that shows no findings suggestive of ischemia or structural heart disease. She does not wish to undergo any invasive procedures currently. What is the next **BEST** step in management?

A. Initiate flecainide.
B. Initiate propafenone.
C. Flecainide with metoprolol
D. Initiate amiodarone.

56.8 A 65-year-old man presents with 3 weeks of palpitations. He also endorses dyspnea on minimal exertion. His examination reveals an irregularly irregular rhythm, tachycardia, no appreciable murmurs, no lower extremity edema, and no rales. The ECG demonstrates atrial fibrillation. What is the **LEAST LIKELY** long-term implication of his tachyarrhythmia?

A. Developing a cardiomyopathy
B. Poor quality of life
C. Risk of syncope
D. Ongoing risk of stroke

56.9 A 35-year-old man with a past medical history of hypertrophic cardiomyopathy, hyperlipidemia, and hypertension presents with palpitations to the cardiology clinic. His screening ECG reveals atrial fibrillation. He is a vegetarian. What is the **MOST** appropriate anticoagulation strategy?

A. Aspirin only
B. No anticoagulation
C. INR-adjusted warfarin
D. Apixaban

56.10 A 70-year-old male with a past medical history of heart failure with preserved ejection fraction, hypertension, and hyperlipidemia presented to his cardiologist with substernal chest pain on exertion that is relieved with rest and sublingual nitroglycerin. He was referred for coronary angiography, which revealed multivessel disease, including a 90% lesion in the proximal left anterior descending (LAD). He subsequently underwent three vessel coronary artery bypass graft surgery, including left internal mammary artery grafting to the LAD and saphenous vein grafts to the first obtuse marginal and posterior descending arteries. On postoperative day 2, he developed 4 hours of atrial fibrillation, and on postoperative day 5, he continues to have daily paroxysms of atrial fibrillation. What is the next **BEST** step in minimizing his risk of cerebral thromboembolism?

A. Aspirin 81 mg daily
B. Apixaban 5 mg twice daily
C. Apixaban 5 mg twice daily and aspirin 81 mg daily
D. Aspirin 81 mg daily and discharge with a 30-day cardiac monitor

ANSWERS

56.1 The correct answer is C.
Rationale: For atypical atrial flutter, prior atrial surgery or ablation is usually a prerequisite. Since the circuits involved with atypical atrial flutter are not anatomic, they are usually caused by scar from prior atrial intervention. The risk factors for both atrial fibrillation and atrial flutter include older age, male sex, genetic predisposition, hypertension, heart failure, valvular or ischemic heart disease, obesity, thyroid dysfunction, obstructive sleep apnea, lung disease, and excessive alcohol consumption.

56.2 The correct answer is C.
Rationale: Catheter ablation is indicated for symptomatic paroxysmal atrial fibrillation as first-line therapy. Although antiarrhythmic therapy is also acceptable, amiodarone would not be the first choice because of the risk of long-term side effects in this young patient. Adding digoxin or diltiazem is unlikely to provide benefit over metoprolol and may cause more side effects. Neither are rhythm control agents. In addition to rhythm control, anticoagulation is indicated, given her hypertension and diabetes.

56.3 The correct answer is B.
Rationale: The patient's physical examination with a loud opening snap appreciated at the apex with radiation to the axilla and history of moving from a country where rheumatic fever is common are consistent with rheumatic mitral stenosis and associated valvular atrial fibrillation. For valvular atrial fibrillation with at least moderate mitral stenosis, anticoagulation with warfarin is indicated, regardless of CHA_2DS_2-VASc score. Aspirin, apixaban, or deferring anticoagulation is not appropriate.

56.4 The correct answer is C.
Rationale: The patient had a clear onset of palpitations within 48 hours and is presumably a very reliable historian. Therefore, a transesophageal echocardiogram is not essential prior to electrical cardioversion. Although his CHA_2DS_2-VASc score is 0, anticoagulation is indicated for a minimum of 30 days following cardioversion, as atrial contractility may be impaired for several weeks despite restoration of sinus rhythm.

56.5 The correct answer is D.
Rationale: There is a clear dose-response relationship between alcohol consumption and atrial fibrillation. In the long-term effect of goal-directed wight management in an atrial fibrillation cohort (LEGACY) trial, optimal risk factor management resulted in freedom from arrhythmias without antiarrhythmic medications in nearly

40% of patients with at least 10% sustained weight loss. Improved cardiorespiratory fitness and reducing or eliminating alcohol consumption also reduces arrhythmia burden. Further randomized data are required for evaluating the optimal strategy and benefit of management of treatment of obstructive sleep apnea, weight loss, exercise, and metabolic risk factors.

56.6 The correct answer is D.

Rationale: Both sotalol and dofetilide would not be appropriate in the setting of chronic kidney disease, as both drugs are renally excreted. Monitoring off amiodarone would not be appropriate because of her symptoms related to atrial fibrillation. She is an appropriate candidate for pulmonary vein isolation for symptomatic atrial fibrillation with limited medical options for rhythm control therapy (**Figure 56.2**).

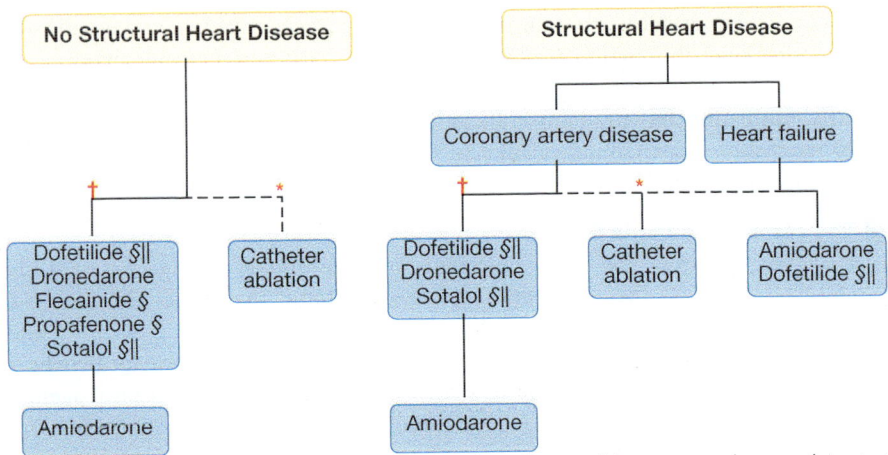

Figure 56.2 Approach to rhythm control strategy in patients with paroxysmal or persistent atrial fibrillation. *Catheter ablation is only recommended as first-line therapy for patients with paroxysmal atrial fibrillation (class IIa recommendation). †Medications are listed alphabetically. §Should not be used in patients with severe left ventricular hypertrophy (>1.5 cm). ‖Should not be used in patients at increased risk of torsades de pointes. (Adapted from January CT, Wann LS, Alpert JS, et al. American College of Cardiology/American Heart Association Task Force on Practice Guidelines. 2014 AHA/ACC/HRS guideline for the management of patients with atrial fibrillation: a report of the American College of Cardiology/American Heart Association Task Force on Practice Guidelines and the Heart Rhythm Society. *J Am Coll Cardiol.* 2014;64(21):e1-e76. Copyright © 2014 American Heart Association, Inc., The American College of Cardiology Foundation, and The Heart Rhythm Society, with permission.)

56.7 The correct answer is C.

Rationale: Class Ic antiarrhythmics, which include flecainide and propafenone, are good first-line options for patients with atrial fibrillation and no structural heart disease or evidence of coronary artery disease, as noted by the patient's normal stress echocardiogram. The patient does not prefer to undergo an invasive procedure, which precludes atrial fibrillation ablation. Therefore, treatment with class 1c agents is reasonable. Because there is a risk of organizing atrial fibrillation into atrial flutter with class Ic drugs, and these drugs slow atrial conduction velocity such that the flutter circuit may be relatively slow, 1:1 atrioventricular (AV) conduction causing very rapid ventricular rates is possible. Therefore, class Ic agents should be used in conjunction with an AV nodal–blocking agent. Amiodarone would not be an appropriate first choice for antiarrhythmic therapy in this relatively young woman with alternative medication options.

56.8 The correct answer is C.
Rationale: Syncope in patients with atrial fibrillation or atrial flutter is uncommon and is only seen if there are conversion pauses following termination of the arrhythmia in the setting of concomitant sick sinus syndrome. Persistent atrial fibrillation or flutter may lead to cardiomyopathy and heart failure in patients without prior evidence of ventricular dysfunction if tachycardia is not controlled. Atrial fibrillation often adversely affects quality of life. Thromboembolism is a serious complication of atrial fibrillation and flutter and may account for up to 15% of ischemic strokes in the United States.

56.9 The correct answer is D.
Rationale: The CHA_2DS_2-VASc score does not apply to patients with atrial fibrillation and thyrotoxicosis, hypertrophic cardiomyopathy, or moderate-to-severe rheumatic mitral stenosis. These populations are at high risk for thromboembolism, warranting anticoagulation regardless of the CHA_2DS_2-VASc score. Apixaban has an improved safety profile over warfarin with similar efficacy in stroke prevention, and it does not have the dietary concerns associated with vitamin K antagonists.

56.10 The correct answer is C.
Rationale: This patient developed postoperative atrial fibrillation, a common occurrence after open heart surgery. His atrial fibrillation has persisted for more than 48 hours. Therefore, anticoagulation is indicated, given his CHA_2DS_2-VASc score of 4 (age >65 years, hypertension, heart failure, and vascular disease). Aspirin is indicated for coronary artery disease, particularly with recent revascularization. A direct oral anticoagulant (DOAC) or warfarin is indicated for stroke prevention in the setting of atrial fibrillation. Aspirin or DOAC monotherapy is not appropriate. Cardiac monitoring has limited proven benefit to date in postoperative atrial fibrillation, although it may prove helpful in this patient after he has fully convalesced.

VENTRICULAR TACHYCARDIA

Jeanwoo Yoo, Evan C. Adelstein, and Alfred M. Loka

CHAPTER 57

QUESTIONS

57.1 When reviewing a 12-lead electrocardiogram (ECG) of a wide complex tachycardia (**Figure 57.1**), which of the following is **NOT** useful in distinguishing between ventricular tachycardia (VT) and supraventricular tachycardia (SVT) with aberrancy?

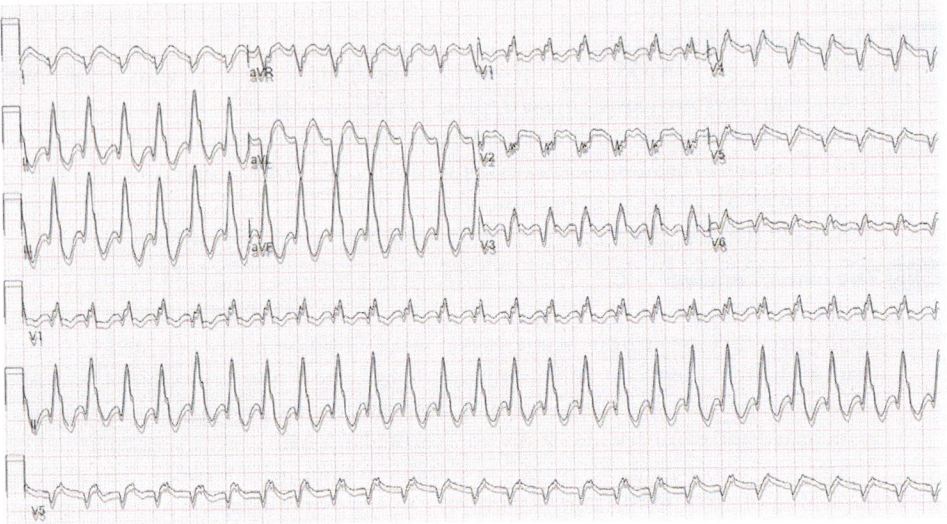

Figure 57.1

- A. Lack of RS complex in any precordial lead
- B. Presence of initial R wave in aVR
- C. Longest R to S interval greater than 100 milliseconds in any precordial lead
- D. Initial R or Q wave less than 40 milliseconds in lead aVR

57.2 A 32-year-old woman with a past medical history of hypertension, hyperlipidemia, obesity, and depression presents with short-lived episodes of palpitations and lightheadedness occurring at rest. She has been taking sertraline for several years and recently was prescribed levofloxacin for bacterial pneumonia. Her ECG is shown in **Figure 57.2**. Subsequent inpatient telemetry monitoring notes several-beat runs of a wide complex tachyarrhythmia with fluctuating QRS amplitude. What is the next **BEST** step in management?

*Questions and Answers are based on Chapter 57: Ventricular Tachycardia by Justin Hayase and Jason S. Bradfield in Cardiovascular Medicine and Surgery, First Edition.

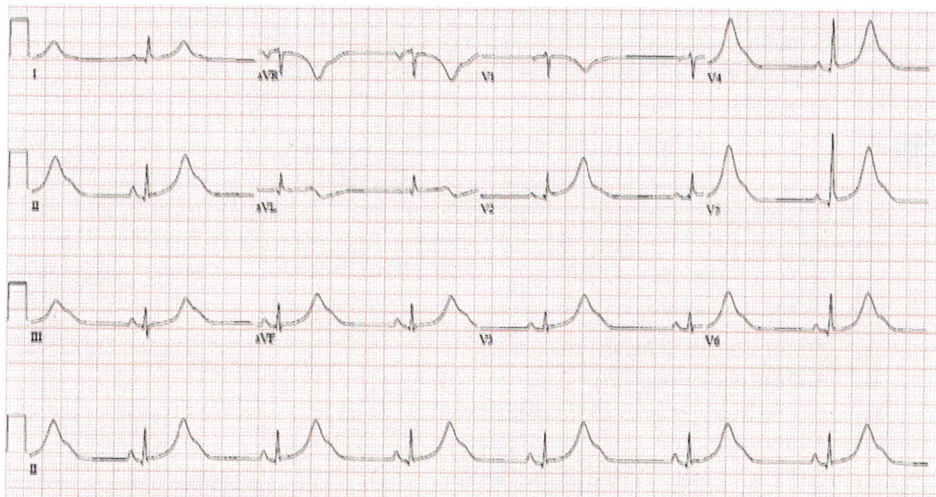

Figure 57.2

A. Intravenous (IV) amiodarone
B. IV magnesium
C. Cardiac catheterization
D. VT ablation

57.3 The patient mentioned in **Question 57.2** receives the proposed therapy. Several hours later, her heart rate increases to 200 beats per minute (bpm), her blood pressure (BP) decreases to 80/40 mm Hg, and she appears lethargic and diaphoretic. There is a thready pulse present. A rhythm strip reveals a wide complex tachycardia with multiple QRS morphologies as shown in **Figure 57.3**. What is the next appropriate step?

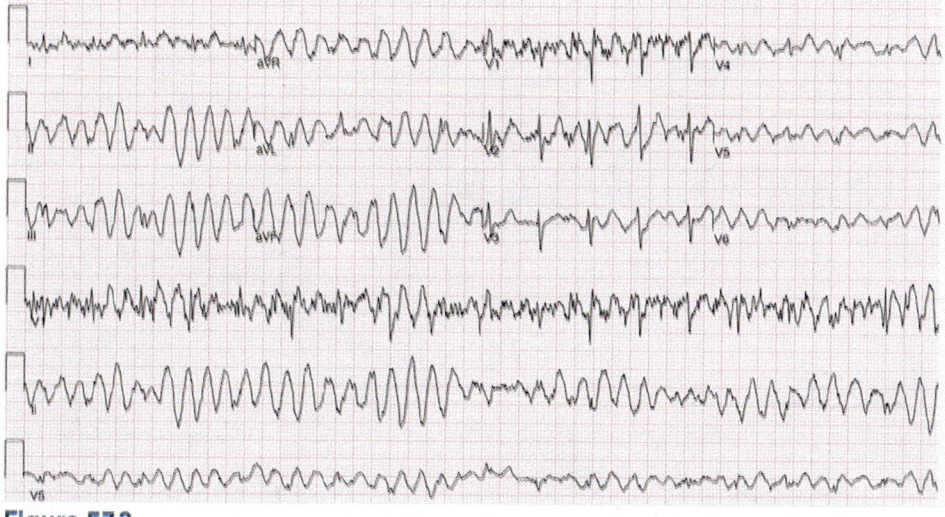

Figure 57.3

A. Unsynchronized cardioversion
B. IV metoprolol
C. Isoproterenol infusion
D. Airway intubation

57.4 A 72-year-old man presents to the hospital via emergency medical services (EMS) because he collapsed after reaching the top of a flight of stairs. His medical history is significant for hypertension, hyperlipidemia, type 2 diabetes mellitus, and active smoking. An ECG obtained by EMS shows a wide complex tachycardia. His vital signs show a heart rate of 220 bpm, BP of 80/40 mm Hg, and agonal respirations. What is the next appropriate step?

A. Administer IV magnesium 2 mg.
B. Administer epinephrine 1 mg.
C. Administer synchronized cardioversion.
D. Administer amiodarone 60 mg/kg.

57.5 The patient mentioned in **Question 57.4** responds to the appropriate therapy, and his mentation improves along with his BP, which is now 120/90 mm Hg. He is in sinus rhythm on telemetry. What is the next step in diagnostic workup?

A. Troponin and ECG assessment
B. Cardiac magnetic resonance imaging (MRI)
C. Transthoracic echocardiogram
D. Pulmonary computed tomography (CT) angiogram

57.6 A 72-year-old man presents with chest pain and dyspnea for 2 days via EMS. He was found to have an anterior ST-segment elevation myocardial infarction (STEMI) and underwent percutaneous coronary intervention to the left anterior descending artery with two drug-eluting stents. His chest pain resolved. An echocardiogram is obtained with notes reduced left ventricular (LV) systolic function with ejection fraction (EF) 30%. Four days after revascularization, he is noted to have the rhythm shown in **Figure 57.4**. What is the most appropriate long-term strategy?

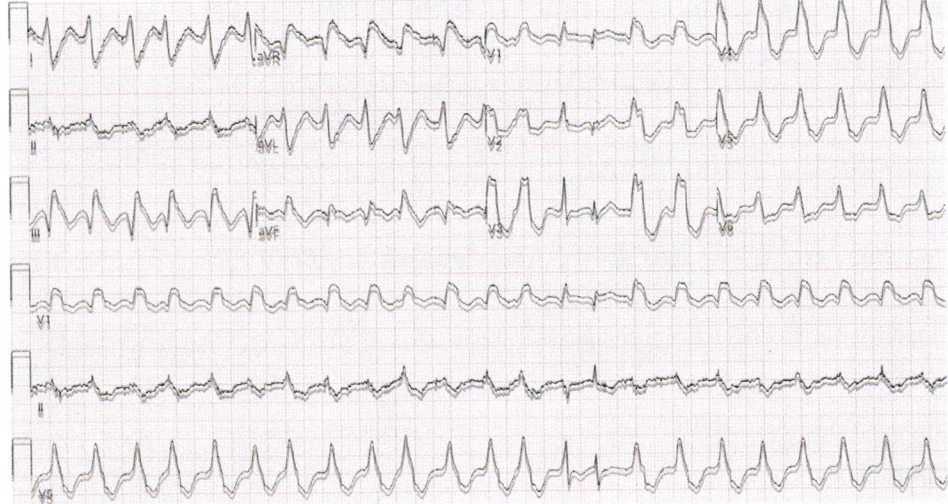

Figure 57.4

A. Implantable cardioverter-defibrillator (ICD) implant
B. Catheter ablation of VT
C. Initiation and continuation of amiodarone
D. Electrophysiology study to assess for inducible arrhythmia

57.7 Which of the following regimens is **NOT** appropriate for suppressing recurrence of VT in the patient **Question 57.6**?

A. Amiodarone
B. Sotalol
C. Mexiletine
D. Flecainide

57.8 A 56-year-old woman with a past medical history of inferior myocardial infarction 5 years ago with subsequent ischemic cardiomyopathy, left ventricular ejection fraction (LVEF) 35% on serial echocardiograms, and a prophylactic ICD presents with progressive shortness of breath and malaise. ECG performed by EMS reveals monomorphic wide complex tachycardia as shown in **Figure 57.5**, for which she is transferred to the emergency department. Examination is notable for BP 98/60 mm Hg, pulse 145 bpm and regular, O_2 saturation 96%, diaphoresis, rales, and lower extremity edema. What is the next appropriate step?

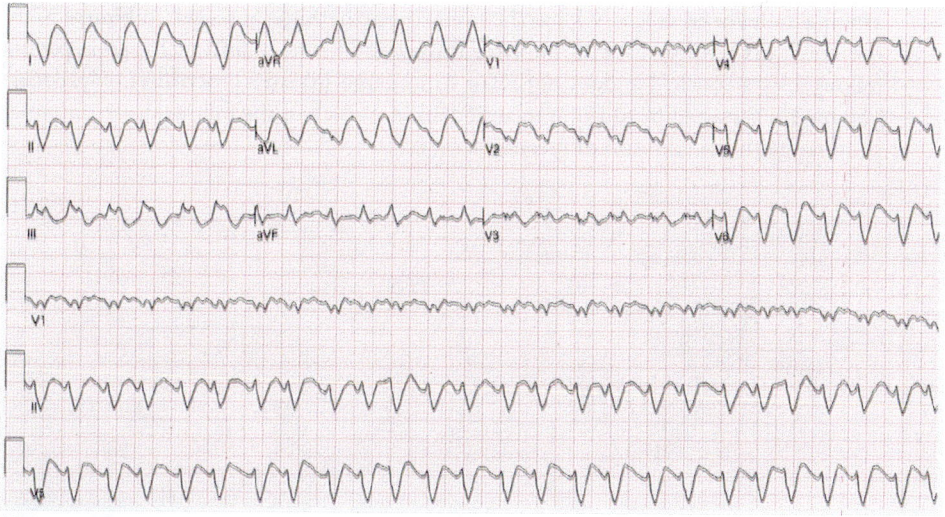

Figure 57.5

A. IV metoprolol
B. IV amiodarone
C. IV lidocaine
D. IV procainamide

57.9 The patient in **Question 57.8** responds to appropriate therapy and converts to sinus rhythm. Which of the following is **TRUE** regarding the mechanism of this patient's arrhythmia?

A. The arrhythmia is likely driven by ongoing ischemia.
B. A prolonged QT interval preceded the arrhythmia.
C. The arrhythmia is likely idiopathic and focal.
D. The arrhythmia is likely the result of macro-reentry with a critical isthmus.

57.10 A 51-year-old woman with a history of ischemic cardiomyopathy, LVEF 30% to 35% secondary to distant myocardial infarction in her 40s, primary prevention ICD for persistently reduced EF, hypertension, and hyperlipidemia presents to the cardiology clinic for device interrogation after complaining of intermittent palpitations. The interrogation notes episodes of monitored VT with heart rates up to 160 bpm for 1 minute duration. She is taking aspirin, atorvastatin, metoprolol succinate, lisinopril, and spironolactone. Her most recent laboratories note normal chemistries. The ECG is notable for inferior Q waves without ST abnormality. Which of the following antiarrhythmic medications is the most appropriate for managing her VT?

A. Amiodarone
B. Sotalol
C. Mexiletine
D. Flecainide

57.11 An 82-year-old patient with prior anterior myocardial infarction, chronic kidney disease stage IV, and peripheral vascular disease who is on chronic amiodarone therapy 400 mg daily for recurrent VT has the following arrhythmia as shown in **Figure 57.6**, for which his ICD treats with multiple unsuccessful runs of anti-tachycardia pacing followed by a shock. He does not want to undergo invasive procedures. Mexiletine 150 mg tid is started in addition to amiodarone. Which of the following are potential concerns with the addition of mexiletine?

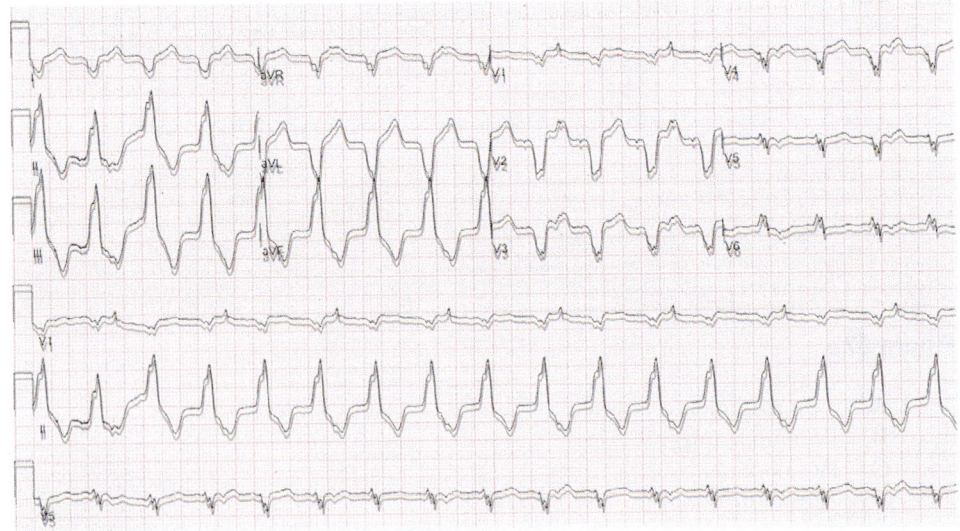

Figure 57.6

A. Negative inotropic effects
B. Decreased defibrillation threshold
C. Central nervous system (CNS) effects (tremor, blurred vision, ataxia)
D. QT prolongation

ANSWERS

57.1 The correct answer is D.

Rationale: According to the Brugada criteria for VT, the absence of an RS complex in all precordial leads or manifesting an RS greater than 100 milliseconds in any precordial lead (ie, time from onset of R wave to nadir of S wave) is indicative of VT. The ECG in **Figure 57.1** demonstrates QR and QS complexes in all precordial leads. According to the aVR criteria for VT, the presence of an R wave in aVR (ie, completely positive QRS complex) or initial R or Q wave greater than 40 milliseconds in lead aVR is indicative of VT. All these findings reflect the activation of myocardium via myocardial cells rather than the His-Purkinje system. Initial ventricular activation in SVT with aberrancy is rapid; delay occurs later in ventricular activation (**Figure 57.7**).

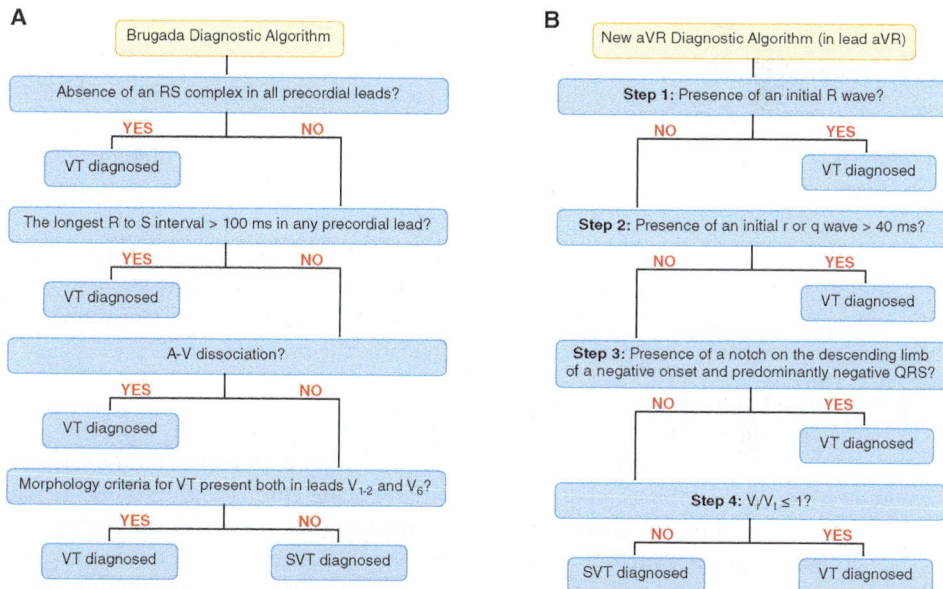

Figure 57.7 Electrocardiographic (ECG) diagnostic algorithms for ventricular tachycardia (VT). **A:** Stepwise Brugada algorithm for diagnosis of VT. Any one of the four criteria can establish the diagnosis of VT. **B:** Stepwise approach for diagnosis of VT using only lead aVR. V_i/V_t represents the ventricular activation velocity ratio, with V_i being the vertical excursion in millivolts during the initial 40 milliseconds of the QRS complex and V_t being the vertical excursion in millivolts during the terminal 40 milliseconds of the QRS complex. SVT, supraventricular tachycardia. (Adapted from Vereckei A, Duray G, Szénási G, et al. New algorithm using only lead aVR for differential diagnosis of wide QRS complex tachycardia. *Heart Rhythm.* 2008;5(1):89-98. Copyright © 2008 Heart Rhythm Society, with permission.)

572. The correct answer is B:
Rationale: A form of polymorphic VT, known as torsades de pointes, may be precipitated by bradycardia and a prolonged QT interval, which is the case for this patient. In patients with torsades de pointes, IV magnesium is first-line therapy. IV amiodarone will further prolong the QT interval and would not be the first choice in this scenario. There are multiple causes of a prolonged QT interval, including electrolyte abnormalities, drug effects (as in this patient), or inherited channelopathies. Cardiac catheterization would be appropriate for polymorphic VT secondary to ischemia not in the setting of a prolonged QT interval. VT ablation would be appropriate for monomorphic VT.

573. The correct answer is A:
Rationale: Management of VT initially should follow the algorithm provided by advanced cardiac life support (ACLS) recommendations, with an emphasis on circulatory support and airway protection. Electrical cardioversion is often recommended if VT does not terminate. Given the patient's hemodynamically deteriorating, cardioversion would be indicated for unstable VT. Synchronization will not be possible for torsades de points.

574. The correct answer is C:
Rationale: This patient has a wide complex tachycardia with hypotension and respiratory distress. Although these characteristics do not rule out SVT with aberrancy or preexcited atrial fibrillation, VT is the most likely diagnosis. The high likelihood of VT and clinical instability warrant prompt action. Prompt synchronized cardioversion should be prioritized according to ACLS protocol for any unstable tachyarrhythmia. Given that the patient has a pulse and BP, epinephrine is not immediately indicated. Similarly, amiodarone may be given after synchronized cardioversion is attempted. IV magnesium is helpful for torsades de pointes but will not terminate the arrhythmia promptly, so cardioversion remains the first logic step.

575. The correct answer is A:
Rationale: Once stabilized, an evaluation for underlying causes of VT should be performed, such as electrolyte imbalances, drug toxicities, endocrine disorders, structural heart disease, inherited channelopathies, or acute coronary syndromes. Given this patient's history of collapse associated with exertion and his risk factors for coronary artery disease, including diabetes, hypertension, gender, age, and smoking, assessment for acute coronary syndromes is most appropriate. A sinus rhythm ECG may also find clues of prior infarction or ventricular preexcitation. Echocardiography is certainly indicated but is not the best next step. Advanced imaging such as cardiac MRI may be performed to assess for myocardial scar or infiltrative disease but is time consuming and of lower yield given the presentation. Pulmonary embolism does not cause VT.

57.6 The correct answer is A.

Rationale: The patient had sustained monomorphic VT more than 72 hours after revascularization, as the ECG shows a wide complex tachycardia with a capture beat indicative of atrioventricular (AV) dissociation. The VT is likely caused by a re-entrant mechanism around nascent myocardial scar. Implantation of an ICD for secondary prevention of sudden cardiac death is indicated. VT ablation does not replace the indication for an ICD, as success rates are variable, and additional VT circuits may occur. Amiodarone may be an adjunctive strategy for recurrent VT, but it is not the first appropriate strategy and does not provide a mortality benefit. An electrophysiology study to assess for inducible sustained monomorphic VT would have been appropriate if the clinical VT was not sustained (ie, <30 seconds).

57.7 The correct answer is D.

Rationale: Class Ic antiarrhythmics are contraindicated in the presence of prior myocardial infarction based upon the results of the Cardiac Arrhythmia Suppression Trial (CAST). Amiodarone is often the primary agent of choice for preventing recurrent VT because of its relatively high efficacy. In the long term, many practitioners prefer to stop this agent or minimize its dose because of myriad potential side effects. Long-term antiarrhythmic medication options for VT in the setting of ischemic cardiomyopathy include amiodarone, sotalol, and mexiletine.

57.8 The correct answer is B.

Rationale: For treatment of hemodynamically stable VT, amiodarone and procainamide are the drugs of choice. Amiodarone is more readily available and has less risk of worsening hypotension during infusion. Procainamide is often less readily available and has the potential for QT prolongation when metabolized to N-acetylprocainamide, particularly in the setting of kidney disease. In this patient with unknown renal function who is stable but has signs of heart failure, amiodarone is preferred. Lidocaine has fallen out of favor as a primary agent for management of VT. However, it still has a role when acute ischemia is suspected or when used as an adjunct in combination with other antiarrhythmic agents such as amiodarone. Intravenous beta-blockers should be avoided in patients with VT as they may worsen the patient's acute heart failure.

57.9 The correct answer is D.

Rationale: This patient with monomorphic VT likely has scar-mediated arrhythmia in the setting of ischemic cardiomyopathy and prior myocardial infarction. The presence of scar promotes a macro-reentrant mechanism for myocardial VT. The heterogeneous conduction properties of scarred myocardium create critical isthmuses, which are zones of slow conduction necessary to sustain a macro-reentrant circuit for monomorphic VT. Torsades de pointes, a form of polymorphic VT, may be precipitated by a long QT interval. Focal mechanisms are often implicated in idiopathic VT, such as outflow tract VT or fascicular VT, which typically occur in the absence of structural heart disease.

57.10 The correct answer is B.
Rationale: Amiodarone is often the agent of choice for preventing ischemic VT because of its higher efficacy compared with other antiarrhythmic drugs. However, it should not be first-line therapy in the long term for patients who are relatively young when alternatives exist, given the multiple potential adverse effects of amiodarone. Sotalol would be a reasonable option because she is not in heart failure and has preserved renal function. Using sotalol may require lowering the dose of metoprolol. Mexiletine is most frequently used as an adjunctive medication with other antiarrhythmic drugs for ventricular arrhythmias and is most effective for ischemia-related ventricular arrhythmias. This patient has prior myocardial infarction and is therefore not a candidate for either flecainide or propafenone.

57.11 The correct answer is C.
Rationale: The most common side effects of mexiletine include CNS (tremor, blurred vision, ataxia) and gastrointestinal (nausea, vomiting, dyspepsia) symptoms. Mexiletine, like lidocaine, does not have significant proarrhythmic effects. All sodium channel–blocking agents may increase defibrillation threshold in long term. Mexiletine is not associated with QT prolongation and does not have negative inotropic effects.

ANTIARRHYTHMIC DRUGS*

Jeanwoo Yoo, Alfred M. Loka, and Evan C. Adelstein

CHAPTER 58

QUESTIONS

58.1 A 74-year-old male presents to the emergency department with palpitations and shortness of breath. His medical history includes stroke, coronary artery disease with the last percutaneous intervention 5 years prior, hypertension, and hyperlipidemia. He has been experiencing palpitations for the past year but has noted increased frequency and duration of his symptoms more recently, along with associated dyspnea and decreased exercise tolerance. His electrocardiogram (ECG) reveals atrial fibrillation (AF) with a ventricular rate of 105 beats per minute (bpm). An echocardiogram reveals left ventricular ejection fraction (LVEF) 45%, mild mitral regurgitation, and mild tricuspid regurgitation. He is taking atorvastatin 80 mg daily, aspirin 81 mg daily, metoprolol succinate 50 mg daily, and amlodipine 5 mg daily. He is started on warfarin and subsequently planned to undergo cardioversion with initiation of amiodarone. Which of the following changes to his medications would be most appropriate?

- A. Increase his dose of metoprolol.
- B. Increase his dose of warfarin.
- C. Decrease his dose of atorvastatin.
- D. Add digoxin to his current regimen.

58.2 A 63-year-old woman is seen in the office for recurrent palpitations. She denies dizziness, lightheadedness, or syncope. She has a history of an anterior myocardial infarction 3 years ago with drug-eluting stents placed in the mid-distal left anterior descending artery, heart failure with LVEF 50%, and type 2 diabetes. She is a former smoker. An outpatient 7-day monitor shows frequent wide ventricular rhythm lasting up to 15 seconds consistent with ventricular tachycardia (VT). Her labs are notable for aspartate aminotransferase (AST) 30, alanine aminotransferase (ALT) 20, creatinine 0.6, hemoglobin 12.0, white blood cell count 6.2, and platelets 220.

Which of the following would you recommend for management of VT?

- A. Amiodarone
- B. Sotalol
- C. Flecainide
- D. Propafenone

---

*Questions and Answers are based on Chapter 58: Antiarrhythmic Drugs by Aadhavi Sridharan and Noel G. Boyle in Cardiovascular Medicine and Surgery, First Edition.

58.3 Select the **CORRECT** contraindications with the appropriate medications.

A. Prior myocardial infarction—amiodarone; prior myocardial infarction—flecainide; acute liver injury—sotalol; acute kidney injury—dronedarone
B. Acute kidney injury—amiodarone; prior myocardial infarction—flecainide; acute liver injury—sotalol; decompensated heart failure—dronedarone
C. Acute liver injury—amiodarone; prior myocardial infarction—flecainide; acute kidney injury—sotalol; decompensated heart failure—dronedarone
D. Decompensated heart failure—amiodarone; prior myocardial infarction—flecainide; acute liver injury—sotalol; acute kidney injury—dronedarone

58.4 A 22-year-old girl had a fainting episode after swim practice. She has no known medical conditions. Her family history is significant for her mother, who died suddenly of unknown cause at the age of 35. An ECG is obtained, and her QTc is 508 milliseconds. What is the most appropriate next step in management?

A. Nadolol
B. Electrophysiology (EP) study
C. Implantable cardioverter-defibrillator (ICD)
D. Sotalol

58.5 A 55-year-old male is seen for post-discharge follow-up after he sustained cardiac arrest with VT noted by emergency medical services. He was successfully resuscitated and underwent urgent left heart catheterization when ST elevations were noted in leads V2 to V5. He had successful stenting of an occluded mid-left anterior descending artery. His predischarge echocardiogram noted an LVEF of 25%. He was started on metoprolol succinate, sacubitril-valsartan, and spironolactone before discharge. His telemetry 4 days after presentation noted several runs of nonsustained VT. In addition to up-titrating metoprolol, which of the following therapies is the next **BEST** step?

A. Flecainide
B. Mexiletine
C. Amiodarone
D. Sodium-glucose cotransporter 2 (SGLT2) inhibitor

58.6 A 43-year-old male with a past medical history of AF and hyperlipidemia had syncope after developing an upper respiratory infection with a fever of 38.2 °C. His medication list includes flecainide, diltiazem, and atorvastatin. His current ECG is shown in **Figure 58.1**. Prior ECGs in sinus rhythm have been unremarkable. Which of the following adjustments should be made to his medication regimen?

A. Decrease the dose of diltiazem.
B. Stop flecainide.
C. Decrease the dose of atorvastatin.
D. Increase the dose of diltiazem.

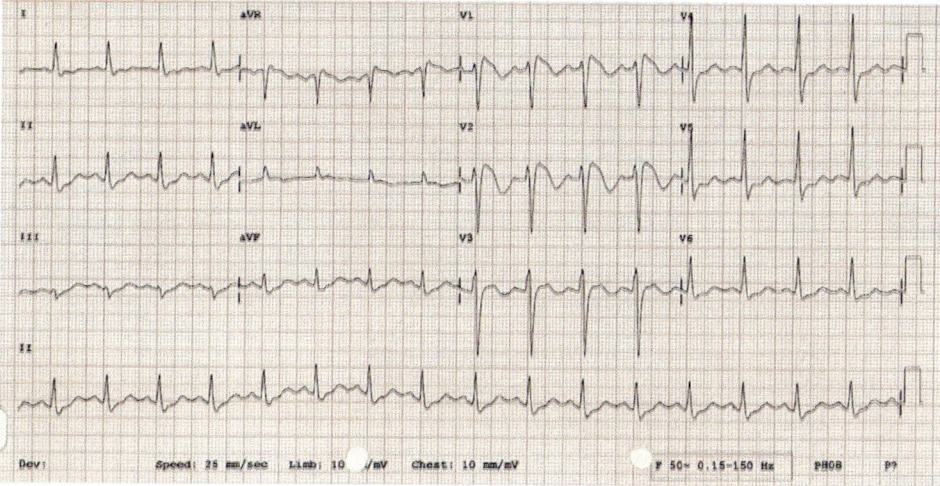

Figure 58.1

58.7 A 48-year-old male presents to the cardiology clinic after endorsing an episode of palpitations with lightheadedness. A screening ECG is obtained as shown in **Figure 58.2**. He is scheduled to undergo catheter ablation as an outpatient. Before his procedure, he presented to the emergency department with palpitations. He has an irregular heart rhythm with rates as high as 182 bpm. His blood pressure is 100/65 mm Hg. The ECG shows an irregular wide complex tachycardia with several QRS morphologies. What is the next appropriate step in management?

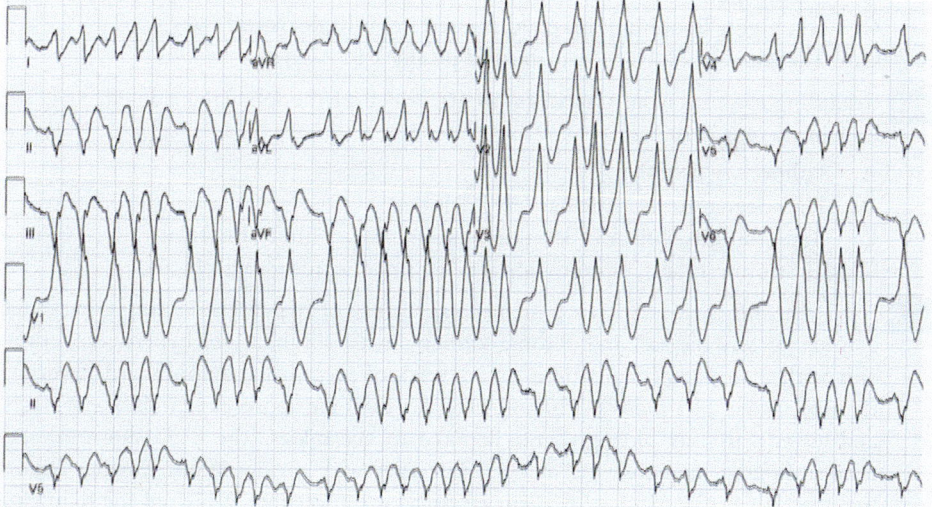

Figure 58.2

    A. Administer amiodarone.
    B. Administer metoprolol.
    C. Administer digoxin.
    D. Administer procainamide.

58.8 For the patient in **Question 58.7**, which of the following labs should be monitored while the patient is on the appropriate regimen?

   A. Liver function test
   B. Liver associated enzymes
   C. Complete blood count
   D. Pulmonary function test

58.9 A 34-year-old woman presents with new onset intermittent palpitations that occur 2 to 3 times a month. A cardiac event monitor records episodes of narrow complex tachycardia with a short RP interval lasting up to 30 minutes. What is the next **BEST** step in management?

   A. Supraventricular tachycardia (SVT) ablation
   B. Mexiletine
   C. Propafenone
   D. Amiodarone

58.10 A 74-year-old woman is evaluated after being noted to have runs of sustained VT with associated palpitations and dizziness. She has a history of ischemic cardiomyopathy with prior myocardial infarction 5 years ago. Her echocardiogram shows an LVEF of 30% and end-diastolic dimension of 6.6 cm. She is on metoprolol succinate, sacubitril-valsartan, spironolactone, and dapagliflozin. She is planned to undergo ICD placement and was started on amiodarone 200 mg daily after a loading dose by her cardiologist.

Which of the following is **NOT TRUE** regarding amiodarone?

   A. The active metabolite is highly protein-bound and has a large volume of distribution.
   B. The onset of action is 1 to 2 hours by IV administration and 2 to 3 days by oral administration.
   C. It is highly lipophilic and concentrated in multiple tissues.
   D. The elimination half-life is short, typically 1 to 2 days.

58.11 Regarding the patient in **Question 58.10**, which of the following side effects is she least likely to experience?

   A. Pulmonary fibrosis
   B. First-degree atrioventricular (AV) delay
   C. Transaminitis with AST levels 2 times the upper limit of normal
   D. Gastrointestinal symptoms when taken on an empty stomach

58.12 A 55-year-old woman with a past medical history of hypertension, hyperlipidemia, coronary artery disease, and chronic kidney disease secondary to hypertension presents with 2 weeks of palpitations and 1 week of progressive dyspnea and lower extremity edema. Her pulse is 120 and irregular, rales are appreciated in bilateral bases, and lower extremity pitting edema is noted to her ankles. The ECG shows AF. An echocardiogram demonstrates an LVEF of 45% with no significant valvular abnormalities. She is planned for inpatient electrical cardioversion. Which of the following medications would be most appropriate to maintain sinus rhythm?

   A. Amiodarone
   B. Sotalol
   C. Digoxin
   D. Dronedarone

ANSWERS

58.1 **The correct answer is C.**
Rationale: This patient is to be initiated on amiodarone, so his medication list needs to be reviewed for potential pharmacokinetic interactions. Amiodarone increases the concentrations of other common cardiac medications, including warfarin, digoxin, and statins. Therefore, this patient's atorvastatin and warfarin may need to be decreased. Metoprolol and amiodarone may cause bradycardia, which may possibly necessitate lowering the dose of metoprolol after cardioversion. Digoxin is not indicated in this patient, as amiodarone increases its levels, and it has a relatively narrow therapeutic window.

58.2 **The correct answer is B.**
Rationale: This patient is found to have a wide complex tachycardia, concerning for VT in the setting of prior myocardial infarction with presumed scarring but overall preserved left ventricular function. Class Ic agents, including flecainide and propafenone, are contraindicated in the setting of prior myocardial infarction because of an increased risk of sudden cardiac death, as seen in the Cardiac Arrhythmia Suppression Trial (CAST). Amiodarone is associated with adverse long-term effects, including pulmonary, thyroid, hepatic, ophthalmic, and neurologic toxicity. Therefore, sotalol would be appropriate for this patient.

58.3 **The correct answer is C.**
Rationale: Amiodarone is contraindicated with acute liver injury because it may cause transaminitis. Flecainide is contraindicated with prior myocardial infarction because of potential proarrhythmia. Sotalol is contraindicated with renal impairment. Dronedarone is contraindicated in acute decompensated heart failure because of the increased risk of mortality.

58.4 **The correct answer is A.**
Rationale: This patient likely has long QT syndrome, possibly long QT syndrome type 1 that is triggered by exertion, for which long-acting beta-blockers would be most suitable. EP study is of limited value in the diagnosis and treatment of patients with long QT syndrome. An ICD would be appropriate for recurrent syncope despite beta-blocker therapy. Despite being a beta-blocker, sotalol is a QT-prolonging class III drug and is contraindicated.

58.5 **The correct answer is D.**
Rationale: There is limited evidence to show the benefit of treating nonsustained VT. The next best step is to optimize guideline medical therapy for heart failure, including SGLT2 inhibitors. Flecainide is contraindicated in the setting of ischemic heart disease. Mexiletine is a class 1b antiarrhythmic agent helpful for ventricular arrhythmias secondary to ischemia. Amiodarone can be effective in managing refractory VT but is not indicated for asymptomatic nonsustained VT.

58.6 The correct answer is B.
Rationale: This patient has a type 1 Brugada pattern suggestive of Brugada syndrome, likely unmasked by the combination of flecainide and a febrile illness. Flecainide is a sodium channel blocker that will elicit a Brugada pattern in patients with genetic predisposition, much like procainamide. The remaining medications do not need to be adjusted, as they will neither help nor harm the patient.

58.7 The correct answer is D.
Rationale: This patient has Wolff-Parkinson-White syndrome (WPW) with concurrent preexcited AF. AF has the potential to conduct rapidly to the ventricles down the accessory pathway. Administering AV nodal blocking agents such as metoprolol and digoxin may cause AF to conduct preferentially down the accessory pathway, resulting in faster ventricular response and precipitating ventricular fibrillation (VF). Procainamide is readily available for rapid intravenous loading in the United States. It will both slow or block accessory pathway conduction and convert AF to sinus rhythm in this situation. Amiodarone has a slower onset of action, so procainamide is the preferred drug.

58.8 The correct answer is C.
Rationale: The most common side effects of procainamide include hypotension with intravenous administration, gastrointestinal effects (nausea, vomiting, and diarrhea), agranulocytosis, and lupus. Complete blood counts should be monitored in patients receiving procainamide, given the ongoing risk of agranulocytosis. Plasma concentrations of procainamide and *N*-acetylprocainamide (NAPA) should also be monitored in patients with renal impairment.

58.9 The correct answer is A.
Rationale: This patient has narrow complex tachycardia with a short RP interval indicative of SVT. Patients with recurrent paroxysmal SVT should be referred for SVT ablation. Mexiletine has no effects on atrial myocardium because of the short action potential duration in atrial myocytes. Amiodarone's potential side effects preclude its use in a young patient with a relatively benign arrhythmia. Propafenone could be used in this situation, but it has the potential for proarrhythmia. This risk is greater than that of SVT ablation.

58.10 The correct answer is D.
Rationale: The onset of action for amiodarone is within 1 to 2 hours after intravenous administration and may take 2 to 3 days (or even longer) after oral administration. It is highly (96%) protein-bound and has a large but variable volume of distribution. It is highly lipophilic and is concentrated in multiple tissues. Consequently, its elimination half-life is long, typically 50 to 60 days.

58.11 The correct answer is A.

Rationale: Amiodarone most commonly causes gastrointestinal side effects, including nausea, vomiting, and anorexia. (Taking amiodarone with food or dividing the dose often obviates these side effects.) Longer-term adverse events include hepatic, thyroid, ocular, cutaneous, and neurologic effects. Hypothyroidism is the most seen long-term side effect but is easily treated with thyroid replacement. Although gastrointestinal and pulmonary toxicities were previously reported in up to 15% to 30% of patients receiving high-dose amiodarone therapy, recent findings suggest that the incidence is much less (<5%). Although amiodarone prolongs the QT interval, the risk of proarrhythmia with amiodarone is lower compared to other class III agents because it has a more uniform effect on endocardial, mid-myocardial, and epicardial myocardium. It commonly causes sinus bradycardia and prolongation of the PR interval because of its calcium channel–blocking activity.

58.12 The correct answer is A.

Rationale: Amiodarone is used for maintenance of sinus rhythm after cardioversion in patients with AF and underlying coronary artery disease. Although sotalol is safe in patients with coronary artery disease, it is contraindicated in the setting of chronic kidney disease. Digoxin is used for rate control and not for maintenance of sinus rhythm, given its vagotonic effects on the AV node. Because of the increased risk of mortality, dronedarone should not be used in patients with acute heart failure (**Table 58.1**).

TABLE 58.1 Singh-Vaughan Williams Classification of Antiarrhythmic Drugs

Class	Drug(s)	Clinical Use	Major Adverse Effects
Ia (sodium channel blocker, intermediate kinetics; potassium channel blocker)	Quinidine, procainamide, disopyramide	AF and ventricular arrhythmias	QT prolongation, torsades de pointes, procainamide: Lupus-like syndrome
Ib (sodium channel blocker, fast kinetics)	Lidocaine, mexiletine	Ventricular arrhythmias (especially ischemic)	Neurologic (tremor, drowsiness, seizures, coma) and gastrointestinal (nausea) effects
Ic (sodium channel blocker, slow kinetics)	Flecainide, propafenone	PSVT, AF, ventricular arrhythmias in the absence of structural heart disease	Proarrhythmic potential in causing reentrant VT
II (beta-adrenoceptor blockers)	Propranolol, nadolol, metoprolol, esmolol, and many others	Ventricular rate control in SVT, AF, AFL, and ventricular arrhythmia in CPVT and LQTS	Beta-adrenergic blocking effects (bronchospasm, bradycardia, fatigue)

(continued)

TABLE 58.1 Singh-Vaughan Williams Classification of Antiarrhythmic Drugs (continued)

Class	Drug(s)	Clinical Use	Major Adverse Effects
III (potassium channel blockers)	Amiodarone (also has class I, II, and IV properties)	Atrial and ventricular arrhythmias	Thyroid, pulmonary, hepatic, cutaneous, and neurologic side effects
	Dronedarone	AF	Increases mortality in heart failure and permanent AF
	Sotalol (also has class II properties)	AF, ventricular arrhythmias	QT prolongation, torsades de pointes
	Dofetilide	AF	QT prolongation, torsades de pointes
	Ibutilide	Acute treatment of AF conversion	QT prolongation, torsades de pointes
IV (calcium channel blockers)	Verapamil, diltiazem	Ventricular rate control in SVT, AF, AFL	Hypotension, negative inotropic effect, bradycardia
Others	Adenosine	Acute treatment of AV node–dependent arrhythmias	Risk of transient asystole
	Digoxin	Ventricular rate control in AF	Common gastrointestinal and neurologic side effects

AF, atrial fibrillation; AFL, atrial flutter; AV, atrioventricular; CPVT, catecholaminergic polymorphic ventricular tachycardia; LQTS, long QT syndrome; PSVT, paroxysmal supraventricular tachycardia; SVT, supraventricular tachycardia; VT, ventricular tachycardia.

CHAPTER 59

CATHETER ABLATION THERAPY*

Jeanwoo Yoo, Alfred M. Loka, and Evan C. Adelstein

QUESTIONS

59.1 A 62-year-old female is planning to undergo catheter ablation with pulmonary vein isolation as an outpatient for her atrial fibrillation (AF). Which of the following imaging modalities is the least helpful in imaging the left atrium and assist in the ablation procedure?

A. Computed tomography (CT) chest
B. Magnetic resonance imaging (MRI) heart
C. Transthoracic echocardiography
D. Intracardiac echocardiography

59.2 A 50-year-old male with a past medical history of non–ST-segment elevation myocardial infarction (NSTEMI) with anterior myocardial infarction status post percutaneous intervention to the mid-left anterior descending (LAD) 6 months prior presents to the cardiology clinic with frequent palpitations and chest discomfort. A cardiac monitor notes sustained ventricular tachycardia (VT). He undergoes cardiac catheterization which shows patent LAD stent and no obstructive coronary artery disease. He is planning to undergo VT ablation. Which of the following is **NOT TRUE** regarding pace mapping?

A. There are limitations to capturing local myocardium at low voltage.
B. There is decreased accuracy if neighboring myocardium is captured at high voltage.
C. Pace mapping is less useful in mapping atrial arrhythmias.
D. Pace mapping requires measurement of voltage to identify areas of scarring.

59.3 A 64-year-old woman presents with frequent symptomatic palpitations. She is found to have AF with episodes lasting as long as several hours on a 7-day cardiac monitor. She is tolerating metoprolol but has breakthrough symptomatic episodes. She states that she wants to be on as few long-term medications as possible. She is open to undergoing catheter ablation. Which of the following is **NOT TRUE** when counseling her regarding cryoablation versus radiofrequency (RF) ablation?

A. The risk of pericardial tamponade is higher with cryoablation than RF ablation.
B. AF recurrence risk is similar with cryoablation and RF ablation for paroxysmal AF.
C. There is a risk of phrenic nerve palsy with both approaches.
D. Cryoablation is generally associated with shorter procedure times as compared to RF ablation.

*Questions and Answers are based on Chapter 59: Catheter Ablation Therapy by Darshan Krishnappa and Kalyanam Shivkumar in Cardiovascular Medicine and Surgery, First Edition.

Section 4: Electrophysiology

59.4 For the patient in **Question 59.3**, which of the following anatomic sites is the **MOST LIKELY** source of triggers for AF?
  A. Cavo-tricuspid isthmus
  B. Pulmonary veins
  C. Left atrial appendage
  D. Coronary sinus

59.5 The patient in **Question 59.3** undergoes successful AF ablation. Post procedure, she is noted to have new onset right-sided weakness. Noncontrast CT of the head followed by CT angiography of the head and neck show acute left middle cerebral artery (MCA) stroke. Which of the following may have helped prevent this procedural complication?
  A. Maintaining a therapeutic activated clotting time (ACT) while ablating in the left atrium
  B. Ensuring continued preprocedural anticoagulation
  C. Safety strategies to avoid air embolization
  D. All of the above

59.6 A 40-year-old man with a past medical history of hypertension and hyperlipidemia presents with palpitations to the cardiology clinic. A Holter monitor is obtained, and frequent premature ventricular contractions (PVCs) and ventricular triplets are noted. A review of the PVCs notes negative QRS complexes in lead V1 and positive QRS complexes in the inferior leads, as shown in the rhythm strip (**Figure 59.1**). The patient endorses frequent symptoms, including chest discomfort and pounding sensation daily for which he is trialed on metoprolol and diltiazem without significant improvement. He is reluctant to take antiarrhythmic agents after reading about potential side effects on the internet. Which of the following is **TRUE** when advising him on the risks and benefits of ablation for his condition?

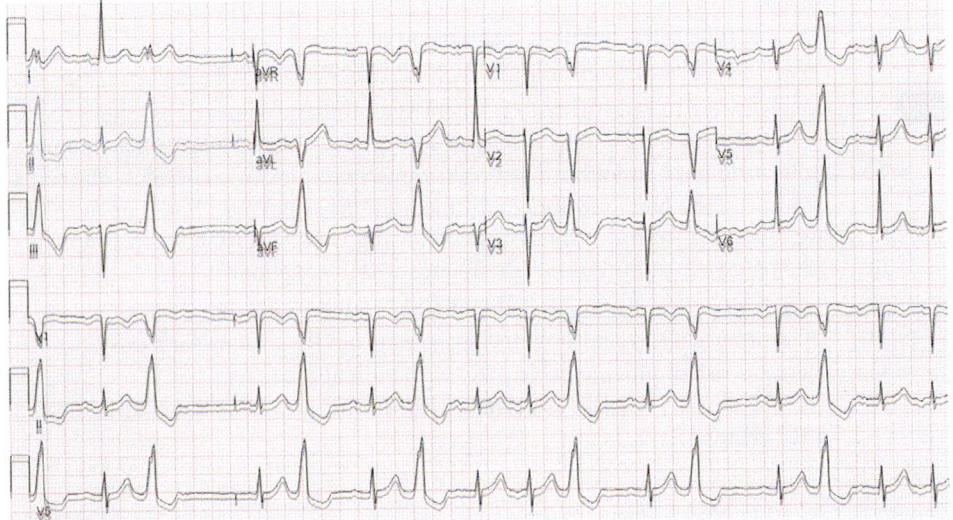

Figure 59.1

A. Catheter ablation is not appropriate.
B. Success rates depend upon anatomic considerations and the frequency of ectopy in the electrophysiology (EP) laboratory.
C. Complete heart block and bundle branch block are not potential complications with ablation.
D. His ventricular ectopy is associated with an increased risk of sudden death.

59.7 A 56-year-old woman with a past medical history significant for inferior ST-elevation myocardial infarction 5 years prior complicated by ventricular fibrillation and cardiac arrest with subsequent dilated ischemic cardiomyopathy. She had persistent severe left ventricular (LV) dysfunction with left ventricular ejection fraction (LVEF) 35%, and an implantable cardioverter defibrillator (ICD) was implanted. She presents to cardiology clinic after recent hospitalization for sustained, slow monomorphic wide complex tachycardia. She was started on amiodarone and cardioverted, and her ICD parameters were adjusted. Guideline medical therapy was optimized before discharge. Which of the following is appropriate in advising her regarding the benefits of ablation for her monomorphic VT?

A. VT ablation reduces recurrence of VT and ICD interventions in the majority of patients.
B. Mortality benefit has been clearly shown with ablation for scar-mediated VT.
C. Success rates of ablation for scar-mediated VT are consistently greater than 90%.
D. Antiarrhythmics must be continued in the long term after VT ablation.

59.8 For the patient in **Question 59.7**, which of the following is appropriate in advising her regarding the risks of ablation for her monomorphic VT?

A. The most frequent complication encountered is related to vascular access.
B. Radiation exposure is minimal for all ablation procedures.
C. Phrenic nerve paralysis is a significant risk during endocardial VT ablation.
D. Cardiac perforation is rare but more common with VT than AF ablation.

ANSWERS

59.1 The correct answer is C.

Rationale: The current practice of catheter ablation of paroxysmal AF generally comprises pulmonary vein isolation. During the procedure, three-dimensional electroanatomic mapping systems are used to construct left atrial and pulmonary vein geometry. Preoperative CT or MRI is often utilized to delineate left atrial and pulmonary venous anatomy, as anatomic variants are common. Intracardiac echocardiography is used for transseptal puncture, real-time assessment of pericardial effusion, and imaging the pulmonary veins. Transthoracic echocardiogram is not useful for AF ablation, although it is critical in the evaluation of patients with paroxysmal AF.

The correct answer is B:
Rationale: Pace mapping involves matching the 12-lead electrocardiogram (ECG) morphology while pacing the ventricle in different locations with the clinical 12-lead ECG during tachycardia. Pacing at the site of tachycardia origin should match the morphology of the clinical tachycardia. Although pace mapping is useful, it has several limitations, including (1) difficulty capturing local myocardium within areas of scarring at lower outputs and (2) capturing neighboring tissue at higher outputs, thus reducing its spatial accuracy. Furthermore, pace mapping is not useful for atrial arrhythmias because surface P waves are often not clearly discernible during atrial tachycardia, which limits any morphologic comparisons. Voltage mapping measures voltage to identify areas of scarring and border zones that may be potential targets for ablation. Activation mapping during a stable tachycardia is the ideal method of arrhythmia mapping.

The correct answer is A:
Rationale: The safety profile for cryoablation and RF ablation for AF is similar. Phrenic nerve injury is reported to have an incidence of 0.2% to 0.5% during AF ablation using either approach, with a higher risk when using the cryoballoon in the right pulmonary veins. Several observational and randomized studies have shown the noninferiority of cryoablation to RF ablation in patients with paroxysmal AF, while being associated with shorter procedural times. Anatomic variation and operator experience are considerations that guide the choice of ablation modality.

The correct answer is B:
Rationale: The antral region of the pulmonary veins, which are invested in myocardial tissue, is the most frequent source of AF triggers. Nonpulmonary vein triggers are seen in 15% to 30% of patients, including from the posterior wall of the left atrium, left atrial appendage, vein (or ligament) of Marshall, the coronary sinus, and the interatrial septum. Right atrial triggers include the crista terminalis, and the superior vena cava. Because pulmonary vein triggers are by far the most common, empiric pulmonary vein isolation is the cornerstone of ablation therapy for paroxysmal AF.

The correct answer is D:
Rationale: Stroke during left-sided catheter ablation is reported in less than 1% of patients, although silent cerebral infarcts have been reported in several imaging-only studies. Uninterrupted anticoagulation and optimal intraprocedural anticoagulation, coupled with safety strategies to avoid air embolization, have led to significant reductions in silent cerebral infarcts.

The correct answer is B:
Rationale: Considerable experience has accrued with catheter ablation of idiopathic ventricular arrhythmias, particularly for those arising from the ventricular outflow tracts. For some patients, ablation may be preferred over antiarrhythmic agents. The outcomes of catheter ablation vary depending on the site of origin, with long-term success rates ranging from 65% to 100%. The three most important determinants of procedural success are frequency of active ectopy during the procedure, depth of the arrhythmia focus within the myocardium, and thorough mapping. Parahisian PVCs are challenging owing to the proximity to the conduction system and the risk for complete heart block and bundle branch blocks. The PVC morphology is consistent with outflow tract origin, which is not associated with sudden cardiac death.

59.7 The correct answer is A.
Rationale: The benefits of catheter ablation of VT have been demonstrated in several randomized, observational, and registry-based studies with reductions in recurrence of VT and ICD therapies, although a mortality benefit has not been consistently demonstrated. Success rates of scar-mediated VT ablation range from 40% to 80%, given the complexity of the substrate, patient comorbidities, and ongoing adverse remodeling over time. Discontinuation of antiarrhythmic drugs may be considered after successful VT ablation in the long term, but this is a tailored decision.

59.8 The correct answer is A.
Rationale: The most frequent complication encountered is related to vascular access, occurring in 1% to 2% of patients, with the most frequent occurrences being bleeding and hematoma formation. Radiation exposure—both to the patient and the interventional electrophysiologist—is a cause for concern particularly for complex cases with long procedural durations, though the advent of 3D electroanatomic mapping has led to significant reductions in the use of fluoroscopy. Phrenic nerve injury is not a risk of endocardial VT ablation because the left phrenic nerve overlies the posterolateral epicardial surface of the heart. Cardiac perforation and tamponade are rare but are more common during catheter ablation of AF owing to the thinner wall of the left atrium.

IMPLANTABLE CARDIOVERTER-DEFIBRILLATORS

Amole Ojo and Casey White

CHAPTER 60

QUESTIONS

60.1 A 56-year-old male presents with a history of former cigarette smoking use, atherosclerotic coronary artery disease, myocardial infarction 5 months ago undergoing percutaneous intervention and placement of a drug-eluting stent to the left anterior descending artery, hypertension, and hyperlipidemia. He has ischemic cardiomyopathy with reduced left ventricular systolic function and calculated ejection fraction of 28%, maintained on maximally tolerated beta-blocker, angiotensin receptor-neprilysin inhibitor, mineralocorticoid receptor antagonist, and diuretic, as well as aspirin and P2Y12 therapies. Recent Holter monitor was notable for nonsustained ventricular tachycardia (VT). He is able to walk one block before having to stop due to exertional dyspnea. Which of the following is the most appropriate next step in management?

- A. Exercise stress test to assess for provocable ventricular ectopy
- B. Referral for implantable cardioverter-defibrillator (ICD)
- C. Referral for dual-chamber permanent pacemaker allowing for further up-titration in beta-blocker therapy
- D. Initiation of antiarrhythmic therapy

60.2 Which of the following clinical scenarios does **NOT** meet the indication for primary prevention ICD therapy?

- A. A 52-year-old patient with ischemic cardiomyopathy and left ventricular ejection fraction (LVEF) 25%, New York Heart Association (NYHA) class I
- B. A 65-year-old patient with nonischemic cardiomyopathy and LVEF 30%, NYHA class III symptoms despite optimized guideline medical therapies
- C. An 84-year-old patient seen in outpatient with nonischemic cardiomyopathy, LVEF 15%, maintained on maximally tolerated guideline medical therapies, NYHA class IV symptoms, not a candidate for left ventricular assist device (LVAD) or cardiac transplant
- D. A 76-year-old patient with ischemic cardiomyopathy, LVEF 38%, nonsustained VT and inducible sustained VT on electrophysiology (EP) study

---

*Questions and Answers are based on Chapter 60: Implantable Cardioverter-Defibrillators by Jonathan Lerner and Noel G. Boyle in Cardiovascular Medicine and Surgery, First Edition.

60.3 Regarding major trials of ICD benefit in primary prevention of sudden cardiac death, which is **CORRECT**?

A. The Sudden Cardiac Death in Heart Failure Trial (SCD-HeFT) included patients with ischemic cardiomyopathy only with NYHA class II-III symptoms and LVEF 35% or less demonstrating no statistical significance in all-cause mortality between ICD and amiodarone groups.

B. The Multicenter Automatic Defibrillator Implantation Trial (MADIT) enrolled patients with LVEF 35% or less, randomized to medical therapy or ICD arms, ultimately demonstrating significant reduction in all-cause mortality in the ICD groups.

C. The Multicenter Unsustained Tachycardia Trial (MUSTT) demonstrated superiority in all-cause mortality in patients undergoing EP study-guided initiation of antiarrhythmic therapy.

D. The MADIT II trial randomized patients with nonischemic cardiomyopathy to conventional medical therapy versus ICD implantation.

60.4 Regarding ICD therapy and nonischemic cardiomyopathy, which of the following statements is most accurate?

A. The Defibrillators in Non-Ischemic Cardiomyopathy Treatment Evaluation (DEFINITE) trial demonstrated statistically significant mortality benefits in patients with nonischemic cardiomyopathy and ICD implantation.

B. In the DANISH (Danish Study to Assess the Efficacy of ICDs in Patients With Nonischemic Systolic Heart Failure on Mortality) trial, there was a high utilization of cardiac resynchronization therapy (CRT) only among patients randomized to the non-ICD arm.

C. There was no significant difference between both ICD and non-ICD groups in the DANISH trial.

D. The SCD-HeFT trial showed ICD benefit in ischemic cardiomyopathy only.

60.5 ICD implantation is recommended in which of the following clinical scenarios?

A. A 68-year-old patient with LVEF 30% status post coronary artery bypass grafting (CABG) 2 weeks ago

B. A 72-year-old patient with LVEF 30% status post percutaneous coronary intervention (PCI) 30-days ago

C. A 56-year-old patient with nonischemic cardiomyopathy with LVEF 25% diagnosed 30-days ago, on guideline-directed therapies

D. A 48-year-old patient with ischemic cardiomyopathy with calculated LVEF 38%, nonsustained VT, and inducible sustained VT on EP study

60.6 Which of the following clinical scenarios is a subcutaneous ICD most indicated?

A. A 22-year-old patient with idiopathic cardiac arrest while running

B. A 50-year-old patient with ischemic cardiomyopathy, LVEF 20%, on maximally tolerated beta-blocker, and resting heart rate of 45 beats per minute (bpm)

C. A 60-year-old patient with nonischemic cardiomyopathy, LVEF 30%, on guideline therapies and amiodarone, recent sustained VT with a heart rate of 170 bpm

D. A 48-year-old patient with nonischemic cardiomyopathy, LVEF 20%, on guideline therapies, NYHA class III symptoms, left bundle branch block with QRS 150 milliseconds

60.7 Which of the following is **TRUE** regarding ICD programming?
- A. Multiple clinical studies have demonstrated the effectiveness of programming a single tachycardia therapy zone.
- B. In most clinical cases, the slowest tachycardia therapy zone in primary prevention patients should include a lower rate of 150 bpm.
- C. Mechanisms of inappropriate ICD therapies include supraventricular tachycardia (SVT) indiscrimination and T-wave oversensing.
- D. ICD programming guidelines recommend shorter tachycardia detection intervals and limiting anti-tachycardia pacing (ATP).

60.8 A 68-year-old patient with ischemic cardiomyopathy, diabetes mellitus, long-standing impaired left ventricular systolic dysfunction with LVEF 25%, VT, and single-chamber ICD with prior appropriate ICD therapies presents during a hospital admission with confirmed *Staphylococcus aureus* bacteremia from a presumed lower extremity ulcer. Which of the following is the appropriate next step in management?
- A. Extraction of complete system including the lead/coil and generator from the device pocket
- B. Obtain a transesophageal echocardiogram to guide strategy for retention versus extraction of device system.
- C. Initiate antibiotic regimen for gram-positive cocci bacteremia with surveillance blood cultures and extraction of complete system if persistently positive after 2 weeks.
- D. Needle aspiration culture of the ICD device pocket

60.9 ICD implantation is a reasonable next step in management for all the following cases **EXCEPT**:
- A. A patient with hypertrophic cardiomyopathy with sustained VT leading to syncope
- B. A patient with type 1 Brugada pattern and ventricular arrhythmia
- C. A patient with asymptomatic long QT syndrome (LQTS) with QTc of 452 milliseconds, on beta-blocker therapy
- D. A patient with cardiac sarcoidosis and sustained VT

60.10 Which of the following statements regarding ICDs is most accurate?
- A. Dual-coil leads are generally preferred over single-coil leads due to a clinically significant decrease in defibrillation thresholds comparatively.
- B. Single-chamber systems, compared to dual-chamber systems, have limited discrimination algorithms leading to comparatively increased rates of inappropriate shocks.
- C. Dual-coil leads have historically higher failure rates with increased technical extraction difficulty.
- D. Compared to cephalic access, subclavian venous access significantly mitigates periprocedural risk of pneumothorax.

ANSWERS

60.1 The correct answer is B.
Rationale: This patient has an ischemic cardiomyopathy with reduced LVEF of 28% and NYHA class II symptoms despite guideline-directed medical therapies. Nonsustained VT is also observed. ICD for primary prevention is indicated. Permanent pacemaker is not indicated. If there is a high likelihood of developing bradycardia, due to further up-titration in medical therapies, a dual-chamber ICD could be considered at the time of implantation. As demonstrated in several major trials, antiarrhythmic therapy did not decrease all-cause mortality compared to ICD groups.

60.2 The correct answer is C.
Rationale: All choices, with the exception of choice C, describe clinical scenarios meeting class I recommendations for ICD therapy for primary prevention. Primary prevention ICD is not recommended in patients with NYHA class IV symptoms who are not candidates for LVAD and cardiac transplantation.

60.3 The correct answer is B.
Rationale: The MADIT trial was the first multicenter trial assessing ICD use for primary prevention of sudden cardiac death. While demonstrating reduction in all-cause mortality in the ICD groups, the trial required EP study and nonsustained VT for inclusion criteria. The MUSTT trial randomized patients to EP study-guided antiarrhythmic therapy; only those with ICD therapy demonstrated reduction in arrhythmic death. The MADIT II included patients with ischemic cardiomyopathy secondary to prior myocardial infarction and LVEF 30% or less. The risk of death from any cause in the ICD group was statistically lower than in the conventional therapy arm. SCD-HeFT included patients with both ischemic and nonischemic cardiomyopathy. The trial revealed reduction in all-cause mortality in the ICD groups.

60.4 The correct answer is C.
Rationale: The DANISH and DEFINITE trials did not show overall mortality benefit. In the DANISH trial, there was high utilization of CRT among both groups. SCD-HeFT, however, showed similar ICD benefits among ischemic and nonischemic cardiomyopathy.

60.5 The correct answer is D.
Rationale: In the setting of CABG or PCI within the last 90 days, ICD is not indicated. Likewise, ICD implantation is not indicated in cases of heart failure treated within 3 months on continuous guideline-directed medical therapies.

60.6 The correct answer is A.
Rationale: Choice A is a likely encountered clinical scenario where implantation of a subcutaneous ICD may be considered. Particularly in younger patients, who may require multiple generator exchanges, possible revisions, and absence of overt need for anti-bradycardia or ATP, subcutaneous ICD is a viable option. Choice B would likely benefit from anti-bradycardia pacing, while choice C would likely benefit from ATP programming, both currently unavailable with subcutaneous ICD systems. Choice D describes indication for an implantable CRT defibrillator.

60.7 The correct answer is C.

Rationale: Studies have demonstrated reduction in inappropriate and appropriate shock burden with programming multiple detection zones, longer detection intervals, and the use of ATP. Burst ATP therapy is preferable with a minimum of eight stimuli at a cycle length of 84% to 88% of the arrhythmia cycle length. In most clinical cases, it is recommended that the slowest tachycardia therapy zone is set between 185 and 200 bpm. Including a lower rate of 150 bpm increases the risk of inappropriate therapy delivery during sinus tachycardia, especially. Choice C correctly identified inappropriate ICD therapies from SVT indiscrimination and T-wave oversensing. Device systems have SVT discriminators and T-wave oversensing algorithms, which in most clinical cases, should be turned on to mitigate inappropriate therapies.

60.8 The correct answer is A.

Rationale: Extraction of the complete ICD system, including lead and generator, in the setting of gram-positive cocci bacteremia, is a class I recommendation. A transesophageal echocardiogram may be clinically indicated to assess for valvular infectious endocarditis, but the absence of definitive valvular lesion(s)/infective endocarditis would not favor retention of the ICD system. Likewise, guideline antibiotic regimen therapy with surveillance blood cultures should be initiated; however, the system should be extracted under class I recommendations. Needle aspiration culture of the ICD device pocket should never be done, even in the presence of fluid under ultrasonography, due to potential introduction of contaminated flora into the device pocket. In this patient scenario, a wearable defibrillator (class IIa) may be considered in the immediate period following extraction before reimplantation of a new ICD.

60.9 The correct answer is C.

Rationale: All choices, apart from choice C, represent class I recommendations for ICD implantation in patients with channelopathies and cardiomyopathies. In choice C, patients with LQTS should be initiated on maximally tolerated beta-blocker therapy. If evidence of high-risk symptomatic features, despite maximally tolerated beta-blocker therapy or if intolerant of beta-blocker therapy, ICD implantation is reasonable. As noted, a class IIb recommendation considers ICD implantation in patients with LQTS with resting QTc greater than 500 milliseconds on beta-blocker therapy. The patient in choice C with LQTS is asymptomatic, on beta-blocker therapy, and QTc is less than 500 milliseconds; ICD implantation is not currently indicated.

60.10 The correct answer is C.

Rationale: Data have demonstrated clinically insignificant defibrillation threshold differences between dual- and single-coil lead systems; however, dual-coils have historically higher lead failure rates compared to single-coil systems. Extraction of dual-coil leads is often technically more challenging than a single-coil lead. A single-chamber ICD system, when compared to a dual-chamber ICD system, has comparable discrimination algorithms to prevent inappropriate shock delivery. Cephalic cut-down access virtually eliminates periprocedural risk of pneumothorax associated with cephalic access.

SYNCOPE

Meet Patel

CHAPTER 61

QUESTIONS

61.1 A 28-year-old woman presents to the emergency department (ED) with complaint of recurrent episodes of fainting. She describes feeling dizzy before losing consciousness, with subsequent spontaneous recovery. Upon further questioning, she reports that these episodes often occur after prolonged standing or during emotionally stressful situations. She worked as a cashier at a **grocery** store and these episodes have resulted in her leaving the job. She denies any associated chest pain, palpitations, or shortness of breath. Her past medical history (PMH) is unremarkable, and she takes no medications. Her vitals are stable and orthostasis is negative. Which of the following **BEST** describes the mechanism underlying the patient's syncopal episodes?

   A. Increased sympathetic tone
   B. Increased vagal tone
   C. Autonomic nervous system dysfunction
   D. Increased cardiac output

61.2 A 45-year-old man presents to his primary care physician with a complaint of recurrent episodes of fainting. He reports that these episodes are preceded by feeling warm all over the body. He denies any chest pain, palpitations, or shortness of breath associated with these episodes. Denies any family history of significant cardiac problems including sudden cardiac death. His medical history is significant for hypertension, for which he takes amlodipine. On further questioning, he mentions that these episodes seem to occur more frequently when he stands up after sitting for a prolonged period. Which of the following is the most appropriate diagnostic test in this patient?

   A. Holter monitor
   B. Exercise stress test
   C. Tilt-table test
   D. Cardiac catheterization

61.3 A 55-year-old woman presents to her primary care physician with complaints of feeling lightheaded and dizzy upon standing up from a sitting or lying position. She reports that these symptoms have been occurring more frequently over the past few weeks and are sometimes accompanied by near-fainting episodes. Her PMH is significant for diabetes mellitus, for which she takes metformin. On physical examination, her blood pressure (BP) is 140/90 mm Hg while sitting and 110/70 mm Hg upon standing. Her heart rate (HR) increases from 70 beats per minute (bpm) while sitting to 100 bpm upon standing. Which of the following conditions is **NOT** commonly associated with this patient's condition?

*Questions and Answers are based on Chapter 61: Syncope by Humberto Butzke da Motta and Olujimi A. Ajijola in *Cardiovascular Medicine and Surgery*, First Edition.

A. Parkinson disease
B. Epilepsy
C. Diabetes mellitus
D. Amyloidosis

61.4 A 47-year-old man came to the ED with complaint of sudden loss of consciousness. He does **NOT** recall the event. Denies any chest pain, chest tightness, or dyspnea. As per wife at the bedside, he was watching television and suddenly passed out on the couch for nearly 15 to 20 seconds. Patient denied having warning symptoms and never had this kind of episode before. Denies any significant family history of sudden cardiac death. He does **NOT** smoke, drink alcohol, or use any recreational drugs. His PMH includes hypertension controlled with amlodipine 5 mg daily. Physical examination was within the normal limit. Which of the following diagnostic tests would be most appropriate for making the diagnosis in this patient?

A. Holter monitor
B. Exercise stress test
C. Tilt-table test
D. Cardiac catheterization

61.5 A 35-year-old man presents to the ED after experiencing an episode of syncope without any warning symptoms. Denies any chest pain, chest tightness, dyspnea, or palpitation. He has no prior history of cardiac disease, and his family history includes the sudden cardiac death in his father at the age of 41. Vitals showed a temperature of 39.1 °C, HR of 93 bpm, and BP of 112/78 mm Hg. Lab work is within normal limits. On initial evaluation, his electrocardiogram (ECG) reveals sinus rhythm with coved-type ST-segment elevation in leads V1 to V3. Which of the following is the **MOST LIKELY** diagnosis?

A. Situational syncope
B. Acute coronary syndrome
C. Brugada syndrome
D. Ventricular tachycardia

61.6 A 45-year-old man presents to the ED with syncope. He did **NOT** have any warning signs or preceding symptoms. His PMH is unremarkable, and he has no family history of cardiac conditions and denied any other symptoms. He undergoes an evaluation, including ECG and transthoracic echocardiography (TTE), both of which are within normal limits. He was discharged home with 14-day Holter monitor. 14-day Holter monitor did **NOT** show any evidence of arrhythmia. A few weeks later, he again had a similar episode of syncope. Which of the following diagnostic modalities is most appropriate for further evaluation of recurrent unexplained syncope in this patient?

A. Transesophageal echocardiogram (TEE)
B. Implantable loop recorder (ILR)
C. Cardiac catheterization
D. Electrophysiologic study (EPS)

61.7 An 82-year-old man presents to the ED with a history of syncope. He reports feeling lightheaded and dizzy before losing consciousness. He also complained of dyspnea especially on exertion for the last 6 months. On physical examination, a crescendo-decrescendo murmur is heard **BEST** at the right upper sternal border, which increases with the Valsalva maneuver. Which of the following diagnostic tests is the most appropriate next step?
  A. Stress echocardiogram
  B. Holter monitoring
  C. TTE
  D. Cardiac catheterization

61.8 A 30-year-old woman presents to the cardiology clinic with a history of recurrent episodes of syncope. She reports feeling lightheaded and dizzy upon standing up from a sitting or lying position, with occasional near-fainting episodes. She has no significant medical history and is **NOT** taking any medications. ECG showed normal sinus rhythm. ECHO shows normal ejection fraction with normal valvular function. Which of the following diagnostic tests is the most appropriate next step in the evaluation of this patient's syncope?
  A. Tilt-table test
  B. Exercise echocardiogram
  C. ILR
  D. EPSs

61.9 A 60-year-old woman presents to the clinic with complaints of feeling lightheaded and dizzy upon standing up from a sitting or lying position. She reports experiencing these symptoms for the past few months, especially when transitioning from lying down to standing. On further inquiry, she mentions that these symptoms have been interfering with her daily activities. Her PMH includes hypertension treated with amlodipine and hydrochlorothiazide. Her BP on sitting is 130/90 mm Hg and on standing, it decreases to 100/70 mm Hg. Which of the following management strategies is recommended for this patient's orthostatic hypotension?
  A. Limit water intake to less than 1.5 L.
  B. Avoidance of salt consumption
  C. Avoidance of diuretics
  D. Dietary Approaches to Stop Hypertension (DASH) diet

61.10 A 52-year-old man presents to the cardiology clinic following an episode of syncope. He reports feeling lightheaded and dizzy before briefly losing consciousness. Upon further inquiry, he mentions experiencing similar episodes in the past, often triggered by pressure on his neck, such as wearing a tight collar or during shaving. On examination, carotid sinus massage reproduces his symptoms and leads to transient asystole on ECG. Which of the following management strategies is recommended for this patient's syncope associated with carotid sinus syndrome?
  A. Initiate treatment with fludrocortisone.
  B. Encourage rapid ingestion of water and salt consumption.
  C. Consider implantable cardiac pacing.
  D. Prescribe midodrine.

ANSWERS

61.1 The correct answer is B.
Rationale: Reflex syncope, also known as neurally mediated syncope or vasovagal syncope (VVS), is characterized by a loss of sympathetic tone or an increase in vagal tone. In the case described, the patient experiences syncopal episodes in situations associated with increased emotional stress or prolonged standing, indicating a predominant increase in vagal tone. This vagal response can result in either a vasodepressive state, with decreased systemic vascular resistance, or a cardioinhibitory state, with bradycardia and low cardiac output. Increased sympathetic tone or increased cardiac output usually doesn't cause syncope; on the contrary, a reduction in sympathetic tone or decreased cardiac output can result in syncope (options A and D). Autonomic nervous system dysfunction usually causes orthostatic hypotension as the compensation mechanism of the sympathetic nervous system to support BP while standing from a sitting position is impaired (option C).

61.2 The correct answer is C.
Rationale: In cases where the diagnosis of reflex syncope is uncertain, a tilt-table test can be used to reproduce the symptoms and confirm the diagnosis. This test involves tilting the patient to different positions on the table while monitoring for changes in HR and **BP**. A positive tilt-table test, characterized by the reproduction of symptoms such as lightheadedness and fainting, supports the diagnosis of reflex syncope, especially when cardiac causes are excluded.

Overall, reflex syncope is considered to have a more benign course compared to cardiac syncope or orthostatic hypotension. It is essential to identify triggers and employ appropriate diagnostic tests to differentiate reflex syncope from other causes of fainting, guiding appropriate management strategies. Holter monitor is an appropriate diagnostic modality when underlying arrhythmia is suspected as the cause of syncope. If the tilt-table test is nondiagnostic and orthostasis is negative, the Holter monitor would be a valid consideration (option A). Exercise stress test and cardiac catheterization are more appropriate options when ischemic heart disease is suspected as the cause of syncope (options B and D).

61.3 The correct answer is B.
Rationale: The patient's symptoms of lightheadedness and dizziness while standing from a sitting position along with a drop in systolic BP of more than 20 mm Hg, a drop in diastolic BP of more than 10 mm Hg, and an increase in HR are indicative of orthostatic hypotension. This condition occurs due to impaired compensatory mechanisms, particularly in states with autonomic failure. Autonomic failure can manifest as a primary phenomenon in neurodegenerative diseases like Parkinson disease, multiple system atrophy, or pure autonomic failure (option A). In addition, it can occur as a secondary effect of systemic illnesses such as diabetes mellitus or amyloidosis (options C and D). Epilepsy, although a neurologic disorder, is not typically associated with orthostatic hypotension or autonomic dysfunction and is one of the most important differential diagnoses that needs to be excluded in patients presenting with syncope due to orthostatic hypotension in ED.

61.4 The correct answer is A.

Rationale: In a patient with sudden loss of consciousness without any warning symptoms, there is a high suspicion for ventricular tachycardia. This patient should be discharged with a Holter monitor. A loop recorder may be considered in the investigation of recurrent unexplained syncope without high-risk criteria, as well as to evaluate the indication for cardiac pacing in patients with reflex syncope. External loop recorders have a better diagnostic performance when compared to Holter monitoring, but also have a low diagnostic yield. Exercise stress tests and cardiac catheterization are more appropriate options when ischemic heart disease is suspected as the cause of syncope. This patient does not have typical symptoms suggestive of ischemic heart disease. Although a noninvasive workup can be considered in the workup, the Holter monitor or loop recorder would be appropriate in the detection of ventricular tachycardia. The most appropriate setting to perform a tilt-table test is in patients with suspected VVS, orthostatic hypotension, postural orthostatic tachycardia syndrome (POTS), or psychogenic pseudo syncope (option C).

61.5 The correct answer is C.

Rationale: This patient with syncope and coveted ST-segment elevation in leads V1 to V3 with a history of sudden cardiac death in first degree relative is consistent with Brugada syndrome. The ECG pattern is unmasked with fever as in this case. Situational syncope is usually associated with specific actions, such as micturition, stimulation of the gastrointestinal tract (swallowing, defecation), cough, post-strenuous exercise, and laughter (option A). This patient does not have any symptoms to suggest acute coronary syndrome (ACS) (option B). Ventricular tachycardia can present with syncope without any warning symptoms but would not have ECG findings of coved-type ST-segment elevation in leads V1 to V3, especially in the setting of fever and family history of sudden cardiac death (option D).

61.6 The correct answer is B.

Rationale: The ILR is indicated in the investigation of recurrent unexplained syncope especially in patients in whom Holter monitor did not show anything. TEE can be useful if there are valvular abnormalities suspected when TTE is nondiagnostic. This patient had a recent normal TTE (option A). Cardiac catheterization is indicated when syncope is suspected due to underlying ACS. These patients do not have symptoms to suggest ACS as the underlying cause of syncope (option C). EPS has a low diagnostic yield when performed in patients with normal ECG and TTE. It would not be indicated at this point (option D).

61.7 The correct answer is C.

Rationale: Given this patient's age, symptoms, or presence of crescendo-decrescendo murmur at right upper sternal border is indicative of severe aortic stenosis. The best next step to diagnose that is TTE to assess the aortic valve structure and function. In addition, TTE can provide valuable information regarding the etiology of the patient's symptoms of dyspnea, particularly if they are related to heart failure secondary to aortic stenosis. Stress echocardiogram is indicated when myocardial ischemia is suspected. Although it may be indicated at some point in the future, it is not the most appropriate next test (option A). Holter monitoring (option B) is used to assess for arrhythmias and is not indicated as the next step in the evaluation of a patient with suspected aortic stenosis and syncope. Cardiac catheterization is an invasive procedure and is typically reserved for cases where noninvasive tests such as TTE or stress echocardiogram are inconclusive or there is evidence of ACS (option D).

61.8 The correct answer is A:
Rationale: In a patient presenting with symptoms suggestive of POTS, such as lightheadedness and dizziness upon standing, the next best step in the evaluation is a tilt-table test. This test is specifically designed to assess autonomic function and orthostatic intolerance. It involves tilting the patient to an upright position and monitoring for changes in HR and BP. The patient is placed in the supine position for at least 20 minutes, with an assessment of baseline HR and BP. The table is then rapidly tilted up to 60° to 80° to the horizontal to place the patient in a head-up position. The end point is to reproduce symptoms alongside a typical hemodynamic pattern (cardioinhibitory, vasodepressive, or mixed). Stress echocardiogram is indicated when myocardial ischemia is suspected (option B). ILR is indicated in the evaluation of recurrent unexplained syncope. EPS has a low diagnostic yield when performed in patients with normal ECG and TTE. It would not be indicated at this point (option D).

61.9 The correct answer is C:
Rationale: Orthostatic hypotension, characterized by a drop in BP upon standing, can significantly impact an individual's quality of life, as experienced by this patient. Intensive treatment for hypertension may exacerbate symptoms, especially when diuretics or beta-blockers are used. Options A and B, limiting water intake and avoiding salt consumption, are not appropriate management strategies for this patient. They are considered in patients with a history of congestive heart failure (options A and B). DASH diet is beneficial for managing hypertension but does not have any role in the management of orthostatic hypotension (option D).

61.10 The correct answer is C:
Rationale: Consideration for pacemaker implantation is warranted for patients with carotid sinus syndrome-associated syncope with a predominant cardioinhibitory response. Carotid sinus massage reproducing symptoms and inducing transient asystole on ECG are characteristic findings in such patients. Encouragement of rapid ingestion of water and salt consumption, fludrocortisone, or midodrine is considered in the management of orthostatic hypotension (options A, B, and D). This patient with classic symptoms of carotid sinus syndrome-associated syncope and dual chamber pacemaker implantation should be considered.

SUDDEN CARDIAC ARREST

Samuel Kim and Mohammad El-Hajjar

CHAPTER 62

QUESTIONS

62.1 What is the most common etiology of sudden cardiac arrest (SCA) in adults in the United States of America?

　A.　Drug overdose
　B.　Coronary artery disease (CAD)/acute coronary syndrome
　C.　Trauma
　D.　Primary arrhythmia syndromes

62.2 You are working in the hospital and respond to a code BLUE paged overhead. You are the first physician to enter the room and observe a patient receiving chest compressions. The patient was noted on telemetry to have ventricular tachycardia (VT). Prompt assessment by the nurse determined the patient to be pulseless and immediately initiated cardiopulmonary resuscitation (CPR). What should you request next?

　A.　Administration of 1 mg of epinephrine intravenously (IV)
　B.　Administration of 1 mg/kg of lidocaine IV
　C.　Defibrillation with 200 J biphasic shock
　D.　Administration of 300 mg of amiodarone IV

62.3 A 53-year-old female presents to the emergency department due to unwitnessed cardiac arrest with nonshockable rhythm. During ongoing resuscitation efforts, one of your team members spoke with her family and elicited a medical history of hypothyroidism and breast cancer undergoing chemoradiation. What test should you obtain specifically for this patient to determine a potential underlying etiology at the earliest possible time?

　A.　Bedside echocardiogram
　B.　Basic metabolic panel
　C.　Chest x-ray
　D.　Computed tomography (CT) chest angiography

62.4 Which one of the following statements is FALSE regarding electrical storm?

　A.　It is defined by three or more episodes of sustained VT within a 24-hour period.
　B.　Incessant VT that lasts for 6 or more hours
　C.　The main medication used in electrical storm is IV beta-blocker.
　D.　Sympathetic activation is a main factor in the pathogenesis of electrical storm and can be potentiated by patient's anxiety, fear, and pain from implantable cardioverter-defibrillator (ICD) shock.

Questions and Answers are based on Chapter 62: Sudden Cardiac Arrest by Yuliya Krokhaleva and Marmar Vaseghi in Cardiovascular Medicine and Surgery, First Edition.

62.5 In which one of the following patients would an ICD **NOT** be indicated?
  A. A 45-year-old male with a medical history of CAD, coronary artery bypass surgery, and heart failure with a left ventricular ejection fraction (LVEF) of 35%
  B. An 18-year-old female who experienced SCA after heroin overdose
  C. A 32-year-old female with a history of sarcoidosis with a left ventricular fraction of 30%
  D. A 25-year-old male who experienced SCA with no etiology discovered

62.6 Which of the following is associated with the highest risk of SCA in the adult population?
  A. Transposition of the great arteries
  B. Fontan physiology
  C. Eisenmenger syndrome
  D. They are all equivalent.

62.7 Which of the following statements regarding SCA is **INCORRECT**?
  A. LVEF is one of the best predictors for risk stratification of SCA.
  B. Shockable rhythms are associated with better outcomes as compared to non-shockable rhythms in SCA.
  C. Presence of monomorphic VT suggests acute ischemia.
  D. Most ventricular tachyarrhythmia are initiated by a premature ventricular contraction (PVC) trigger.

62.8 A 41-year-old female with a past medical history significant for hypertension presented to the emergency department with SCA and return of spontaneous circulation (ROSC) achieved after defibrillation for polymorphic VT. An electrocardiogram (ECG) showed prolonged QTc, which you suspect is the likely etiology of this event. What additional information would be important to obtain?
  A. List of home and recent medication usage
  B. Basic metabolic panel
  C. Family history
  D. All of the above

62.9 An unidentified 65-year-old male is brought in by emergency medical service (EMS) for SCA with initial rhythm reported as VT and defibrillation was performed with ROSC achieved. The patient remained unresponsive and did not follow commands and thus intubation was performed. Which of the following is **NOT** indicated currently?
  A. Targeted temperature management
  B. 12-lead ECG
  C. ICD implantation
  D. Hemodynamic monitoring

62.10 Which of the following statements regarding SCA is **TRUE**?
  A. Many risk factors for CAD and SCA are similar.
  B. At any given age, SCA is more common in women.
  C. Most cardiac arrest survivors are unlikely to report any symptoms hours to weeks before event.
  D. Impaired cardiac autonomic activity (eg, decreased heart rate) has no association with SCA.

ANSWERS

62.1 The correct answer is B.

Rationale: The age of the individual affects the likelihood of a certain etiology of sudden cardiac death. Younger patients are more likely to have structurally normal hearts with predominant cardiac causes to be considered are congenital channelopathies, inherited cardiomyopathies (eg, dilated, hypertrophic, arrhythmogenic), and coronary artery anomalies. Older victims are more likely to have structural heart disease with CAD accounting for 70% of the cases.

Noncardiac causes (eg, trauma, drug overdose, pulmonary embolism [PE]) account for 5% to 25% of the cases and primary arrhythmia syndromes have been identified as the etiology in 1% to 2% of the cases.

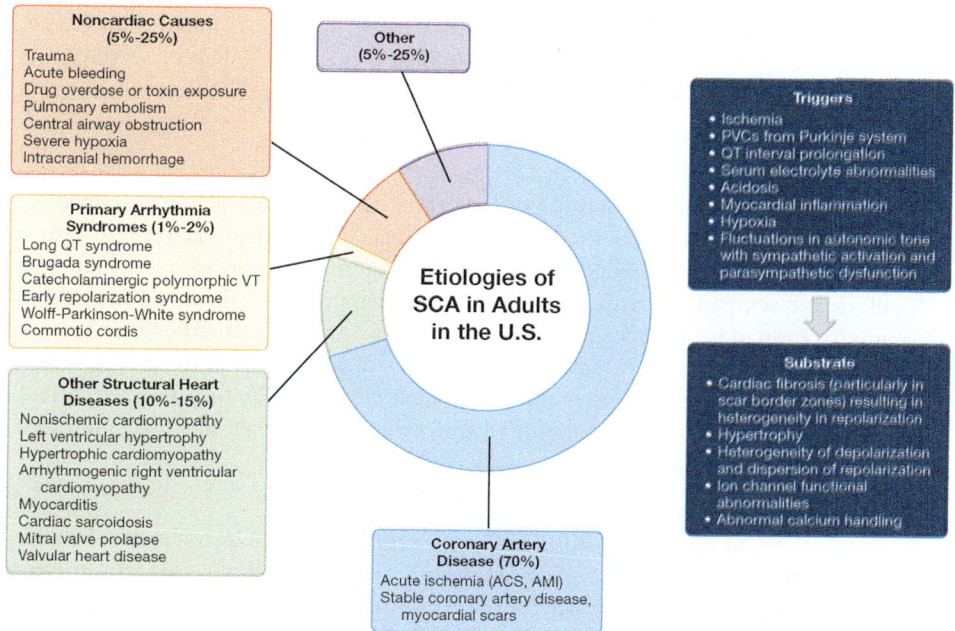

62.2 The correct answer is C.

Rationale: This patient experienced a cardiac arrest with a shockable rhythm (VT) and thus prompt defibrillation with 200 J biphasic shock should be delivered as soon as possible followed by CPR. If the patient continues to remain in shockable rhythm, additional defibrillation should be performed that is followed by CPR and administration of 1 mg of epinephrine.

Amiodarone and lidocaine can be administered if the patient continues to remain in shockable rhythm despite defibrillation attempts. At this time, prompt defibrillation should take place first.

62.3 The correct answer is A:

Rationale: This is a patient with a relevant past medical history of malignancy and radiation and thus should be alert to the possibility of cardiac tamponade. Additional risk factors include a recent history of invasive cardiac procedures or surgery. The diagnosis can be confirmed with a bedside echocardiogram and the patient should then undergo emergent pericardiocentesis.

Electrolyte abnormalities rarely lead to SCA independently but can potentiate another primary cause, such as QT prolongation or ischemia. Attempts at metabolic derangement correction should be made: potassium IV can be administered for hypokalemia; magnesium infusion for hypomagnesemia; and calcium, bicarbonate, and insulin with glucose for hyperkalemia.

Tension pneumothorax should be considered in those who recently underwent internal jugular or subclavian venous line placement, pacemaker implantation, thoracentesis, chest trauma, and those with severe chronic obstructive pulmonary disease (COPD)/emphysema.

PE should be suspected in those with a recent history of long-distance travel and prolonged immobilization, recent surgical procedures (especially orthopedic), central venous access with indwelling catheter, recent cardiac catheter ablation, and history of hypercoagulable state.

62.4 The correct answer is B:

Rationale: Electrical storm is defined by three or more episodes of sustained VT or incessant VT that lasts for 12 hours or longer. Sympathetic activation leads to ventricular tachyarrhythmia, and thus the medications and procedures are aimed to block the sympathetic activation on several different levels. These can include administration of beta-blocker, deep sedation, thoracic epidural anesthesia, and stellate ganglion block. IV beta-blocker is the main medication used with data indicating that nonselective beta-blocker propranolol may be superior to a selective beta-1-blocker (ie, metoprolol) in patients with electrical storm when it is used simultaneously with IV amiodarone.

62.5 The correct answer is B:

Rationale: ICD implantation for secondary prevention of SCA has a class I indication according to the ACC/AHA (American College of Cardiology/American Heart Association) guidelines only when a reversible cause is not discovered.

ICD is recommended for primary prevention of SCA in all patients with both ischemic and nonischemic cardiomyopathy with LVEF of less than or equal to 30% and 35%, respectively. These data were established in two seminal randomized controlled trials, MADIT-II (Multicenter Automatic Defibrillator Implantation Trial) and SCD-HeFT (Sudden Cardiac Death in Heart Failure Trial), by demonstrating a reduction in all-cause mortality by 23% to 28% in the ICD group compared to the medical therapy group.

62.6 The correct answer is C:

Rationale: The congenital heart disease adult population is associated with higher risk of SCA as compared to the general adult population and increases depending on the complexity of the heart defect. Eisenmenger syndrome has the highest incidence of SCA.

62.7 The correct answer is C.
Rationale: Ventricular tachyarrhythmia can be further subdivided into monomorphic VT, polymorphic VT, and ventricular fibrillation. Monomorphic VT is generally associated with a scar from a previous ischemic injury or fibrosis from other pathologies. Polymorphic VT generally occurs in the setting of inflammation, acute ischemia, serum electrolyte abnormalities, QT prolongation, or an imbalance of the autonomic nervous system. Both types of VT can degenerate into ventricular fibrillation.

A number of parameters have been investigated and are suggested to be part of the risk stratification for SCA but none have been superior to LVEF and thus it remains the key parameter currently used.

While overall survival is poor in those who experience SCA, those with shockable rhythms generally have better outcomes when compared to nonshockable rhythms (survival rates 25%-40% vs <5%, respectively).

62.8 The correct answer is D.
Rationale: QT prolongation is a risk factor for SCA with presentation of polymorphic VT that may or may not degenerate into ventricular fibrillation. It can be subdivided into congenital or acquired categories and requires careful investigation. A family history of SCA in a first-degree relative is a well-known risk factor for sudden cardiac death. Common cardiac channelopathies, such as long QT syndrome and Brugada syndrome, are not associated with any morphologic abnormalities on postmortem examination. There are several medications that precipitate QT prolongation (eg, azithromycin, ketoconazole, methadone, lithium). There are several internet sites listing these medications and can be used as a reference (eg, www.crediblemeds.org). Serum electrolyte abnormalities, particularly hypokalemia, hypomagnesemia, and hyperkalemia, can potentiate effects of other conditions (eg, ischemia, prolonged QT interval) and result in SCA and/or death as well.

62.9 The correct answer is C.
Rationale: ICD implantation is indicated for secondary prevention of SCA when not due to an identifiable reversible cause. In patients presenting with SCA, search for culprit substrate, triggers, and acute conditions that resulted in SCA should be started promptly once ROSC is achieved if it has not been performed already.

Targeted temperature management was introduced for the management of SCA victims after ROSC was achieved with noted better neurologic recovery in avalanche victims. It has been demonstrated to improve survival and thus should be initiated as soon as possible when indicated.

12-Lead ECG is important to obtain as CAD accounts for 70% of SCA and can assist in diagnosing a cardiac etiology and determining the need for emergent intervention (eg, STEMI [ST-segment elevation myocardial infarction] noted on the electrocardiogram).

Many patients who experience SCA require advanced airway, sedation, and hemodynamic support which can be achieved with infusion of inotropic and/or vasopressor medications.

62.10 The correct answer is A:

Rationale: CAD and SCA share many similar risk factors that include hypertension, hyperlipidemia, diabetes mellitus type 2, smoking, obesity, and a sedentary lifestyle.

SCA is more common in males with data suggesting that they are 2 to 3 times more likely to experience this event than females at any given age.

While majority of SCAs are not witnessed, and thus it is difficult to ascertain symptoms immediately before the index event, literature suggests that half of the survivors experienced nonspecific symptoms preceding the event by 24 hours and up to 4 weeks. The most common of these symptoms are reportedly chest pain and dyspnea.

Impaired cardiac autonomic activity has been shown to predict cardiovascular mortality with increased risk of SCA and ventricular tachyarrhythmia, specifically after myocardial infarction and in the setting of congenital heart disease (**Table 62.1**).

TABLE 62.1 Triggers for Sudden Cardiac Arrest

Trigger	Clinical Significance
Ischemia	• Acute ischemia should be suspected in all SCA victims. • May range from ACS to transient ischemia in an otherwise stable patient with CAD to coronary spasm • Acute ischemia is associated with polymorphic VT, VF, or rapid monomorphic VT (ventricular flutter). • Chronic CAD with myocardial scar usually leads to slower monomorphic VT.
Serum electrolyte abnormalities	• Particularly hypokalemia, hypomagnesemia, and hyperkalemia • Unlikely to cause VA but usually potentiate effects of other conditions (eg, ischemia, prolonged QT interval)
Acidosis	• Either metabolic or respiratory acidosis • Unlikely to cause VA, usually potentiates effects of other conditions
QT interval prolongation	• Congenital or acquired • Often precipitated by QT-prolonging medications (azithromycin, levofloxacin, ketoconazole, metoclopramide, sertraline, lithium, methadone, etc) • Many internet sites list QT-prolonging medications (www.crediblemeds.org). • Bradycardia potentiates QT prolongation. • Usually associated with polymorphic VT, VF, and TdP
Antiarrhythmic medications	• All antiarrhythmics may cause proarrhythmia, especially in patients with SHD. • May be challenging to differentiate if SCA is caused by underlying condition that antiarrhythmic is prescribed for or because of proarrhythmia

TABLE 62.1 Triggers for Sudden Cardiac Arrest (*continued*)

Trigger	Clinical Significance
Myocardial inflammation	• Myocarditis, active inflammatory phase of cardiac sarcoidosis, inflammatory cardiomyopathy
Heart failure	• Risk of SCA is elevated in all patients with CHF but particularly during CHF exacerbation.
Severe hypoxemia	• More commonly associated with PEA arrest but may lead to VA caused by exacerbating underlying ischemia
Fluctuations in the autonomic tone	• Sympathetic activation, parasympathetic withdrawal • Often implicated in SCA occurring during exercise, physical or emotional stress • Associated with LQT1, catecholaminergic polymorphic VT, ARVC, polymorphic VT, VF, and monomorphic VT with faster tachycardia rates

ACS, acute coronary syndrome; ARVC, arrhythmogenic right ventricular cardiomyopathy; CAD, coronary artery disease; CHF, congestive heart failure; LQT1, long QT 1 syndrome; PEA, pulseless electrical activity; SCA, sudden cardiac arrest; SHD, structural heart disease; TdP, torsades de pointes; VA, ventricular tachyarrhythmia; VF, ventricular fibrillation; VT, ventricular tachycardia.

PERMANENT PACEMAKER*
Amole Ojo and Casey White

CHAPTER 63

QUESTIONS

63.1 When programming a permanent pacemaker, VVIR is most appropriate in which of the following clinical scenarios?

  A. A 65-year-old patient with sick sinus syndrome
  B. An 84-year-old patient with permanent atrial fibrillation and symptomatic bradycardia
  C. A 45-year-old patient with intermittent high-grade atrioventricular (AV) block
  D. A 70-year-old patient with symptomatic second-degree AV block Mobitz I

63.2 Which of the following patient scenarios is implantation of a permanent pacemaker **NOT** recommended?

  A. A patient with symptomatic chronotropic incompetency
  B. Recurrent syncope with greater than 3-second asystole during carotid sinus massage
  C. Asymptomatic cardioinhibitory response to carotid sinus massage
  D. Neurocardiogenic syncope with symptomatic bradycardia/asystole during tilt table testing

63.3 A 57-year-old patient with dual-chamber permanent pacemaker presents with sustaining tachycardia at 140 beats per minute (bpm), which is also the upper tracking rate limit. Device interrogation of electrogram (EGMs) reveals ventricularly paced activity with apparent shortly coupled atrially sensed retrograde P waves occurring at regular, fixed intervals. Pacemaker-mediated tachycardia (PMT) is confirmed. Which of the following statements regarding PMT is INACCURATE?

  A. Initiation of this mechanism most commonly occurs with a ventricular extrasystole and is contingent on retrograde ventriculoatrial (VA) conduction.
  B. PMT can occur with single- or dual-chamber permanent pacemakers.
  C. Mitigation of PMT is often achieved with extension of the postventricular atrial refractory period (PVARP).
  D. PMT can be terminated with placement of a 90-gauss magnet over the device.

63.4 A 63-year-old patient with a history of nonischemic cardiomyopathy (left ventricular ejection fraction [LVEF] 45%), chronic left bundle branch block (LBBB) with QRS duration 150 milliseconds presents with a recent history of exertional fatigue and lightheadedness. Workup is ultimately revealing for high-grade AV block.

Questions and Answers are based on Chapter 63: Permanent Cardiac Pacemakers by Carlos Macias in Cardiovascular Medicine and Surgery, First Edition.

Reversible etiologies are not identified. Implantation of a permanent pacemaker is planned. Which of the following system configurations is recommended?

A. Single-chamber transvenous pacemaker
B. Dual-chamber transvenous pacemaker with apically placed right ventricular (RV) lead
C. Consideration for biventricular pacemaker or left bundle area pacing
D. Dual-chamber implantable cardioverter-defibrillator (ICD)

63.5 Which of the following clinical scenarios is a leadless permanent pacemaker most reasonably indicated?

A. A 76-year-old patient with high-grade AV block and history of inferior vena cava filter
B. An 82-year-old patient with symptomatic sinus bradycardia and a history of mechanical tricuspid valve
C. A 70-year-old patient with symptomatic sick sinus syndrome
D. A 72-year-old patient with permanent atrial fibrillation and a history of chronic kidney disease who has been found to have symptomatic bradycardia

63.6 A 65-year-old patient presents with symptomatic bradycardia. Subsequent workup and diagnosis are consistent with sinus node dysfunction. The patient undergoes successful placement of a dual-chamber permanent pacemaker, programmed DDDR. At the time of implant, right atrial lead capture threshold is 1.7 V at a pulse width of 0.4 milliseconds, P-wave sensing at 2.1 mV, and impedance of 650 Ω. An immediate post-procedural anteroposterior (AP) chest radiograph confirms the expected atrial and ventricular lead position. There is no pneumothorax. There are no perceived complications. On interrogation the following morning, right atrial lead capture threshold is significantly elevated with intermittent capture at an output of 6.0 V, sensing is 7.1 mV, and impedance of 300 Ω. The patient is asymptomatic. What is the next appropriate step in management?

A. Continued observation with follow-up interrogation in 24 hours
B. Posteroanterior (PA) and lateral chest radiograph
C. Reprogram device to AAI (atrial pacing, atrial sensing, inhibition)
D. Decrease device sensitivity for long-term battery optimization

63.7 A 52-year-old male previously underwent implantation of a dual-chamber permanent pacemaker. He has noted intermittent lightheadedness and fatigue over the past several days. He further has noted a sensation from the left-sided device pocket since implantation, which improves with palpation and "moving" the device within the pocket. Device remote transmissions have revealed variable capture thresholds and undersensing, later confirmed on in-office interrogation. Which of the following is **MOST** likely?

A. Lead micro-dislodgement
B. Pacemaker crosstalk
C. PMT
D. Runaway pacemaker

Section 4: Electrophysiology

63.8 Which of the following is CORRECT regarding device sensing?
   A. Oversensing is a failure of the pacemaker system to recognize true cardiac potentials resulting in inappropriate pacing output.
   B. Undersensing is a failure of the pacemaker system to detect extracardiac potentials resulting in inappropriate pacing behavior.
   C. Myopotential interference, especially in unipolar pacing, can trigger oversensing and symptoms from pacing inhibition.
   D. Oversensing can occur secondary to acid-base disorders, ischemia, or with programmed sensitivity above intrinsic sensing.

63.9 A 67-year-old patient has a history of complete heart block with subsequent left-sided dual-chamber permanent pacemaker and lung carcinoma. The patient is scheduled to undergo video-assisted thoracoscopic lung lobectomy. Use of electrocautery is anticipated. The device is currently programmed with bipolar DDDR with an upper tracking rate of 160 bpm. Which of the following programming changes, if any, should be made at the time of surgery?
   A. No device programming changes are necessary.
   B. Reprogram to AAI.
   C. Reprogram from bipolar to unipolar mode; DDDR.
   D. Reprogram to asynchronous mode (DOO).

63.10 Which of the following, regarding permanent pacemakers, is most accurate?
   A. Atrial mode switch is not recommended in patients with paroxysmal atrial fibrillation.
   B. Rate-response programming requires dual-chamber configuration.
   C. AAIR⇔DDDR is a programmable mode most ideal for sinoatrial nodal dysfunction and intact AV nodal conduction.
   D. Anti-PMT algorithms target shortening of the PVARP.

ANSWERS

63.1 The correct answer is B.
Rationale: Of the listed choices, choice B describes a clinical case appropriate for VVIR pacing. Atrial pacing, sensing, and response are not desired in permanent atrial fibrillation; ventricular-based pacing is therefore indicated. The remaining choices would likely benefit from a dual-chamber system configuration (ie, DDD or DDDR). AAI single-chamber could be considered in choice A; however, AAI⇔DDD is encountered perhaps more in clinical practice.

63.2 The correct answer is C.
Rationale: All choices, with the exception of choice C, detail class I and IIa indications for permanent pacemaker implantation. Asymptomatic cardioinhibitory response during carotid sinus massage does not warrant permanent pacemaker implantation and is considered a contraindication.

63.3 The correct answer is B.

Rationale: PMT occurs when a ventricular extrasystole conducts retrogradely (via atrioventricular node [AVN] or bypass tract) to the atrium. The retrograde atrial activity is thereby sensed by the atrial lead, with subsequently timed and paced ventricular activity, thereby continuing the cycle. This mechanism is contingent on retrograde V-A conduction, as well as dual-chamber system. The absence of an atrial lead disallows this process; thus, choice B is incorrect. Mitigation of PMT is achieved by extending the PVARP, which effectively prevents further timing and pacing off of retrogradely conducted atrial activity in the cycle. PMT, in this sense, can be terminated. Many programmed algorithms attempt to detect PMT, followed by serial extension of the PVARP to terminate the tachycardia. Another mechanism to terminate PMT can be accomplished by placing a magnet over the device, effectively placing the system into DOO mode.

63.4 The correct answer is C.

Rationale: In this patient scenario, there is baseline left ventricular systolic dysfunction with LVEF falling in the 36% to 50% range. In the presence of high-grade AV block, LBBB with QRS 150 milliseconds or more, and predicted pacing requirement greater than 40%, cardiac resynchronization therapy should be considered. Data are currently evolving with ongoing studies assessing long-term outcomes regarding conduction system pacing. At present, left bundle area pacing is a reasonable alternative in this outlined clinical scenario and if placement of a coronary sinus lead for CRT-P (cardiac resynchronization therapy with a pacemaker device) is not technically feasible. A single-chamber pacemaker would disallow atrial-ventricular synchrony and could further result in further worsening of the patient's cardiomyopathy. Likewise, apical RV lead placement should be avoided to mitigate pacemaker-induced dyssynchrony, and in turn, worsening cardiomyopathy. In this clinical scenario, there is no indication for ICD therapy in this patient.

63.5 The correct answer is D.

Rationale: In this clinical scenario, a leadless cardiac pacemaker may be reasonably selected for the patient in choice D. At present time, there is not an approved dual-pacing leadless system. One of the current leadless devices is able to sense atrial activity, in addition to ventricular pacing. Therefore, at present patients without sinoatrial nodal dysfunction, or with permanent atrial fibrillation, should be optimally considered for a leadless system. The patient in choice D also has chronic kidney disease, making future vascular access and potential infection risks of paramount consideration. The patients in choices B and C would both require and benefit from atrial pacing, which at present, is not supported by current leadless systems. In addition, as in patients in choices A and B, there are contraindicated conditions present, namely the presence of an inferior vena cava filter and mechanical tricuspid valve. Though there have been reported cases of leadless pacemakers implanted in patients with inferior vena cava (IVC) filters, there is no strong indication for a leadless pacemaker in choice A.

63.6 The correct answer is B.

Rationale: The patient in this clinical scenario depicts a known complication of pacemaker implantations, namely lead dislodgement. Right atrial lead dislodgement, especially, is encountered more frequently (compared to ventricular leads). As described in this scenario, initial parameters were notable for a higher capture threshold at the time of implantation. Although not described in the scenario, an assessment of the injury pattern is particularly helpful. The presence of an injury profile during intraprocedural assessment indicates myocardial penetration. P-wave sensing and impedance, however, are otherwise acceptable. At follow-up interrogation, capture threshold has increased substantially and capture is intermittent at high output, likely depicting dislodgement of the atrial lead into the RV cavity. The first step is obtainment of a PA and lateral chest x-ray, which will confirm dislodgement. The atrial lead should be turned off with the device reprogrammed to VVI mode. The right atrial lead should promptly be revised before discharge.

63.7 The correct answer is A:
Rationale: The patient in this clinical scenario displays features of Twiddler syndrome. The intentional or unintentional "flipping" or "twisting" of the device results in coiling and twisting of the leads, which over time result in lead micro- or macro-dislodgement or further mechanical breakdown of the leads (ie, insulation breaks). Pacemaker crosstalk can occur in dual-chamber systems whereby the paced activity in one chamber is detected in the other chamber leading to subsequent inhibition. Runaway pacemaker is a rare dysfunction caused by generator battery depletion in older systems. Essentially, this results in aberrant pacemaker behavior characterized by mode switching and intermittent capture failure leading to the induction of potential ventricular arrhythmias. PMT, as described in **Question 63.3**, is less likely in this clinical scenario.

63.8 The correct answer is C:
Rationale: Undersensing is a failure of the pacemaker system to recognize true cardiac potentials resulting in appropriate pacing output. This can be potentially proarrhythmic, particularly if pacing during the relative refractory period leads to "R on T" phenomenon. Choice D describes conditions that can lead to undersensing. Oversensing is the detection of electrical signals that the device erroneously considers cardiac in origin, resulting in inappropriate inhibition of pacing, which can come from electromagnetic interference (ie, electrocautery) or myopotentials, not infrequently encountered with unipolar pacing, particularly in older devices or algorithms. Choice C appropriately describes myopotential interference leading to oversensing and pacing inhibition.

63.9 The correct answer is D:
Rationale: The close proximity of the surgical site and the anticipated use of unipolar electrocautery can result in potential electromagnetic interference. This in turn can potentially result in pacemaker oversensing, leading to inappropriate inhibition of pacemaker activity. In complete heart block, this phenomenon could lead to hemodynamic instability intraoperatively. To mitigate this phenomenon, reprogramming from unipolar to bipolar (if possible) is first preferential, while reprogramming to an asynchronous pacing mode. AAI is not appropriate in this situation due to (a) the anticipated use of electrocautery and potential oversensing and (b) baseline complete heart block.

63.10 The correct answer is C.

Rationale: AAIR⇔DDDR is a programmable mode most ideal for sinoatrial nodal dysfunction. This mode provides necessary backup antibradycardia atrial pacing. If there is no sensed ventricular activity, as well, the device will mode switch to DDDR providing ventricular pacing. Once native ventricularly sensed activity is discovered, the device will mode switch back to AAIR. Atrial mode switch is a programmable mode in dual-chamber systems recommended for tachy-atrial arrhythmias (ie, atrial fibrillation). The program allows for a nontracking mode, triggered by exceeding an atrial upper rate threshold. Rate-response is a programmable feature in single- or dual-chamber systems, whereby rates are incrementally increased according to level of activity. Depending on device manufacturer, this is achieved with accelerometers and biophysical data (ie, minute ventilation, thoracic impedance). As discussed, mitigation of PMT is dependent on the extension, not shortening, of the PVARP.

LEAD EXTRACTION

Nathan Gentybear and Evan C. Adelstein

CHAPTER 64

QUESTIONS

64.1 A 38-year-old male with a history of hypertrophic cardiomyopathy and dual chamber implantable cardioverter-defibrillator (ICD) placement 10 years ago presents to the hospital emergency department with 2 weeks of intermittent fevers, palpitations, and cough. Labs are notable for a white blood cell (WBC) level of 18, a hemoglobin (Hgb) level of 10, platelets of 123, and a serum creatinine level of 0.9. A computed tomography (CT) scan of the patient's chest is consistent with multiple septic pulmonary emboli. A transesophageal echocardiogram reveals a vegetation on the right ventricular lead. Blood cultures are drawn. Treatment with antibiotics and complete device removal, including lead extraction, are planned. Which of the following does not increase the risk of major complications from transvenous lead extraction for this patient?

  A. Age at the time of device implantation
  B. Hgb level
  C. The patient's sex
  D. How many years have passed since the device was placed

64.2 A 45-year-old patient with a pacemaker and endocarditis is found to have a 2.8-cm vegetation on the right ventricular lead. Appropriate treatment is **MOST LIKELY** to involve:

  A. Only treatment with antibiotics
  B. Transvenous lead extraction using a telescoping sheath and device removal
  C. Transvenous lead extraction with a laser sheath and device removal
  D. Surgical lead and device removal

64.3 Transvenous lead extraction is planned in a patient. Imaging is suggestive of extensive calcifications and fibrous tissue around the leads targeted for extraction. Which type of sheath may be needed during the extraction procedure to address the imaging findings?

  A. Simple traction
  B. Rotational mechanical cutting sheath
  C. Telescoping sheath
  D. Laser sheath

---

*Questions and Answers are based on Chapter 64: Lead Extraction by Munish Kannabhiran and Noel G. Boyle in *Cardiovascular Medicine and Surgery*, First Edition.

64.4 When pertaining to lead extraction, "ghosts" refer to:
A. Fibrinous material in the right atrium and superior vena cava (SVC) following lead extraction
B. Retained lead fragments seen on echocardiogram
C. Ectopic electrical activity originating from the implantation site following lead extraction
D. All of the above

64.5 Which of the following statements is **TRUE**?
A. Performing lead extraction with both a cardiologist and cardiothoracic surgeon present has not been associated with a change in complication rates.
B. Performing lead extraction with both a cardiologist and cardiothoracic surgeon present is associated with increased complication rates.
C. Most transvenous lead extractions are performed in catheterization laboratories.
D. Most transvenous lead extractions are performed in hybrid laboratories.

64.6 The most common indication for lead extraction is:
A. Lead fracture
B. Infection
C. Severe tricuspid regurgitation
D. Thrombosis

64.7 Transvenous lead extraction is planned in a patient. The device was implanted 2 months ago. The leads move freely within the vein. The device **MOST LIKELY** to be used for extraction is:
A. Simple traction
B. Rotational mechanical cutting sheath
C. Telescoping sheath
D. Laser sheath

64.8 You are counseling a patient with sick sinus syndrome regarding planned lead and device removal for pocket infection. Which statement is **ACCURATE** with respect to her procedure?
A. She is at lower risk because she is female.
B. Her replacement device should be placed in the same location.
C. Venous thrombosis requiring medical intervention is the most common complication.
D. Overall mortality with transvenous lead extractions is lower than 2%.

64.9 Which of the following statements is **TRUE**?
A. Use of laser sheaths versus telescopic extraction is not associated with a difference in success rate.
B. The advantage of laser sheaths is that they may be used to cut the lead tip free of the myocardium.
C. The complication rate of coronary sinus lead removal is much higher than that of noncoronary sinus leads.
D. Fibrous adhesions are not commonly seen in the coronary sinus as compared to other venous structures.

64.10 The purpose of a SVC balloon during lead extraction is:
   A. To open calcified valves and allow for better access
   B. To tamponade a SVC tear
   C. To provide additional lead traction
   D. To aid in freeing leads from venous adhesions

ANSWERS

64.1 The correct answer is C.
Rationale: Female sex, not male sex, is associated with increased risk of major complications. Hgb less than 11.5, a sum of the dwell times of leads greater than 16.5 years, and patient age of first implantation under 30 years are all associated with increased risk of major complications (**Table 64.1**).

64.2 The correct answer is D.
Rationale: Surgical removal is indicated for leads with a vegetation or thrombus greater than 2.5 cm. These masses are more likely to embolize during transvenous extraction and cause complications, such as pulmonary embolism, septic emboli, or systemic inflammatory response.

TABLE 64.1 Calculator of Probability of Major Complications of Transvenous Lead Extractions

No.	Predictors of the Risk of Major Complications			Score
1	Sum of dwell times of leads planned for extraction (>16.5 y)			6.0
2	Young patient (first implantation under the age of 30 y)			2.2
3	Hemoglobin concentration <11.5 g/dL			2.3
4	Female gender			2.7
5	Number of previous CIED procedures per patient			1.4
	Total score			—
Total score	0-4.0	4.1-10	10.1-16	>16
Complications	0.2%-0.5%	0.5%-2.5%	2.5%-11.8%	>11.8%
Risk	Low risk	Intermediate risk	High risk	Very high risk

CIED, cardiovascular implantable electronic device.
From Jacheć W, Polewczyk A, Polewczyk M, et al. Transvenous lead extraction SAFeTY score for risk stratification and proper patient selection for removal procedures using mechanical tools. *J Clin Med.* 2020;9(2):361. https://creativecommons.org/licenses/by/4.0/.

64.3 The correct answer is B.
Rationale: Although multiple types of cutting tools may be used in a single procedure, mechanical cutting tools are the most efficient at traversing densely calcified fibrotic lesions.

64.4 The correct answer is A.
Rationale: "Ghosts" refer to small fibrinous sheaths, strands, or vegetations in the right atrium or SVC following lead extraction.

64.5 The correct answer is B.
Rationale: This is an example of selection bias. Although studies have shown increased complication rates when both a cardiologist and surgeon are present compared with procedures in which a cardiologist is alone, this reflects the high-risk profile and complexity of cases that warrant performing in an operating room with a surgeon present.

64.6 The correct answer is B.
Rationale: Infection remains the most common indication (48% of cases in the Patient-Related Outcomes of Mechanical lead Extraction Techniques [PROMET] study published in 2020), followed by lead dysfunction, abandoned functional leads, thrombosis/vascular access issues, and severe tricuspid regurgitation.

64.7 The correct answer is A.
Rationale: Explantation for relatively recent leads that move freely in the vein may be performed by simple traction of the lead after its distal helix has been unscrewed.

64.8 The correct answer is D.
Rationale: Overall mortality with lead extraction is less than 2%. Female sex is associated with increased risk of complications. Replacement devices are ideally placed in a different location from the original device in cases of localized infection. Hematoma requiring evacuation is the most common complication (**Table 64.2**).

64.9 The correct answer is D.
Rationale: Fibrous adhesions are less common in the coronary sinus. The pacemaker lead extraction with the excimer sheath (PLEXES) trial demonstrated the superiority of excimer laser over standard telescopic extraction sheaths with success rates of 94% compared to 64% for 465 leads. Laser application should stop 0.5 cm from the lead tip to prevent myocardial damage. The complication rate of coronary sinus lead removal is similar to that of other leads.

64.10 The correct answer is B.
Rationale: SVC balloons are used as a rescue device that may be deployed quickly in case of an SVC tear. In high-risk extractions, they are placed in the inferior vena cava prophylactically over a wire extending into and beyond the SVC and quickly advanced into the SVC over the wire if needed.

TABLE 64.2 Periprocedural Complications of Lead Extraction

Complications	Incidence (%)
Major complications	**0.19-1.80**
Death	0.19-1.20
Cardiac avulsion	0.19-0.96
Vascular laceration	0.19-0.96
Respiratory arrest	0.20
Pericardial effusion requiring intervention	0.23-0.59
Hemothorax requiring intervention	0.07-0.20
Massive pulmonary embolism	0.08
Minor complications	**0.60-6.20**
Hematoma requiring evacuation	0.90-1.60
Pneumothorax requiring chest tube	1.10
Bleeding requiring blood transfusion	0.08-1.00
Worsening tricuspid valve function	0.32-0.59
Pulmonary embolism	0.24-0.59
Venous thrombosis requiring medical intervention	0.10-0.21
Migrated lead fragment without sequelae	0.20
Pericardial effusion without intervention	0.07-0.16

Reprinted from Kusumoto FM, Schoenfeld MH, Wilkoff BL, et al. 2017 HRS expert consensus statement on cardiovascular implantable electronic device lead management and extraction. *Heart Rhythm.* 2017;14(12):e503-e551. Copyright © 2017 Heart Rhythm Society, with permission.

SECTION 5 HEART FAILURE

HEART FAILURE: EPIDEMIOLOGY, CHARACTERISTICS, AND PROGNOSIS*

CHAPTER 65

Robert L. Carhart and Anojan Pathmanathan

QUESTIONS

65.1 A 65-year-old female with a history of coronary artery disease, hypertension, type 2 diabetes mellitus, and rheumatoid arthritis presents to the emergency department with complaints of shortness of breath on exertion and lower extremity swelling that has been worsening over the last week. She states that she is finding it harder to climb her stairs at home and carry out her daily activities such as doing the laundry or outdoor gardening. She is also needing one extra pillow to sleep at night and denies any symptoms while at rest. Physical examination shows elevated jugular venous pulse and 2+ pitting edema in bilateral lower extremities. S3 is significant on auscultation. Chest x-ray shows bilateral pleural edema. Transthoracic echocardiogram was obtained and demonstrated an ejection fraction of 35% with no valvular abnormalities. Her ejection fraction has decreased when compared to prior studies. What New York Heart Association (NYHA)/American Heart Association (AHA) functional class does this patient fall under?

A. NYHA I/stage A
B. NYHA I/stage B
C. NYHA III/stage C
D. NYHA IV/stage D

65.2 A 79-year-old female with a history of hypertension, type 2 diabetes, and morbid obesity presents to the emergency department with shortness of breath. She states that she was walking her dog today and needed to rest multiple times on the way. She denies any chest pressure or palpitations but feels like her legs are more swollen. Workup in the emergency department revealed elevated natriuretic peptide levels with normal troponin T levels. An echocardiogram demonstrated an ejection fraction of 52% with valvular or regional wall motion abnormalities. Doppler studies of mitral inflow showed an *E*/*e′* ratio of 16, a septal *e′* velocity of 5 cm/s, and a tricuspid regurgitation (TR) velocity of 3.0 cm/s. Which one of the following statements is **TRUE**?

A. The prevalence of her diagnosis has decreased over the last two decades.
B. The prevalence of her diagnosis is highest in North America and lowest in Eastern Europe and Russia.
C. For her diagnosis, ischemic heart disease is responsible for two-thirds of cases.
D. Incidence rates of her diagnosis have increased since the mid-1990s.

---

*Questions and Answers are based on Chapter 65: Heart Failure: Epidemiology, Characteristics, and Prognosis by Justin Ezekowitz in Cardiovascular Medicine and Surgery, First Edition.

65.3 A 67-year-old female with known heart failure with reduced ejection fraction (HFrEF) presents to the cardiology clinic for follow-up. She has been on optimal guideline-directed therapy for 2 months and a repeat echocardiogram today shows a left ventricular ejection fraction of 45%. The patient denies any shortness of breath or extremity swelling. She does report occasional palpitations at rest which resolve within 3 minutes. Which of the following statements is **TRUE**?

A. Atrial fibrillation is the most common cardiac rhythm abnormality in patients with heart failure (HF).
B. A combination of atrial fibrillation and HF has no significant increase in morbidity and mortality when compared to each disorder alone.
C. Palpitations are an expected symptom of HF and this patient needs no further evaluation or treatment changes.
D. The presence of atrial fibrillation is used in the Boston criteria for diagnosis of patients with HF.

65.4 A 59-year-old male with a history of hypertension, type 2 diabetes was referred to the cardiology clinic after seeing his family doctor for worsening swelling in both of his feet. He reports dyspnea on exertion and an inability to sleep flat on his bed without the use of two extra pillows. Physical examination reveals jugular venous distension, an S3 heart sound, bilateral rales, and bilateral lower extremity edema to the level of the ankles. According to what criteria can this patient be diagnosed with definite HF?

A. Gothenburg criteria
B. European Society of Cardiology (ESC) criteria
C. Framingham criteria
D. Boston criteria

65.5 A 49-year-old Aboriginal male presents to the outpatient cardiology clinic for evaluation of his congestive HF. He has been hospitalized numerous times over the past year needing optimization of his medical therapy. Which one of the following statements on HF is **TRUE**?

A. The total direct and indirect cost associated with HF in the United States is expected to decrease by 2030.
B. Since the mid-1990s, the incidence of heart failure with preserved ejection fraction (HFpEF) has declined faster than HFrEF.
C. Many studies have reported a higher incidence of HF in Whites as compared to Blacks.
D. In Canadian-based studies, Aboriginal patients with HF were shown to have increased mortality when compared to their White counterparts.

ANSWERS

65.1 **The correct answer is C.**
Rationale: This patient presents with significant limitations of ordinary activity with a resolution of her symptoms on rest. Her physical examination is evidence of clinical HF confirmed by her chest x-ray and transthoracic echocardiogram. Patients with cardiac disease resulting in marked limitations in ordinary activity due to fatigue, palpitations, dyspnea, or chest pain and without symptoms at rest fall under the NYHA class III classification. The presence of clinical HF on examination categorizes patients into AHA stage C.

NYHA class I functional classification signifies cardiac disease without limitations or symptoms. NYHA class II classification is for patients with slightly limited time during ordinary physical activity but comfortable at rest. NYHA class IV patients are unable to conduct any physical activity without discomfort and symptoms are also present at rest. As per AHA functional classifications, stage A are patients at risk of HF. Stage B are those with structural heart disease without symptoms. Stage D are patients with advanced HF requiring advanced interventions such as cardiac resynchronization therapy, left ventricular assist device, or heart transplantation.

KEY POINTS

✔ The NYHA/AHA functional classifications of HF help assess the severity of patient symptoms, disease progression, and possible need for escalation of care. Of note, patients can move back and forth between the different classes based on their response to therapy.

65.2 **The correct answer is B.**
Rationale: Based on her clinical symptoms and echocardiogram results, this patient's diagnosis is HFpEF. Data from a multinational randomized controlled trial showed the prevalence of HFpEF to be highest in North America, intermediate in Western Europe, and lowest in Eastern Europe and Russia. The prevalence of HFpEF has increased over the last two decades but the incidence peaked over in the mid-1990s and has subsequently stabilized and decreased. Ischemic heart disease is responsible for one-third of HFpEF cases and two-thirds of HFrEF cases.

KEY POINTS

✔ The prevalence of HF (both HFpEF and HFrEF) has increased over the last two decades with incidence rates peaking and decreasing since the mid-1990s.

65.3 The correct answer is A.

Rationale: Atrial fibrillation is the most common cardiac rhythm abnormality in patients with HF. One-third of patients with HF have been shown to have atrial fibrillation as a comorbidity in community-based studies. A combination of atrial fibrillation and HF has a significant increase in morbidity and mortality when compared to each disorder alone. This patient should be evaluated with electrocardiogram (ECG) or remote monitoring to evaluate her likely arrhythmia. The presence of atrial fibrillation contributes to the cardiac score of the Gothenburg criteria in diagnosing patients with HF

KEY POINTS

- Atrial fibrillation is the most common cardiac rhythm abnormality in patients with HF. A combination of both HF and atrial fibrillation shows significant increase in morbidity and mortality when compared to each disorder alone. Thus, adequate rate control of atrial fibrillation is essential to prevent decompensated HF.

65.4 The correct answer is C.

Rationale: According to the Framingham criteria, this patient can be diagnosed with HF. The Framingham criteria require two or more major criteria (acute pulmonary edema, jugular vein distension, hepatojugular reflux, paroxysmal nocturnal dyspnea or orthopnea, pulmonary rales, S3 heart sound, weight loss >4.5 kg in 5 days in response to treatment, cardiomegaly on chest x-ray) or one major and two or more minor criteria (ankle edema, dyspnea on exertion, hepatomegaly, nocturnal cough, pleural effusion, tachycardia, weight loss >4.5 kg in 5 days with diuretics).

The Gothenburg criteria take into account history of cardiac disease, pulmonary disease, and digoxin or diuretic use in the past to determine a grade. The ESC criteria use clinical history, physical examination, ECG or echocardiography abnormalities, and elevated B-type natriuretic peptide (BNP) for determination of HF diagnosis. Finally, the Boston criteria evaluate history, physical examination, and chest radiography to determine the likelihood of HF (definite, possible, unlikely). This patient does not meet the criteria for a definite diagnosis when using these other three diagnostic criteria.

KEY POINTS

- Several criteria—including the Framingham, Boston, Gothenburg, Duke, and ESC criteria—have been developed over several decades to help us with the task of diagnosing HF, with variable performances in the validation studies.

65.5 The correct answer is D.

Rationale: In a population-based study from Canada, Aboriginal patients with HF were shown to have increased mortality at 1 and 5 years compared to Caucasians, even after adjusting for demographic and clinical cofounders. Studies from Australia have also shown higher incidence rates among Aboriginals as compared to White patients.

The total direct and indirect cost associated with HF in the United States is expected to increase by 2030. Since the mid-1990s, the incidence of HFrEF has declined faster than HFpEF. Studies have reported a higher incidence of HF in Blacks as compared to Caucasians.

> **KEY POINTS**
>
> ✔ With the increase and prevalence of HF, providing long-term, evidence-based care for patients is a necessity and becomes more challenging and complex, especially in underserved regions and minorities.

PATHOPHYSIOLOGY OF HEART FAILURE

Phillip Olsen and Dmitri Belov

CHAPTER 66

QUESTIONS

66.1 Which of the following statements is **TRUE** regarding the pathophysiology of heart failure with reduced ejection fraction (HFrEF)?

A. It is characterized by cardiomyocyte dysfunction and neurohormonal activation leading to disease progression.
B. It is characterized by comorbid proinflammatory conditions leading to myocyte hypertrophy.
C. It is characterized by elevated filling pressures and increased left ventricular (LV) compliance.
D. It is characterized by endothelial dysfunction and reduced nitric oxide bioavailability.

66.2 A 62-year-old man with a history of ST-elevation myocardial infarction and ischemic cardiomyopathy 1 year ago is seen in the heart failure clinic for routine follow-up. He was diagnosed with ischemic cardiomyopathy and symptomatic heart failure during his hospitalization with an ejection fraction of 25% on echocardiogram. After 1 year of treatment with guideline-directed medical therapy, a repeat transthoracic echocardiogram shows LV ejection fraction has increased to 40%. Which of the following terms is most appropriate to describe his heart failure?

A. Heart failure with preserved ejection fraction (HFpEF)
B. HFrEF
C. Heart failure with mid-range ejection fraction
D. Heart failure with improved ejection fraction

66.3 The initial hemodynamic adaptive response is characterized by:

A. Activation of renin-angiotensin-aldosterone system (RAAS) and sympathetic nervous system resulting in increased circulatory volume and reduced vasoconstriction
B. Activation of the RAAS and sympathetic nervous system resulting in increased circulatory volume and increased vasoconstriction
C. Activation of RAAS and inhibition of the parasympathetic nervous system resulting in reduced circulatory volume and increased peripheral vasoconstriction
D. Inhibition of RAAS and activation of the sympathetic nervous system resulting in increased circulatory volume and increased peripheral vasoconstriction

---

*Questions and Answers are based on Chapter 66: Heart Failure Pathophysiology by Luise Holzhauser and Paul J. Mather in Cardiovascular Medicine and Surgery, First Edition.

66.4 Which of the following is **TRUE** regarding beta-receptor signaling in heart failure?
- A. Chronic heart failure leads to upregulation of beta-1-receptors thus causing increased cardiomyocyte sensitivity to catecholamine stimulation.
- B. Beta-receptor activation reduces calcium overload to inhibit apoptosis.
- C. Chronic beta-receptor stimulation has not been found to correlate with mortality or LV function.
- D. Downregulation of beta-1 as a result of chronic sympathetic nervous system activation leads to downstream excitation-contraction uncoupling.

66.5 Which of the following is **FALSE** regarding calcium in cardiac function and the failing heart?
- A. Mechanical unloading of the LV with assist devices has been shown to improve calcium homeostasis.
- B. Reduction of energy consumption through beta-blockade improves calcium homeostasis and signaling.
- C. Sarcoplasmic-endoplasmic reticulum Ca^{2+} ATPase (SERCA) is upregulated in heart failure leading to enhanced calcium sequestration and reduced contractility.
- D. Impairment in calcium signaling leads to decreased contractility through impaired myofilament cross-bridging formation and release.

66.6 Which of the following is **FALSE** regarding sodium-glucose cotransporter-2 inhibitors (SGLT2i) and energy metabolism?
- A. SGLT2i reduce cardiac metabolic efficiency.
- B. SGLT2i reduce glycosylation and free fatty acid (FFA) oxidation.
- C. SGLT2i improve mitochondrial respiratory function.
- D. SGLT2i increase ketone levels and ketone oxidation resulting in net increase in adenosine triphosphate (ATP) production.

66.7 Which of the following is **FALSE** regarding heart failure, insulin resistance, and glucose homeostasis?
- A. In advanced heart failure, myocardium develops insulin resistance and is reliant on FFA metabolism.
- B. Insulin resistance is associated with reduced mitochondrial uptake of FFAs, leading to FFA accumulation and mitochondrial-mediated cell death.
- C. Hyperglycemia and hyperinsulinemia are caused by increased gluconeogenesis and glycolysis in response to the compensatory increased adrenergic state in heart failure.
- D. Beta-blockers prevent metabolic shift from FFA utilization to glucose metabolism, thereby improving myocardial energy efficiency.

66.8 You are counseling your patient in the advanced heart failure clinic on the metabolic benefits of left ventricular assist devices (LVADs) in combination with guideline-directed medical therapy. Which of the following statements is **FALSE**?

A. LVAD implantation leads to improved myocardial function by upregulating cardiac beta-1-receptors and increasing adrenergic tone.
B. LVAD implantation with medical therapy has been shown to improve metabolic dysfunction.
C. LVAD mechanical unloading reduces toxic lipid metabolites in the myocardium and improves insulin signaling within the myocardium.
D. Mechanical unloading with LVADs improves calcium homeostasis to support myocardial function.

66.9 End-systolic elastance (EES) slope on a pressure-volume loop (**Figure 66.1**):
A. Is independent of preload and afterload
B. A load-independent marker of contractility
C. Increases with inotropic therapy
D. All of the above

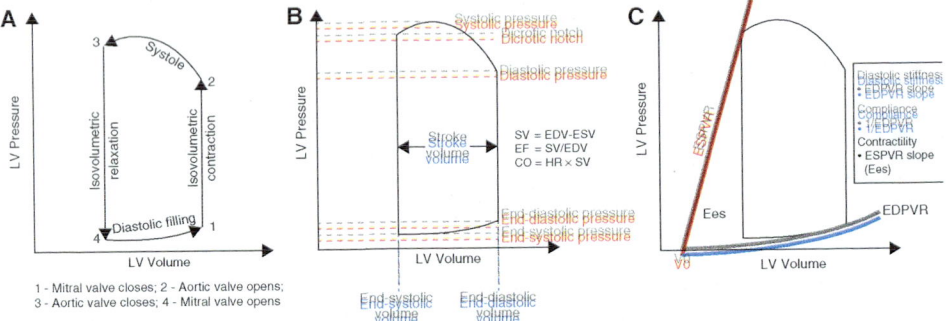

Figure 66.1 Pressure-volume loops. The four phases of the cardiac cycle are depicted in the pressure-volume loop by plotting left ventricular (LV) pressure against LV volumes **(A)**. These time points correlate with distinct pressures and volumes **(B)**. The end-diastolic pressure-volume relationship (EDPVR) is nonlinear and is descriptive of the diastolic properties of the LV **(C)**. The end-systolic pressure-volume relationship (ESPVR) is linear and load independent, and its slope (Ees) describes the LV contractility **(C)**. CO, cardiac output; EDV, end-diastolic volume; Ees, end-systolic elastance; EF, ejection fraction; ESV, end-systolic volume; HR, heart rate; SV, stroke volume; V0, volume at end-systolic pressure of 0 mm Hg. (Adapted from Burkhoff D, Wang J. Mechanical properties of the heart and its interaction with the vascular system. 2002.)

66.10 A 72-year-old woman with HFrEF is seen in clinic, 1 year since her last hospitalization for heart failure exacerbation. The pressure-volume loop describing her LV hemodynamics (**Figure 66.2**) can be described by which of the following?
A. Afterload independent
B. Preload sensitive
C. End-diastolic pressure-volume relationship (EDPVR) is shifted up and to the right.
D. EES slope is increased compared to normal.

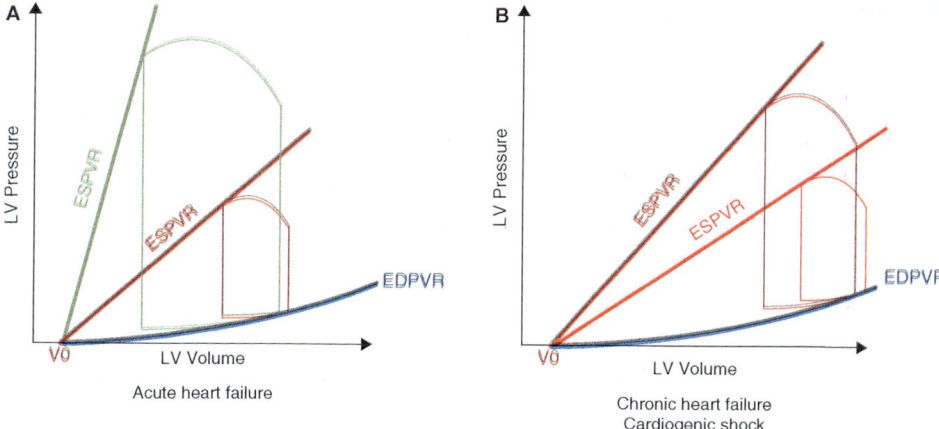

Figure 66.2 Acute and chronic heart failure. An acute decrease in contractility lowers blood pressure and stroke volume but will only have a minor effect on the end-diastolic pressure-volume relationship (EDPVR) **(A)**. In contrast, in chronic heart failure, the EDPVR moves up and to the right reflective of gradual increase in diastolic stiffness of the failing heart **(B)**. EDPVR, end-diastolic pressure-volume relationship; ESPVR, end-systolic pressure-volume relationship; LV, left ventricular; V0, volume at end-systolic pressure of 0 mm Hg. (Adapted from Burkhoff D, Wang J. Mechanical properties of the heart and its interaction with the vascular system. 2002.)

ANSWERS

66.1 The correct answer is A.
Rationale: HFrEF is characterized by a primary event (eg, ischemic infarct) or heritable condition that results in cardiomyocyte death and loss of function which in turn leads to neurohormonal activation and further loss of cardiac function. Increased LV compliance does not characterize heart failure, but all are characterized by elevated filling pressures. The remainder of answers describes HFpEF which is believed to be more causatively linked to proinflammatory states.

66.2 The correct answer is D.
Rationale: Heart failure with improved ejection fraction. Heart failure categorization was updated with the 2020 Universal Definition of Heart Failure and provides greater specifications as to categorization of heart failure. Heart failure with improved ejection fraction identifies patients with symptomatic heart failure with baseline ejection fraction less than 40% and an increase of at least 10% from baseline and ejection fraction of greater than or equal to 40% on a second echocardiogram. HFrEF indicates patient with an ejection fraction less than 40%. Heart failure with mid-range ejection fraction refers to a patient with LV ejection fraction between 41% and 49%. Heart failure with preserved ejection refers to patients with heart failure and an ejection fraction greater than 50%.

66.3 The correct answer is B.

Rationale: The initial adaptive response in heart failure is triggered by a reduced cardiac output leading to peripheral baroreceptor neurohormonal activation of RAAS and sympathetic nervous systems. In tandem, these systems work to preserve cardiac output by increasing contractility and heart rate as well as circulatory volume expansion via renin activation ultimately leading to increased sodium and water retention (**Figure 66.3**).

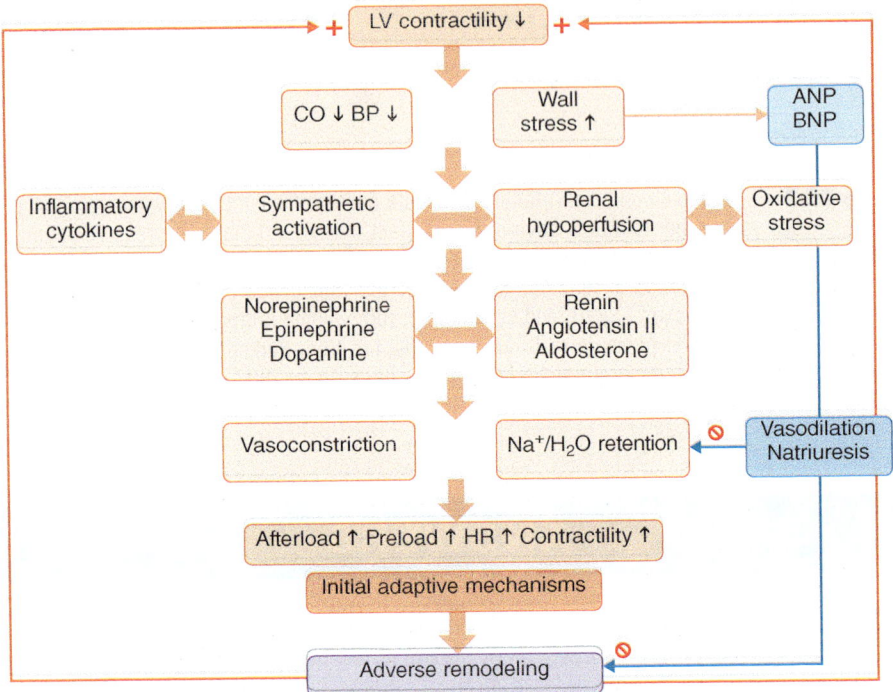

Figure 66.3 The vicious cycle of neurohormonal activation in HFrEF. A decrease in cardiac output and blood pressure leads to activation of the sympathetic nervous system and the RAAS. The resulting increase in preload and afterload as well as heart rate and contractility maintain cardiac output and perfusion. However, this initially adaptive process leads to adverse remodeling and sets off the vicious cycle of neurohormonal activation in chronic HF. ANP, atrial natriuretic peptide; BNP, B-type natriuretic peptide; BP, blood pressure; CO, cardiac output; HFrEF, heart failure with reduced ejection fraction; HR, heart rate; H_2O, water; LV, left ventricular; Na, sodium.

66.4 The correct answer is D.

Rationale: Beta-receptor activity plays many roles in the failing heart that cannot be clearly labeled as protective or damaging to the heart. Chronic heart failure and high adrenergic tone lead to downregulation of beta-1-receptors, calcium overload, and eventual uncoupling of the excitation-contraction pathway. This facilitates beta-arrestin and mitogen-activated protein kinase (MAP-K) activity, which lead to adverse remodeling cardiomyocyte apoptosis. Beta-2-receptors have been found to activate cell survival pathways in contrast to the deleterious effects of chronic beta-1 activity.

66.5 The correct answer is C.
Rationale: Calcium regulation is vital for cardiomyocyte function. Calcium binds to the tropomyosin on actin filaments allowing for crossbridge formation and myocyte contraction. SERCA is downregulated in heart failure resulting in reduced sarcoplasmic reticulum calcium release and impaired myocyte function. Heart failure is an energy-deficient state which impairs normal ATPase activity and intracellular handling of calcium.

66.6 The correct answer is B.
Rationale: SGLT2i affect energy metabolism by improving mitochondrial respiratory function and increasing ketone oxidation. This effect is independent of glycosylation and FFA oxidation, working to increase overall ATP production, thus increasing the available source of energy for the failing heart without an intrinsic improvement to cardiometabolic efficiency.

66.7 The correct answer is D.
Rationale: Beta-blockers improve myocardial energy efficiency by reducing oxygen consumption by inducing metabolic shift toward increased glucose utilization. High sympathetic nervous system tone increases corticosteroids and FFA levels leading to increased insulin resistance by increasing gluconeogenesis and glycolysis. A shift toward FFA-dependent energy utilization requires high oxygen utilization and increases demand on the already failing myocardium.

66.8 The correct answer is A.
Rationale: Mechanical unloading of the LV with LVADs and medical therapy has been shown to improve calcium homeostasis, and improves myocardial insulin signaling and metabolic dysfunction. LVADs have not been shown to upregulate beta-receptors. β-adrenergic stimulation increases demand in the failing heart and reduces myocardial efficiency.

66.9 The correct answer is D.
Rationale: End-systolic elastance is defined as the slope between the end-systolic pressure-volume relationship and the volume axis intercept. It reflects LV contractility independent of LV preload or afterload conditions. Inotropic agents will augment EES.

66.10 The correct answer is C.
Rationale: EDPVR is shifted right and up reflecting increased diastolic stiffness resulting in increased diastolic filling volumes and pressure in HFrEF. The LV in HFrEF is relatively preload independent but very afterload sensitive, with small increases in afterload greatly reducing stroke volume. EES is decreased in HFrEF (**Figure 66.2**).

GENETICS OF CARDIOMYOPATHY

Nathan Gentybear, Edward F. Philbin III, and Naveed M. Akhtar

CHAPTER 67

QUESTIONS

67.1 All of the following conditions can involve sarcomeric proteins **EXCEPT**:
  A. Brugada syndrome
  B. Dilated cardiomyopathy (DCM)
  C. Hypertrophic cardiomyopathy (HCM)
  D. Left ventricular noncompaction (LVNC)

67.2 A 23-year-old male patient comes to your office after a first-degree relative was diagnosed with a familial type of HCM. If a pathogenic gene mutation were to be identified, it would **MOST LIKELY** be a gene that encodes for:
  A. A desmosomal component
  B. A sarcomeric protein
  C. An ion channel
  D. A transmembrane signaling protein

67.3 The patient's family member from **Question 67.2** was found to carry a TNNT2 gene mutation. What correlation has been linked to this genotype?
  A. Early-onset disease
  B. Late-onset disease
  C. A more severe phenotype
  D. High incidence of sudden cardiac death

67.4 A 19-year-old is evaluated after a syncope event during a soccer game. An electrocardiogram (ECG) shows T-wave inversion in V1 to V3 and an epsilon wave. An echocardiogram reveals a dilated right ventricle with systolic dysfunction. He subsequently undergoes a cardiac magnetic resonance imaging (MRI) which shows wall thinning and fatty replacement of the myocardium. Which of the following genes might be linked to his condition?
  A. Dystrophin
  B. Lysosomal-associated membrane protein 2
  C. Plakophilin-2
  D. Titin

*Questions and Answers are based on Chapter 67: Genetics of Cardiomyopathies by Gary S. Beasley, Hugo Martinez, and Jeffrey A. Towbin in Cardiovascular Medicine and Surgery, First Edition.

675 Which of the following statements is **TRUE** regarding arrhythmogenic cardiomyopathy (ACM)?
   A. It typically follows an autosomal recessive pattern.
   B. The majority of cases only involve the right ventricle.
   C. Arrhythmogenic left ventricular cardiomyopathy (ALVC) is associated with low-QRS voltage.
   D. The majority of cases involve non-desmosomal proteins.

676 The most commonly mutated genes detected in patients with LVNC cardiomyopathy encode for:
   A. Components of desmosomes
   B. Sarcomeric proteins
   C. Ion channels
   D. Transmembrane signaling proteins

677 A family is discovered to have a genetic condition that is associated with cardiomyopathy and has a maternal pattern of inheritance. All female and male children of the affected mother appear to develop cardiomyopathy. The father does not carry the trait. Of the following, which fits this pattern of inheritance:
   A. Mitochondrial
   B. X-linked recessive
   C. Both A and B
   D. Neither A nor B

678 A 30-year-old patient comes to your office for counseling after having seen a report about cardiomyopathy on the news. He lives a healthy lifestyle and has no significant medical problems, but he wants to have genetic testing to "make sure my heart is ok." He has no cardiac symptoms, a normal examination, and a blood pressure of 118/76. Basic labs and a lipid panel are normal. As far as he knows, none of his relatives have heart problems. Which of the following is the **BEST** approach to advising this patient?
   A. Perform a calcium score and echocardiography before considering genetic testing.
   B. Send a genetic panel to screen for known gene mutations implicated in cardiomyopathy.
   C. Perform a cardiac MRI before considering genetic testing.
   D. Genetic testing is not indicated as an initial test.

679 Of the inherited causes of restrictive cardiomyopathy, the most common involves a gene that encodes which protein:
   A. Alpha-actin
   B. Filamin C
   C. Myopalladin
   D. Desmin

67.10 Which of the following genes has been implicated in both HCM and LVNC cardiomyopathy?
- A. MYH7 (myosin heavy chain 7)
- B. MYBPC3 (myosin-binding protein C)
- C. DSP (desmoplakin)
- D. TAZ (tafazzin)

ANSWERS

67.1 The correct answer is A.
Rationale: Brugada syndrome is a channelopathy and involves gene mutations that encode for ion channels, not genes that involve sarcomeres. The other choices may all be associated with genes that code for sarcomere proteins or genes involving sarcomere pathways (see **Figure 67.1**).

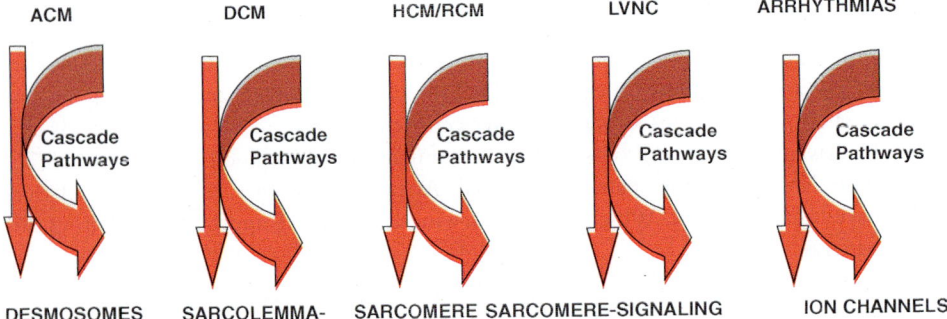

Figure 67.1 Primary pathways responsible for the different cardiomyopathy and arrhythmia phenotypes. The cascade pathways include interacting proteins, medications, mitochondrial disturbance, or other modifying factors. ACM, arrhythmogenic cardiomyopathy; DCM, dilated cardiomyopathy; HCM, hypertrophic cardiomyopathy; LVNC, left ventricular noncompaction; RCM, restrictive cardiomyopathy.

67.2 The correct answer is B.
Rationale: Approximately 80% of familial HCM cases are caused by mutations in four sarcomere genes: beta-myosin heavy chain, myosin-binding protein C, cardiac troponin T, and cardiac troponin I.

67.3 The correct answer is B.
Rationale: The TNNT2 gene mutation is associated with a high incidence of sudden cardiac death.

67.4 The correct answer is C.

Rationale: This patient's diagnostic findings are consistent with arrhythmogenic right ventricular cardiomyopathy (ARVC). Of the choices listed, only plakophilin-2, a desmosome protein gene, is associated with ARVC.

67.5 The correct answer is C.

Rationale: Fibro-fatty myocardial replacement of a significant portion of the left ventricle results in a low-QRS voltage in ALVC. Although some variants are autosomal recessive, the majority are autosomal dominant. The left ventricle is involved in 65% to 85% of cases. Non-desmosomal genes have been reported in only 1% to 3% of patients with ACM.

67.6 The correct answer is B.

Rationale: Mutations in cytoskeletal, sarcomeric, ion channel, and mitochondrial genes have been implicated in LVNC, with sarcomeric genes being the most common (**Figure 67.1**).

67.7 The correct answer is A.

Rationale: This inheritance pattern reflects a mitochondrial genetic disorder, as mitochondrial DNA is only inherited from the mother and may be passed to both male and female children. Since the father does not carry the trait, female children would not express the disease phenotype if the disease were X-linked recessive, as they would only receive one copy of the trait from the mother and would need two copies to express the disease phenotype. An example of mitochondrial disease is myoclonus epilepsy with ragged-red fibers (MERRF) syndrome. Duchenne muscular dystrophy is an example of an X-linked recessive condition, which primarily affects male children, and only rarely do female carriers have symptoms of the disease.

67.8 The correct answer is D.

Rationale: Associated genes are identified in less than half of patients with cardiomyopathies. Many of these genes demonstrate incomplete penetrance and variable expressivity, making the clinical significance uncertain. Without any evidence of a familial condition or symptoms of cardiomyopathy, it is best to recommend against any genetic screening as an initial test. Based on the information provided in the question, this patient does not have any risk factors or symptoms related to coronary disease, and therefore a calcium score is not indicated. A cardiac MRI is an expensive and time-consuming test, and should not be recommended for this patient who does not have any known risk factors or evidence of disease.

67.9 The correct answer is A.

Rationale: Although some cases of restrictive cardiomyopathy are inherited, in the majority of cases no specific cause is identified. All of the answer choices listed have been reported in inherited restrictive cardiomyopathy, but variants in the alpha-actin gene are the most common.

67.10 The correct answer is A.

Rationale: MYH7 is the only listed option implicated in both HCM and LVNC. MYBPC3 is associated with DCM and HCM. DSP is associated with ARVC, ALVC, and DCM. TAZ is associated with Barth syndrome, which can exhibit varying levels of DCM and LVNC (**Table 67.1**).

TABLE 67.1 Genes Associated With Cardiomyopathies and Their Allelic Disorders

Gene	OMIM[a]	Locus	Gene Name[b]	Associated Phenotypes[b]
ABCC9	601439	12p12.1	ATP-binding cassette, sub-family C (CFTR/MRP), member 9	DCM
ACTC1	102540	15q14	Actin, alpha, cardiac muscle 1	DCM HCM RCM
ACTN2	102573	1q42-q43	Actinin, alpha 2	DCM HCM
BAG3	603883	10q25.2-q26.2	BCL-2-associated athanogene 3	MFM DCM
CSRP3	600824	11p15.1	Cysteine and glycine-rich protein 3 (cardiac LIM protein)	DCM LVNC HCM
DES	125660	2q35	Desmin	MFM DCM RCM
DMD	300377	Xp21.2	Dystrophin	DMD BMD DCM
DSC2	125645	18q12.1	Desmocollin 2	ARVC
DSG2	125671	18q12.1	Desmoglein 2	ARVC ALVC DCM
DSP	125647	6p24	Desmoplakin	ARVC ALVC DCM
DTNA	601239	18q12.1	Dystrobrevin, alpha	LVNC
EMD	300384	Xq28	Emerin	EDMD DCM
EYA4	603550	6q23-q24	Eyes absent homolog 4 (Drosophila)	DFNA DCM
FKTN	607440	9q31	Fukutin	FCMD DCM
HCN4	605206	15q24.1	Hyperpolarization activated cyclic nucleotide-gated potassium channel 4	LVNC CD MVP
HSPB7	610692	1p36.13	Heat shock 27 kDa protein family, member 7	DCM

TABLE 67.1 Genes Associated With Cardiomyopathies and Their Allelic Disorders (*continued*)

Gene	OMIM[a]	Locus	Gene Name[b]	Associated Phenotypes[b]
JUP	173325	17q21	Junctional plakoglobin	ARVC ND
LAMP2	309060	Xq24	Lysosomal-associated membrane protein 2	DD HCM DCM
LDB3	605906	10q22-q23	LIM-domain binding 3	DCM ± LVNC MFM
LMNA	150330	1q21.2	Lamin A/C	DCM ± CD CMT2B1 EDMD HGPS LGMD MADA FPLD2
MYBPC3	600958	11p11.2	Myosin-binding protein C, cardiac	DCM HCM
MYH6	160710	14q12	Myosin, heavy chain 6, cardiac muscle, alpha	DCM HCM
MYH7	160760	14q12	Myosin, heavy chain 7, cardiac muscle, beta	DCM HCM RCM LVNC
MYL2	160781	12q23-q24	Myosin, light chain 2, regulatory, cardiac, slow	HCM
MYL3	160790	3p21.3-21.2	Myosin, light chain 3, alkali light chain; ventricular isoform, skeletal isoform, slow	HCM
MYPN	608517	10q21.1	Myopalladin	DCM RCM HCM
NEBL	605491	10p13-p12	Nebulette	DCM
NEXN	613121	1p31.1	Nexilin (F-actin binding protein)	DCM HCM
PKP2	602861	12p11	Plakophilin 2	ARVC
PKP4	604276	2q23-q31	Plakophilin 4	ARVC
PLN	172405	6q22.1	Phospholamban	DCM
PRKAG2	602743	7q36.1	Protein kinase, AMP-activated, gamma 2 noncatalytic subunit	HCM ± WPW FCNCG

(*continued*)

TABLE 67.1 Genes Associated With Cardiomyopathies and Their Allelic Disorders (continued)

Gene	OMIM[a]	Locus	Gene Name[b]	Associated Phenotypes[b]
PSEN1	104311	14q24.3	Presenilin 1	AD DCM FAI
PSEN2	600759	1q31-q42	Presenilin 2 (Alzheimer disease 4)	AD-4 DCM
RBM20	613171	10q25.2	RNA binding motif protein 20	DCM
RYR2	180902	1q43	Ryanodine receptor 2 (cardiac)	ARVC CPVT1
SCN5A	600163	3p21	Sodium channel, voltage-gated, type V, alpha subunit	BRS LQTS DCM ± CD
SGCB	600900	13q12	Sarcoglycan, beta	LGMD2E DCM
SGCD	601411	5q33-q34	Sarcoglycan, delta	LGMD2F DCM
TAZ	300394	Xq28	Tafazzin	BTS LVNC DCM
TCAP	604488	17q12	Titin-cap (telethonin)	LGMD2G HCM DCM
TGFB3	190230	14q24	Transforming growth factor, beta 3	ARVC
TMEM43	612048	3p25.1	Transmembrane protein 43	ARVC
TMPO	188380	12q22	Thymopoietin	DCM
TNNC1	191040	3p21.1	Troponin C type 1 (slow)	DCM HCM
TNNI3	191044	19q13.4	Troponin I type 3 (cardiac)	DCM HCM RCM
TNNT2	191045	1q32	Troponin T type 2 (cardiac)	DCM HCM RCM
TPM1	191010	15q22.1	Tropomyosin 1 (alpha)	DCM HCM

TABLE 67.1 Genes Associated With Cardiomyopathies and Their Allelic Disorders (*continued*)

Gene	OMIM[a]	Locus	Gene Name[b]	Associated Phenotypes[b]
TTN	188840	2q31	Titin	TMD LGMD2J EOMFC DCM HCM HMERF
VCL	193065	10q22.1-q23	Vinculin	DCM HCM

[a]OMIM, online Mendelian inheritance in man (http://www.ncbi.nlm.nih.gov/omim)
[b]Genetic Home References (http://ghr.nlm.nih.gov/)

AD, Alzheimer disease; ALVC, arrhythmogenic left ventricular cardiomyopathy; ARVC, arrhythmogenic right ventricular cardiomyopathy; ATP, adenosine triphosphate; BCL-2, B-cell lymphoma 2; BMD, Becker muscular dystrophy; BRS, Brugada syndrome; BTS, barth syndrome; CD, conduction defects; CFTR, cystic fibrosis transmembrane conductance regulator; CMT2B1, Charcot-Marie-Tooth disease type 2B1; CPVT, catecholaminergic polymorphic ventricular tachycardia; DCM, dilated cardiomyopathy; DD, Danon disease; DFNA, autosomal dominant late-onset progressive nonsyndromic deafness; DMD, Duchenne muscular dystrophy; EDMD, Emery-Dreifuss muscular dystrophy; EOMFC, early-onset myopathy with fatal cardiomyopathy; FAI, familial acne inverse; FCMD, Fukuyama congenital muscular dystrophy; FCNCG, fatal congenital nonlysosomal cardiac glycogenosis; FPLD2, familial partial lipodystrophy of the Dunnigan type; HCM, hypertrophic cardiomyopathy; HGPS, Hutchinson-Gilford progeria syndrome; HMERF, myopathy with early respiratory muscle involvement; LGMD, limb-girdle muscular dystrophy; LIM, lin-11, islet-1, mec-3; LQTS, long-QT syndrome; LVNC, left ventricular noncompaction; MADA, mandibuloacral dysplasia type A with partial lipodystrophy; MFM, myofibrillar myopathy; MRP, multidrug resistance-associated protein; MVP, mitral valve prolapse; ND, Naxos disease; nNOS, neuronal nitric oxide synthase; RCM, restrictive cardiomyopathy; TMD, tibial muscular dystrophy, tardive; WPW, Wolff-Parkinson-White syndrome

HEART FAILURE WITH PRESERVED EJECTION FRACTION

CHAPTER 68

John Tremblay and Mikhail Toroseff

QUESTIONS

68.1 An 84-year-old female presents to the emergency department with dyspnea on exertion and orthopnea which have become progressively worse over the last 2 to 3 weeks. The patient has a past medical history of coronary artery disease (CAD), obesity, atrial fibrillation, and hypertension (HTN). Which of the following is the most common risk factor for developing heart failure with preserved ejection fraction (HFpEF)?

A. CAD
B. Obesity
C. Atrial fibrillation
D. HTN
E. A and D

68.2 A 76-year-old female with a past medical history of HFpEF presents to the clinic for a yearly follow-up. The patient is accompanied by her daughter who is a pharmacist. Her daughter is curious about her mother's condition and asks what are some of the causes of the rise in end-diastolic pressure in patients with HFpEF?

A. Atrial and left ventricular (LV) stiffness
B. Reduction in arterial compliance
C. Diastolic dysfunction
D. Systolic dysfunction
E. All the above

68.3 A 72-year-old woman with a past medical history of type 2 diabetes mellitus (DMT2), obesity, HTN, and atrial fibrillation presents to the clinic concerned for her recent change in exercise capability. The patient has been inactive since she underwent total right knee arthroplasty 2 years ago, but after being educated on her health risk decides to start exercising again. She states she becomes very winded after walking only a half mile before she must stop to rest. She initially attributed her symptoms to her current state of health. Over the last 4 weeks, the patient can only walk roughly one-tenth of a mile before having to catch her breath. The patient is having difficulty losing weight and has noticed worsening lower extremity edema. She consumes two to three glasses of wine per week and was a previous smoker with a 40-pack-year history but quit 20 years ago. Brain natriuretic peptide (BNP) was 716 ng/L and echocardiogram left ventricular ejection fraction (LVEF) was greater than 55%. Which of the following conditions and mechanisms resulted in endothelial inflammation contributing to her HFpEF?

*Questions and Answers are based on Chapter 68: Heart Failure with Preserved Ejection Fraction by Tyler Moran, Anita Deswal, and Arunima Misra in Cardiovascular Medicine and Surgery, First Edition.

A. Diabetes and nitric oxide availability
B. Obesity and cyclic guanosine monophosphate content
C. HTN and protein kinase G (PKG)
D. All of the above
E. None of the above

68.4 A 54-year-old African American male with a past medical history of tobacco use, chronic obstructive pulmonary disease (COPD), and HTN presents to the clinic for dyspnea. He does not take any medications. The patient is a carpenter and previously was able to work throughout the day without any shortness of breath. Starting 1 year ago, he noticed he would become increasingly short of breath carrying lumber around the job site. Initially, he was not concerned and attributed his symptoms to old age but now presents due to concerns of his wife. The patient does not have a primary care doctor but does follow up with a pulmonologist who prescribes him Anoro ellipta (umeclidinium/vilanterol). Which of the following is **LEAST LIKELY** based on this patient's H_2FPEF score?

A. Constrictive pericarditis
B. Severe valvular disease
C. Hypertrophic cardiomyopathy
D. Amyloid heart disease
E. HFpEF

CASE 1

Questions 68.5 and 68.6 are based on the following case.

A 57-year-old female with a past medical history of obesity, diabetes, HTN, and chronic kidney disease (CKD) stage III presents to the clinic for evaluation of dyspnea with exertion. The patient states that when she enters her third-story apartment, she becomes short of breath when reaching the top of the first flight of stairs. Roughly 1 year ago, the patient was able to climb two flights of stairs before becoming short of breath. Her current medications include chlorthalidone 25 mg daily, amlodipine 5 mg daily, metformin 1,000 mg tid, and semaglutide1 mg weekly. On physical examination, the patient's body mass index (BMI) is 52 kg/m², blood pressure (BP) is 128/86 mm Hg, and heart rate (HR) 72 beats per minute (bpm).

68.5 In **Case 1**, the patient's echocardiogram and blood work are pending. What is the patient's H_2FPEF score?

A. 2
B. 3
C. 4
D. 5
E. 6

68.6 In **Case 1**, the patient's echocardiogram shows LVEF greater than 55%, global longitudinal strain (GLS) of 12%, LV wall thickness is 13 mm, and BNP of 90. What is her heart failure association diagnostic algorithm of heart failure with preserved ejection fraction (HFA-PEFF) score and what is the next **BEST** diagnostic test?

A. 1 point and no further diagnostic testing
B. 2 points and cardiac magnetic resonance imaging (MRI)
C. 3 points and right heart catheterization
D. 5 points and no further diagnostic testing
E. None of the above

68.7 A 73-year-old male presents to the hospital with worsening dyspnea on exertion. He now must rest while performing his daily 5-mile walk. The patient has a past medical history of atrial fibrillation, HTN, and CAD status post stenting to the left anterior descending (LAD) artery 3 years ago. The patient is compliant with his medications including atorvastatin 40 mg at bedtime, aspirin 81 mg daily, metoprolol succinate 50 mg tid, apixaban 5 mg tid, and lisinopril 40 mg daily. Labs are significant for BNP greater than 800, hemoglobin 14.5 g/dL, serum creatinine (SCr) 1.2 mg/dL, and potassium 5.2 mmol/L. Patient's echocardiogram shows LVEF greater than 55%. Patient is started on intravenous (IV) furosemide 40 mg daily with the improvement of symptoms and is discharged from the hospital. Which of the following interventions has the **BEST** data for morbidity and mortality in HFpEF in this patient?

A. Fluid restriction
B. Adding a beta-blocker
C. Adding an angiotensin-converting enzyme inhibitor (ACEI)
D. Adding a loop diuretic
E. None of the above

68.8 A 65-year-old male presents to the clinic for BP management. The patient smokes 2 packs of cigarettes daily and does not take any medications at home. The patient's BP on initial evaluation 1 month ago was 165/92 mm Hg. The patient quit smoking and was started on losartan with good improvement in his BP. On BP recheck, the patient's BP is 128/80 mm Hg. What is the mechanism of uncontrolled HTN leading to HFpEF and what would be the percent reduction in incidence of heart failure (HF) with adequate BP control?

A. Reduced preload, 20%
B. Increased preload, 30%
C. Reduced afterload, 40%
D. Increased afterload, 50%

68.9 A 73-year-old male with atrial fibrillation and HFpEF presents to the clinic for evaluation. The patient states that he is compliant with his medications, which include metoprolol succinate 50 mg bid and apixaban 5 mg bid. His atrial fibrillation is paroxysmal. Which is the **BEST** atrial fibrillation strategy to prevent progression of the HF and what factors contribute to this patient's development of permanent atrial fibrillation?

A. Rate control, HFpEF worsens atrial function
B. Rhythm control, CAD worsens atrial function
C. Rate control, CAD worsens atrial function
D. Rhythm control, HFpEF worsens atrial function
E. None of the above, HFpEF worsens atrial function

68.10 A 61-year-old male with a past medical history of obesity, DMT2, HTN, and HFpEF presents to the clinic for medication reconciliation and BP check. The patient is currently taking metformin 1,000 mg bid, losartan 50 mg daily, and chlorthalidone 25 mg daily. The patient was recently diagnosed with gout and his chlorthalidone was discontinued. The patient's BP today is 126/78 mm Hg. He states that he has lost 25 lb in the last 3 months with an improved diet and his BMI has dropped from 36 to 31. Which of the following medication recommendations would reduce this patient's number of hospitalizations and cardiovascular (CV) death?

A. Start furosemide 20 mg po daily.
B. Start metoprolol succinate 25 mg bid.
C. Start hydralazine 10 mg tid.
D. Start dapagliflozin 5 mg daily.

ANSWERS

68.1 The correct answer is E.
Rationale: There are several risk factors that are associated with the development of HFpEF including CAD, HTN, DM, obesity, and smoking. HTN is the most common cause of HFpEF and is present in the majority of patients with HFpEF regardless of age, gender, or racial group. CAD is also a strong risk factor as it is noted in 35% to 60% of patients with HFpEF and is also associated with the greatest risk of developing HFrEF. Obesity and atrial fibrillation are risk factors of HFpEF but carry a reduced risk compared to HTN (**Table 68.1**).

TABLE 68.1 Potential Etiologies of HFpEF

Abnormalities of the myocardium	
Ischemic	Coronary artery disease with a scar or active ischemia Microvascular disease and endothelial dysfunction
Toxic	Drugs: alcohol, cocaine, anabolic steroids Metals: iron, lead Medications: chemotherapy, immunomodulators
Immune and inflammatory	Radiation: high cardiac radiation doses Infectious: HIV, Chagas Noninfectious: lymphocytic myocarditis, autoimmune diseases, eosinophilic myocarditis, immune checkpoint inhibitor therapy
Infiltrative	Malignant: direct involvement or metastases Nonmalignant: amyloidosis, sarcoidosis, hemochromatosis, storage diseases including Fabry disease
Metabolic	Thyroid, growth hormone diseases, adrenal hormone diseases, pregnancy, diabetic cardiomyopathy

(continued)

TABLE 68.1 Potential Etiologies of HFpEF (continued)

Genetic	Hypertrophic cardiomyopathy, muscular dystrophy
Endomyocardial	Endocardial fibroelastosis, hypereosinophilic syndrome, carcinoid
Abnormalities of loading conditions	
Hypertension	Primary and secondary forms of hypertension
Valvular/structural disease	Heart valve disease Septal defects
Pericardial disease	Constrictive pericarditis
High output states	Severe anemia, sepsis, thyrotoxicosis, AV fistula, pregnancy
Volume overload	Renal failure
Obesity-related HFpEF	Metabolic/inflammatory with microvascular dysfunction/volume expansion/pericardial and chest wall, abdominal restraint
Abnormalities of cardiac rhythm	
Rhythm disorders	Atrial or ventricular arrhythmias, eg, atrial fibrillation, pacing, conduction disorders

AV, arteriovenous; HFpEF, heart failure preserved ejection fraction.
Modified from How to diagnose heart failure with preserved ejection fraction: the HFA-PEFF diagnostic algorithm: a consensus recommendation from the Heart Failure Association (HFA) of the European Society of Cardiology. *Eur Heart J.* 2019;40(40):3297-3317. Reproduced by permission of Oxford University Press.

68.2 The correct answer is E.

Rationale: In HFpEF, the rise in end-diastolic pressure is caused by multiple factors. The complex relationship between diastolic dysfunction, underlying minimal systolic dysfunction, atrial and LV stiffness, and reduced arterial compliance are all factors contributing to LV dysfunction. This is usually caused by a systemic proinflammatory state which causes microvascular inflammation. This ultimately leads to a reduction in nitric oxide bioavailability causing myocardial hypertrophy. This can progress to cardiomyocyte stiffness and interstitial fibrosis. Overall, it's the combination of atrial and LV stiffness, reduction in arterial compliance, systolic and diastolic dysfunction that contributes to the rise in the end-diastolic pressure.

68.3 The correct answer is D.

Rationale: The paradigm proposed by Paulus and Tschope suggests that HFpEF is the result of a proinflammatory state which leads to endothelial dysfunction, coronary microvascular dysfunction, and abnormal cardiac structure and function. The proinflammatory states of HTN, diabetes, and obesity lead to endothelial inflammation which reduces nitric oxide bioavailability, cyclic guanosine monophosphate content, and PKG activity. These pathways result in LV hypertrophy. In addition, the hypophosphorylation of titin has been shown to lead to stiff cardiomyocytes and interstitial fibrosis. Overall, anti-inflammatory strategies may hold promise in the treatment of HFpEF phenotype.

68.4 The correct answer is E.

Rationale: The H$_2$FPEF score is a diagnostic approach for patients with suspected HFpEF. It was established from the 2019 recommendations per the European Society of Cardiology (ESC) with an evidence-based approach. The H$_2$FPEF score helps categorize the probability of HFpEF based on a patient's current risk factors. In the acronym, H$_2$ represents BMI greater than 30 kg/m^2 and HTN which scores 2 points and 1 point, respectively. F stands for atrial fibrillation and is worth 3 points. P represents pulmonary HTN with a pulmonary artery systolic pressure greater than 35 mm Hg on an echocardiogram worth 1 point. E represents the elderly with an age above 60 years, worth 1 point, and the second F represents filling pressure with an *E/e* ratio greater than 9 on echo. If the H$_2$FPEF score is between 0 and 1, there is a low probability of the patient having HFpEF. A H$_2$FPEF score of 2 to 5 is an intermediate probability of HFpEF, and a H$_2$FPEF of 6 to 9 is a high probability and likely HFpEF. This patient has a score of 1 and is unlikely HFpEF.

Once the HFpEF diagnosis is confirmed, the etiology of the HFpEF should guide specific therapy. These common underlying conditions that can cause HFpEF are CAD, HTN, valvular disease, infiltrative disease, autoimmune disease, glycogen storage disease, certain medications, radiation toxicity, metabolic and hormonal causes. Mimickers of HFpEF include but are not limited to constrictive pericarditis, hypertrophic cardiomyopathy, congenital heart disease, primary pulmonary HTN, or cor pulmonale.

68.5 The correct answer is B.

Rationale: The H$_2$FPEF score helps categorize the probability of HFpEF based on a patient's current risk factors. In the acronym, H$_2$ represents BMI greater than 30 kg/m^2 and HTN which scores 2 points and 1 point, respectively. F stands for atrial fibrillation and is worth 3 points. P represents pulmonary HTN with a pulmonary artery systolic pressure greater than 35 mm Hg on echocardiogram worth 1 point. E represents elderly with an age above 60 years, worth 1 point, and the second F represents filling pressure with an *E/e* ratio greater than 9 on echo. If the H$_2$FPEF score is between 0 and 1, there is a low probability of the patient having HFpEF. A H$_2$FPEF score of 2 to 5 is an intermediate probability of HFpEF, and a H$_2$FPEF of 6 to 9 is a high probability and likely HFpEF. The patients H$_2$FPEF score would be 3. She would score 2 points for BMI greater than 30 kg/m^2 and 1 point for HTN. This would place the patient at an intermediate probability and possible HFpEF.

68.6 The correct answer is C.

Rationale: Patients with dyspnea should have an echocardiography performed. Echocardiography can evaluate for heart failure with reduced ejection fraction (HFrEF), valvular disease, pulmonary HTN, and pericardial effusion. HFpEF is consistent with concentric remodeling or LV hypertrophy and left atrial enlargement. In addition, abnormal diastole and longitudinal strain can also be seen on echocardiography. The European Society of Cardiology/Heart Failure Association (ESC/HFA) suggests the calculation of the HFA-PEFF score. The function morphology found on the echocardiogram would be allotted points which would be converted into a scoring system to predict the likelihood of HFpEF. Septal e less than 7, lateral e less than 10, average E/e greater or equal to 15, or tricuspid regurgitation (TR) velocity greater than 2.8 m/s would be worth 2 points while average E/e 9 to 14 and GLS less than 16% would be worth 1 point. The measurement of early diastolic tissue velocity, left atrial volume indexed (LAVI) to body surface area (BSA), and TR velocity to assess pulmonary artery systolic pressure can all lead to the suggestion of HFpEF but are not definitive.

This patient's HFA-PEFF score is 3. She would get 1 point for GLS, 1 point for LV wall thickness, and 1 point for BNP greater than 80. This would be nondiagnostic and further invasive assessments are needed. A right heart catheterization result of a pulmonary capillary wedge pressure (PCWP) greater than or equal to 15 would be diagnostic of HFpEF. Cardiac MRI would be able to assess the ejection fraction (EF) and infiltrative cardiac disease but is unlikely to aid in the diagnosis of HFpEF. A score of 5 to 6 is a high probability of HFpEF and no further test is needed.

68.7 The correct answer is E.
Rationale: None of the following medications or interventions have been shown to improve morbidity and mortality in this patient without being contraindicated. Fluid restriction has limited data and is recommended only for patients with severe HF with hyponatremia. Beta-blockers could be used for the treatment of HTN but did not show any improvement in HF or CV death according to the Japanese diastolic heart failure (J-DHF) trial with concerns of worsening chronotropic incompetence. Renin-angiotensin-aldosterone system (RAAS) antagonists (ACEI and ARBs [angiotensin receptor blockers]) did not show any improvement in CV death or HF hospitalizations in the CHARM (Candesartan in heart failure: assessment of reduction in mortality and morbidity)-Preserved trial. Loop diuretics improve symptoms but do not improve CV death of HF hospitalizations. Mineralocorticoid receptor antagonists (MRAs), based on the TOPCAT (treatment of preserved cardiac function heart failure with an aldosterone antagonist) trial, showed that MRAs may be considered to reduce HF hospitalization in patients with LVEF greater than 45% and elevated BNP levels with HF admission within 1 year. MRAs would be contraindicated in this patient due to the patient's potassium being greater than 5 mEq/L. SGLT2 (sodium-glucose cotransporter 2) inhibitors appear to be beneficial and have been approved for use in patients with HFpEF (**Tables 68.2 and 68.3**).

68.8 The correct answer is D.
Rationale: Elevated arterial pressure due to smoking and vasoconstriction increases afterload which impairs LV relaxation and filling. In addition, impaired LV relaxation and elevated filling pressure can reduce coronary vascular reserve without epicardial coronary disease. ARBs ameliorate arterial vasoconstriction and decrease afterload. Trials suggest that BP control is more important than the class of medication used to achieve BP control. The patient's BP is within goal (<130/80 mm Hg), but there is evidence suggesting intensive BP control further reduces the incidence of HF. Those who are adequately treated for HTN have a 50% reduction in the incidence of HF.

TABLE 68.2 Treatment of HFpEF From ACC/AHA/HFSA and ESC/HFA Guidelines

COR	LOE	Recommendation ACC/AHA/HFSA	Recommendation ESC/HFA
I	B	Systolic and diastolic blood pressure should be controlled in accordance with clinical practice guidelines to prevent morbidity.	Diuretics are recommended in congested patients to alleviate symptoms and signs of HF.
I	C	Diuretics should be used for relief of symptoms owing to volume overload.	Treatment of all cardiac and noncardiac comorbidities is recommended to improve symptoms, well-being, and/or prognosis.
IIa	C	Coronary revascularization is reasonable in patients with CAD in whom angina or demonstrable ischemia is adversely affecting HFpEF symptoms.	In ESC/HFA guidelines, above applies for HFpEF and HFmEF.
IIa	C	Management of AF according to published clinical practice guidelines in patients to improve symptoms of HF.	
IIa	C	Use of BBs, ACEIs, and ARBs in patients with hypertension is reasonable to control blood pressure.	
IIb	B-R	In select patients with HFpEF (LVEF ≥45%), elevated BNP levels or HF admission within 1 y, eGFR >30 mL/min, creatinine <2.5 mg/dL, potassium <5.0 mEq/L, MRAs may be considered to reduce hospitalizations.	
IIb	B	Use of ARBs may be considered to decrease hospitalizations for patients with HFpEF.	
III	B-R	Routine use of nitrates or phosphodiesterase-5 inhibitors to increase the activity of QoL in patients with HFpEF is ineffective.	

ACC, American College of Cardiology; ACEI, angiotensin-converting enzyme inhibitor; AF, atrial fibrillation; AHA, American Heart Association; ARB, angiotensin receptor blocker; BB, beta-blocker; BNP, brain natriuretic peptide; CAD, coronary artery disease; COR, class of recommendation; eGFR, estimated glomerular filtration rate; ESC, European Society of Cardiology; HF, heart failure; HFA, Heart Failure Association; HFmEF, heart failure with midrange ejection fraction; HFpEF, heart failure with preserved ejection fraction; HFSA, Heart Failure Society of America; LOE, level of evidence; LVEF, left ventricular ejection fraction; MRA, mineralocorticoid receptor antagonist; QoL, quality of life.
From ACC/AHA/HFSA guidelines reprinted from Yancy CW, Jessup M, Bozkurt B, et al. 2017 ACC/AHA/HFSA focused update of the 2013 ACCF/AHA guideline for the management of heart failure: a report of the American College of Cardiology/American Heart Association task force on clinical practice guidelines and the Heart Failure Society of America. *J Card Fail.* 2017;23(8):628-651. Copyright © 2017 Elsevier. With permission. ESC/HFA guidelines adapted from Baumgartner H, Falk V, Bax JJ, et al. 2017 ESC/EACTS guidelines for the management of valvular heart disease. *Eur Heart J.* 2017;38(36):2739-2791.

TABLE 68.3 Drug Classes, Study Results, and Recommended Treatment of HFpEF

Drug Class	Mechanism	Clinical Trials	Results	Recommendations
Nitrates and nitrites	Preload lowering agents, nitric oxide donors, venodilators	**NEAT-HFpEF:** isosorbide mononitrate vs placebo **INDIE-HFpEF:** inhaled inorganic nitrite vs control	No difference, in activity, quality of life, or NT-proBNP in either trial	Data do not support the routine use of nitrates or nitrites.
RAAS antagonists	Improve systemic blood pressure, myocardial relaxation, myocardial fibrosis	**CHARM-Preserved:** candesartan vs placebo **PEP-CHF:** perindopril in older adults vs placebo **I-PRESERVE:** irbesartan vs placebo	No significant difference in CV death or HF hospitalization Borderline significant benefit on reduction in HF hospitalization No difference in all-cause mortality or HF hospitalization No difference in all-cause mortality or CV hospitalization	In CHARM-Preserved: Data do not support routine use of ACEI or ARBs specifically for HFpEF; can be used to control underlying hypertension or if indicated in select patients with diabetes
Mineralocorticoid receptor antagonists	Less sodium and more potassium retention, attenuating endothelial dysfunction, reducing vascular inflammation and fibrosis	**Aldo-DHF:** spironolactone vs placebo **RAAM-PEF:** eplerenone vs placebo **TOPCAT:** spironolactone vs placebo	Improved echo diastolic parameters E/e', LV mass index, and NT proBNP; no change in QoL or functional capacity Improved E/e', reduced collagen turnover, but no change in functional capacity No difference in CV death/HF hospitalization/aborted cardiac arrest; HF hospitalization was lower but not total hospitalizations, more hyperkalemia, and renal failure; post hoc analysis showed reduced HF hospitalizations/CV death/aborted cardiac arrest in the Americas.	Based on **TOPCAT** showing improved outcomes in North America, updated ACC/AHA HF Guideline 2017 Focused update: MRA may be considered to reduce HF hospitalizations in patients with: LVEF ≥45% Elevated BNP levels HF admission within 1 y eGFR >30 mL/min, creatinine <2.5 mg/dL, and potassium <5 mEq/L

TABLE 68.3 Drug Classes, Study Results, and Recommended Treatment of HFpEF (*continued*)

Drug Class	Mechanism	Clinical Trials	Results	Recommendations
Angiotensin receptor-neprilysin inhibitors	Elevate circulating natriuretic peptides to improve sodium excretion, vasodilation, and inhibit RAAS	**PARAMOUNT:** sacubitril/valsartan vs valsartan alone **PARAGON-HF:** sacubitril/valsartan vs valsartan	Reduced NT-proBNP levels No significant difference in HF hospitalizations or CV death	No recommendations for use of ARNIs yet although some suggest that select populations including women, those with recent HF hospitalizations, and mildly reduced EF may benefit; more studies are needed.
Beta-blockers and ivabradine (I$_f$ channel blocker)	Increase diastolic filling time with reduced heart rate	**J-DHF:** carvedilol vs placebo **ELANDD:** nebivolol vs placebo **EDIFY:** ivabradine vs placebo	Underpowered study but no differences in HF hospitalization or CV death No difference in 6-min walk test or oxygen consumption No difference in *E/e'*, 6-min walk test, or NT-proBNP	No recommendations for beta-blockers in HFpEF; concern for worsening chronotropic incompetence in some patients; may be used for coexisting indications of angina, post-myocardial infarction, rate control in atrial fibrillation, and in some for hypertension No recommendations for ivabradine
Selective phosphodiesterase type 5 inhibition (PDE-5 inhibition)	Enhance nitric oxide–mediated vasodilation as well as effects on pulmonary artery pressure and right ventricular hypertrophy	**RELAX:** sildenafil vs placebo	No change in peak oxygen consumption, exercise tolerance, diastolic parameters, or pulmonary artery pressure	Not recommended routinely for HFpEF
Endothelin antagonists	To reduce pulmonary hypertension in HFpEF	**BADDHY:** bosentan and sitaxsentan	No benefit	Not recommended for pulmonary hypertension owing to HFpEF
Lusitropic agents	Improve relaxation	**RALI-DHF:** ranolazine	No change in echo parameters or NT-proBNP	
Soluble guanylate cyclase stimulator	Generate cyclic guanosine monophosphate and restore sensitivity of soluble guanylate cyclase to endogenous nitric oxide	**VITALITY-HFpEF:** vericiguat	No improvement in QoL	

(*continued*)

TABLE 68.3 Drug Classes, Study Results, and Recommended Treatment of HFpEF (continued)

Drug Class	Mechanism	Clinical Trials	Results	Recommendations
Partial adenosine A1 receptor agonist	Improve mitochondrial function, enhance sarcoplasmic reticulum 2a activity, optimize energy substrate metabolism, reverse cardiac remodeling	PANACHE: neladenoson	No initial benefit noted on 6-min walk distance, QoL, NT-proBNP levels	Early clinical phase IIb trial data not encouraging

ACC, American College of Cardiology; ACEI, angiotensin-converting enzyme inhibitor; AHA, American Heart Association; ARB, angiotensin receptor blocker; ARNI, angiotensin receptor neprilysin inhibitors; BNP, brain natriuretic peptide; CV, cardiovascular; eGFR, estimated glomerular filtration rate; EF, ejection fraction; HF, heart failure; HFpEF, heart failure preserved ejection fraction; HFSA, Heart Failure Society of America; LV, left ventricular; LVEF, left ventricular ejection fraction; MRA, mineralocorticoid receptor antagonist; NT-proBNP, N-terminal pro-brain natriuretic peptide; QoL, quality of life; RAAS, renin-angiotensin-aldosterone system.

68.9 The correct answer is E.
Rationale: Atrial fibrillation is common and is associated with worse outcomes. The progression of the HFpEF leads to worsening atrial dysfunction. This can lead to severe atrial dysfunction with abnormal right ventricular (RV) pulmonary vascular congestion compared to sinus rhythm. At this time, it is unclear if there is a benefit between rate control versus rhythm control in atrial fibrillation.

68.10 The correct answer is D.
Rationale: SGLT2 inhibitors work by reducing the glucose reuptake in the kidney. This leads to improvement in glycemic control, BP, and weight loss. In addition, a 30% reduction in HF hospitalization was noted in randomized trials. The mechanisms unrelated to glycemic control are most likely responsible for the CV benefit including natriuresis, BP lowering, reduction in arterial stiffness or preserved renal function, or cardiac metabolism with a shift from fatty acids to ketones. Loop diuretics, beta-blockers, and afterload reducers do not have any data to support improvement in CV death and HF hospitalizations.

HEART FAILURE WITH REDUCED EJECTION FRACTION*

John Tremblay and Mikhail Torosoff

CHAPTER 69

QUESTIONS

CASE 1

Questions 69.1 and 69.2 are related to the following stem:

A 48-year-old male presents to a health fair with questions about heart failure (HF). The gentleman states that his father was recently diagnosed with HF and is concerned about his risk. He works a sedentary job as an accountant for a health insurance company. He tries to have a healthy lifestyle including weekly exercise and a low-fat, low-carbohydrate diet.

69.1 For the patient in **Case 1**, what is his lifetime risk of developing heart failure with reduced ejection fraction (HFrEF)?

- A. 6.8%
- B. 15.1%
- C. 10.6%
- D. 21.3%
- E. 18.8%

69.2 The patient in **Case 1** works as an accountant for a health insurance company and is curious about the economic burden of HF. He is also concerned about his father's recent HF diagnosis and prognosis. What is the 5-year mortality of HFrEF and what is the economic burden of HF in the United States?

- A. 40%, 20 billion dollars per year
- B. 45%, 25 billion dollars per year
- C. 50%, 30 billion dollars per year
- D. 55%, 35 billion dollars per year
- E. 60%, 40 billion dollars per year

CASE 2

Questions 69.3 and 69.4 are based on the following question stem:

A new animal model for testing pharmaceutical therapies for HFrEF is being developed. In these models, mice are genetically modified to overactivate the neurohormonal response to hypotension.

Questions and Answers are based on Chapter 69: Heart Failure with Reduced Ejection Fraction by John M. Suffredini and Savitri E. Fedson in Cardiovascular Medicine and Surgery, First Edition.

Section 5: Heart Failure

69.3 For the patient in **Case 2**, which of the following is **NOT** a result of stimulation of the neurohormonal axes?
  A. Increased catecholamines released from the myocardium
  B. Increased stimulation of alpha-1 leading to increased left ventricular (LV) afterload
  C. Increased sodium channels in the ascending loop of Henle
  D. Promotion of collagen synthesis and fibrosis within the myocardium
  E. None of the above

69.4 For the patient in **Case 2**, a second generation of the genetically modified mice was found to overexpress a compensatory mechanism in response to the overactivation of the renin-angiotensin-aldosterone system (RAAS). The compensatory mechanism in these mice will cause a release of what hormone with increased expression of which receptor?
  A. BNP (brain natriuretic peptide), natriuretic peptide receptor NPR-B
  B. ANP (atrial natriuretic peptide), natriuretic peptide receptor NPR-A
  C. Angiotensin, angiotensin receptor
  D. Aldosterone, tyrosine kinase receptor
  E. A and B

69.5 A 68-year-old African American female with a past medical history of diabetes, hypertension, and obesity presents to the clinic with 3 weeks of progressively worsening dyspnea on exertion. The patient's BNP is 133. Which of the following factors does **NOT** affect BNP?
  A. African American race
  B. Obesity
  C. Age
  D. Sepsis
  E. Gender

69.6 A 65-year-old female presents to the emergency department with worsening dyspnea with exertion for the last 2 months. The patient has a past medical history of type 2 diabetes mellitus (DMT2), hypertension, and chronic kidney disease. The patient denies any palpitations but states she will occasionally feel fluttering in her chest with exertion in addition to the dyspnea. Patient's vital signs are significant for a blood pressure (BP) of 136/92 mm Hg, pulse O_2 of 96% on room air, and heart rate (HR) of 98 beats per minute (bpm). Electrocardiogram (ECG) performed in the emergency department revealed sinus tachycardia. High-sensitivity troponins were elevated. Which of the following etiology is responsible for the elevated troponin?
  A. Acute coronary syndrome
  B. Atrial fibrillation
  C. LV strain
  D. Pulmonary embolism
  E. None of the above

CASE 3

Questions 69.7 and 69.38 are based on the following question stem:

A 48-year-old male with a past medical history of HFrEF presents to the cardiology clinic for guideline-directed medical therapy. He denies chest pain, shortness of breath, palpitations, or dyspnea on exertion. The patient has a 20-year history of cocaine abuse. The patient has recently graduated from rehab and has not been using any illicit drugs for the past year. The patient's most recent echocardiogram shows an ejection fraction (EF) of 30% to 35%. Patient's vitals are taken and his BP is 132/74 mm Hg and his HR is 60 bpm.

69.7 In consideration of the patient from **Case 3**, which of the following mechanisms has been shown to improve mortality in patients with HFrEF?

- A. NPR agonist
- B. NPR antagonist
- C. Neprilysin enzyme inhibitor
- D. Renin inhibitor
- E. None of the above

69.8 For the patient in **Case 3**, follow-up echocardiogram showed EF greater than 50%. What is the definition of LV recovery?

- A. Normalization of left ventricular ejection fraction (LVEF) to greater than 50%
- B. Normalization of the molecules and gross structure changes of the heart
- C. LV end-systolic pressure-volume relationship to normal
- D. Decrease in left ventricular end-diastolic dimension (LVEDD) of 10%
- E. A and B

CASE 4

Questions 69.9 and 69.10 are related to the following question stem:

A 54-year-old male presents to the cardiology clinic for his annual appointment. The patient has been following up with his cardiologist since his diagnosis of HFrEF 4 years ago. The patient works as a CEO for an investment banker and lives a sedentary lifestyle. The patient drinks five to six drinks about five times a week but denies any tobacco use. He is very stressed at work due to the current economic situation. His BP was previously elevated, but since starting his HF medications, it has been well controlled. The patient only experiences symptoms with exertion after one flight of stairs which has been stable for the last 2 years. The patient's initial echocardiogram showed an EF of 30% to 35%. The patient's most recent echocardiogram showed an EF of 50% to 55%.

69.9 For the patient in **Case 4**, which of the following etiologies is **NOT** associated with better outcomes for LV recovery?

- A. Hypothyroidism
- B. Chemotherapy-related toxicity
- C. Alcohol
- D. Viral myocarditis
- E. None of the above

Section 5: Heart Failure

69.10 For the patient in **Case 4**, which of the following clinical factors are associated with LV recovery?
A. NYHA (New York Heart Association) class
B. Ethnicity/race
C. Hypertension
D. Less fibrosis
E. All of the above

ANSWERS

69.1 The correct answer is C.
Rationale: The lifetime risk for the development of HFrEF is 10.6% in males. Approximately 6% of the population will have asymptomatic LV dysfunction without clinical symptoms consistent with HF. It is estimated that 750,000 new cases of HF will be diagnosed each year by 2040. This is due to the incidence of HF doubling each decade of life.

69.2 The correct answer is C.
Rationale: HF is associated with a 5-year mortality of approximately 50% and accounts for 5% of all cardiovascular deaths. Other strong predictors of mortality include renal function, serum sodium concentration, age, and systolic BP. The health care cost burden for HF is significant. The total cost associated with the health care services and lost worker productivity are estimated to be more than 30 billion a year and represent 2% of all health care spending. This includes new pharmacologic agents and device therapy which have improved outcomes but significantly contributed to the rising cost of care. By 2030, the direct health care cost of HF will exceed 50 billion dollars.

69.3 The correct answer is E.
Rationale: The neurohormonal axis helps regulate BP and perfusion and responds to a fall in the cardiac output through various hormonal compensatory mechanisms. The sympathetic nervous system (SNS) activation results in the release of catecholamines by the adrenal medulla and from the myocardium (A). This increases myocardial oxygen demand and causes downregulation of the cardiac beta-adrenergic receptors. In the peripheral vasculature, the alpha receptor activation causes vasoconstriction and increased LV afterload (B). In the kidneys, there is an increased production of renin due to decreased blood flow through the juxtaglomerular apparatus in addition to direct activation of renin on the juxtaglomerular apparatus which triggers the RAAS. Angiotensin increases the expression of sodium channels in the ascending loop of Henle (C) and induces the release of aldosterone from the zona glomerulosa in the adrenal cortex and antidiuretic hormone (ADH) from the posterior pituitary gland. Aldosterone increases sodium reabsorption and promotes collagen synthesis and fibrosis within the myocardium (D). ADH leads to the insertion of aquaporin-2 channels in the collecting duct allowing for increased water reabsorption.

The short-term compensation for declining cardiac output leads to increased neurohormonal axes activation leading to increased blood volume, increased cardiac contractility, and peripheral vasoconstriction.

69.4 The correct answer is E.
Rationale: BNP and ANP will be released as a direct result of increased wall strain on the atrium and ventricle. In general, BNP and ANP will cause excretion of water and sodium which will lower systemic BP and slow the progression of LV remodeling. These peptides bind to NPRs A and B, which are found in the kidneys, vascular smooth muscles, adrenal gland, and myocardium. Once stimulated, this causes an increase in cyclic guanosine monophosphate (cGMP), which will inhibit the Na/Cl transporter and inhibit RAAS activation in the juxtaglomerular apparatus. cGMP will also inhibit the secretion of aldosterone in the adrenal cortex. In the smooth muscle, it will cause smooth muscle dilation. Finally, it protects cardiac myocytes against apoptosis and cardiac fibroblast proliferation. These enzymes are degraded by neprilysin.

69.5 The correct answer is E.
Rationale: The diagnosis of HF can be aided by serum biomarkers with the most used biomarkers being BNP and N-terminal prob-type natriuretic peptide (NT-proBNP). Noncardiac factors of obesity and African American race may decrease serum BNP. Other factors that may increase serum BNP include significant pulmonary disease, pulmonary edema, older age, renal disease, and sepsis. Gender has not been described to affect BNP. This patient's BNP is above 100 which is 90% sensitive for the diagnosis of HF but may be falsely lowered given a history of obesity and ethnicity (**Table 69.1**).

TABLE 69.1 Noncardiac Influence on Natriuretic Peptides

Diagnosis of Heart Failure	
BNP >100 pg/mL NT-proBNP >900 pg/mL	90% sensitivity
Noncardiac factors that decrease BNP/ NT-proBNP	**Obesity African American race**
Noncardiac factors that increase BNP/ NT-proBNP	Significant pulmonary disease Pulmonary embolism Older age Renal disease Sepsis

BNP, brain (or b-type) natriuretic peptide; NT-proBNP, N-terminal pro b-type natriuretic peptide.

69.6 The correct answer is C.
Rationale: Troponin elevation can occur in several cardiac conditions. This patient is presenting with signs and symptoms of HF. The elevated troponin in this patient is most likely related to LV strain and myocardial injury. The ECG shows sinus tachycardia which could also further contribute to increased myocardial oxygen demand.

The patient's ECG was negative for atrial fibrillation but would still need to be ruled out given her history of chest fluttering. Acute coronary syndrome is less likely given the clinical context and lack of ischemia found on ECG. Pulmonary embolism can cause elevated troponin secondary to right heart strain; however, hypoxia is not identified (normal pulse O_2).

69.7 The correct answer is C:
Rationale: This patient has a history of HFrEF. His EF is reduced, but he does not show any signs or symptoms of decompensated HF. NPRs are the receptors that BNP and ANP bind to and there are currently no medications that have targeted these receptors and improved HFrEF outcomes. Renin inhibitors have also been investigated but have failed to demonstrate any significant improvement in HF outcomes and are not currently recommended. A new medication class that has been recently approved for congestive heart failure (CHF) management is neprilysin inhibitors. Neprilysin is the enzyme responsible for the breakdown of ANP and BNP. These receptors act as a counter regulatory mechanism to RAAS and SNS. Sacubitril is the only medication in this class and is sold as a combination with an angiotensin receptor blocker (ARB, valsartan) under the brand name Entresto.

69.8 The correct answer is E:
Rationale: There is a debate over whether the LV can recover or whether there is reverse remodeling of the myocardial maladaptation. The definition of LV recovery has been accepted as the normalization of the LVEF to more than 50% with additional normalization of the molecular, cellular, and gross structure changes of the heart (A and B). Reversely, a remodeled left ventricle is defined as a shift in LV end-diastolic pressure-volume relationship to normal, an absolute increase in LVEF of 10% to 35%, and a decrease in LVEDD of 10%. Approximately 40% of patients receiving guideline-directed medical therapy will demonstrate an improvement in LVEF. There is a correlation between the dosage of the medical therapy and the improvement in LVEF.

69.9 The correct answer is A:
Rationale: Some etiology of HF is associated with better outcomes. HFrEF etiologies that have been shown to be associated with better outcomes and recovered EF include stress-induced, chemotherapy-related, tachycardia-induced, alcohol, viral myocarditis, peripartum, and recent onset dilated cardiomyopathy. Hypothyroidism etiology is not associated with a better prognosis in the recovery of the LVEF.

69.10 The correct answer is E:
Rationale: Clinical factors that determine LV recovery include hypertension, non-African American race, less fibrosis, and lower NYHA class. Magnetic resonance imaging (MRI) may help identify patients without mid-wall late gadolinium enhancement who are most likely to have recovery. Patients who experience LV recovery have a 49% reduction in mortality and improvement in quality of life. Once these patients recover, they should remain on guideline-directed medical therapy indefinitely.

DILATED CARDIOMYOPATHY*

John Tremblay and Mikhail Torosoff

CHAPTER 70

QUESTIONS

70.1 Which of the following is characterized by dilated cardiomyopathy (DCM)?

  A. Hypertension
  B. Valvular disease
  C. Congenital disease
  D. Ischemic heart disease
  E. None of the above

70.2 Which of the following statements is most accurate in describing the incidence of DCM in the United States?

  A. 36 cases per 100,000 population, women greater than men, fifth and sixth decade of life
  B. 36 cases per 100,000 population, women greater than men, third and fourth decade of life
  C. 1:2,500 individuals, men greater than women, third and fourth decade of life
  D. 1:2,500 individuals, men greater than women, fifth and sixth decade of life
  E. None of the above

70.3 A 49-year-old male presents to the clinic for a heart murmur evaluation. The patient was undergoing an evaluation for a right total knee replacement by his primary care who detected a systolic murmur. On evaluation today, the physical examination is significant for a mitral regurgitation murmur and displacement of the point of maximum impulse (PMI) laterally. Due to the patient's knee pain, he has been sedentary for the last 1 to 2 years. The patient denies any symptoms besides right knee pain. A follow-up echocardiogram was ordered and showed a newly reduced left ventricular ejection fraction (LVEF) of 30% to 35%. During the preoperative evaluation, the patient underwent basic blood work, which included a normal complete blood count (CBC), comprehensive metabolic panel (CMP), magnesium, thyroid-stimulating hormone (TSH), and hemoglobin A1c (A1c). Which of the following is the next **BEST** test for this patient?

  A. Left heart catheterization
  B. Coronary computed tomography
  C. Nuclear stress test
  D. Echocardiography stress test
  E. All of the above

---

*Questions and Answers are based on Chapter 70: Dilated Cardiomyopathy by Reema Hasan, Taylor Alexander Lebeis, Supriya Shore, and Monica Mechele Colvin in Cardiovascular Medicine and Surgery, First Edition.

CASE 1

Questions 70.4 and 70.5 are related to the following question stem.

A 74-year-old male with a past medical history of osteoarthritis and DCM re-presents to the clinic for further evaluation. The patient had previously undergone a left heart cardiac catheterization which showed nonobstructive coronary disease. Prior echocardiography revealed left ventricular (LV) dilation and an ejection fraction (EF) of 35% to 40%. Electrocardiogram (ECG) performed in the office was significant for decreased QRS amplitude. There were no bundle branch blocks, atrioventricular (AV) blocks, or ST changes. The patient denies any history of autoimmune disease, recent infections, or illicit drug use.

70.4 Cardiac magnetic resonance imaging (MRI) was ordered for the patient in **Case 1**. Which of the following would **MOST LIKELY** be seen on cardiac MRI?
- A. Global subendocardial late gadolinium enhancement (LGE)
- B. Early after injection enhancement of LGE
- C. Late enhancement in T2-weighted gadolinium in the mid-myocardial basal segment
- D. Increased epicardial signal intensity of T1-weighted post-gadolinium contrast sequence in a noncoronary distribution
- E. None of the above

70.5 The diagnosis of amyloidosis is suspected for the patient in **Case 1**. Which of the following studies can differentiate between transthyretin and light-chain amyloidosis?
- A. Positive emission tomography imaging with fluorodeoxyglucose
- B. Technetium pyrophosphate
- C. Tc-3,3-diphosphono-1,2-propanodicarboxylic acid
- D. All of the above
- E. None of the above

70.6 A 63-year-old woman with a past medical history of metastatic breast cancer complicated by DCM presents to the clinic for follow-up. The patient is being treated with high dose doxorubicin (400 mg/m^2) for her breast cancer. Currently, she is asymptomatic, denies any dyspnea on exertion, chest pain, paroxysmal nocturnal dyspnea (PND), or palpitations. The patient's most recent echocardiogram revealed an EF of 35% to 40%. Her current medications include carvedilol 12.5 mg bid, lisinopril 20 mg daily, and tamoxifen 20 mg daily. Which of the following medication changes would benefit this patient?
- A. Change lisinopril 20 mg to losartan 100 mg daily.
- B. Change carvedilol 12.5 mg to atenolol 50 mg daily.
- C. Add dexrazoxane 50 mg/m^2 infusion.
- D. None of the above

70.7 A 68-year-old African American male presents to the cardiology clinic for evaluation of his persistent symptoms of dyspnea. The patient has persistent symptoms of dyspnea on exertion and becomes short of breath when performing his daily activities, including when he cooks and cleans. The patient is currently on carvedilol 25 mg bid, sacubitril/valsartan (Entresto) 49/51 mg, spironolactone 25 mg daily, bumetanide

1 mg daily, and empagliflozin 10 mg daily. The patient's vitals were obtained, and his heart rate (HR) is 68 beats per minute (bpm) (sinus rhythm), blood pressure (BP) is 128/72 mm Hg, and pulse oxygenation is 98% room air. Which of the following medications should be added to this patient's current therapeutic regimen?

A. Lisinopril 40 mg daily
B. Hydralazine 10 mg tid
C. Isosorbide dinitrate 40 mg bid
D. Ivabradine 5 mg bid
E. B and C

70.8 A 61-year-old male is following up in the cardiology clinic for management of his DCM. The patient was hospitalized 9 months ago with acute decompensated heart failure (HF) exacerbation. Recent left heart catheterization showed nonobstructive coronary arteries. His medications have slowly been titrated up to improve his symptoms. His symptoms have been stable, and he remains in New York Heart Association (NYHA) class II. Which of the following interventions would be recommended for implantable cardioverter-defibrillator (ICD) or cardiac resynchronization therapy (CRT)?

A. 1 month of guideline-directed medical therapy (GDMT), with greater than 1 year expected survival
B. 3 months on GDMT, with greater than 6 months of expected survival
C. 6 months on GDMT, with greater than 6 months of expected survival
D. Left bundle branch block (LBBB) with QRS duration greater than 120 milliseconds, with 1 year expected survival
E. None of the above

70.9 An 83-year-old male with a past medical history of DCM secondary to amyloidosis presents to the cardiology office for follow-up. The patient suffered from complete heart block 2 years ago status post permanent pacemaker (PPM). Over the last 3 months, the patient has had difficulty tolerating his HF medications. The patient was unable to tolerate any beta-blockers due to episodes of presyncope and syncope. He experienced angioedema secondary to angiotensin-converting enzyme (ACE) inhibitor treatment. The patient's diuretics have also been reduced from furosemide 40 mg daily to furosemide 20 mg daily. His BP today was 94/56 mm Hg. Which of the following medications is contraindicated in this patient?

A. Diflunisal
B. Tafamidis
C. Patisiran
D. Digoxin
E. Doxycycline

70.10 A 34-year-old African American female presents 37 weeks gestation to the hospital for worsening shortness of breath and right calf pain. The patient was in her usual state of health and her pregnancy had been uncomplicated until about 2 weeks ago when she started developing dyspnea on exertion and shortness of breath. The patient had an echocardiogram performed which showed an LVEF of 40%. Vital signs are BP 92/58 mm Hg, HR 86 bpm, and pulse oxygenation 90% on 2 L. Physical examination is significant for bibasilar inspiratory crackles R>L. Jugular vein distention

(JVD) measured 8 cm. The right lower extremity has 3+ edema and tenderness to palpation compared to 1+ edema on the left. Venous Doppler was performed which was significant for a deep venous thrombosis. Which of the following medications should be initiated at this time?

A. Heparin, losartan, metoprolol succinate
B. Unfractionated heparin, hydralazine, dinitrate
C. Low-molecular weight heparin, nadolol
D. Low-molecule weight heparin bridge to warfarin, lisinopril, carvedilol
E. None of the above

ANSWERS

70.1 The correct answer is E:
Rationale: DCM refers to a spectrum of heterogeneous myocardial disorders that are characterized by depressed myocardial performance and ventricular dilation in the absence of hypertension, valvular disease, congenital disease, or ischemic heart disease. According to the American Heart Association (AHA) guidelines, their classification schemes are divided into two major groups based on predominant organ involvement with these two groups being primary and secondary cardiomyopathy. In primary cardiomyopathy, the disease is solely or predominantly confined to the heart versus in secondary cardiomyopathy where myocardial involvement is part of a generalized systemic disease.

70.2 The correct answer is C:
Rationale: Incidence and prevalence of DCM worldwide are affected by geographic differences, diagnostic criteria, and socioeconomic factors. In the United States, the age-adjusted prevalence of DCM is approximately equal to 36 cases per 100,000 population or 1:2,500 individuals. DCM is more commonly seen in men than women and typically occurs in the third or fourth decade of life.

70.3 The correct answer is E:
Rationale: The diagnosis of DCM begins with a clinical history and physical examination. This patient's knee pain is limiting his function and may prevent the HF symptoms from being revealed. On physical examination, mitral or tricuspid regurgitation can be present due to ventricular enlargement and annular dilation in DCM. After completing the general clinical examination, an ischemic evaluation should be performed to determine whether coronary artery disease is the cause. Ischemic evaluation is not required in patients under the age of 40.

70.4 The correct answer is A:
Rationale: This patient's ECG was significant for low voltage and with previous left heart catheterization (LHC) showing nonobstructive coronary artery disease, the most likely diagnosis is cardiac amyloidosis. On cardiac MRI, amyloidosis can be seen as global subendocardial LGE. Early enhancement of LGE can be seen in other

autoimmune diseases, most specifically systemic lupus erythematosus (SLE). This patient's age, sex, and no previous history of autoimmune disease make SLE unlikely. Late enhancement in T2-weighted gadolinium in the mid-myocardial basal segment is commonly seen in patients with cardiac sarcoidosis. Cardiac sarcoidosis is often accompanied by ECG findings including bundle branch blocks, AV blocks, Q or epsilon waves. Increased epicardial signal intensity in a noncoronary distribution is seen with myocarditis. This patient denies any recent viral infections making this less likely. Cardiac MRI utilization is limited by the cost, availability, and incompatibility with some implanted cardiac devices.

70.5 The correct answer is C.

Rationale: The diagnosis of some cardiomyopathies can be aided with nuclear medicine studies. Increased technetium pyrophosphate uptake can be seen with amyloid infiltration but will not be able to distinguish between light-chain and transthyretin amyloidosis (ATTR). Tc-3,3-diphosphono-1,2-propanodicarboxylic acid is a highly sensitive technique for imaging cardiac ATTR and can be used to differentiate between transthyretin and light-chain amyloidosis. Positive emission tomography is considered the gold standard imaging criteria for the diagnosis of amyloidosis.

70.6 The correct answer is C.

Rationale: The cardiotoxic effects of anthracycline are dose dependent. When higher doses of anthracyclines are needed, cardiotoxicity may be reduced by addition of U.S. Food and Drug Administration (FDA)-approved dexrazoxane, an EDTA (ethylenediaminetetraacetic acid) derivative iron chelator, which decreases formation of the superoxide radicals. Dexrazoxane is available for prevention of anthracycline-mediated cardiomyopathy for patients receiving over 300 mg/m^2 of doxorubicin. In this patient, it would be important to assess the risk/benefits of chemotherapy versus cardiotoxicity.

In patients with chemotherapy-related DCM, guidelines recommend treatment with ACE inhibitors in addition to beta-blockers. There are data to support the use of an angiotensin receptor blocker (ARB) if the patient is unable to tolerate ACE inhibitors, but this patient currently is tolerating all her medications. Changing this patient's beta-blocker from a beta-blocker that has shown to have mortality benefit (carvedilol, bisoprolol, metoprolol succinate) in HF to a different beta-blocker (atenolol) is not recommended.

70.7 The correct answer is E.

Rationale: Patients who are already on an evidence-based HF regimen that includes evidence-based beta-blockes, ARNI (angiotensin receptor neprilysin inhibitor)/ARB, aldosterone antagonist, and sodium-glucose cotransporter 2 (SGLT2) inhibitors should have afterload reducing agents added. Despite his current regimen, the patient is still having symptoms secondary to his HF. The patient at this time would benefit from the addition of hydralazine and isosorbide dinitrate (E). This patient's resting HR is less than 70 bpm and would not benefit from the addition of ivabradine. The addition of an angiotensin-converting enzyme inhibitor (ACEI) and ARB combination has not shown any benefit, but increased side effects when used in combination (**Figure 70.1**).

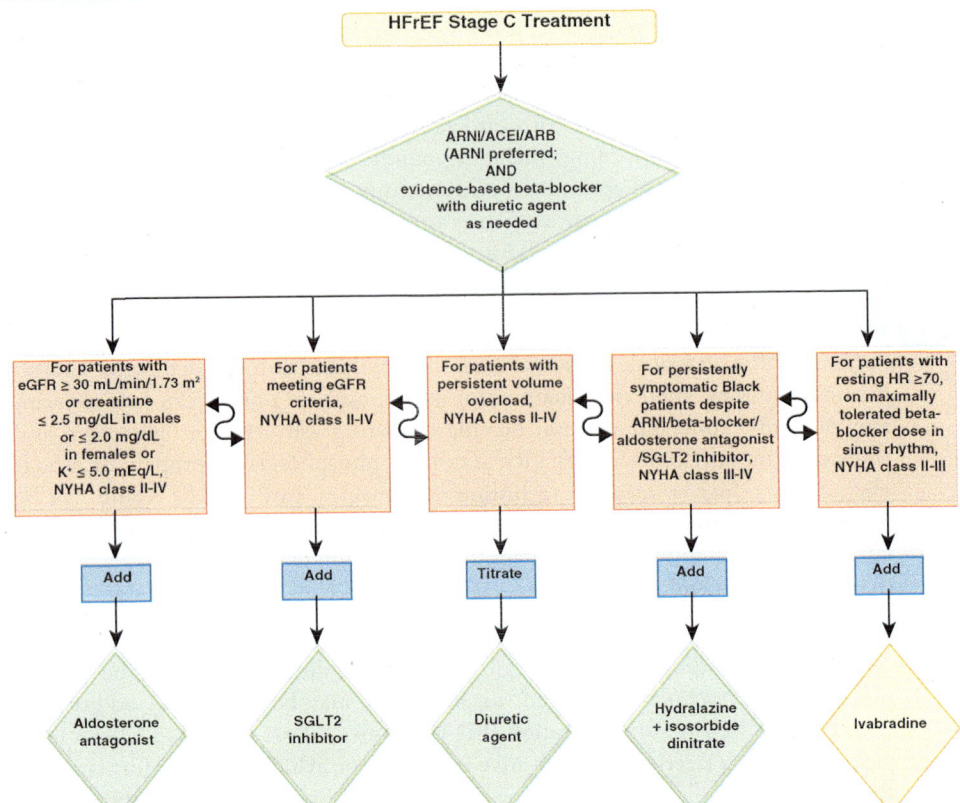

Figure 70.1 Guideline-directed management of symptomatic heart failure. ACEI, angiotensin-converting enzyme inhibitor; ARB, angiotensin receptor blocker; ARNI, angiotensin receptor neprilysin inhibitor; eGFR, estimated glomerular filtration rate; HFrEF, heart failure with reduced ejection fraction; HR, heart rate; NYHA, New York Heart Association; SGLT2, sodium-glucose cotransporter 2. (Reprinted from Maddox TM, Januzzi JL Jr, Allen LA, et al. 2021 update to the 2017 ACC expert consensus decision pathway for optimization of heart failure treatment: answers to 10 pivotal issues about heart failure with reduced ejection fraction: a report of the American College of Cardiology Solution Set Oversight Committee. *J Am Coll Cardiol.* 2021;77(6):772-810. Copyright 2021 by the American College of Cardiology Foundation, with permission.)

70.8 The correct answer is E.

Rationale: In patients with DCM with an LVEF less than or equal to 35%, ICD has been shown to reduce the incidence of sudden cardiac death. Guidelines recommend ICD placement in all patients with LVEF less than 35% secondary to nonischemic DCM despite maximally tolerated GDMT for at least 3 months with NYHA class II symptoms or worse and at least 1 year of expected survival. CRT is also recommended in patients with NYHA class II to IV symptoms and LBBB with a QRS duration of greater than or equal to 150 milliseconds. CRT is associated with improved LV systolic function and remodeling with reduced mitral regurgitation leading to improved symptoms and survival. Patients who receive CRT should be on at least 3 months of GDMT before initiation.

70.9 The correct answer is D.

Rationale: Digoxin is contraindicated in patients with amyloidosis as it has a high affinity for amyloid fibrils, which will predispose the patient to digoxin cardiotoxicity. The standard use of GDMT therapy is challenging in patients with amyloidosis due to the patient's hypotension with diuretics. In addition, vasodilators should be used with caution due to amyloidosis' restrictive cardiac physiology. Beta-blockers should also be used cautiously since the cardiac output is HR dependent. Both diflunisal and tafamidis stabilize the transthyretin tetramer and reduce the formation of transthyretin amyloid (ATTR). In a randomized trial, tafamidis reduced mortality and symptom burden in patients with ATTR cardiomyopathy. Tafamidis is now recommended and has been approved by the FDA for patients with ATTR cardiac disease and NYHA class I-III symptoms, although the cost may be prohibitive for some patients. While there are no randomized clinical trials for diflunisal and ATTR cardiac disease, single center and retrospective studies suggest tolerability. Tafamidis has shown to reduce mortality and symptom burden in patients with ATTR cardiomyopathy. Diflunisal currently has no randomized clinical trials, but single center studies suggest its use. New agents such as patisiran are anti-TTR interfering ribonucleic acid, which lower serum protein levels. Doxycycline therapy in amyloidosis is currently under investigation.

70.10 The correct answer is B.

Rationale: Peripartum cardiomyopathy is defined as cardiomyopathy with LVEF less than 45% that presents during the last month of pregnancy or within the first 5 months postpartum in the absence of other causes of HF and cardiomyopathy. Risk factors include age greater than 30 years, African descent, multiparity, preeclampsia, or hypertension. Peripartum cardiomyopathy is associated with higher rates of thromboembolism. Anticoagulation with heparin is recommended during pregnancy and the first 2 months after delivery. In addition, ACE inhibitors and ARBs are contraindicated during pregnancy, and hydralazine combined with nitrates are favored. Beta-blockers are safe in pregnancy, but beta-one selective agents are preferred during pregnancy as nonselective beta-blockers may promote uterine contractions. Most women will recover within 6 months. Women with persistent LV dysfunction before subsequent pregnancy are associated with a 16% mortality.

HYPERTROPHIC CARDIOMYOPATHY*

Robert L Carhart, Mostafa Vasigh and Muhammad Malik

CHAPTER **71**

QUESTIONS

71.1 What are the most common mutations known to cause hypertrophic cardiomyopathy (HCM)?

- A. ACTC1, TPM1
- B. MYL2, MYL3
- C. TNNT2, MYH7
- D. MYH7, MYBPC3

71.2 What are the histopathologic features of HCM?

- A. Myocyte hypertrophy, disarray, and interstitial fibrosis
- B. Noncaseating granuloma formation
- C. Organized parallel myocyte hypertrophy
- D. Interstitial amyloid fibril deposits

71.3 A 34-year-old male is brought to the emergency department (ED) after he loses consciousness when he is out for his daily jog. Currently, his vitals are within normal limits. A grade 2/6 systolic murmur is **BEST** heard at the left sternal border. The intensity of the murmur increases when he stands up from a seated position. An echocardiogram was done which identified HCM with left ventricular outflow tract obstruction (LVOTO). Which of the following hemodynamic changes causes decreased LVOTO in this patient?

- A. Increased inotropy and increased preload
- B. Increased afterload and decreased preload
- C. Decreased inotropy and increased preload
- D. Increased afterload and increased inotropy

71.4 What are the most common functional defects identified in sarcomeres containing mutant proteins in HCM?

- A. Impaired K sensitivity and increased force generation
- B. Impaired Ca sensitivity, altered actin-myosin cross-bridge cycling, and inefficient force generation
- C. Impaired Na sensitivity with maintained actin-myosin bridge cycling
- D. Increased ATP/ADP-independent association and dissociation of actin and myosin

*Questions and Answers are based on Chapter 71: Hypertrophic Cardiomyopathy by Ali J. Marian in Cardiovascular Medicine and Surgery, First Edition.

CHAPTER 71 | Hypertrophic Cardiomyopathy

71.5 What are the most common arrhythmias detected in symptomatic patients with HCM?
   A. Supraventricular tachycardia (SVT) and different degrees of atrioventricular (AV) blocks
   B. Atrial fibrillation and atrial flutter
   C. Nonsustained ventricular tachycardia (NSVT), SVT, and atrial fibrillation
   D. NSVT and different degrees of AV blocks

71.6 What are the hallmark findings of echocardiogram in patients with HCM?
   A. Decreased left ventricular ejection fraction (LVEF) along with symmetric septal wall thickness greater than 13 mm
   B. Increased/normal LVEF with left ventricular wall thickness greater than 20 mm
   C. Increased/normal LVEF with asymmetric left ventricular wall thickness greater than 13 mm
   D. Decreased LVEF with asymmetric left ventricular wall thickness greater than 13 mm

71.7 What are the hallmark electrocardiogram (ECG) findings in HCM?
   A. Increased QRS voltage, ST/T-wave changes, left atrial enlargement, and deep Q waves in inferior and lateral leads
   B. Increased QRS voltage, right bundle branch block (RBBB), and ST/T-wave changes
   C. Increased QRS voltage, left bundle branch block (LBBB), and ST/T-wave changes
   D. Decreased QRS voltage, ST/T-wave changes, left atrial enlargement, and deep Q waves in inferior and lateral leads

71.8 What are the clinical utilities of genetic testing in patients suspected of having HCM?
   A. No role in diagnosis but may assist in risk stratification of family members
   B. Can assist with diagnosis, risk stratification of family members, and guide management in phenocopy conditions
   C. Can assist with diagnosis and risk stratification of family members but no role in treatment
   D. Only used for family risk stratification

71.9 A 35-year-old female visits the clinic for evaluation after an episode of syncope. She was out running in the afternoon when she felt lightheaded and lost consciousness. The patient explains that she has had other episodes of feeling lightheaded during her runs in the past year. She is in good shape and has no other past medical history. She explains that her father died suddenly at the age of 32. A physical examination reveals the presence of a harsh systolic murmur. An echocardiogram is performed and reveals asymmetric interventricular septal hypertrophy left side. What are the common pharmacologic therapies used for this patient?
   A. Beta-blockers, calcium channel blockers, and angiotensin-converting enzyme (ACE) inhibitors
   B. Beta-blockers, ACE inhibitors, and propafenone
   C. Calcium channel blockers, flecainide, and disopyramide
   D. Beta-blockers, calcium channel blockers, and disopyramide

71.10 During her stay in the hospital, the patient in **Question 71.9** is found to have a 2-minute run of ventricular tachycardia on telemetry which resolves spontaneously. What would you recommend next?

   A. Start patient on amiodarone.
   B. Start 1-month Holter monitoring before discharge.
   C. Refer for an implantable cardioverter-defibrillator (ICD) placement.
   D. Since this episode only lasted 2 minutes and resolved spontaneously, the patient can be discharged with close follow–up.

ANSWERS

71.1 The correct answer is D:
Rationale: Mutations in the *MYH7* and *MYBPC3* genes, the latter coding for myosin-binding protein C3, are the most common causes for HCM, being responsible for 40% to 50% of HCM. Mutations in the *TNNT2* (cardiac troponin T), *TNNI3* (cardiac troponin I), *TPM1* (a-tropomyosin), *ACTC1* (cardiac-actin), *MYL2* (myosin light chain), *MYL3* (myosin light chain 3), and *CSRP3* (muscle LIM domain protein) genes are responsible for less than 10% of the HCM cases.

71.2 The correct answer is A:
Rationale: Myocyte hypertrophy, disarray, is defined as the disorganized orientation of myocytes, and interstitial fibrosis comprises histologic features of HCM. Although myocyte hypertrophy and interstitial fibrosis are common to various myocardial diseases, disarray, typically involving greater than 10% of the myocardium, is the pathologic hallmark of HCM. Interstitial fibrosis, clinically assessed by detection of late gadolinium enhancement (LGE) on cardiac magnetic resonance (CMR) imaging, is common in patients with HCM.

71.3 The correct answer is C:
Rationale: A unique characteristic of HCM is the presence of LVOTO, which occurs because of encroachment of the hypertrophic septum on the left ventricular outflow tract (LVOT) and systolic anterior motion of the mitral valve anterior leaflet owing to the Venturi effect induced by the hyperdynamic contraction. LVOTO is typically detected by Doppler echocardiography or cardiac catheterization upon documentation of a systolic pressure gradient between the left ventricular cavity and the subaortic valve region. LVOTO varies with changes in contractility, preload, and afterload. Increased contractility or reduced left ventricular volume increases LVOTO. Conversely, negative inotropic agents and increased left ventricular volume reduce LVOTO. The Valsalva maneuver provokes or increases LVOTO during the straining phase.

71.4 The correct answer is B:
Rationale: Sarcomeres containing the mutant proteins exhibit a diverse array of functional effects, such as impaired Ca^{2+} sensitivity, altered actin-myosin cross-bridge

cycling, and inefficient force generation. Functional effects of the mutations vary among different mutations and the involved genes. Mutations in the MYH7 and MYBPC3 proteins typically affect adenosine diphosphate/adenosine triphosphate (ADP/ATP)-dependent association and dissociation of actin and myosin molecules during a cardiac cycle and consequently, inefficient force generation. Likewise, increased Ca^{2+} sensitivity of the myofilaments is the main effect of mutations involving the thin filament proteins. The net effect of this functional phenotype at the molecular level is an increased number of myosin molecules bound to actin at any given moment during a cardiac cycle.

71.5 The correct answer is C.

Rationale: Palpitations, often caused by SVT or NSVT, is a common symptom in patients with HCM. NSVT is present in 20% to 30% of the patients and is a risk factor for sudden cardiac death (SCD), particularly in the symptomatic young patients. Syncope is relatively uncommon but a serious manifestation of HCM, as it is usually caused by cardiac arrhythmias and less commonly by severe LVOTO or autonomic dysfunction. The annual incidence of atrial fibrillation in patients with HCM is approximately 2% to 3%. A quarter of patients with HCM experience atrial fibrillation, which is poorly tolerated by most patients because of the shortening of the left ventricular filling period resulting from the rapid ventricular rate and loss of the atrial contribution to ventricular filling. Atrial fibrillation is particularly common in patients with LVOTO, heart failure with preserved ejection fraction (HFpEF), and left atrial enlargement. It is also a major risk factor for thromboembolic stroke, and when detected, an oral anticoagulant should be administered to prevent stroke.

71.6 The correct answer is C.

Rationale: Unexplained cardiac hypertrophy, typically detected on an echocardiogram, is the clinical diagnostic hallmark of HCM. The diagnosis is commonly based on detection of a left ventricular wall thickness of 13 mm or greater, unexplained by the loading conditions, and a preserved or increased LVEF. Using a cutoff point of 15 mm or greater increases the specificity of the diagnosis but reduces the sensitivity of the echocardiographic diagnosis. A Z score representing a deviation from the expected values in a matched group is used to detect cardiac hypertrophy in children.

Cardiac hypertrophy is often asymmetric with a predominant involvement of the interventricular septum, which is referred to as asymmetric septal hypertrophy (ASH). However, hypertrophy may involve the apex of the left ventricle only, which is denoted as apical HCM. Rarely, hypertrophy is restricted to other regions of the left ventricle, including the lateral or posterior wall. The expression of cardiac hypertrophy is age dependent. It is infrequent in childhood, typically develops during adolescence, and seldom initially manifests after the fifth decade of life. A unique phenotypic feature of HCM is the presence of LVOTO, which is present at rest in about one-third of the patients and inducible by exercise or inotropic stimulation in another third.

71.7 The correct answer is A.

Rationale: The ECG often provides the first clue to the diagnosis of HCM by showing evidence of cardiac hypertrophy. ECG abnormalities, found in most patients with HCM, often precede expression of cardiac hypertrophy on the echocardiogram.

The ECG findings are notable for the presence of increased QRS voltage, secondary ST and T changes, left atrial enlargement, and deep Q waves in the inferior and lateral leads that mimic myocardial infarction. Apical HCM has characteristic electrocardiographic manifestations with deep T-wave inversions in the precordial leads. In addition, preexcitation and delta wave, resembling Wolff-Parkinson-White, is detected in 2% to 3% of patients with HCM. The presence of preexcitation findings on ECG suggests a phenocopy condition.

71.8 The correct answer is B.
Rationale: Clinical utilities of genetic testing include accurate diagnosis of HCM from the phenocopy conditions and the preclinical diagnosis and stratification of the family members at risk. Family members who carry the pathogenic variant are at increased risk and require periodic phenotypic evaluation to detect HCM early and intervene to prevent major events such as SCD. This is clinically impactful because SCD is often the first manifestation of HCM. Conversely, family members who have not inherited the pathogenic variants are not at an increased risk of HCM and do not require frequent clinical evaluation. Moreover, identification of the causal gene/mutation might enable gene/mutation-specific therapies, as they become available. Finally, genetic testing could lead to the identification of the phenocopy conditions that mimic HCM, which encompasses about 3% to 5% of the adult patients with HCM. The distinction is clinically valuable as the natural history and treatment of the phenocopy conditions differ and specific therapies might be available, such as enzyme replacement therapy for Anderson-Fabry disease, a lysosomal storage disorder.

71.9 The correct answer is D.
Rationale: For symptomatic patients with HCM, the first and likely cornerstone of therapy is a beta-adrenergic receptor blocker (beta-blocker), specifically, one without intrinsic sympathetic activity. Beta-blockers are useful for relieving or attenuating symptoms of palpitations, chest pain, and dyspnea as well as exercise-induced LVOTO. The benefits of beta-blockers in reducing the risk of SCD are unclear. Their typical side effects, such as excessive fatigue, exercise intolerance, and central nervous system symptoms, are the main hindrance to the use of beta-blockers in patients with HCM. The second line of therapy—and the first line in those who do not tolerate beta-blockers—are the L-type calcium channel blockers, such as verapamil or diltiazem. The potential beneficial effects of the L-type calcium channel blockers are in accord with our understanding of the role of altered Ca^{2+} currents in diastolic dysfunction in HCM. Calcium channel blockers are also helpful in the management of SVT and possibly in slowing the development of HCM in those who carry pathogenic variants in the MYBPC3 gene.

Disopyramide, a negative inotropic agent, in conjunction with a beta-blocker—the latter to reduce the parasympatholytic effects of disopyramide—is used to reduce LVOTO. Diuretics are useful in a subset of patients who have symptoms of heart failure, elevated left ventricular filling pressure, and elevated serum N-terminal pro-brain natriuretic peptide (NT-proBNP) levels. The risk associated with the use of diuretics includes hypovolemia and consequently hypotension and syncope. Antiarrhythmic drugs are used judiciously in the treatment of SVT or NSVT because of the risk of proarrhythmias in the background of a pathologic ventricular substrate.

71.10 The correct answer is D.

Rationale: Although none of the known risk factors reliably predict the risk of SCD, several algorithms have been developed to stratify and identify the individuals at high risk. Implantation of an ICD is indicated in those with a prior episode of cardiac arrest or SVT. A history of recurrent syncope, suggestive of arrhythmias as the cause, as well as the presence of symptomatic NSVT, identifies individuals at high risk. Indication for an ICD is less clear in asymptomatic patients with recurrent NSVT. A history of SCD in more than one family member also denotes a genetic background that is susceptible to cardiac arrhythmias and hence, increased risk of SCD. An ICD is the first choice in symptomatic patients with recurrent NSVT or SVT. The intervention is often complemented with radiofrequency ablation and the use of antiarrhythmic drugs to prevent or reduce the frequency of arrhythmias.

RESTRICTIVE CARDIOMYOPATHY*

Robert L. Carhart, Subash Nepal, and Muhammad Malik

CHAPTER 72

QUESTIONS

72.1 A 68-year-old White male presented with dyspnea on exertion, lower extremities swelling, and orthopnea for a month. Past medical history was significant for bilateral carpel tunnel syndrome and lumbar spinal canal stenosis. The general examination was remarkable for elevated jugular venous pressure (JVP) of 14 cm above the sternal angle, and bilateral 2+ pitting pedal edema. Auscultation of precordium revealed the normal S1 and S2 along with grade 2 mid-to-late-ejection systolic murmur in the aortic area which accentuated on standing to squat position. There were bilateral diffuse crackles on lung auscultation.

Electrocardiogram (ECG) was remarkable for low-voltage QRS complexes. Basic metabolic panel (BMP) and serum troponin levels were normal and serum proBNP (B-type natriuretic peptide) was 1,600 pg/mL. Chest x-ray showed hilar prominence, cephalization of pulmonary vessels, and moderate pleural effusion. A transthoracic echocardiogram showed a normal systolic function with a left ventricular (LV) ejection fraction of 54%, with normal regional wall motion. The interventricular wall thickness was measured to be 1.5 cm, the posterior wall thickness of 1.6 cm, a relative wall thickness of 0.45, and the LV mass index of 115 g/m^2. Severe biatrial enlargement was present with moderate tricuspid regurgitation (TR) with a TR jet velocity of 3 m/s. No systolic anterior motion (SAM) of anterior mitral leaflet or dynamic left ventricular outflow tract (LVOT) obstruction was present. Mitral inflow spectral Doppler showed an *E/A* ratio of 2.5. The tissue Doppler showed reduced septal and lateral mitral annular diastolic velocity. The inferior vena cava measured 2.5 cm in diameter and did not collapse with inspiration. Mild pericardial effusion without tamponade physiology was present. Strain analysis showed base to apex gradient with preserved apical global longitudinal strain.

Which of the following is the **MOST LIKELY** diagnosis?

A. Restrictive cardiomyopathy
B. Hypertrophic cardiomyopathy
C. Idiopathic dilated cardiomyopathy
D. Ischemic cardiomyopathy
E. Chronic constrictive pericarditis

72.2 A 45-year-old African American woman with a past medical history of diabetes mellitus and sickle cell trait presented to the emergency department with palpitations and recurrent syncopal episodes. Her review of systems was remarkable for dyspnea with normal activities for 2 months. General physical examination was unremarkable **EXCEPT** for the left-sided Bell palsy. The cardiovascular system examination was normal. ECG showed the right bundle branch block and was negative for any

Questions and Answers are based on Chapter 72: Restrictive Cardiomyopathies by Gurusher Panjrath and Joseph M. Krepp in Cardiovascular Medicine and Surgery, First Edition.

ischemic ST-segment changes or Q waves. Her BMP was within normal limits and serum troponin was not elevated. Complete blood count (CBC) was remarkable for hemoglobin of 10 and hematocrit of 35%. Iron panels showed a serum ferritin level of 350 ng/mL and transferrin saturation of 25%.

The patient was admitted for further workup. She had another syncopal episode overnight and telemetry showed episodes of nonsustained ventricular tachycardia, 20 beats long at a heart rate of 140/min. Two-dimensional transthoracic echocardiography showed a normal LV cavity size, LV ejection fraction of 45%, thin and akinetic basal septal and lateral walls, and grade I diastolic dysfunction. Chest x-ray revealed hilar prominence and scattered infiltrates bilaterally. Cardiac magnetic resonance (CMR) imaging was performed, which revealed myocardial edema in T2-weighted images and delayed gadolinium enhancement localized to the epicardial and mid-myocardial region of the basal septum and lateral wall with endocardial sparing.

Which of the following is the **MOST LIKELY** diagnosis and **BEST** treatment option for this patient?

A. Myocarditis and expectant management with short-term antiarrhythmics
B. Cardiac sarcoidosis and treatment with steroids and implantable cardioverter-defibrillator (ICD) placement
C. Ischemic cardiomyopathy and treatment with aspirin, statins, and beta-blockers
D. Iron overload cardiomyopathy and treatment with phlebotomy
E. Idiopathic dilated cardiomyopathy and treatment with beta-blockers and renin-angiotensin-aldosterone system (RAAS) inhibitors

72.3 A 20-year-old female with a history of chronic wrist joint pain and mild cognitive impairment presented to the clinic with palpitations and New York Heart Association (NYHA) class III dyspnea for 5 months. She also complained of progressive swelling of the legs, easy fatigability, and yellowish discoloration of the sclera. She had been an avid marathon runner and had stopped running due to poor stamina. Her family history is positive for congestive heart failure in her older sister diagnosed when she was in her 30s. Vitals showed a blood pressure (BP) of 140/90 mm Hg and a pulse rate of 80/min. General physical examination was remarkable for 2+ pitting pedal edema bilaterally and scleral icterus. A cardiovascular system examination revealed a normal S1 and S2, without any murmur. Gastrointestinal system examination was remarkable for mild hepatomegaly.

ECG was normal. BMP was remarkable for random blood glucose of 300 mg/dL and hemoglobin A1C (HBA1C) 7.5%. Hepatic function panels showed aspartate aminotransferase (AST) of 150 U/L, alanine aminotransferase (ALT) of 200 U/L, alkaline phosphatase (ALP) of 300 IU/mL, total bilirubin of 2 mg/dL, and indirect bilirubin of 1.5 mg/dL.

Two-dimensional transthoracic echocardiography showed a mildly dilated interventricular cavity, an interventricular septal diameter of 0.8 cm, a posterior wall diameter of 0.9 cm, and a relative wall thickness of 0.42. The ejection fraction was 45% with diffuse hypokinesis. Both atria were moderately dilated, and a restrictive LV filling pattern was present. No significant valvular heart disease was noted. She was sent home on 2 weeks Holter, which showed episodes of paroxysmal atrial fibrillation, the longest one lasting for about an hour.

Which of the following is the **MOST LIKELY** diagnosis and what is the next **BEST** test?

A. Hereditary hemochromatosis
B. Fabry disease
C. Cardiac amyloidosis
D. Hypertensive heart disease with metabolic syndrome
E. Athlete's heart

72.4 A 40-year-old migrant woman from Nigeria presented to the emergency department with dyspnea on exertion and palpitations for 6 months. She arrived in the United States 2 months ago. Her symptoms began with a fever, chest pain, and periorbital swelling but they have subsided now. Her vitals were remarkable for a pulse rate of 140/min with irregularly irregular rhythm and BP of 120/80 mm Hg. A general physical examination revealed 2+ pitting pedal edema bilaterally and JVP of 14 cm above the sternal angle. Cardiovascular system examination revealed normal S1 and S2 with holosystolic murmur at the apex. Abdominal percussion was positive for moderate ascites.

ECG showed atrial fibrillation with a heart rate of 146/min. Lab work showed proBNP of 1,600 pg/mL with normal serum troponins and BMP. CBC showed a serum total eosinophil count of 1,200/μL. Chest x-ray showed bilateral moderate pleural effusion and cardiomegaly. Two-dimensional transthoracic echocardiography showed a normal ejection fraction, thickened right ventricular, and LV walls, retracted apex, small biventricular cavities, and endomyocardial plaques in LV posterior wall, tethering of mitral valve and tricuspid valve chordal apparatus, moderate mitral and TR, moderate biatrial enlargement, and absent septal bounce. Doppler study showed a restrictive filling pattern with reduced septal and lateral e′ velocities (but with higher lateral e′ compared with septal e′ velocity) and absent significant mitral inflow respirophasic mitral variation. Moderate pericardial effusion was present without tamponade physiology. Echocardiography with contrast showed a filling defect in the LV apex with normal wall motion.

Which of the following is the **MOST LIKELY** diagnosis?

A. Endomyocardial fibrosis
B. Chagas cardiomyopathy
C. Cardiac amyloidosis
D. Constrictive-effusive pericarditis
E. Carcinoid heart disease

72.5 A 30-year-old Caucasian male presented to the clinic with exertional dyspnea, chest pain, and episodes of syncope for about 6 months. The patient endorses burning pain in his feet since his childhood. Family history is positive for sudden cardiac death on the maternal uncle. On examination, vitals and cardiovascular system examination were unremarkable.

BMP, serum troponins, and proBNP were within normal limits. Two-dimensional transthoracic echocardiography showed a diastolic interventricular septal diameter of 2 cm, posterior wall thickness of 2.1 cm, a relative wall thickness of 0.55, and a LV mass index of 125 g/m². Systolic anterior movement of the anterior mitral leaflet and dynamic LVOT obstruction were absent at baseline and with the Valsalva maneuver. Mitral and aortic valves are moderately thickened with moderate aortic and mitral regurgitation, and mild dilation of the ascending aorta. Doppler study showed a restrictive filling pattern. Two-week Holter showed episodes of nonsustained ventricular tachycardia and paroxysmal atrial fibrillation correlating with syncopal episodes. CMR imaging showed delayed gadolinium enhancement predominantly in basal and mid-anterolateral and inferolateral areas. Vasodilator myocardial perfusion single photon emission computed tomography (SPECT) study showed multiple small-sized fixed as well as reversible perfusion defects, and coronary angiogram showed normal coronary arteries with a slow flow.

Which of the following is the **MOST LIKELY** diagnosis?
A. Hypertrophic cardiomyopathy
B. ATTR (amyloidosis transthyretin related) cardiac amyloidosis
C. Fabry disease
D. Ischemic cardiomyopathy
E. Hypertensive heart disease

72.6 A 62-year-old man with a past medical history of carpal tunnel syndrome, lumbar spinal canal stenosis, early satiety, and constipation was admitted to the hospital with progressive dyspnea for 2 months. This is his third admission this year for heart failure exacerbation. He also complains of orthopnea, paroxysmal nocturnal dyspnea, and bilateral moderate pedal edema. General physical examination is remarkable for JVP 15 cm above the sternal angle, 3+ pitting pedal edema, and ascites. Vitals showed a pulse of 105/min, BP of 160/80 mm Hg, respiratory rate of 24/min, and temperature of 36.6 °C.

ECG was remarkable for low-voltage QRS complexes. Lab work showed proBNP of 1,500 pg/mL, normal BMP, and CBC. Chest x-ray showed bilateral moderate pleural effusions, bilateral hilar opacities, and cephalization of pulmonary vessels. Echocardiography showed a normal LV systolic function with moderate concentric hypertrophy with speckling, no dynamic LVOT gradient, moderate aortic stenosis, mild TR, moderate biatrial dilatation, and dilated and noncollapsible inferior vena cava. The transmitral Doppler study showed a restrictive filling pattern. The strain study showed reduced global longitudinal strain with preserved strain in the apex. CMR imaging showed transmural late gadolinium enhancement (LGE). The serum κ/λ free light chain ratio was 0.5, and the serum and urine immune protein immunofixation study was negative.

Which of the following is the next appropriate step in diagnosis?
A. Nuclear scintigraphy/SPECT with Technetium-99m pyrophosphate (Tc 99m pyrophosphate)
B. Cardiac amyloidosis is unlikely as immune electrophoresis is negative, and start treatment for heart failure with preserved ejection fraction (HFpEF)
C. Myocardial biopsy and Congo red stain
D. Genetic testing for ATTR
E. Abdominal fat pad biopsy

72.7 A 55-year-old Caucasian man presented to the clinic with NYHA class IV dyspnea for 6 months along with bilateral lower extremities swelling, chronic cough, and paroxysmal nocturnal dyspnea. He visited urgent care multiple times and was treated with intravenous (IV) diuretics with symptomatic improvement. He has a long-standing history of peripheral neuropathy and has been seeing a neurologist. General physical examination is remarkable for respiratory distress, JVP of 15 cm above the sternal angle, and 3+ bilateral pitting pedal edema. Vitals showed a pulse of 100/min, BP of 130/80 mm Hg, respiratory rate of 30/min, and temperature of 36.6 °C. First and second heart sounds were normally heard without any murmurs. Diffuse crackles were present over all the lung fields.

Lab work showed normal BMP, serum troponins, and proBNP of 2,000 pg/mL. ECG showed low-voltage QRS complexes. Two-dimensional transthoracic echocardiography showed normal LV systolic function, moderate LV concentric hypertrophy without dynamic LVOT gradient, small right ventricular and LV cavity size, and moderately thickened aortic valve with moderate aortic stenosis. Doppler study showed a restrictive LV filling pattern. The global longitudinal strain was reduced with apical sparing. CMR imaging showed a global transmural LGE. The serum κ/λ ratio was normal and the serum and urine protein immunofixation tests were negative. Nuclear scintigraphy and SPECT study with Tc 99m pyrophosphate showed grade 3 myocardial uptake. The patient was treated with IV diuretics with a good response.

Which of the following is the **BEST** treatment option?
A. Tafamidis
B. Supportive management with diuretics as amyloidosis has been ruled out
C. Orthotopic heart transplantation
D. Sacubitril-valsartan
E. Left ventricular assist device (LVAD)

72.8 A 60-year-old man with a past medical history of essential hypertension and hyperlipidemia presented with palpitations and syncope for 2 months. The review of systems is positive for early satiety, chronic back pain, and easy fatigability. He is on hydrochlorothiazide 25 mg daily. A general physical examination showed periorbital purpura and macroglossia, and systemic examination was remarkable for hepatomegaly.

ECG showed low-voltage QRS complexes. BMP and proBNP were within normal limits. Urinalysis was positive for proteinuria. Two-week Holter showed nonsustained ventricular tachycardia. Two-dimensional transthoracic echocardiography showed moderate LV concentric hypertrophy without obstruction. Vasodilator SPECT myocardial perfusion scan showed a normal rest and stress perfusion with normal LV systolic function. The patient was discharged on metoprolol. He came back to the clinic in 2 months with persistent symptoms. His heart rate was 40. Cardiac amyloidosis was suspected.

Which of the following is the next appropriate test?
A. Serum protein electrophoresis (SPEP)
B. Serum-free light chains
C. Beta-2 microglobulin
D. 5-Hydroxyindoleacetic acid (5-HIAA)
E. None of the above

72.9 Which of the following is **TRUE** regarding nuclear Tc 99m pyrophosphate scintigraphy/SPECT scan in the diagnosis of cardiac amyloidosis?

A. In the presence of typical echocardiography and CMR findings, the absence of monoclonal gammopathy with positive Tc 99m pyrophosphate scintigraphy/SPECT scan is diagnostic of ATTR, tissue diagnosis is not required
B. Myocardial biopsy is a must for the diagnosis of ATTR even with positive nuclear scintigraphy/SPECT
C. Positive nuclear scintigraphy rules out AL (amyloidosis light chain) amyloidosis
D. Tc 99m pyrophosphate is a bone radiotracer and uptake is high in AL amyloidosis because the density of microcalcifications is higher in AL amyloid fibrils than in ATTR amyloid.
E. None of the above

72.10 A 55-year-old man with a past medical history of carpal tunnel syndrome, peripheral neuropathy, and nephrotic syndrome presented with recurrent palpitations for 2 months. The review of systems is positive for easy fatigability and dyspnea on exertion. He had multiple hospital admissions due to congestive heart failure exacerbations in the last year. He is currently euvolemic and symptomatically better on diuretics. General physical examination and vitals were normal. Cardiovascular system examination was remarkable for mid-systolic ejection murmur in the aortic area with radiation to bilateral common carotid arteries. Abdominal palpation revealed hepatomegaly.

Echocardiography showed a normal LV systolic function and moderate concentric LV hypertrophy without any obstruction, and moderate calcific aortic stenosis. The transmitral Doppler study showed a restrictive filling pattern. Two-week Holter monitoring showed episodes of paroxysmal atrial fibrillation, the longest one lasting for 15 minutes at a heart rate of 150. His CHA2DS2VASC score is 0. CMR showed transmural LGE and the absence of thrombus in the left atrial appendage. Lab work showed a normal BMP, elevated serum-free light chain assay with κ/λ ratio of 2, and positive serum and urine protein electrophoresis with immunofixation. Urinalysis showed 3+ proteinuria. Nuclear scintigraphy was ordered which was indeterminate.

Which of the following is the next **BEST** step?
A. Cardiac biopsy for Congo red staining
B. Start tafamidis.
C. Referral to a hematologist for chemotherapy and possible stem cell transplantation and start long-term anticoagulation
D. Beta-blocker, angiotensin-converting enzyme inhibitor (ACEI), and sacubitril/valsartan
E. None of the above

ANSWERS

72.1 The correct answer is A.
Rationale: This patient presented with acute decompensated HFpEF with volume overload as suggested by elevated JVP, 2+ pedal edema, and crackles in the lung field. Lab work was remarkable for elevated proBNP, cephalization of pulmonary vessels with hilar prominence, and pleural effusion. All the options listed can cause

acute heart failure with volume overload. The echocardiography showed a normal LV ejection fraction, moderate concentric hypertrophy, and restrictive filling pattern with (*E/A* ratio of >2, severe biatrial enlargement, and reduced both medial and lateral mitral annular tissue velocity). Low-voltage ECG along with preserved LV apical global longitudinal strain with reduced basal and mid strain ("Cherry on top pattern") suggest cardiac amyloidosis as the likely diagnosis. Cardiac amyloidosis is an evolving etiology of restrictive cardiomyopathy. Hypertrophic cardiomyopathy can present in a similar way but an augmentation of a late systolic murmur in an aortic area with increased afterload (standing to squat), and the absence of SAM or LVOT gradient makes it less likely. Idiopathic dilated cardiomyopathy would cause a reduction in LV systolic function and eccentric LV hypertrophy. Ischemic cardiomyopathy is a less likely diagnosis due to normal LV ejection fraction and normal regional wall motion. Chronic constrictive pericarditis would also cause a restrictive filling but with increased medial mitral annular tissue velocity and reduced lateral annular velocity due to tethering of lateral mitral annulus with calcified pericardium (annulus reversus).

KEY POINTS

✔ End-stage cardiomyopathy due to coronary artery disease, chronic pericardial disease, hypertrophic cardiomyopathy, and dilated cardiomyopathy all can cause acute or chronic decompensated heart failure with restrictive filling. Differentiation is important because treatment is different. Cardiac amyloidosis is an evolving cause of restrictive cardiomyopathy in the middle-aged and older adults. An initial ECG followed by echocardiography gives important clues to the diagnosis. The findings suggestive of cardiac amyloidosis are low-voltage ECG, thickened LV walls with biatrial enlargement, restrictive filling pattern, and apical sparing in a global longitudinal strain study. Sometimes, the speckled appearance of the LV walls in nonharmonic echocardiographic imaging can be seen, but this finding is neither sensitive nor specific for the diagnosis of cardiac amyloidosis. This must be followed by CMR imaging, serum-free light chain assays, and serum and urine protein electrophoresis with immunofixation.

72.2 The correct answer is B.

Rationale: This patient of African American descent presented with cardiogenic syncope due to ventricular tachyarrhythmias. She was found to have a syncope due to nonsustained ventricular tachycardia in the hospital. She has Bell palsy on examination, possible hilar lymphadenopathy, and pulmonary infiltrates on chest x-ray, basal septal akinesis with mildly reduced LV ejection fraction in echocardiography, and right bundle branch block in ECG likely due to cardiac sarcoidosis. She likely has a history of undiagnosed pulmonary and nervous system sarcoidosis with hilar lymphadenopathy and bilateral interstitial infiltrates in chest x-ray, and Bell palsy. Cardiac sarcoidosis was confirmed by CMR, which showed delayed gadolinium enhancement suggestive of fibrosis in noncoronary artery distribution as well as myocardial edema in T2-weighted images suggestive of active sarcoidosis. Treatment of active cardiac sarcoidosis is steroids and as she had recurrent cardiogenic syncope due to ventricular tachyarrhythmias and has a LV ejection fraction of less than 50%, she is a candidate for an ICD. Although myocarditis can present with LV systolic dysfunction as well as ventricular tachyarrhythmias, myocarditis causes global hypokinesis and regional wall motion abnormalities are unlikely. Ischemic cardiomyopathy would cause regional wall motion abnormalities in coronary artery distribution patterns and would not spare endocardium as shown in CMR in this patient. Although this patient has a history of sickle cell trait and diabetes mellitus and is prone to recurrent hemolysis leading to an iron overload state, this patient has normal serum ferritin and transferrin saturation making hemochromatosis an unlikely diagnosis. Treatment of dilated cardiomyopathy is beta-blockers and RAAS inhibitors, but dilated cardiomyopathy causes LV dilatation with globally reduced LV systolic function, unlike cardiac sarcoidosis.

KEY POINTS

- ✔ Cardiac sarcoidosis presents with ventricular tachyarrhythmias and predominantly causes akinetic or aneurysmal basal septum and lateral wall. Suspected cardiac sarcoidosis should be worked up by initial ECG, Holter, chest radiographs, transthoracic echocardiography, and confirmed by CMR. Evidence of concomitant extracardiac sarcoidosis should be sought. Treatment of active sarcoidosis is steroids, and prophylactic ICD should be placed in patients with ejection fraction less than 50%.

72.3 The correct answer is A.

Rationale: This patient presented with cardiomyopathy with multisystem involvement. She had wrist arthropathy, cognitive impairment, hepatitis, diabetes mellitus, and cardiomyopathy most likely due to hereditary hemochromatosis and organ damage due to iron overload. The classic echocardiographic features of early cardiac hemochromatosis are normal LV wall thickness with a dilated cavity, reduced LV systolic function, and restrictive filling pattern. It can cause atrial arrhythmias due to dilated atria. Serum ferritin and transferrin saturation are markedly elevated. Fabry disease is an X-linked disease due to a deficiency of alpha-galactosidase enzyme that classically affects males in early life with clinical onset in early childhood. Deposition of glycosphingolipids causes concentric LV hypertrophy, preserved LV systolic function, and restrictive filling pattern. Cardiac amyloidosis generally presents between the ages of 40 and 70 years with concentric LV hypertrophy and restrictive filling pattern in echocardiography and HFpEF. Although hypertension, diabetes mellitus, metabolic syndrome, and concomitant nonalcoholic steatohepatitis (NASH) can cause an elevation in liver enzymes and bilirubin, hypertensive heart disease classically presents with LV concentric hypertrophy. An athlete's heart can cause mild LV dilation, but hallmark features are mild-moderate concentric LV hypertrophy, normal systolic and diastolic function, and normal atrial sizes.

KEY POINTS

- ✔ Hereditary hemochromatosis often involves the heart and presents with cardiomyopathy, and manifests with exertional dyspnea and atrial and ventricular arrhythmias. Classical echocardiographic findings of early hereditary hemochromatosis are normal LV wall thickness with a dilated LV cavity, reduced systolic function, restrictive filling pattern, and dilated atria. Concomitant extracardiac manifestations also give clues to the diagnosis.

724. The correct answer is A.

Rationale: This patient is from a tropical area and presented initially with febrile illness with periorbital swelling and chest pain which later progressed to congestive heart failure. Echocardiography showed preserved LV systolic function with thickened ventricular walls with small cavity size and tethering of atrioventricular valves leading to regurgitation, biatrial dilatation, restrictive filling pattern, apical thrombus, and pericardial effusion. This is typical of endomyocardial fibrosis. Peripheral eosinophilia and atrial fibrillation are commonly seen. Chagas disease is due to *Trypanosoma cruzi* and is endemic in Latin America. Chagas cardiomyopathy also presents with congestive heart failure, arrhythmias, and LV apical mural thrombus but its classic echocardiographic finding is apical aneurysm with mural thrombus. Valve apparatus tethering, small biventricular cavities, and endomyocardial plaques are not seen in Chagas cardiomyopathy. Although cardiac amyloidosis can cause a restrictive LV filling pattern, it does present with a retracted apex, tethering of the mitral valve, and apical thrombus formation. Constrictive-effusive pericarditis presents with pericardial effusion, but the echocardiography classically shows a septal bounce, an increased septal and reduced lateral mitral annulus tissue Doppler velocities, and significant respirophasic mitral inflow variation. Carcinoid heart disease predominantly causes the thickening and retraction of the tricuspid valve. Left-sided valves are not commonly involved unless the patient has large right to left shunts or bronchial carcinoids. Carcinoid heart disease causes enlarged right atrial and ventricular cavity due to TR.

KEY POINTS

- Endomyocardial fibrosis is commonly seen in tropical regions and classically presents with prodromal symptoms of acute febrile illness, chest pain, periorbital swelling, and eosinophilia. This may progress to chronic HFpEF and present with classical echocardiographic findings of apical fibrosis, apical retraction, small biventricular cavities, tethering of atrioventricular valves with secondary regurgitation, restrictive filling pattern, biatrial enlargement, atrial arrhythmias, apical thrombus formation with normal wall motion, and pericardial and pleural effusion.

725. The correct answer is C.

Rationale: A male patient in his third decade of life with a positive history of acroparesthesia presented with chronic exertional dyspnea and syncope attributable to non-sustained ventricular tachycardia. A positive family history of sudden cardiac death, probably due to malignant ventricular arrhythmias in his maternal uncle, suggests an X-lined transmission. Echocardiography showed severe concentric hypertrophy without LVOT gradient, thickened aortic and mitral valves, and restrictive filling pattern. CMR showed fibrosis in the basal and mid-anterolateral areas. Myocardial SPECT perfusion and coronary angiogram were suggestive of small vessel disease. These features are classical for Fabry disease which is a lysosomal storage disease due to deficiency of alpha-galactosidase deficiency. Although hypertrophic cardiomyopathy can cause concentric hypertrophy, cardiac arrhythmias, and a positive family history of cardiac death, the absence of systolic anterior motion of the mitral leaflet and LVOT gradient make hypertrophic cardiomyopathy a less likely diagnosis. Amyloidosis generally causes global subendocardial LGE in CMR and presents predominantly with congestive heart failure and not chest pain and cardiac arrhythmias. Although coronary artery disease can cause diastolic dysfunction, and this patient presented with chest pain, the SPECT myocardial perfusion study showed reversible perfusion defects due to small vessel disease caused by fibrosis. However, the coronary angiogram did not reveal epicardial coronary artery disease. Ischemic cardiomyopathy in the absence of epicardial coronary artery disease and with normal ejection fraction is unlikely. Hypertensive heart disease can cause concentric LV hypertrophy, aortic root dilatation, and secondary aortic regurgitation, but it does not cause small vessel disease and fibrosis of basal and mid-anterolateral and inferolateral areas. X-linked transmission and a positive family history of sudden cardiac death make this diagnosis unlikely.

KEY POINTS

✓ Fabry disease is an X-linked disease that affects multiple systems and presents with severe concentric LV hypertrophy, restrictive cardiomyopathy, angina with positive stress test due to small vessel disease from fibrosis, and positive family history of sudden cardiac death due to malignant ventricular arrhythmias. Treatment is enzyme replacement therapy with recombinant IV alpha-galactosidase A infusion every 2 weeks.

72.6 The correct answer is A.

Rationale: This patient presented with acute or chronic congestive HFpEF. Low-voltage ECG, moderate concentric LV hypertrophy with a speckling pattern, moderate aortic stenosis, apical sparing pattern in global longitudinal strain study, and global transmural LGE in CMR are suggestive of cardiac amyloidosis. There are two major types of cardiac amyloidosis. AL amyloidosis consists of immunoglobulin light chain deposition and ATTR with deposition of the destabilized quaternary protein structure of transthyretin. Once clinical features, initial echocardiography, and CMR findings are suspicious for amyloidosis, lab work should begin with the workup for monoclonal gammopathy with serum κ/λ ratio, serum and urine protein immunofixation. If these are elevated, AL amyloidosis is likely. If these tests are negative, a workup for ATTR should begin with nuclear scintigraphy and SPECT study with Tc 99m pyrophosphate. Sometimes, AL amyloidosis can have a positive nuclear scintigraphy study, hence the initial test for monoclonal gammopathy is mandatory. Negative monoclonal gammopathy rules out AL amyloidosis and a workup of ATTR should begin with nuclear scintigraphy as the initial workup for cardiac amyloidosis is strongly positive. Myocardial biopsy and Congo red stain are performed for suspected ATTR cardiac amyloidosis but only with an indeterminate nuclear scintigraphy study. Genetic testing for the subtypes of ATTR (ATTR-hereditary [ATTRh] and ATTR-wild type [ATTRwt]) is performed in patients with absent monoclonal gammopathy but with abnormal nuclear scintigraphy. There has been a marked shift over the last decade in how ATTR cardiac amyloidosis is being diagnosed with increasing use of noninvasive testing in preference to biopsy. Abdominal fat pad biopsy is performed in patients who are screened positive for AL amyloidosis by elevated plasma free light chains and positive urine protein electrophoresis and SPEP with immunofixation. We resort to myocardial biopsy for suspected ATTR only with an indeterminate nuclear scintigraphy study.

KEY POINTS

✓ Workup of suspected cardiac amyloidosis should always begin with tests for monoclonal gammopathy with free light chain assay and serum and urine protein electrophoresis with immunofixation. Patients with monoclonal gammopathy should be worked up for AL amyloidosis and its presence rules out ATTR. Patients with suspected cardiac amyloidosis but negative monoclonal gammopathy should undergo nuclear scintigraphy and SPECT study with Tc 99m pyrophosphate study to assess for ATTR. This differentiation is important because patients with ATTR cardiac amyloidosis can be treated with drug therapy with good outcomes.

72.7 The correct answer is A.

Rationale: This patient has ATTR cardiac amyloidosis based on negative monoclonal gammopathy and suspicious echocardiographic and CMR findings confirmed by strongly positive nuclear scintigraphy and SPECT study with Tc 99m pyrophosphate. Tafamidis is a TTR amyloid fibril stabilizer and is U.S. Food and Drug Administration (FDA)-approved for the treatment of both ATTRh and ATTRwt cardiomyopathy. AL amyloidosis has been ruled out with negative monoclonal gammopathy and workup for ATTR should be initiated with nuclear scintigraphy. Orthotopic heart transplantation is the treatment for end-stage amyloid cardiomyopathy nonresponsive to drug therapy. Sacubitril-valsartan has no role in the treatment of HFpEF in amyloidosis as these patients are prone to hypotension due to autonomic neuropathy, small LV cavity size, and small-fixed cardiac output. Mechanical circulatory support with ventricular assist device (VAD) as a bridge to transplantation is ineffective with poor outcomes due to small LV chamber size, concentric LV hypertrophy, and restrictive physiology leading to suction events and right ventricular failure.

KEY POINTS

✓ Tafamidis is an ATTR amyloid fibril stabilizer and is FDA approved in the treatment of both ATTRh and ATTRwt cardiac amyloidosis. It has been shown to significantly improve survival and reduce mortality and hospitalization in patients with ATTR.

72.8 The correct answer is B.

Rationale: Serum-free light chains assay is an easily available test for screening cardiac amyloidosis. Serum-free light chains and serum and urine protein electrophoresis with immunofixation and not SPEP alone are used for screening cardiac amyloidosis. Beta-2 microglobulin is associated with dialysis-related amyloidosis (DRA). 5-HIAA is the product of serotonin metabolism and is elevated in carcinoid heart disease and not cardiac amyloidosis.

> **KEY POINTS**
>
> ✓ Serum and urine protein electrophoresis with immunofixation and serum-free light chain assays are the recommended screening tests for suspected cardiac amyloidosis. Positive screening tests for AL amyloidosis with typical echocardiography and CMR findings should be followed by a noncardiac or heart biopsy. Patients with cardiac amyloidosis don't tolerate beta-blockers due to autonomic dysfunction, hypotension, and low and fixed stroke volume due to small LV cavity size.

72.9 The correct answer is A.

Rationale: Nuclear scintigraphy with positive Tc 99m pyrophosphate and SPECT study and negative monoclonal gammopathy diagnose cardiac ATTR with 100% specificity and positive predictive value. There has been a paradigm shift in diagnosing cardiac ATTR with positive nuclear scintigraphy/SPECT in patients with suspicious echocardiographic and CMR findings and without monoclonal gammopathy, thus obviating the need for cardiac biopsy. Positive nuclear scintigraphy does not rule out AL amyloidosis as some patients with AL amyloidosis may have false positive nuclear scintigraphy. Hence, an initial test for monoclonal gammopathy is a must. Tc 99m pyrophosphate is a bone radiotracer and uptake is high in cardiac ATTR and not in AL amyloidosis as the density of microcalcifications is higher in ATTR amyloid fibrils.

> **KEY POINTS**
>
> ✓ Nuclear scintigraphy/SPECT with Tc 99m pyrophosphate scan may replace cardiac biopsy in the diagnosis of cardiac ATTR biopsy in patients with absent monoclonal gammopathy and suspicious echocardiographic and CMR findings.

72.10 The correct answer is C.

Rationale: This patient with a history of recurrent HFpEF exacerbations presented with symptomatic atrial fibrillation. Echocardiography and CMR findings are consistent with cardiac amyloidosis. Elevated serum-free light chains and positive serum and urine protein electrophoresis with immunofixation are suggestive of AL amyloidosis. These patients are very prone to forming left atrial appendage thrombus and hence should be anticoagulated for atrial fibrillation even with the CHA_2DS_2VASC score of 0. Tissue diagnosis of AL amyloidosis is first obtained with bone marrow or abdominal fat pad biopsy. Tafamidis is an ATTR amyloid fibril stabilizer and is FDA approved for the treatment of ATTR and not AL amyloidosis. Beta-blockers, ACEI/angiotensin receptor blocker (ARB), and sacubitril/valsartan have no role in the treatment of heart failure in patients with cardiac amyloidosis even with low ejection fraction as these patients are prone to hypotension due to underlying autonomic neuropathy from the disease process and fixed and low stroke volume due to restrictive filling and small LV cavity size.

KEY POINTS

- Early differentiation of types of cardiac amyloidosis is important as treatment and prognosis are different. ATTR/ACT trial has shown a statistically significant reduction in all-cause mortality and all-cause hospitalization with tafamidis in patients with ATTRwt and ATTRh. Cardiac AL amyloidosis is treated with chemotherapy targeted for multiple myeloma and stem cell transplantation. Mortality is higher with AL amyloidosis whereas outcome is better with ATTR due to availability of drug therapy.

MYOCARDITIS

Hamza Oglat, William Alderisio, and Sulagna Mookherjee

CHAPTER 73

QUESTIONS

73.1 What percentage of patients with myocarditis develop chronic dilated cardiomyopathy (DCM)?

A. 10%
B. 20%
C. 30%
D. 40%

73.2 Which of the following statements regarding myocarditis is **TRUE**?

A. Myocarditis occurs more frequently in females than males.
B. There is no gender difference in the severity of myocarditis.
C. A male patient with severe myocarditis requiring mechanical circulatory support has a higher likelihood of bridge to recovery compared to a female patient.
D. There is a bimodal age distribution in myocarditis.

73.3 Which of the following is one of the most common causes of myocarditis?

A. Viruses
B. Bacteria
C. Parasites
D. Toxins

73.4 A 35-year-old male is seen in the emergency department (ED) for shortness of breath, orthopnea, and palpitations. The physical examination is significant for bilateral crackles on lung auscultation, elevated jugular venous pressure as well as lower extremity edema. While in the ED, the patient developed wide-complex tachycardia with hypotension and underwent successful cardioversion with restoration of sinus rhythm. The patient is suspected of having acute myocarditis. Which of the following is the **MOST LIKELY** etiology of myocarditis in this patient?

A. Enterovirus infection
B. Adenovirus infection
C. Bacterial infection
D. Giant cell myocarditis (GCM)

73.5 A 26-year-old male presents with 10 days of worsening fatigue and shortness of breath. Echocardiogram reveals severely depressed left ventricular systolic function. He is suspected of having acute myocarditis. Which of the following findings would make endomyocardial biopsy (EMB) strongly indicated in this patient?

*Questions and Answers are based on Chapter 73: Myocarditis by Melissa A. Lyle, Lori A. Blauwet, and Leslie T. Cooper in Cardiovascular Medicine and Surgery, First Edition.

A. Cardiogenic shock
B. Ventricular arrhythmia
C. High-grade atrioventricular (AV) block
D. All of the above

73.6 Which of the following medications should **NOT** be used in patients with acute myocarditis and DCM?

A. Carvedilol
B. Digoxin
C. Entresto
D. Spironolactone

73.7 Which of the following conditions is **LEAST LIKELY** to respond to immunosuppressive therapy?

A. Acute lymphocytic myocarditis and DCM
B. Chronic virus-negative DCM
C. GCM
D. Eosinophilic necrotizing myocarditis

73.8 A 39-year-old male developed cardiogenic shock in setting of GCM. He is requiring multiple inotropes and mechanical circulatory support is being considered as a bridge to cardiac transplantation. Compared to patients who undergo cardiac transplantation for other indications, patients with GCM who undergo cardiac transplantation have:

A. Higher rates of early rejection
B. Lower rates of early rejection
C. Higher survival rates
D. Lower survival rates

73.9 The use of interferon-beta leads to improvement in the New York Heart Association functional class and clearance of viral genome in patients with chronic viral cardiomyopathy caused by which of the following viruses?

A. Enterovirus
B. Parvovirus B19
C. Adenovirus
D. A and C

73.10 High level of clinical suspicion is necessary to make the appropriate clinical diagnosis of myocarditis. Which of the following is **NOT TRUE** regarding the diagnosis of myocarditis?

A. There are no pathognomonic electrocardiographic findings.
B. Chest radiography may reveal cardiomegaly secondary to chamber dilatation or pericardial effusion.
C. Cardiac biomarkers, if elevated, are helpful in the diagnosis of myocarditis.
D. Cardiac magnetic resonance imaging (MRI) should be considered if the patient has high-grade heart block on electrocardiogram.

ANSWERS

73.1 The correct answer is B.
Rationale: The clinical presentation of myocarditis can range from subclinical disease to fulminant myocarditis that requires inotropic or mechanical circulatory support. The host immune response can downregulate after clearance of damage with little scar or result in more persistent or extensive inflammation that permanently damages heart tissue. Usually, the process is self-limited, but if the immune response persists, then cardiac remodeling can lead to chronic DCM. Up to 20% of patients with myocarditis develop chronic DCM.

73.2 The correct answer is D.
Rationale: There is a bimodal age distribution in myocarditis. The prevalence of myocarditis as a cause of cardiomyopathy is high in the first year of life. It is thought that the increased rate and more fulminant presentation in infants can be attributed to an immature immune system. Myocarditis is responsible for approximately 2% of infant sudden cardiovascular deaths. The prevalence of myocarditis relative to all heart failure declines between ages 1 and 12 years, then the risk again increases after puberty. The mean age of adults with the most forms of myocarditis ranges between 20 and 51 years, while the mean age of patients with GCM is 42 years.

Most cases of myocarditis illustrate a male predominance, which is strongly influenced by sex hormones. Males are more likely to have a more severe disease and have a lower likelihood of bridge to recovery if requiring mechanical circulatory support for myocarditis.

73.3 The correct answer is A.
Rationale: Viral infection is one of the most common causes of myocarditis. From the 1950s to the 1990s, enterovirus species, specifically coxsackievirus, were the most frequently identified viruses in patients with myocarditis. Molecular studies during the late 1980s and 1990s utilizing polymerase chain reaction (PCR) from heart biopsies, identified an enterovirus genome in 15 to 30% of patients with acute myocarditis.

The incidence of adenovirus and patients with myocarditis varies between a high of 23% and a low of 2%. The most commonly detected viral genomes on EMB samples are now parvovirus B19 and human herpes virus 6.

Myocarditis is the most common cardiac pathologic finding at autopsy in patients with severe HIV. The incidence of myocarditis, in addition to cardiomyopathy and pericardial disease, correlates with the severity of HIV infection as measured by a low CD4+ count or high viral titers. Since the introduction of highly active antiretroviral therapy (HAART), the incidence of myocarditis in patients who are infected with HIV has dramatically decreased in developed countries.

Influenza A and B viruses are known causes of myocarditis, with H1N1 having a particularly severe clinical syndrome. The incidence of myocarditis and severe influenza A infections may be as high as 5% with reports of electrocardiographic changes suggestive of subclinical cardiac involvement as high as 11%. Some cases of influenza A resulted in fulminant myocarditis with a high rate of recovery after supportive medical care.

In the setting of the COVID-19 pandemic, it has been demonstrated that patients admitted with COVID-19 had a 13% to 41% incidence of myocardial injury, but classic lymphocytic myocarditis was relatively uncommon.

73.4 The correct answer is D.

Rationale: Sustained arrhythmias are more common in patients with GCM compared with lymphocytic myocarditis. Idiopathic GCM is a rare, autoimmune form of myocarditis histologically defined by the presence of multinucleated giant cells, lymphocytic inflammatory infiltrate, and myocyte necrosis. Usually occurring in young adults, GCM carries a high risk of death without cardiac transplantation. Initially, cardiac rhythm disturbances, such as premature ventricular contractions (PVCs), are very common as the initial presentation. The prevalence of ventricular arrhythmias varies by histologic type of myocarditis, with sustained or symptomatic arrhythmias more common in GCM and hypersensitivity myocarditis compared with lymphocytic myocarditis.

73.5 The correct answer is D.

Rationale: EMB remains essential in more severe cases of acute myocarditis. Two scenarios exist in which both the American College of Cardiology (ACC) and European Society of Cardiology (ESC) give EMB class I or equivalent recommendation: (1) unexplained new-onset heart failure symptoms less than 2 weeks in duration with hemodynamic compromise concerning for fulminant myocarditis and (2) unexplained new-onset heart failure with symptoms of 2 weeks to 3 months duration associated ventricular arrhythmias or high-grade AV block (Mobitz type II second-degree or third-degree AV block), concerning for GCM. In addition, an EMB is reasonable in the setting of suspected eosinophilic myocarditis or myocarditis associated with systemic conditions such as rheumatoid arthritis, lupus, or scleroderma (**Figure 73.1**).

73.6 The correct answer is B.

Rationale: Patients with acute myocarditis who present with DCM should be treated according to the current heart failure guidelines (ACC, American Heart Association [AHA], Heart Failure Society of America [HFSA], and ESC). Guideline-directed medical therapy including beta-blockers, angiotensin-converting enzyme inhibitor/angiotensin receptor blockers/angiotensin receptor–neprilysin inhibitors, mineralocorticoid receptor antagonists, and diuretics, if needed, should be implemented in these (and other patients with heart failure). Digoxin should generally be avoided in acute myocarditis; digoxin was found to have increased mortality in mice with viral myocarditis.

73.7 The correct answer is A.

Rationale: In a randomized controlled trial immunosuppression (prednisone with either azathioprine or cyclosporine) did not improve left ventricular ejection fraction at 28 weeks or transplant-free survival at 5 years in patients with acute lymphocytic

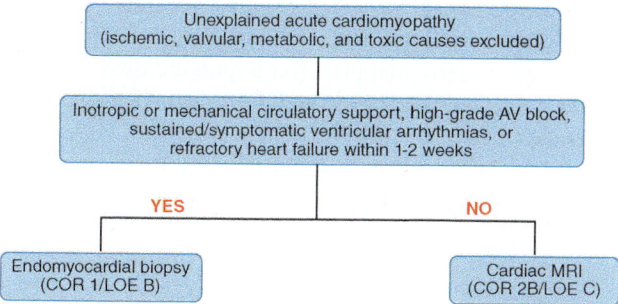

Figure 73.1 Approach to diagnosis in unexplained acute cardiomyopathy. AV, atrioventricular; COR, class of recommendation; LOE, level of evidence; MRI, magnetic resonance imaging.

myocarditis and DCM. Three studies have shown that treatment of patients with chronic virus-negative DCM with azathioprine and prednisone may improve left ventricular ejection fraction and New York Heart Association functional class. Immunosuppressive therapy in patients with GCM and less than 3 months of symptoms increases transplant-free survival. Eosinophilic necrotizing myocarditis is responsive to immunosuppression.

73.8 The correct answer is A.
Rationale: Patients with GCM who undergo cardiac transplantation have higher rates of early rejection but similar survival rates compared to patients who undergo cardiac transplantation for other indications.

73.9 The correct answer is D.
Rationale: In the Betaferon in Chronic Viral Cardiomyopathy (BICC) trial, the use of interferon-beta in patients with chronic DCM and enterovirus or adenovirus genomes identified on heart biopsy using PCR led to improvement in New York Heart Association functional class and clearance of viral genome. However, in patients with parvovirus B19, the use of interferon-beta was not associated with clearance of the genome.

73.10 The correct answer is D.
Rationale: There are no pathognomonic electrocardiographic findings, but nonspecific T-wave abnormalities and sinus tachycardia frequently occur. Low voltage can suggest diffuse edema seen in fulminant myocarditis. PR-segment depression may signal associated pericarditis. High-degree heart block or ventricular arrhythmias suggest a higher risk of specific disorders such as GCM, and EMB is recommended. Cardiac MRI should only be considered if the patient is asymptomatic and has no evidence of sustained or symptomatic ventricular arrhythmias, high-grade heart block, responds to guideline-directed medical therapy, and has no need for inotrope or mechanical circulatory support. Cardiac MRI can distinguish between ischemic and nonischemic cardiomyopathy and can evaluate intracellular and interstitial edema, hyperemia, capillary leakage, necrosis, and fibrosis. The international consensus group on cardiovascular magnetic resonance and myocarditis suggests that a cardiac MRI could be performed in patients with clinical suspicion of myocarditis if

the MRI results affect management. MRI is most accurate for the diagnosis of acute myocarditis within the first several weeks of symptom onset. Accuracy is increased when T1 and T2 parametric mapping techniques are used in addition to standard late gadolinium enhancement (LGE) and T2-weighted imaging. Recent data suggest that the persistence or increase of LGE at 6 months is associated with a worse prognosis following acute myocarditis and that risk increases as the extent of LGE increases. Resolution of LGE was associated with a better prognosis.

TOXIN-INDUCED CARDIOMYOPATHIES*

Robert L. Carhart and Teni Olatunde

CHAPTER 74

QUESTIONS

74.1 A 50-year-old male with no medical history presents with worsening shortness of breath at rest and exertion for 2 months. He reports a weight gain of 20 lbs, inability to lay flat in bed, and orthopnea. He presents to the emergency department for further evaluation. He denies any family history of cardiomyopathy, and he drinks ½ a pint of Vodka daily since the age of 42 but denies any other substance use.

His vital signs include blood pressure 100/60 mm Hg, heart rate 75 beats per minute (bpm), jugular venous pressure (JVP) is distended, S3 is audible, and bibasilar crackles are present. He has 3+ pitting edema extending to his thigh. Pro-B-type natriuretic peptide (ProBNP) is greater than 10,000. Chest x-ray confirms pulmonary edema. He is admitted to the hospital for decompensated heart failure (HF). An echocardiogram is performed during hospitalization which shows ejection fraction (EF) of 15% with dilated chambers.

What is the likely etiology of his cardiomyopathy?

A. Ischemic cardiomyopathy
B. Alcoholic cardiomyopathy
C. Cocaine induced cardiomyopathy
D. Methamphetamine induced cardiomyopathy

74.2 A 46-year-old woman with a history of familial hyperlipidemia presents for further evaluation of sudden onset dyspnea which woke her up from sleep. She describes a "drowning" sensation. Her vital signs include blood pressure 220/110 mm Hg, heart rate 80 bpm, audible S3 on cardiac auscultation, and bibasilar crackles on lung examination. A chest x-ray showed pulmonary edema. She denies a history of hypertension, however, reports a prior intravenous drug use (IVDU) history which prompts a urine toxicology which is positive for cocaine and cannabinoids. An echocardiogram is performed which shows left ventricular ejection fraction (LVEF) 35% with left ventricular hypertrophy.

She is diagnosed with flash pulmonary edema secondary to hypertensive emergency thought to be related to cocaine use.

What is the mechanism of action of cocaine on the cardiovascular system?

A. Excessive stimulation of dopaminergic sympathetic nervous systems and platelet activation
B. Direct toxic effects on cardiac myocytes, increased beta-adrenergic tone, and inappropriate activation of renin-angiotensin-aldosterone system (RAAS) axis
C. Disruption of sarcoplasmic reticulum causing inappropriate calcium release and derangement of calcium metabolism
D. Mitochondrial dysfunction and increased arrhythmogenic potential

*Questions and Answers are based on Chapter 74: Toxin-Induced Cardiomyopathies by Omar Jawaid, Suparna C. Clasen, Abhishek Khemka, and Maya Guglin in Cardiovascular Medicine and Surgery, First Edition.

74.3 A 52-year-old male with a history of nonischemic cardiomyopathy, hypertension, and a drug abuse history involving marijuana and methamphetamine presents for further evaluation of progressive dyspnea for 1 week. He noticed shortness of breath climbing one flight of stairs which was **NOT** an issue 2 weeks before. He also reports lower extremity edema bilaterally and feeling "full."

His home medications include Entresto 24/26 mg, metoprolol succinate 50 mg daily, furosemide 40 mg daily, and spironolactone 12.5 mg daily.

He adheres to a low-salt diet and reports compliance with his medication with the exception of furosemide which he takes every other day instead of daily as prescribed. He also admits to methamphetamine use recently.

On physical examination, his blood pressure is 132/80 mm Hg, heart rate is 70 bpm, jugular venous pulse distension is noted, S3 audible on cardiac examination, and 2+ bilateral lower extremity edema. Chest x-ray showed bibasilar crackles, proBNP is greater than 10,000. Echocardiogram from 1 month before showed EF 38%. She was diagnosed with HF exacerbation and admitted to the hospital for further evaluation and management.

Which of the following is the **MOST LIKELY** cause of HF exacerbation in this patient?

A. Medication noncompliance
B. Diet noncompliance
C. Marijuana use
D. Methamphetamine use

74.4 A 55-year-old female recently diagnosed with rheumatoid arthritis 3 months ago presents with complaints of fatigue and lethargy. She noticed shortness of breath and easy fatiguability with climbing one flight of stairs. She also reports lower extremity pitting edema and recent difficulty lying flat in bed. She now requires two pillows when she required only one pillow previously.

She takes medication for rheumatoid arthritis; however, does **NOT** recall the name of the medication.

Vital signs reveal blood pressure 110/70 mm Hg, heart rate 70 bpm, physical examination unremarkable **EXCEPT** minimal crackles in lung bases with decreased air entry in the left lower lobe, and 1+ pitting edema in her lower extremities bilaterally.

Chest x-ray shows left-sided pleural effusion. An echocardiogram is performed which shows EF 40% with grade 3 diastolic dysfunction concerning for restrictive filling.

Which of the following is the next step to determine the possible etiology of cardiomyopathy?

A. Nuclear stress test
B. Heart catheterization
C. Thorough review of medication list
D. Endomyocardial biopsy

74.5 A 35-year-old female was recently diagnosed with stage 3 breast cancer. She is currently undergoing further testing and evaluation to determine the course of treatment. There are ongoing discussions about double mastectomy and chemotherapy. The exact choice of chemotherapeutic agents has **NOT** been decided. She is sent for further cardiac evaluation due to a family history of early coronary artery disease (CAD) in her father at the age of 45 and an implantable defibrillator in her mother. Before starting chemotherapy, which of the following should be performed?

A. Stress echocardiogram
B. Electrocardiogram (ECG)
C. 2D echocardiogram
D. Coronary calcium score

74.6 A 68-year-old female with recently diagnosed leukemia is currently managed on doxorubicin for chemotherapy. She has a history of hypertension and hyperlipidemia managed with amlodipine 10 mg, 50 mg of chlorthalidone daily, and 40 mg of atorvastatin nightly. An echocardiogram was performed before starting chemotherapy which showed EF 65% and left ventricular hypertrophy. She has received two cycles of chemotherapy and is sent by her hematologist for cardiac monitoring with an echocardiogram.

Based on the patient's risk factors and current treatments, which of the following would likely increase the incidence of anthracycline-induced chemotherapy?

A. Age above 65 and female sex
B. Hypertension and hyperlipidemia
C. Doxorubicin dose
D. All of the above

74.7 A 40-year-old female undergoing chemotherapy with doxorubicin for stage 3 breast cancer is sent by her oncologist due to reported symptoms of lower extremity edema, shortness of breath with one flight of stairs, and difficulty sleeping at night. She takes no daily medication apart from vitamins.

Vital signs showed blood pressure 125/80 mm Hg, heart rate 80 bpm. She has 2+ bilateral lower extremity edema, jugular venous distension, and lung crackles. An echocardiogram performed before beginning treatment showed EF 55%. You performed an echocardiogram today which shows a decline in EF by 39%. You are suspicious of anthracycline-induced cardiomyopathy.

What is the next step in management?

A. Initiate therapy for decompensated HF.
B. Initiate therapy for decompensated HF and continue therapy with anthracycline at current dose.
C. Decrease dose of anthracycline therapy and repeat echocardiogram after completion of next cycle of chemotherapy.
D. Initiate therapy for decompensated HF and advise cessation of anthracycline therapy.

74.8 A 58-year-old female with a history of hypertension and type 2 diabetes was recently diagnosed with stage 2 breast cancer. She met with an oncologist who discussed starting chemotherapy with anthracyclines; however, she read online about the dangers of chemotherapy to the heart and cardiovascular system and therefore she presented to your office to discuss further.

She is on amlodipine 10 mg and lisinopril 20 mg daily for blood pressure control and metformin for type 2 diabetes. Her last A1c was 7. Her blood pressure is 135/80 mm Hg, heart rate is 75 bpm. The rest of her physical examination is unremarkable.

She asks if you have a plan to ensure she does **NOT** develop HF from chemotherapy.

How frequently would she undergo echocardiographic surveillance while on chemotherapy?

- A. Baseline echocardiogram before starting treatment
- B. Dose-dependent surveillance during therapy
- C. A and B
- D. Every 3 months during treatment

CASE 1

A 68-year-old female with stage 3 HER2-breast cancer is started on trastuzumab after doxorubicin therapy. Her echocardiograms before starting therapy with doxorubicin showed EF 60%, and subsequent imaging during therapy and at completion of therapy showed EF 55% to 60%.

She has a history of hypertension managed on lisinopril 40 mg daily and chlorthalidone 25 mg daily, and type 2 diabetes on metformin.

She presents for evaluation at her oncologist's office before cycle 2 of chemotherapy regimen with trastuzumab where she reports fatigue, dyspnea on exertion, and pedal edema for 2 weeks. She is sent to your office for further evaluation and a repeat echocardiogram.

With further questioning, she reveals orthopnea and paroxysmal nocturnal dyspnea. Vital signs include blood pressure 120/85 mm Hg, heart rate 72 bpm. There is no jugular venous distension; however, S3 is audible on auscultation, and she has bibasilar crackles as well as 1+ pitting edema in her lower extremities.

An echocardiogram is performed in your office which shows a decline in EF to 40% from 58%.

74.9 For the patient in **Case 1**, which of the following risk factors is associated with the highest risk of developing trastuzumab-induced cardiomyopathy?

- A. Age above 50 years
- B. Obesity
- C. Decreased LVEF
- D. Previous concurrent use of anthracyclines

74.10 You suspect trastuzumab cardiotoxicity and begin goal-directed medical therapy for HF. What is your recommendation regarding further trastuzumab therapy?

- A. Stop trastuzumab therapy completely.
- B. Hold trastuzumab therapy for 4 weeks and reassess EF.
- C. Continue trastuzumab therapy since patient is on goal-directed medical therapy for HF.
- D. Hold trastuzumab therapy for 2 weeks until HF therapy reaches a steady state and then restart.

ANSWERS

74.1 **The correct answer is B.**
Rationale: He has no other medical history concerning for underlying CAD; therefore, ischemic cardiomyopathy is an unlikely etiology. Considering he denies any other substance use but admits to alcohol use, alcoholic cardiomyopathy is the likely etiology.

KEY POINTS

- Patients with alcohol consumption of greater than 90 g/day of ethanol for more than 5 years are at the highest risk for developing cardiomyopathy. As ethanol exposure increases, so does the risk of cardiomyopathy, with those ingesting greater than 200 g/day of ethanol having the highest risk of developing cardiomyopathy

74.2 **The correct answer is A.**
Rationale: Cocaine exerts its effects by excessively stimulating the dopaminergic and sympathetic nervous systems. This in turn has multiple effects on the heart through hypertension, tachyarrhythmias, cardiomyocyte toxicity, coronary vasospasm, and dissection. It also causes accelerated atherosclerosis as well as microvascular ischemia through inappropriate platelet activation, which contributes to myocardial dysfunction. Hypertension is a well-documented effect of sympathetic activation.

Options B, C, and D are the pathogenesis of alcoholic cardiomyopathy.

KEY POINTS

- Cocaine has multiple effects on the heart through hypertension, tachyarrhythmias, cardiomyocyte toxicity, coronary vasospasm, and dissection.

74.3 **The correct answer is D.**
Rationale: Patient is compliant with all medication except furosemide which he takes every other day and adheres to a low-salt diet. Marijuana is not known to cause HF exacerbation.

Data from hospital diagnosis codes reveal that up to 5% of admissions for HF exacerbations are caused by methamphetamine use.

Methamphetamine exerts numerous effects on the cardiovascular system, which in turn promote aberrant remodeling, myocardial loss, and ultimately cardiomyopathy.

KEY POINTS

- Methamphetamine exerts effects on the cardiovascular system which ultimately can lead to cardiomyopathy. Its use can also cause HF exacerbation.

74.4 The correct answer is C.

Rationale: Ischemic workup with a nuclear stress test and heart catheterization are reasonable to determine the etiology of her new cardiomyopathy; however, they should not precede a thorough review of her medication list in this patient who likely could be on chloroquine which has been recognized as a cardiotoxic agent leading to drug-induced cardiomyopathy.

A thorough history always provides additional information useful for diagnosis.

Although endomyocardial biopsy is the gold standard for diagnosis of drug-induced cardiomyopathy, it is an invasive procedure that can be explored if the etiology of the cardiomyopathy cannot be determined by less invasive methods.

KEY POINTS

- Chloroquine (used for the treatment of rheumatoid arthritis) and derivatives are increasingly recognized as cardiomyocyte toxic agents leading to drug-induced cardiomyopathy. Frequently, a restrictive cardiomyopathy occurs, although dilated and hypertrophic variants have been described as well.

74.5 The correct answer is C.

Rationale: Chemotherapy has the potential for adverse cardiac side effects; therefore, baseline cardiac structure and function should be known before starting chemotherapy. An ECG or coronary calcium score is suboptimal to a 2D echocardiogram in providing more information on cardiac structure and function. She does not report any angina symptoms, so a stress echocardiogram is not needed.

KEY POINTS

- Treatment of breast cancer involves chemotherapy with anthracycline-containing regimens, targeted therapy with antihuman epidermal growth factor receptor 2 (HER2) agents, and radiation therapy. The use of these agents may result in treatment-associated cardiotoxicity. Furthermore, the presence of concomitant cardiovascular risk factors and comorbidities can affect the timing, severity, and potentially the reversibility of cancer therapy–related cardiotoxicities. Cardiotoxic effects of chemotherapeutics can occur immediately upon exposure or years later depending on the anticancer therapy. It is important that before chemotherapy induction, a baseline echocardiogram is obtained in patients due to the risk of chemotherapy-induced cardiotoxicity.

74.6 The correct answer is D.

Rationale: All of the factors listed are associated with increased incidence of anthracycline-induced cardiomyopathy.

KEY POINTS

- Factors associated with an increased incidence of anthracycline-induced cardiomyopathy include total dose, dose fractions, concomitant therapies (ie, other chemotherapy or radiotherapy), female sex, cardiovascular risk factors (including tobacco use, hypertension, dyslipidemia, obesity, diabetes mellitus, underlying left ventricular dysfunction), and age (>65 years).

74.7 The correct answer is D.

Rationale: Since the patient has developed anthracycline-induced chemotherapy, chemotherapy should be stopped, and therapy for decompensated HF should be initiated, including guideline-directed medical therapy. A discussion between the cardiologist and oncologist should be had to determine the cumulative dose the patient has received so far and other chemotherapy regimens should be considered.

KEY POINTS

- Anthracycline-induced cardiomyopathy is treated according to guideline-directed management of HF, with no specific interventions for this etiology. The focus should be on prevention. Because anthracycline-induced cardiotoxicity is dose-dependent, dose limitation plays a major role. The generally accepted safe cumulative dose is less than 400 mg/m^2 as there is an estimated 5% risk of HF at a cumulative dose of 400 mg/m^2.

74.8 The correct answer is C.

Rationale: Due to the cardiotoxic effects of anthracyclines, patients on this chemotherapy medication should obtain a baseline echocardiogram to determine baseline cardiac structure and function. If cumulative dose is greater than 240 mg/m^2, imaging before each additional dose of 50 mg/m^2 should be performed. For patients with cumulative dose less than 240 mg/m^2, a subsequent echocardiogram should be obtained at the completion of therapy and 6 months later.

Patients on HER2 targeted breast cancer chemotherapy require an echocardiogram at baseline, every 3 months during treatment and 6 months post therapy also due to cardiotoxic effects of this group of medication.

KEY POINTS

- Echocardiographic surveillance before (at baseline), during, and after treatment with anthracycline therapy or HER2 targeted therapy is important due to their cardiotoxic effects. The cumulative dose the patient receives is a determining factor for the timing of echocardiogram surveillance during therapy with anthracyclines.

74.9 The correct answer is D.

Rationale: Clinical risk factors associated with an increased risk of developing trastuzumab-induced cardiomyopathy include age above 50 years, decreased LVEF, obesity, and previous or concurrent anthracycline use, particularly those receiving concurrent anthracyclines at a dose greater than 300 mg/m^2. For this reason, trastuzumab is typically given in sequential therapy after anthracycline-containing regimens.

74.10 The correct answer is A:

Rationale: This patient has a newly diagnosed cardiomyopathy and has symptomatic HF on therapy; therefore, further trastuzumab cycles should be stopped.

If the LVEF absolute decline is greater than 15% from baseline to below the lower limit of normal (50%), trastuzumab is withheld for 4 weeks, and LVEF is reassessed. If the LVEF remains below these levels after treatment interruption, then typically trastuzumab is discontinued.

KEY POINTS

✓ Patients with prior/concurrent anthracycline use are at increased risk for trastuzumab toxicity. If trastuzumab cardiotoxicity is suspected and the decline in LVEF is more than 15% from baseline to below 50%, therapy should be withheld for 4 weeks and LVEF reassessed. If the LVEF remains below these levels after treatment interruption, then typically trastuzumab is discontinued. In addition, those who develop symptomatic HF on therapy (such as this patient) should stop further trastuzumab cycles.

ACUTE HEART FAILURE

Matthew Derakhshesh and Dmitri Belov

CHAPTER 75

QUESTIONS

75.1 Which of the following is **TRUE** regarding heart failure in women?
   A. The lifetime risk of heart failure is greater in women than in men.
   B. Compared to men, women who are hospitalized for acute decompensated heart failure (ADHF) are more likely to present with heart failure with preserved ejection fraction (HFpEF).
   C. Compared to men, women with heart failure are more likely to have coronary artery disease.
   D. Compared to men, women with heart failure are less likely to have hypertension and diabetes.
   E. Compared to men, women hospitalized with ADHF are more likely to be younger.

75.2 A 62-year-old male with a history of coronary artery disease, diabetes, and hypertension presents with 2 weeks of progressive shortness of breath with exertion along with orthopnea and lower extremity swelling. Labs are notable for a troponin I of 2.3 µg/L, a brain natriuretic peptide (BNP) of 535 pg/mL, and a creatinine of 1.9 mg/dL. All of the following are mechanisms that may contribute to his presentation **EXCEPT**:
   A. High left ventricular (LV) diastolic pressure leading to decreased coronary artery perfusion
   B. Elevated right atrial pressure causing increased renal vascular resistance
   C. Peripheral artery vasoconstriction causing central redistribution of blood flow
   D. High coronary diastolic blood pressure leading to decreased coronary artery perfusion
   E. None of the above

75.3 Which of the following clinical examination findings in ADHF has the highest specificity?
   A. S3 gallop
   B. 2+ pitting edema
   C. Proportional pulse pressure less than 25%
   D. Cool extremities
   E. None of the above

75.4 A 66-year-old female with a history of heart failure with reduced ejection fraction (HFrEF) and hypertension presents to the emergency department with a week of shortness of breath, orthopnea, and weight gain. Her vitals include a blood pressure of

*Questions and Answers are based on Chapter 75: Acute Heart Failure by Nicholas S. Hendren, Justin L. Grodin, and Mark H. Drazner in Cardiovascular Medicine and Surgery, First Edition.

82/47 mm Hg, a heart rate of 92 beats per minute (bpm), and an SpO_2 of 92% on 6 L of supplemental oxygen. On auscultation, there is an S4 gallop along with rales at the bases of the lung. Her extremities are cool to touch with 2+ pitting edema bilaterally. What is this patient's Stevenson clinical profile and what is the most appropriate management?

A. Profile A; start intravenous (IV) diuretics only.
B. Profile B; start IV diuretics and adjust vasodilators.
C. Profile L; start IV diuretics and consider cardiac resynchronization therapy.
D. Profile C; start IV diuretics and add inotropes.
E. None of the above

75.5 A 79-year-old male with a past medical history significant for HFrEF in the setting of nonischemic cardiomyopathy, hypertension, and hyperlipidemia presents with 3 days of shortness of breath, weight gain, and lower extremity swelling despite increasing his home dose of outpatient diuretics. His heart rate is 75 bpm, his blood pressure is 112/79 mm Hg, and his SpO_2 is 93% on a 2-L nasal cannula. His creatinine is 1.1 mg/dL; potassium is 4.1 mEq/L. Aside from taking furosemide 40 mg daily, his other medications include sacubitril-valsartan 24 to 26 mg tid, metoprolol succinate 50 mg daily, and spironolactone 12.5 mg daily. He is started on IV diuretics for ADHF. Which of his outpatient medications should be held while he is being treated?

A. Sacubitril-valsartan
B. Metoprolol succinate
C. Spironolactone
D. All of the above
E. None of the above

75.6 Which of the following is **NOT** a factor contributing to diuretic resistance?

A. Impairment by uremic toxins
B. Neurohormonal activation
C. High-renal blood flow
D. Reduced glomerular filtration
E. None of the above

75.7 A 56-year-old male with a past medical history significant for ischemic cardiomyopathy presents with a week of progressive shortness of breath with associated paroxysmal nocturnal dyspnea and orthopnea. He states that the week before he had gone on cruise and consumed foods high in salt. His N-terminal probrain natriuretic peptide (NT-proBNP) level is 820 pg/mL, and his chest x-ray shows diffuse cephalization with small bilateral pleural effusions. Which diuretic is **NOT** an appropriate treatment option for relieving his pulmonary congestion?

A. Spironolactone
B. Acetazolamide
C. Furosemide
D. Bumetanide and metolazone
E. None of the above

75.8 A 58-year-old male with a past medical history significant for dilated cardiomyopathy presents with weakness, shortness of breath, weight gain, and lower extremity swelling for the past 5 days. He was hospitalized for ADHF less than 1 month ago in the setting of medication nonadherence. Her vitals include a heart rate of 101 bpm, a blood pressure of 82/55 mm Hg, a respiratory rate of 20 breaths/min, and an Spo$_2$ of 92% on a-6 L nasal cannula. On physical examination, he has diffuse crackles posteriorly with diminished breath at the bases as well as a jugular venous pressure (JVP) of 12 cm and 2+ pitting edema tracking to the sacrum. His extremities are cool to touch. Which of the following would **NOT** be an inappropriate vasoactive medication to initiate?

A. Norepinephrine
B. Phenylephrine
C. Dobutamine
D. Milrinone
E. None of the above

75.9 Choose the **CORRECT** answer that matches the following trials with their corresponding results:

A. PIONEER-HF (Comparison of Sacubitril-Valsartan versus Enalapril on Effect on NT-proBNP in Patients Stabilized from an Acute Heart Failure Episode)
B. ESCAPE (Evaluation Study of Congestive Heart Failure and Pulmonary Artery Catheterization Effectiveness)
C. EVEREST (Efficacy of Vasopressin Antagonism in Heart Failure Outcome Study with Tolvaptan)
D. ROSE (Renal Optimization Strategies Evaluation)

> I. No difference in 72-hour urine output for low-dose dopamine or nesiritide versus placebo in those hospitalized with ADHF.
>
> II. No difference in mortality between tolvaptan and placebo in those hospitalized with ADHF.
>
> III. No difference in mortality or number of hospitalized days for patients hospitalized with ADHF and pulmonary artery catheters versus those who underwent standard care.
>
> IV. A greater reduction in death and hospitalization at 16-week follow-up in those hospitalized with ADHF who took sacubitril-valsartan versus those who took enalapril.

A. IV, B-III, C-II, D-I
B. IV, A-III, C-II, D-I
C. IV, B-III, A-II, D-I
D. IV, B-III, C-II, A-I
E. None of the above

75.10 Which of the following is **TRUE** regarding rehospitalization for ADHF?

A. The rehospitalization rate for HFpEF is roughly equal to that of HFrEF.
B. The rehospitalization rate for HFrEF within 60 to 90 days of discharge is approximately 45%.
C. Early post discharge follow-up within 14 days is associated with a lower risk of hospitalization.
D. Approximately 10% of older patients admitted for ADHF are rehospitalized within 30 days.
E. None of the above.

ANSWERS

75.1 The correct answer is B.
Rationale: In general, women who are hospitalized for ADHF are more likely to present with HFpEF (choice B) and more likely to be older when compared to men (choice E). In comparison to men, women with heart failure are less likely to have coronary artery disease (choice C) but are more likely to have other hypertension and diabetes as comorbidities (choice D). Finally, the lifetime risk of heart failure is similar in men and in women though when coronary artery disease is excluded, the lifetime risk is slightly higher in women than in men (choice A).

75.2 The correct answer is B.
Rationale: Myocardial injury due to increased myocardial oxygen demand and decreased supply can lead to ADHF. This mismatch can be exacerbated by decreased coronary artery perfusion which may be a result of low coronary diastolic blood pressure (choice D) or high LV diastolic pressure (choice A). Increased afterload can also cause elevated filling pressure, which can redistribute blood flow centrally (choice C). This patient's acute kidney injury is likely due to cardiorenal syndrome, which can be due to either low cardiac output or elevated right atrial pressure that leads to increased vascular resistance and pressure in the Bowman capsule (choice B).

75.3 The correct answer is C.
Rationale: Extra heart sounds (S3 or S4) are present in at least 30% of the patients admitted for ADHF with a specificity of 32%, though there is poor interobserver agreement (choice A). Lower extremity edema, which is typically pitting and symmetric, is present in half to two-thirds of patients with ADHF (choice B). Because of hypertrophy of the lymphatic system, peripheral edema may also be absent, especially in patients with chronic heart failure. Cool extremities are indicative of poor perfusion and low cardiac output; however, assessing for cool extremities can be highly subjective with a specificity of 88% (choice D). Proportional pulse pressure which is defined as the pulse pressure divided by the systolic blood pressure is an indirect crude assessment of LV stroke volume and in turn, cardiac index. A proportional pulse pressure of less than 25% is associated with a cardiac index of less than 2.2 L/min/m^2, carrying a specificity of 96% (choice C, **Table 75.1**).

75.4 The correct answer is D.
Rationale: This patient's symptoms and physical examination are consistent with abnormal perfusion and hemodynamic congestion which corresponds to Stevenson profile C ADHF. Given her hypotension which is likely contributing to being "cold" on examination, she would benefit from inotropes to augment her perfusion and supplement diuretics which are needed for her congestion (choice D). In Stevenson profile A and L, filling pressures are normal, and therefore patients appear "dry" on examination (choices A and C). Patients under the category of Stevenson profile B have normal perfusion and are therefore "warm" on examination (choice B) (**Figure 75.1**).

TABLE 75.1 Utility of Clinical Examination Findings in ADHF

	Examination Findings	Sensitivity	Specificity	PPV	NPV	(+) LR	(−) LR
Perfusion[a]	S3 gallop	62	32	61	33	0.92	0.85
	SBP <100 mm Hg	42	66	77	29	1.24	1.14
	PPP <25%	10	96	88	28	2.54	1.07
	Cool extremities	20	88	82	28	1.68	1.10
	"Cold" profile	33	86	87	32	2.33	1.28
Congestion[b]	Ascites	21	92	81	40	2.44	1.15
	Rales >1/3	15	89	69	38	1.32	1.04
	Edema >2+	41	66	67	40	1.20	1.11
	Orthopnea >2 pillows	86	25	66	51	1.15	1.80
	JVP >12 mm Hg	65	64	75	52	1.79	1.82
	HJR	83	27	65	49	1.13	1.54

ADHF, acute decompensated heart failure; HJR, hepatojugular reflux; JVP, jugular venous pressure; LR, likelihood ratio; NPV, negative predictive value; PPP, proportional pulse pressure; PPV, positive predictive value; SBP, systolic blood pressure.
[a]Cardiac index less than 2.2 L/min/m².
[b]Pulmonary capillary wedge pressure greater than 22 mm Hg.
Adapted with permission from Drazner MH, Hellkamp AS, Leier CV, et al. Value of clinician assessment of hemodynamics in advanced heart failure: the ESCAPE trial. *Circ Heart Fail.* 2008;1(3):170-177.

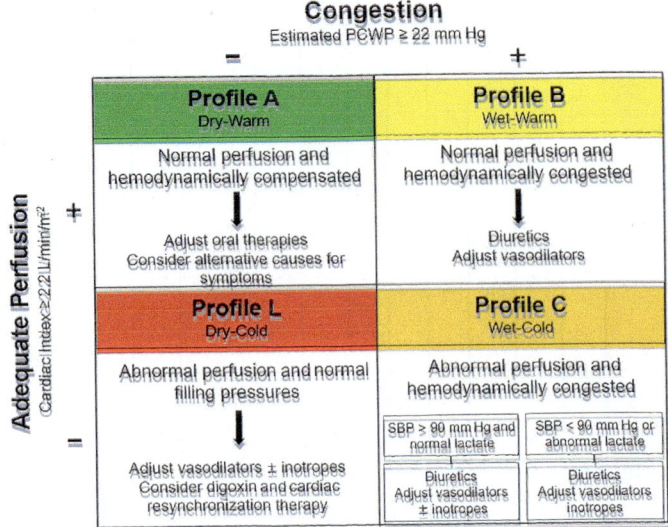

Figure 75.1 Stevenson clinical profiles and suggested clinical therapies. PCWP, pulmonary capillary wedge pressure.

75.5 The correct answer is E.

Rationale: This patient's symptoms along with normal blood pressure are consistent with Stevenson clinical profile B ADHF. He is perfusing well without evidence of renal dysfunction or electrolyte derangements. His guideline-directed medical therapies need not be held while he is being treated with IV diuretics. Thus, he can continue to take sacubitril-valsartan, metoprolol succinate, and spironolactone (choice D). All of these medications, along with the recently studied sodium-glucose transporter 2 (SGLT2) inhibitors carry a class I indication for use in HFrEF.

75.6 The correct answer is C.

Rationale: There are a multitude of reasons for diuretic resistance which range from an insufficient diuretic dose to the use of nonsteroidal anti-inflammatory drugs. Many of the etiologies for diuretic resistance stem from either impaired renal function or increased activation of the renin-angiotensin-aldosterone system. With regard to reduced renal function which can be represented by a reduced glomerular filtration (choice D), loop diuretics and thiazide diuretics may not be able to exert their action on the ascending loop of Henle and distal convoluted tubule, respectively, due to suboptimal nephron function. Impaired renal function is often associated with worsening uremia, which can contribute to reduced tubular uptake of the diuretics (choice A). Neurohormonal activation of the renin-angiotensin-aldosterone system in the setting of repeated diuretic use can result in increased tubular reabsorption at sites that are not particularly sensitive to diuretics, a concept known as the "braking phenomenon" (choice B). Decreased rather than increased renal blood flow can result in compromised kidney function as well as increased neurohormonal activation, which can contribute to diuretic resistance overall (choice C).

75.7 The correct answer is A.

Rationale: This patient has signs and symptoms of ADHF as evidenced by orthopnea, paroxysmal nocturnal dyspnea, liberal salt intake, elevated NT-pro-BNP levels, and signs of pulmonary congestion on his chest x-ray. Loop diuretics such as furosemide are one of the mainstay therapies for achieving a net negative fluid balance and ultimately relieving pulmonary congestion (choice C). The initial dose of loop diuretics in ADHF is typically 2.5 times the oral outpatient dose. If diuretic resistance is observed despite an escalating dose of loop diuretics, a thiazide diuretic can be added to augment diuresis and improve pulmonary edema (choice D). Acetazolamide is under investigation in ADHF with recent literature demonstrating that it improves natriuresis and promotes pulmonary decongestion (choice B[1]). The ATHENA-HF (Aldosterone Targeted Neurohormonal Combined with Natriuresis Therapy in Heart Failure) trial that evaluated the addition of daily spironolactone as an adjusted diuretic in ADHF did not show a significant difference in pulmonary decongestion or reduction in NT-proBNP levels when compared to placebo (choice A, See **Table 75.2**).

75.8 The correct answer is B.

Rationale: This patient has evidence of hypervolemia and congestion. When combined with his lower extremities which are cool to touch and his low blood pressure, he likely fits in the category of Stevenson profile C, which is concerning for cardiogenic shock. Suspecting that the cardiac output is low, a vasopressor or inotrope that increases inotropy would be the best option to augment cardiac hemodynamics. Although norepinephrine stimulates a_1 receptors, it also binds to B_1 receptors to increase inotropy (choice A). Dobutamine stimulates both B_1 and B_2 receptors to help increase inotropy, chronotropy, as well as cause mild vasodilation (choice B). Milrinone is a phosphodiesterase inhibitor that stimulates the cyclic adenosine monophosphate (cAMP) pathway to increase inotropy, chronotropy, and lusitropy (choice D). Both dobutamine and milrinone can cause arrhythmias and therefore should be used with caution in patients who are already prone to arrhythmias (ie, cardiogenic shock). Phenylephrine is a selective a_1 receptor agonist which causes vasoconstriction. It increases afterload without increasing inotropy and is therefore a poor choice in cardiogenic shock (choice B).

75.9 The correct answer is A. A-IV, B-III, C-II, D-I.

Rationale: PIONEER-HF was a multicenter, double-blind, randomized control trial that compared sacubitril-valsartan and enalapril in patients hospitalized with ADHF and a left ventricular ejection fraction (LVEF) of less than 40%. Results showed a greater reduction on NT-proBNP, death, and heart failure hospitalization at 16-week follow-up in the sacubitril-valsartan arm versus the enalapril arm (choice IV). ESCAPE was a multicenter, open-label, randomized control trial that evaluated survival in patients hospitalized with ADHF and an LVEF of less than 30% who underwent placement of a pulmonary artery catheter versus standard of care. Overall, there was no difference in mortality or length of stay between the two groups (choice III). Notably, patients with Stevenson profile C were not included in this trial. EVEREST was a multicenter, double-blinded, placebo-controlled trial that evaluated the benefits of tolvaptan versus placebo when given for 60 days in patients hospitalized with ADHF and an LVEF of less than 40%. There was no difference in mortality,

TABLE 75.2 Major Clinical Trials for Patients with Acute Decompensated Heart Failure

Trial for ADHF	Treatment	Cohort	Results
VMAC (2002, $N = 489$)	Double-blind IV nitroglycerin vs IV nesiritide (recombinant human B-type natriuretic peptide) vs placebo	Hospitalized with ADHF and SBP >90 mm Hg	Greater reduction of PCWP with IV nesiritide vs nitroglycerin at 24 h (-8.2 mm Hg, -6.3 mm Hg, -2 mm Hg; $P = .04$). No difference in patient-reported dyspnea at 24 h ($P = .13$)
OPTIME-CHF (2003, $N = 949$)	Double-blind, IV milrinone (0.5 µg/kg/min) vs placebo for 48-72 h	Hospitalized ADHF without cardiogenic shock	No difference in number of days hospitalized within 60 d ($P = .20$)
ESCAPE (2005, $N = 433$)	Unblinded pulmonary artery catheter vs standard care	Hospitalized ADHF with LVEF <30% and SBP <125 mm Hg	No difference in mortality ($P = .35$) or number of hospitalized days ($P = .67$) at 180 d
REVIVE-2 (2005, $N = 600$)	Double-blind, IV levosimendan or placebo	Hospitalized with ADHF, LVEF <35% and dyspnea at rest despite IV diuretics	Mild improvement of clinical course at 5 d with levosimendan; however, numerically more deaths
EVEREST (2007, $N = 4,133$)	Double-blind, tolvaptan (vasopressin V_2 receptor blocker) vs placebo	Hospitalized ADHF and LVEF <40% without cardiogenic shock	No difference in mortality ($P = .68$) or composite of CV death and HF hospitalization ($P = .55$) during 9.9-mo median follow-up
SURVIVE (2007, $N = 1,327$)	Double-blind, IV dobutamine vs IV levosimendan (calcium-sensitizing inodilator)v	Hospitalized ADHF, LVEF <30% and required inotropic support	No difference in all-cause mortality at 31 ($P = .29$) or 180 d ($P = .40$)
UNLOAD (2007, $N = 200$)	Unblinded ultrafiltration vs usual care for 48 h	Hospitalized with ADHF and serum creatinine <3.0 mg/dL	At 48 h greater weight loss in ultrafiltration arm ($P = .001$), but no difference in dyspnea improvement

Trial	Design	Population	Outcome
VERITAS (2007, $N = 1,435$)	Double-blind, IV tezosentan (endothelin receptor A/B antagonist) vs placebo	Hospitalized with ADHF and LVEF <40%	No difference in patient-reported symptoms at 24 h ($P > .50$) or the incidence of death or worsening HF at 7 d ($P = .95$)
PROTECT (2010, $N = 2,033$)	Double-blind, rolofylline (adenosine A_1-receptor antagonist) vs placebo	Hospitalized with ADHF and eGFR 20-80 mL/min/1.73 m²	No difference in clinical improvement ($P = .35$) or renal function ($P = .44$) at 60 d
ASCEND-HF (2011, $N = 7,141$)	Double-blind, IV nesiritide (recombinant human B-type natriuretic peptide) vs placebo	Hospitalized with ADHF and SBP <100 mm Hg	No difference in composite end point of HF and all-cause death at 30 d ($P = .31$) or 24-h improvement in dyspnea
DOSE (2011, $N = 308$)	Double-blind, 1:1:1:1 low-dose (intermittent vs continuous IV) or high-dose (intermittent vs continuous IV) furosemide	Hospitalized with ADHF and SBP <90 mm Hg	No difference in symptoms at 70 h between treatment arms. Mild increase in weight loss in high-dose arm at 72 h ($P = .01$)
SMAC-HF (2011, $N = 1,771$)	Single-blind, hypertonic saline solution (150 mL 1.4%-4.6% NaCl) tid and 120 mmol vs 80 mmol Na restriction	Single center, hospitalized for ADHF, LVEF <40% and NYHA class III	Primary outcome of all-cause death ($P < .001$) or HF rehospitalization ($P < .001$) at mean 57-mo follow-up favoring hypertonic saline arm
CARRESS-HF (2012, $N = 188$)	Ultrafiltration (200 mL/h) vs usual care with diuretics to resolution of congestion	Hospitalized with ADHF and increase in serum creatinine of at least 0.3 mg/dL within 12 wk	Increase of composite end point of change in weight and increase of creatinine at 96 h for ultrafiltration arm ($P = .003$)
ROSE (2013, $N = 360$)	Double-blind, IV dopamine (2 µg/kg/min) vs nesiritide (recombinant human B-type natriuretic peptide) vs placebo	Hospitalized with ADHF and eGFR 15-60 mL/min/1.73 m²	No difference in 72-h urine output for low-dose dopamine ($P = .59$) or nesiritide ($P = .49$) vs placebo

(continued)

TABLE 75.2 Major Clinical Trials for Patients with Acute Decompensated Heart Failure (*continued*)

Trial for ADHF	Treatment	Cohort	Results
ATHENA (2017, $N = 360$)	Double-blind, daily spironolactone 100 mg vs spironolactone 25 mg vs placebo	Hospitalized with ADHF and eGFR >30 mL/min/1.73 m²	No difference in the change in NT-proBNP at 96 h ($P = .57$) or secondary 30-d mortality or HF rehospitalization rate
TRUE-AHF (2017, $N = 2,157$)	Double-blind, IV Ularitide (urodilatin) vs placebo for 48 h	Hospitalized ADHF with SBP >115 mm Hg	No difference in CV death at 2 y ($P = .75$) or median length of stay at 30 d ($P = .16$)
PIONEER-HF (2019, $N = 881$)	Double-blind, sacubitril-valsartan vs enalapril	Hospitalized with ADHF with an LVEF <40%	Greater reduction of NT-proBNP ($P <.001$) and death or HF hospitalization ($P = .007$) at 16-wk follow-up in sacubitril-valsartan arm
RELAX-AHF-2 (2019, $N = 6,545$)	Double-blind, IV serelaxin (recombinant human relaxin-2) vs placebo for 48 h	Hospitalized with ADHF and SBP >125 mm Hg	No difference in CV death at 180 d ($P = .77$) or worsening HF at 5 d ($P = .19$)

ADHF, acute decompensated heart failure; CV, cardiovascular; eGFR, estimated glomerular filtration rate; HF, heart failure; IV, intravenous; LVEF, left ventricular ejection fraction; NYHA, New York Heart Association; PCWP, pulmonary capillary wedge pressure; SBP, systolic blood pressure.

cardiovascular death, and heart failure hospitalizations between the two groups (choice II). ROSE was a multicenter, double-blinded, placebo-controlled trial that evaluated decongestion with IV dopamine and nesiritide versus placebo in patients with ADHF and an estimated glomerular filtration rate (eGFR) between 15 and 60 mL/min/1.73 m². Ultimately, there was no difference in 72-hour urine output both between low-dose dopamine and placebo as well as nesiritide versus placebo (see **Table 75.2**).

75.10 The correct answer is A.
Rationale: Rehospitalization for heart failure has imposed a significant burden in the health care industry. Approximately 25% of older patients admitted for ADHF are rehospitalized within 30 days (choice D). The rehospitalization rate for HFrEF within 60 to 90 days is approximately 30% and is equal to HFpEF (choices A and B). To combat these hospitalization rates, a Medicare rehospitalization reduction program was initiated with literature demonstrating that early post discharge follow-up within 7 to 10 days and promoting the use of guideline-directed medical therapy can decrease hospitalization rates (choice C, **Table 75.2**).

REFERENCES

1. Mullens W, Dauw J, Martens P, et al. Acetazolamide in acute decompensated heart failure with volume overload. *N Engl J Med.* 2022;387(13):1185-1195.

CHRONIC HEART FAILURE MANAGEMENT

Kellsey Peterson

CHAPTER 76

QUESTIONS

76.1 Which of the following is **NOT** a **TRUE** statement regarding loop diuretics?
  A. Loop diuretics have venodilatory effects and have been shown to decrease right atrial and pulmonary venous wedge pressure within minutes of intravenous (IV) infusion.
  B. Furosemide has greater bioavailability than bumetanide and torsemide and may be more effective in patients with significant volume overload and intestinal edema.
  C. The Diuretic Optimization Strategies Evaluation (DOSE) study demonstrated that there was no difference in the co-primary end points of global assessment of symptoms or a change in creatinine at 72 hours in either the bolus versus continuous infusion group of IV furosemide.
  D. Loop diuretics initiate a renal homeostatic mechanism that increases distal solute and water reabsorption, which can be overcome with coadministration of a thiazide-like diuretic to increase diuretic effectiveness.

76.2 Which of the following is **NOT** a mechanism of angiotensin receptor neprilysin inhibitors (ARNI)?
  A. Inhibition of neprilysin increases levels of atrial natriuretic peptide, B-type natriuretic peptide, C-type natriuretic peptide, and adrenomedullin which results in increased venodilation.
  B. Inhibition of neprilysin results in increased natriuresis and decreased left ventricular fibrosis and hypertrophy.
  C. Neprilysin breaks down angiotensin II and its inhibition can lead to venodilation and decreased afterload.
  D. Neprilysin is a zinc-dependent membrane endopeptidase and cleaves a variety of peptides including natriuretic peptides, bradykinin, and adrenomedullin.

76.3 Which of the following was a pivotal finding in the PARADIGM-HF (Prospective Comparison of ARNI with ACEIs [angiotensin-converting enzyme inhibitors] to Determine Impact on Global Mortality and Morbidity in Heart Failure) trial?

*Questions and Answers are based on Chapter 76: Chronic Heart Failure Management by Ray Hu, Edo Y. Birati, and Lee R. Goldberg in Cardiovascular Medicine and Surgery, First Edition.

A. The use of sacubitril/valsartan resulted in a 20% relative risk reduction (RRR) as compared to enalapril in the combined end point of cardiovascular mortality and heart failure hospitalizations in stable patients who are classified as NYHA (New York Heart Classification) class I to II with left ventricular ejection fraction (LVEF) less than 35%.
B. The use of sacubitril/valsartan resulted in a 20% RRR as compared to enalapril in the combined end point of cardiovascular mortality and heart failure hospitalizations in stable patients who are classified as NYHA class II to IV with LVEF less than 25%.
C. A significant decrease in all-cause mortality was observed in the sacubitril/valsartan arm compared to enalapril.
D. A significant decrease in acute kidney injury (AKI) was observed in the sacubitril/valsartan arm compared to enalapril.

76.4 Which of the following statements regarding the side effects of renin-angiotensin-system (RAS) antagonists is **NOT TRUE**?

A. Angiotensin receptor blockers (ARBs) have no effect on bradykinin activity and thus avoid some of the adverse effects of ACEIs.
B. An ARB can be used for patients who have a history of cough and angioedema with an ACEI.
C. The combination of an ACEI and a neprilysin inhibitor significantly increases the risk of angioedema.
D. A 12-hour washout period is required when transitioning from an ACEI to ARNI.

76.5 Which of the following strategies should be employed in the use of beta-blockers (BB) in heart failure?

A. Initiate BB when patients are euvolemic or dry.
B. Initiate BB after patients have achieved the maximum tolerated dose of renin-angiotensin-aldosterone-system (RAAS) blockade.
C. BB should be continued in acute heart failure exacerbation when patients are in cardiogenic shock requiring inotropic support.
D. BB should be up-titrated every 24 to 48 hours to maximally tolerated doses.

76.6 A 68-year-old African American male with an ischemic cardiomyopathy (LVEF of 32%) presents to your office for routine heart failure follow-up. He has chronic kidney disease, hypertension, and type 2 diabetes (DMII). Blood pressure is 146/78 mm Hg, pulse 58 beats per minute (bpm), oxygen saturation 98% on room air. His physical examination demonstrates a well-appearing male resting comfortably, and lungs are clear to auscultation bilaterally. Neck is supple without jugular venous distension. Cardiac examination with a regular rhythm, normal S1 and S2 without any appreciable murmurs. Extremities are warm without any evidence of jugular venous distension. Labs are notable for Na 134, K 5.2, Cr 2.7 (baseline 1.8), and BNP 64. His cardiac medications include carvedilol 6.25 mg bid, lisinopril 10 mg, and Lasix 40 mg daily. Which of the following medication changes should be made to optimize his heart failure regimen?

A. Add spironolactone 25 mg.
B. Increase carvedilol to 12.5 mg bid.
C. Discontinue lisinopril, allow for a 36-hour washout period then start Entresto 24 to 26 mg bid.
D. Discontinue lisinopril and start isosorbide dinitrate (Isordil) 10 mg tid along with hydralazine 10 mg tid.

76.7 Which of the following patients would **NOT** benefit from ivabradine?
A. A 58-year-old female with LVEF of 33%, NYHA class III symptoms with blood pressure of 110/70 mm Hg, and heart rate (HR) of 90 bpm on carvedilol 25 mg bid, Entresto 24 to 26 mg bid, Aldactone 50 mg, and Jardiance 10 mg.
B. A 68-year-old female with LVEF of 28% who cannot tolerate beta-blockade due to severe asthma and bronchospasm with a resting pulse of 75 bpm.
C. A 71-year-old male with LVEF of 30%, paroxysmal atrial fibrillation (AF) with sick sinus syndrome requiring a dual chamber pacemaker, on maximally tolerated guideline-directed medical therapy (GDMT) with persistent NYHA class III symptoms.
D. All of the above are correct.

76.8 All of the following statements regarding sodium-glucose cotransporter 2 inhibitors (SGLT2i) are correct **EXCEPT**:
A. The DAPA-HF (Dapagliflozin and Prevention of Adverse Outcomes in Heart Failure) trial showed a significant reduction in heart failure hospitalizations and mortality in patients who are classified as NYHA II to III with LVEF less than 40% treated with dapagliflozin independent of the presence of diabetes.
B. SGLT2i produce favorable changes in blood pressure, weight loss, uricosuria, intravascular volume, and ketosis.
C. Patients with diabetes, particularly type 1 diabetics, gain more benefit from SGLT2i than nondiabetic patients.
D. SGLT2i may need to be held before surgery, during periods of fasting, or during major illnesses.

76.9 Which of the following heart failure therapies has demonstrated improvements in NYHA functional class, 6-minute walk test, and quality of life?
A. Finerenone
B. IV iron
C. Ivabradine
D. Digoxin

76.10 Routine evaluation and management of patients with heart failure include all the following **EXCEPT**:
A. Regular assessment of left ventricular size and function with serial echocardiograms
B. Frequent follow-ups to assess for adherence to medical and lifestyle changes
C. Regular assessment for the ability to increase target doses of GDMT even in the absence of symptoms
D. Regular surveillance labs and serum drug levels

CHAPTER 76 | Chronic Heart Failure Management

ANSWERS

76.1 The correct answer is B.
Rationale: Torsemide and bumetanide have bioavailability greater than 80% compared to furosemide which can be as low as 40%. Patients with significant right-sided heart failure and congestion may therefore benefit from switching to torsemide or bumetanide. Loop diuretics do not just help to achieve proper fluid balance via diuretic effect. They also have venodilatory effects as outlined in the question stem that helps to relieve congestion instantaneously. The DOSE study was a randomized double-blind trial that compared diuretic strategies in acute heart failure with IV furosemide using either twice daily bolus dosing or continuous infusion and demonstrated that there was no difference in symptoms or kidney function at 72 hours in either the low- versus high-dose groups or the bolus versus infusion groups. Notably, there was a trend toward greater relief of symptoms and fluid loss in the high-dose group. The practice of adding a thiazide-like diuretic (ie, metolazone or chlorthalidone) can often precipitate a brisk diuresis.

76.2 The correct answer is C.
Rationale: ARNI has been shown to have beneficial effects in heart failure via its inhibition of neprilysin which cleaves and breaks down numerous peptides that have positive effects on heart failure. Its inhibition thus promotes venodilation and natriuresis, and decreases left ventricular hypertrophy and fibrosis. Neprilysin does, however, break down angiotensin II, which has detrimental effects leading to venoconstriction and increased afterload. Therefore, neprilysin inhibitors are combined with RAAS inhibitors to prevent the deleterious potentiation of angiotensin II.

76.3 The correct answer is C.
Rationale: The PARADIGM-HF was a pivotal trial demonstrating the benefit of ARNI. The use of sacubitril/valsartan resulted in a 20% RRR in the combined end point of cardiovascular mortality and heart failure hospitalizations in stable patients who are classified as NYHA class II to IV with LVEF less than 35%. Statement C is the correct answer. These findings helped to inform current guidelines which recommend replacement with ARNI in patients who are classified as class II to III tolerating ACEI or ARB therapy. More recent guidelines suggest that ARNI can be the initial de novo therapy for systolic heart failure in place of ACEI or ARB.

76.4 The correct answer is D.
Rationale: The kinin effects of ACEIs can lead to side effects including dry cough in up to 10% of patients and angioedema. ARBs function by antagonizing the angiotensin type 1 receptor to inhibit the adverse biologic effects of angiotensin II on cardiac remodeling and have no effect on bradykinin levels and therefore avoid cough and angioedema. The combination of ACEIs and neprilysin inhibitors can lead to high levels of bradykinin and therefore a sufficient transitional washout period of 36 hours (not 12 hours) following discontinuation of ACEIs is required to avoid the risk of angioedema.

76.5 The correct answer is A:
Rationale: BB should not be initiated or rapidly titrated in the setting of volume overload or borderline-low cardiac output as the inhibition of the adrenergic system can exacerbate acute heart failure. The majority of patients enrolled in BB trials were not on high-dose ACEIs and findings from trials suggest that there is greater mortality benefit to be gained by adding moderate- to high-dose BB to lower dose ACEIs as opposed to maximizing ACEIs and introducing low-dose BB only. BB should be held in cardiogenic shock; however, in the absence of this, there is evidence that acute withdrawal of BB can lead to worse outcomes. Studies have, therefore, suggested that most patients with acute heart failure should be continued on BB therapy. Lastly, BB should be initiated in low doses and titrated slowly, ideally no more than every 2 weeks.

76.6 The correct answer is D:
Rationale: This patient has evidence of AKI with hyperkalemia. Lisinopril should be discontinued, and he would benefit from the addition of Isordil/hydralazine as he is hypertensive as well. This combination has shown to be beneficial in African American patients with NYHA class III to IV symptoms with an LVEF of less than 40%, who are already receiving RAAS and beta-blockade. They can also be used in patients who cannot RAAS blockade due to kidney injury and hyperkalemia. He is already bradycardic; therefore, increasing beta-blockade would be inadvisable. While a 36-hour washout period when transitioning from an ACEI to Entresto is necessary, his AKI and hyperkalemia preclude this as well as the addition of spironolactone.

76.7 The correct answer is C:
Rationale: Ivabradine is a class IIa recommendation in those with an LVEF of 35% or less, NYHA class II to III symptoms who are on maximum tolerated BB therapy in sinus rhythm whose HR remains above 70 bpm; therefore, choice A is incorrect. In clinical practice, ivabradine is useful in patients who are unable to tolerate maximal BB due to adverse side effects of bronchospastic pulmonary disease. Ivabradine should not be used in patients who are in persistent AF since the mechanism involves the sinoatrial (SA) node. Furthermore, since its mechanism has been shown to increase the incidence of AF, it should not be used in patients with paroxysmal AF. Ivabradine should also not be used in patients with pacemakers as further reduction in HR could render patients pacemaker dependent which could lead to worsening of their cardiomyopathy.

76.8 The correct answer is C:
Rationale: DAPA-HF is a landmark trial for SGLT2i that has paved the way for its use in patients with heart failure. The mechanism of the clinical impact of SGLT2i in heart failure is not well understood; however, there is likely a significant contribution from the favorable physiologic changes described in statement B. SGLT2i have demonstrated benefit in adults with heart failure with reduced ejection fraction (HFrEF) independent of the presence of diabetes, prompting the approval of dapagliflozin by the U.S. Food and Drug Administration in patients with HFrEF with or without diabetes to reduce the risk of cardiovascular death or hospitalization. In fact, SGLT2i should be avoided in type 1 diabetics as their use can be associated with euglycemic ketoacidosis. This phenomenon is also observed in the setting of surgery,

infection, trauma, major illness, or decreased oral intake, and SGLT2i may need to be held in these settings.

76.9 The correct answer is B.

Rationale: Trials of IV iron therapy in patients with heart failure who are symptomatic and classified as NYHA class II to III with LVEF 40% or less and evidence of iron deficiency (ferritin <300 ng/mL, transferrin saturation ≤20%) demonstrated an increase in functional class, 6-minute walk test, and quality of life. Iron deficiency leads to impaired oxygen delivery and thus aerobic performance. Furthermore, its incidence is increased in patients with heart failure. It is important to recognize that oral iron formulation is less effective at replenishing iron stores than parenteral formulations. Finerenone is a nonsteroidal, selective mineralocorticoid recepter antagonist (MRA) that has been shown to have a similar efficacy profile as steroidal MRAs and to reduce chronic kidney disease progression and cardiovascular events in patients with kidney disease and DMII. Ivabradine has demonstrated a reduction in heart failure hospitalizations and mortality in HFrEF 35% or less and HR greater than 70 bpm on standard GDMT, including a BB. Despite digoxin's long history, considerable debate exists about its clinical utility.

76.10 The correct answer is A.

Rationale: Current guidelines recommend against routine echocardiograms in the absence of clinical or therapeutic changes. Management of patients with heart failure requires adherence to a complex medical regimen, daily self-monitoring, and maintaining specific lifestyle modifications. Patients should, therefore, be followed closely to allow for adherence to these regimens and to evaluate for symptoms and side effects, and monitor for disease progression. GDMT should be maximized to the highest tolerated strength in an effort to reach target doses used in clinical trials (see Tables 76.1-76.4 in *Cardiovascular Medicine and Surgery Textbook*). Numerous heart failure medications affect renal function and electrolytes, and therefore surveillance labs should be obtained routinely.

CARDIAC RESYNCHRONIZATION THERAPY*

Phillip Olsen and Alfred M. Leka

CHAPTER **77**

QUESTIONS

77.1 A 68-year-old man is seen in follow-up 3 months after a myocardial infarction (MI) with stent placement to the left anterior descending artery. Left ventricular ejection fraction (LVEF) during the index hospitalization was estimated at 20% to 25%. He was noted to have recurrent episodes of nonsustained ventricular tachycardia (NSVT) on telemetry monitoring while hospitalized. He was discharged on guideline-directed medical therapy including beta-blocker, angiotensin receptor neprilysin inhibitor (ARNI), mineralocorticoid antagonist, and sodium-glucose cotransporter 2 (SGLT2) inhibitor. He reports mild dyspnea and limitation of his physical activity after cardiac rehabilitation. Electrocardiogram (ECG) demonstrates normal sinus rhythm with a left bundle branch block and a QRS duration of 150 milliseconds. What is the most appropriate next step in his care?

- **A.** Schedule for electrophysiology study (EPS)
- **B.** Repeat transthoracic echocardiogram
- **C.** 30 days mobile telemetry monitoring
- **D.** Schedule for cardiac resynchronization therapy with defibrillator (CRT-D) implantation

77.2 A 72-year-old woman with a medical history including inferior MI occurring 1 year ago is seen in follow-up for palpitations. Holter monitoring showed recurrent episodes of NSVT lasting up to 7 seconds. She is on maximally tolerated guideline-directed medical therapy including beta-blocker, angiotensin receptor blocker, and mineralocorticoid antagonist. She has persistent New York Heart Association (NYHA) class II heart failure symptoms, and echocardiogram 3 months ago demonstrated an LVEF of 35%. What is the most appropriate next step?

- **A.** EPS
- **B.** Repeat transthoracic echocardiogram
- **C.** Initiation of amiodarone
- **D.** Initiation of sotalol

77.3 A 59-year-old man with a past medical history of paroxysmal atrial fibrillation and nonischemic cardiomyopathy with a severely reduced ejection fraction of 30% is seen in follow-up. He has been on maximally tolerated guideline-directed medical therapy for 9 months and reports persistent dyspnea with minimal exertion. ECG is unchanged and shows sinus rhythm with a left bundle branch block and QRS of 155 milliseconds. What is the next **BEST** step?

*Questions and Answers are based on Chapter 77: Cardiac Electronic Implantable Device Therapy by Yang, Irakli Giorgberidze, and Lorraine Cornwell in Cardiovascular Medicine and Surgery, First Edition.

A. Left ventricular assist device (LVAD) placement
B. Implantable cardioverter-defibrillator (ICD) implantation
C. Atrioventricular (AV) node ablation and implantation of dual chamber pacemaker
D. CRT-D implantation

77.4 A 67-year-old woman with a medical history of ischemic cardiomyopathy with reduced ejection fraction of 35% on guideline-directed medical therapy for the past 2 years is seen in the hospital for heart failure exacerbation and is diagnosed with sick sinus syndrome. ECG shows sinus bradycardia with a rate of 48 beats per minute (bpm) with a QRS of 100 milliseconds. Repeat transthoracic echocardiogram shows no change from her last study 1 year ago. Which of the following is the **BEST** next step in treatment after treatment of her current heart failure exacerbation?
A. Ivabradine initiation
B. Dual chamber ICD placement
C. CRT-D placement
D. No change in treatment

77.5 A 60-year-old man is hospitalized for the fourth time this year for a heart failure exacerbation despite maximally tolerated medical therapy. He reports severe fatigue and dyspnea with all activities at home. Recent echocardiogram demonstrates an LVEF of less than 25%. ECG demonstrates sinus rhythm with a left bundle branch block and a QRS of 160 milliseconds. During a hospitalization last month, he was found to have colon cancer with lung and liver metastases. Which of the following is the **BEST** next step in treatment?
A. Palliative care consultation
B. Transplant evaluation
C. LVAD evaluation
D. CRT-D implantation

77.6 Which of the following statements regarding CRT is **FALSE**?
A. CRT has demonstrated mortality benefits in appropriate patients.
B. CRT has demonstrated a reduction in heart failure hospitalizations.
C. CRT has been shown to reduce the number of medications needed for long-term management of heart failure with reduced ejection fraction (HFrEF).
D. CRT has been shown to reverse left ventricular (LV) dilatation.

77.7 Which of the following is **FALSE** regarding complications or ICD and CRT placement?
A. Pneumothorax is a possible complication of lead insertion.
B. Subclavian crush phenomenon occurs when leads are inserted too far laterally.
C. Atrial lead dislodgement is the most common site for lead dislodgement.
D. Lead perforation is rare and estimated to occur in less than 0.5% of cases.

77.8 A 45-year-old man with a past medical history including poorly controlled hypertension, hyperlipidemia, and alcohol abuse presents to the emergency department (ED) after a witnessed out-of-hospital cardiac arrest. The patient's presenting rhythm after Emergency Medical Services (EMS) arrival was ventricular fibrillation. After advanced cardiovascular life support (ACLS), return of spontaneous circulation is achieved, and the patient makes a good recovery during the hospitalization. ECG shows normal sinus rhythm with first-degree AV block, a QRS of 100 milliseconds, and evidence of LV hypertrophy. He undergoes a cardiac catheterization that shows nonobstructive coronary artery disease. Transthoracic echocardiogram shows a LVEF of 30%. Which of the following is the **BEST** next step?

A. ICD placement for primary prevention
B. ICD placement for secondary prevention
C. CRT-D placement for primary prevention
D. CRT-D placement for secondary prevention

77.9 A 75-year-old woman with a past medical history significant for hypertension and HFrEF status post CRT-D placement was hospitalized after a mechanical fall. While admitted, she was observed to have painless abdominal contractions which the patient reported had been going on for many months but were not painful, so she never mentioned them. Chest x-ray shows normal device positioning and cardiomegaly similar to the prior x-ray 1 year ago. Device interrogation reveals no arrhythmias. Basic metabolic profile was normal. Which of the following is the **MOST LIKELY** cause?

A. Benign fasciculation syndrome
B. Abdominal aortic aneurysm
C. Phrenic nerve stimulation
D. Lead perforation

77.10 A 56-year-old woman presents to the ED after out-of-hospital cardiac arrest with the return of spontaneous circulation and is found to have anterior ST-segment elevation myocardial infarction (STEMI) on ECG. She is brought to the cath lab and undergoes stent placement to the left anterior descending artery. On day 1 of her hospitalization, she has intermittent accelerated idioventricular rhythms (AIVR), which spontaneously resolve over the next 24 hours. ECG shows normal sinus rhythm with anteroseptal Q waves and a QRS of 110 milliseconds. Transthoracic echocardiogram shows LVEF of 25%. She is initiated on guideline-directed therapy and prepared for hospital discharge. Which of the following is the **BEST** next step?

A. Discharge on guideline-directed medical therapy (GDMT) with close follow-up.
B. Begin amiodarone to prevent further arrhythmia.
C. Begin dofetilide to prevent further arrhythmia.
D. Implant ICD for prevention of sudden cardiac death.

ANSWERS

77.1 **The correct answer is B.**
Rationale: This patient is seen 3 months after a primary ischemic event leading to cardiomyopathy with an ejection fraction of 20% to 25% now with persistent NYHA class II symptoms. He was discharged from the hospital on complete guideline medical therapy and enrolled in cardiac rehabilitation. The next most appropriate step is to reassess LV function on repeat echocardiogram to evaluate for appropriateness of ICD or CRT-D implantation. If LVEF has recovered to 35% or more, ICD therapy

TABLE 77.1 Class I and IIa Indications for Implantable Cardioverter-Defibrillator Therapy

CLASS I INDICATIONS FOR ICD THERAPY

Survivors of cardiac arrest due to VF or hemodynamically unstable sustained VT after evaluation to determine the cause and to exclude any completely reversible causes (LOE: A)

Structural heart disease and spontaneous sustained VT, whether hemodynamically stable or unstable (LOE: B)

Syncope of undetermined origin with clinically relevant, hemodynamically significant sustained VT/VF induced at EPS (LOE: B)

LVEF ≤35% due to prior MI who are at least 40 days post-MI and are in NYHA class II or III heart failure (LOE: A)

Left ventricular dysfunction due to prior MI who are at least 40 d post-MI, have an LVEF ≤30%, and are in NYHA functional class I heart failure (LOE: A)

Nonsustained VT due to prior MI, LVEF ≤40%, and inducible VF or sustained VT at EPS

CLASS IIA INDICATIONS

Sustained VT and normal or near-normal ventricular function (LOE: C)

Catecholaminergic polymorphic VT who has syncope and documented sustained VT while receiving beta-blockers (LOE: C)

Brugada syndrome who have had syncope or documented VT that has not resulted in cardiac arrest (LOE: C)

Unexplained syncope, significant LV dysfunction, and nonischemic dilated cardiomyopathy (LOE: C)

Hypertrophic cardiomyopathy that has one or more major risk factors for SCD (LOE: C)

Cardiac sarcoidosis, giant cell myocarditis, or Chagas disease (LOE: C)

EPS, electrophysiology study; ICD, implantable cardioverter-defibrillator; LOE, level of evidence; LVEF, left ventricular ejection fraction; MI, myocardial infarction; NYHA, New York Heart Association; SCD, sudden cardiac death; VF, ventricular fibrillation; VT, ventricular tachycardia.
Adapted from Epstein AE, DiMarco JP, Ellenbogen KA, et al. ACC/AHA/HRS 2008 guidelines for device-based therapy of cardiac rhythm abnormalities: a report of the American College of Cardiology/American Heart Association Task Force on Practice Guidelines (Writing Committee to Revise the ACC/AHA/NASPE 2002 Guideline Update for Implantation of Cardiac Pacemakers and Antiarrhythmia Devices) developed in collaboration with the American Association for Thoracic Surgery and Society of Thoracic Surgeons. *J Am Coll Cardiol.* 2008;51(21):e1-e62. Copyright © 2008 American College of Cardiology Foundation, the American Heart Association, Inc., and the Heart Rhythm Society, with permission.

would not be indicated. Telemetry monitoring may be considered to assess for persistent episodes of NSVT after his ischemic event but would not be the most appropriate next step (**Table 77.1**).

77.2 The correct answer is A.

Rationale: EPS is the most appropriate next step in the treatment of this patient. The Multicenter Unsustained Tachycardia Trial (MUSTT) evaluated the use of EPS to guide decision-making for antiarrhythmic therapy or ICD implantation in patients with ischemic cardiomyopathy with LVEF 40% or less and NSVT. The study found mortality benefit to ICD implantation in patients with inducible sustained ventricular tachycardia on EPS. This recommendation is further supported by the SCD-HeFT (Sudden Cardiac Death in Heart Failure Trial) which found mortality benefit with ICD implantation as compared to amiodarone therapy in patients with LVEF 35% or less and NYHA class II or III symptoms. Recent transthoracic echocardiogram demonstrated persistent reduced LVEF well over 40 days after MI on guideline-directed therapy, and a repeat study would not be the most beneficial step at this time. The MUSTT found a significant relative risk reduction with ICD therapy as compared to antiarrhythmic therapy, and sotalol is contraindicated in heart failure.

77.3 The correct answer is D.
Rationale: This patient presents with persistent NYHA class III heart failure symptoms on optimal medical therapy and with evidence of a widened QRS with left bundle branch block morphology. It is a class I indication for CRT-D placement in this setting by the 2022 ACC/AHA/HFSA (the American College of Cardiology/ American Heart Association/ Heart Failure Society of America) guidelines. The CARE-HF (Cardiac Resynchronization in Heart Failure) trial demonstrated benefit of CRT to medical therapy alone in patients with prolonged QRS, LVEF 35% or less, and NYHA class III/IV symptoms. Further expounding on CARE-HF was MADIT-CRT (Multicenter Automatic Defibrillator Implantation Trial With Cardiac Resynchronization Therapy), which demonstrated mortality benefit with CRT-D as opposed to ICD-only therapy in patients with NYHA class I or II heart failure, LVEF 30% or less, and a QRS greater than 130 milliseconds (**Table 77.2**).

TABLE 77.2 Indications for Cardiac Resynchronization Therapy

NYHA Functional Class			
LEFT BUNDLE BRANCH BLOCK			
	QRS 120-129 ms	QRS 130-149 ms	QRS >150 ms
II	COR IIa (LOE B)	COR IIa (LOE B)	COR I (LOE B)
III and IV	COR IIa (LOE B)	COR IIa (LOE B)	COR I (LOE A)
NON-LEFT BUNDLE BRANCH BLOCK			
	QRS 120-129 ms	QRS 130-149	QRS >150 ms
II	COR III (LOE B)	COR III (LOE B)	COR IIb (LOE B)
III and IV	COR IIb (LOE B)	COR IIb (LOE B)	COR IIa (LOE B)

COR, classification of recommendation; LOE, level of evidence; ms, milliseconds; NYHA, New York Heart Association.
Adapted from Epstein AE, DiMarco JP, Ellenbogen KA, et al. 2012 ACCF/AHA/HRS focused update incorporated into the ACCF/AHA/HRS 2008 guidelines for device-based therapy of cardiac rhythm abnormalities: a report of the American College of Cardiology Foundation/American Heart Association Task Force on Practice Guidelines and the Heart Rhythm Society. *J Am Coll Cardiol*. 2013;61(3):e6-e75.

77.4 The correct answer is B.

Rationale: This patient has a history of ischemic cardiomyopathy with persistently reduced ejection fraction despite maximally tolerated medical therapy. Her ECG shows a narrow QRS of less than 120 milliseconds. ICD implantation is a class I recommendation in patients with prior MI with LVEF 35% or less at least 40 days post-MI and with class II/III heart failure symptoms. CRT is not recommended in patients with a narrow QRS complex. Ivabradine can be considered in patients with persistent symptoms and elevated heart rates on GDMT but should be avoided in this patient with sick sinus syndrome.

77.5 The correct answer is A.

Rationale: Palliative care consultation would be the most appropriate next step in this patient with class IV heart failure symptoms. Advanced therapies including cardiac transplantation and ventricular assist device (VAD) placement are contraindicated in this patient with metastatic cancer. Similarly, ICD therapy is not recommended in patients with a life expectancy of less than 1 year, NYHA class IV heart failure who are not candidates for transplantation or VADs, or with incessant ventricular tachycardia.

77.6 The correct answer is C.

Rationale: CRT has been shown to improve mortality, heart failure hospitalizations, and reverse LV dilatation when used in appropriate patients with widened QRS complexes and NYHA class II/III/IV heart failure symptoms. CRT has not been studied independently of medical therapy and is not recommended as a therapy to reduce the pharmacologic burden for patients.

77.7 The correct answer is B.

Rationale: Subclavian crush phenomenon describes a mechanism of early lead failure due to compression of the lead between the clavicle and first rib and most commonly occurs if leads are inserted in too medially. There is increased risk of pneumothorax with lateral lead insertion, but appropriate use of ultrasonography and fluoroscopy can reduce the risk. Lead dislodgement has reduced in frequency with the introduction of active fixation leads but still occurs most commonly in the atrial lead. Lead perforation is a very rare complication with active fixation leads, occurring in only 0.1% to 0.4% of cases. Perforation is typically self-limited and not require operative intervention.

77.8 The correct answer is B.

Rationale: In this case of a patient with sudden cardiac death in the setting of ventricular fibrillation without a clear reversible cause (ie, ischemia), a defibrillator is indicated during the index hospitalization. CRT is not indicated as the QRS is normal. Device insertion in this case would be for *secondary* prevention as he has already survived an initial event and is at high risk for recurrent events. Primary prevention refers to device placement in patients who are at high risk for life-threatening arrhythmias and have not had sudden cardiac death.

77.9 The correct answer is C.
Rationale: Phrenic nerve stimulation is a rare complication of CRT with the LV lead traversing the coronary sinus and cardiac vein along the LV wall. It should be excluded at the time of initial device implantation before lead securement. Lead perforation is unlikely to cause abdominal fasciculation and the unchanged cardiomegaly in this case makes it less likely.

77.10 The correct answer is A.
Rationale: In this case of a patient presenting with out-of-hospital arrest due to myocardial ischemia and developing acute HFrEF, the first priority is initiation of GDMT. AIVR is a benign arrhythmia sometimes present after myocardial reperfusion and does not require antiarrhythmic therapy. Transthoracic echocardiogram should be repeated 40 days after MI to assess for improvement in LVEF on GDMT. If LVEF remains less than 35%, ICD would be indicated.

MECHANICAL CIRCULATORY SUPPORT*

Phillip Olsen and Dmitri Belov

CHAPTER 78

QUESTIONS

78.1 A 60-year-old man with a past medical history significant for end-stage renal disease (ESRD) on thrice weekly hemodialysis and ischemic cardiomyopathy with a left ventricular ejection fraction (LVEF) of 30% is hospitalized for hypervolemia and NYHA (New York Heart Association) class IV heart failure symptoms. His condition deteriorates on the second day of his hospitalization, requiring transfer to the Coronary Care Unit (CCU) for vasopressor and inotropic support. He has rapidly rising vasopressor requirements requiring high doses of norepinephrine, vasopressin, and epinephrine. Which one of the following INTERMACS (Interagency Registry for Mechanically Assisted Circulatory Support) profiles **BEST** describes the patient?

  A. INTERMACS 1
  B. INTERMACS 2
  C. INTERMACS 3
  D. INTERMACS 4

78.2 A 55-year-old woman with a past medical history significant for hypertension, diabetes mellitus complicated by osteomyelitis and above-the-knee amputation of the left leg, ESRD recently initiated on hemodialysis, and obesity (body mass index [BMI] 32) is admitted to the CCU with decompensated heart failure and cardiogenic shock. Her status deteriorates with worsening shock, hypoxic respiratory failure, and ischemic hepatitis. Eventually, she stabilizes and remains dependent on inotropes. She is evaluated by the advanced heart failure team for consideration of ventricular assist device (VAD) placement. Which of the following is an absolute contraindication to VAD implantation?

  A. Obesity
  B. Hepatic dysfunction
  C. Baseline mobility impairment
  D. ESRD on dialysis

78.3 Which of the following valvulopathies **DOES NOT** require surgical intervention with left ventricular assist device (LVAD) implantation?

  A. Moderate aortic regurgitation
  B. Severe aortic stenosis
  C. Severe mitral stenosis
  D. Severe tricuspid regurgitation

Questions and Answers are based on Chapter 78: Mechanical Circulatory Support by Anju Bhardwaj, Alexis Shafii, Andrew Civitello, and Ajith Nair in Cardiovascular Medicine and Surgery, First Edition

78.4 Which of the following is the **MOST IMPORTANT** risk factor for death after implantation of LVADs?

A. Intraoperative coagulopathy
B. Acute renal failure
C. Right ventricular failure
D. Degree of left ventricular failure

78.5 A 62-year-old woman with a history of ischemic cardiomyopathy status post single chamber implantable cardioverter-defibrillator (ICD) and severe heart failure stage D symptoms despite guideline-directed medical therapy undergoes LVAD implantation. She tolerates the procedure well and is discharged home. When seen in follow-up, which of the following treatments is **NOT** required?

A. Warfarin
B. Afterload reduction therapy for hypertension management
C. Diuretics as needed
D. Cardiac resynchronization therapy

78.6 A 58-year-old man with a history of hypertension, diabetes mellitus, and ischemic cardiomyopathy with stage D heart failure symptoms undergoes LVAD implantation with significant improvement. He does well and is maintained on warfarin for therapeutic anticoagulation for his device. He presents to the hospital 9 months after implantation with complaints of a week of persistent nausea, vomiting, diarrhea, and sudden onset arm weakness. On examination, LVAD hum is heard well, jugular venous pressure (JVP) is **NOT** elevated, and neurologic examination shows 1/5 strength in his left arm. LVAD interrogation shows frequent low pulsatility index alarms. Which of the following is the **BEST** next step?

A. Complete blood count (CBC)
B. International normalized ratio (INR)
C. Computed tomography (CT) of the head
D. Fluid bolus

78.7 Which of the following is **NOT** a risk factor for LVAD driveline infections?

A. Trauma to driveline site
B. Older age
C. Obesity
D. Poor driveline care

78.8 Which of the following is **NOT TRUE** regarding gastrointestinal (GI) bleeding in patients with LVADs?

A. Arteriovenous malformations are a common cause of bleeding.
B. Routine reversal of anticoagulation is recommended in patients on LVAD with suspected GI bleeding.
C. Acquired von Willebrand factor deficiency is a common contributor to bleeding.
D. Octreotide may be used in recurrent GI bleeding in patients on LVAD.

78.9 Which of the following factors contribute to the risk for LVAD thrombosis?
A. Pump speed
B. Outflow graft stenosis
C. Antiplatelet selection
D. Driveline infection

78.10 A 78-year-old man presents to the hospital with profound shortness of breath and palpitations. After extensive evaluation, he is found to have fulminant myocarditis with profound cardiogenic shock, ischemic hepatitis, pulmonary hypertension, and acute renal failure. He requests continued aggressive care early in his hospitalization. He has worsening shock on multiple vasopressors and inotropes but is eventually stabilized on inotropes and temporary VAD with improvement in right ventricular (RV) function. You are asked to evaluate the patient on the advanced heart failure team. What is the most appropriate recommendation?
A. Palliative care with withdrawal of care
B. LVAD implantation for destination therapy
C. LVAD implantation for bridge to decision
D. Cardiac transplantation

ANSWERS

78.1 The correct answer is A.
Rationale: INTERMACS profiles are used to categorize patients and assist in the selection of patients who may benefit from mechanical circulatory support. INTERMACS 1 represents severe cardiogenic shock, and INTERMACS 3 represents patients who are hemodynamically stable but inotrope dependent. Select patients in INTERMACS profiles 1 and 2 may be considered for VAD therapy. All INTERMACS 3 patients may be considered for LVAD. Only severely symptomatic patients with profiles 4 to 7 should be considered for LVAD implantation. LVAD therapy is indicated in patients with end-stage heart failure and severe left ventricular dysfunction (**Table 78.1**).

TABLE 78.1 INTERMACS Ventricular Assist Device Placement According to INTERMACS Profiles

INTERMACS Profile	Description	% VAD implants
7	Advanced NYHA class III symptoms	0.5
6	Exertion limited	0.9
5	Exertion intolerant	2.3
4	Resting symptoms (home on oral therapy)	13.0
3	Stable but inotrope dependent	31.7
2	Progressive decline on inotropic support	36.5
1	Critical cardiogenic shock	15.1

INTERMACS, Interagency Registry for Mechanically Assisted Circulatory Support; NYHA, New York Heart Association; VAD, ventricular assist device.

78.2 The correct answer is D.

Rationale: Many patient-specific factors and comorbidities need to be considered when evaluating patients for VAD therapy. ESRD requiring hemodialysis is an absolute contraindication to LVAD implantation. Obesity with BMI 35 or more is considered a relative contraindication and patients may be considered with weight loss. Hepatic dysfunction that is attributable to ischemic hepatitis is expected to improve with VAD therapy; however, if it is unclear whether there is an additional cause of hepatic dysfunction further investigation may be required. Advanced age and debilitation are not absolute contraindications but require careful patient screening to best select patients who will benefit. Lastly, similar to heart transplantation, the intensive requirements of VAD therapy require strong social support and thorough psychosocial assessments before device implantation (**Table 78.2**).

TABLE 78.2 Absolute and Relative Contraindications to Left Ventricular Assist Devices

Absolute	Relative
Sepsis or current active infection	Morbid obesity
Right heart failure	Chronic renal dysfunction, not on dialysis
Untreated and severe carotid artery disease	Malnutrition
Severe pulmonary disease	Severe or untreated mitral stenosis
Severe irreversible cerebral injury	
Dialysis-dependent renal failure	
Elevated INR from liver failure	
Disseminated intravascular coagulation	
Severe end-organ failure	
Noncardiac illness with survival <2 y	

INR, international normalized ratio.

78.3 The correct answer is B.

Rationale: Valvular disease plays an important role in preoperative testing for planned LVAD implantation. Severe aortic stenosis does not require any intervention at the time of device insertion as systemic blood flow bypasses the aortic valve via the VAD. Moderate aortic regurgitation requires bioprosthetic valve replacement or oversewing of the native valve to prevent regurgitant flow from reducing effective cardiac output. Severe mitral stenosis impairs left ventricular filling thereby reducing device flow, so it must be repaired if present. Tricuspid valve repair should be considered in cases of severe tricuspid regurgitation to reduce the risk of postoperative right heart failure and thus the overall morbidity and mortality after VAD implantation.

78.4 The correct answer is C.

Rationale: Right heart failure has been found to be the most significant risk factor for death after VAD implantation. Complete assessment and prediction of RV failure is challenging and despite multiple predictive measures, no definitive measure has been identified to serve as an absolute marker for VAD placement. Predictive assessments include pulmonary hypertension, pulmonary artery pulsatility index (PAPI) less than 2, RV dilation, and impaired contractility. In cases of impaired RV function, planned right heart support at the time of VAD insertion has been found to have improved mortality.

78.5 The correct answer is D.
Rationale: Warfarin is indicated to maintain a target INR range of 2 to 3 to prevent pump thrombosis. Angiotensin receptor blockers (ARBs) and angiotensin-converting enzyme (ACE) inhibitors for afterload reduction are beneficial for blood pressure management and have been shown to reduce the GI bleed incidence. Diuretics are appropriate to continue to prevent volume overload. Benefit of continued cardiac resynchronization therapy after VAD insertion is not clear as the majority of cardiac output is supplied by the VAD and not dependent on ventricular synchrony.

78.6 The correct answer is C.
Rationale: In this patient with a VAD and recent GI illness symptoms now presenting with new onset left arm weakness, there is high concern for a neurologic complication of LVAD therapy. Hemorrhagic and ischemic stroke contribute significantly to the morbidity and mortality in patients with LVADs, with an annual incidence of about 9%. In this case of inability to tolerate oral intake including warfarin, the patient likely has a subtherapeutic INR and is at increased risk of thrombotic and cardioembolic events. A CT head would allow for rapid detection and distinction of hemorrhagic versus ischemic stroke to guide further workup. CBC, INR, and fluid bolus would all be beneficial in this case, but CT is the most appropriate next test for rapid diagnosis (**Table 78.3**).

TABLE 78.3 Assessment and Treatment of Left Ventricular Assist Device Complications

Neurologic emergencies
Activate stroke team.
Hold anticoagulation until imaging and INR obtained.
Obtain head CT.
Ischemic stroke—order CT angiogram head and neck, MAP optimization to ensure perfusion, endovascular thrombectomy if indicated
Hemorrhagic stroke—INR reversal, neurosurgery evaluation

LVAD infection
Obtain driveline drainage cultures and blood cultures.
CT or PET scan imaging
Intravenous antibiotics followed by chronic suppressive antibiotics
Surgical debridement with or without antibiotic bead placement
Transplant in eligible candidates if advanced local infection but no evidence of active bacteremia

GI bleeding
Assessment of hemodynamic status
Hold aspirin and warfarin.
Consider reversal of anticoagulation if hemodynamically unstable.
Transfuse as needed.

(continued)

TABLE 78.3 Assessment and Treatment of Left Ventricular Assist Device Complications (continued)

GI consult for colonoscopy for lower GI bleeding and EGD/enteroscopy for upper GI bleeding.
If rapid bleeding, tagged RBC scan recommended
If source identified and massive bleeding present may consider IR embolization
Lowering goal INR and/or decreasing/discontinuing antiplatelet therapy for recurrent bleeding
Long-term agents like octreotide (somatostatin analogue), thalidomide (antiangiogenic agent), and danazol may be considered.

Ventricular arrhythmias
Assessment of hemodynamic status
Defibrillation if hemodynamically unstable
If stable, obtain echocardiogram and speed optimization for a reversible cause.
Antiarrhythmic drugs
Catheter ablation for select cases of scar VT

Heart failure
Assess left-sided vs right-sided or biventricular HF
For left-sided or biventricular HF
- Systemic vasodilators for hypertension
- If aortic insufficiency present, diuresis, increasing LVAD support, inotropic support, TAVR in select cases
- Pump speed optimization for inadequate unloading

For right-sided HF
- Diuretics
- Inotropic agents
- Pulmonary vasodilators
- Right VAD, if indicated

LVAD malfunction
Assessment of hemodynamic status and check if VAD dependent
Evaluate device connections.
Evaluate driveline for tear/fracture.
Review LVAD flows and alarms.
Check batteries and controller.
Consult LVAD engineer.

Pump thrombosis
Assessment of hemodynamic status
Laboratory evaluation for markers of hemolysis
Echocardiography with ramp study (LVEDD is recorded at increasing LVAD speeds.)
CT angiogram if concern for outflow graft thrombus

Intravenous heparin or direct thrombin inhibitors depending on INR
Pump exchange is definitive therapy and should be done promptly to avoid renal failure/end-organ damage.
Increase goal INR and intensify antiplatelet therapy if preceding INRs are therapeutic.

CT, computed tomography; EGD, esophagogastroduodenoscopy; GI, gastrointestinal; HF, heart failure; INR, international normalized ratio; IR, interventional radiology; LVAD, left ventricular assist device; LVEDD, left ventricular end-diastolic diameter; MAP, mean arterial pressure; PET, positron emission tomography; RBC, red blood cells; TAVR, transcatheter aortic valve replacement; VAD, ventricular assist device; VT, ventricular tachycardia.

78.7 The correct answer is B.
Rationale: LVAD infections occur in 15% to 30% of patients and are most commonly caused by *Pseudomonas* or *Staphylococcus* organisms. Risk factors for infection include trauma to the driveline, obesity, exposure of the driveline velour, and younger age. The mainstay of LVAD infection treatment involves intravenous antibiotics and debridement followed by suppressive oral antibiotics. Pump exchange is not curative and is associated with recurrent infection.

78.8 The correct answer is B.
Rationale: Gastrointestinal bleeding is a common complication in patients with LVADs leading to frequent admission. Arteriovenous malformation due to continuous flow from the LVAD and acquired von Willebrand factor deficiency due to pump shear stress are common contributors to significant bleeding. Anticoagulant reversal is only recommended in hemodynamically unable cases. Identification of a bleeding source frequently requires endoscopy, video capsule endoscopy, or push enteroscopy. Octreotide and thalidomide can be considered in cases of recurrent GI bleeding and embolization in refractory cases.

78.9 The correct answer is C.
Rationale: LVAD thrombosis can occur in the pump, outflow graft, or inflow cannula and can be detrimental to device functioning, leading to hemolysis and symptomatic anemia, cardiogenic shock, and multiorgan failure. Low pump speed, outflow graft stenosis, and driveline infections all increase the risk of LVAD thrombosis. Antiplatelet selection has not been shown to affect the risk for LVAD thrombosis, but the interruption in or subtherapeutic anticoagulation clearly increases risk. Pump thrombosis can be treated with thrombolytic therapy in stable cases or with device replacement in more critical cases.

78.10 The correct answer is B.
Rationale: In this case of fulminant myocarditis and cardiogenic shock that was successfully stabilized on temporary mechanical circulatory support, the most appropriate recommendation for a patient wishing for continued aggressive care would be for LVAD implantation for destination therapy. The patient is not appropriate for transplantation due to advanced age and thus both C and D are incorrect. Palliative care with the withdrawal of support would not be the most appropriate decision as the patient's wishes were clear to proceed with aggressive care. Destination therapy refers to LVAD implantation for treatment in patients who are not suitable for transplant.

SECTION 6 VASCULAR MEDICINE

CHAPTER 79

AORTIC DISEASES*

Brian Conway and William Bachman

QUESTIONS

79.1 A 56-year-old female with a history of bicuspid aortic valve presents to the hospital with acute onset tearing chest pain. Workup is consistent with an acute type B aortic dissection. All of the following are concerning possible complications of this **EXCEPT**:
  A. Renal insufficiency
  B. Aortic aneurysm
  C. Retroperitoneal bleed
  D. Acute cerebrovascular accident (CVA)

79.2 A 62-year-old male with a history of hypertension presents to the hospital with symptoms of crushing chest pain radiating to both arms with associated diaphoresis. Blood pressure is elevated on arrival to 210/140 mm Hg. Electrocardiogram (ECG) demonstrates 2 mm ST-segment elevations in leads II, III, and aVF and reciprocal ST depressions in leads I and aVL. Basic labwork is drawn including high-sensitivity troponins and is currently pending. What is the **BEST** next step in the management of this patient?
  A. Medical management for acute coronary syndrome (ACS), await troponin
  B. Emergent computed tomography (CT) scan to rule out pulmonary embolism (PE) or aortic dissection
  C. Transfer immediately to the coronary catheterization laboratory.
  D. Initiate intravenous (IV) antihypertensive treatment.

79.3 A 75-year-old male with a history of Marfan syndrome, hypertension, and hyperlipidemia presents to the emergency department with severe, sharp lower back pain. Symptoms began abruptly an hour ago while exercising at the gym. The patient recently restarted weight lifting exercises. Blood pressure on arrival is elevated at 175/110 mm Hg on the right arm and 170/100 mm Hg on the left. ECG demonstrates normal sinus rhythm without significant ST or T-wave abnormalities. A CT scan of the entire aorta is obtained showing an aortic dissection appearing to originate 2 cm distal to the left subclavian artery and extending throughout the aorta, terminating in the iliac arteries bilaterally. What is the **BEST** next step in the management of this patient?
  A. Emergent surgical consultation
  B. Start an infusion of clevidipine with goal reduction in systolic blood pressure less than 120 mm Hg.
  C. Start an infusion of labetalol with goal reduction in systolic blood pressure less than 120 mm Hg.
  D. Start oral carvedilol with PRN (pro re nata, as needed) IV hydralazine pushes to reach goal systolic blood pressure less than 120 mm Hg.

*Questions and Answers are based on Chapter 79: Aortic Diseases by Dawn S. Hui, Lalithapriya Jayakumar, and Andrea J. Carpenter in Cardiovascular Medicine and Surgery, First Edition.

Section 6: Vascular Medicine

79.4 A 70-year-old white male with a history of hypertension, hyperlipidemia, diabetes mellitus, prior deep vein thrombosis (DVT) on apixaban, and an active 50-pack year smoking history presents to the clinic to establish care with a new provider since relocating to Florida for retirement. He has **NOT** been followed for some time as he did **NOT** believe his medications were noticeably improving his quality of life. He denies any new symptoms, only presenting to the clinic at the insistence of his wife. His primary care doctor performs a detailed history and physical examination and ultimately orders an abdominal ultrasound for abdominal aortic aneurysm (AAA) screening purposes. A 5.0-cm infrarenal aortic aneurysm is noted. What is the **BEST** next step in this patients' management?

A. Serial imaging with repeat CT scan in 12 months
B. Duplex ultrasound imaging in 6 months
C. Referral to vascular surgery
D. Medical optimization of his chronic comorbidities

79.5 An 85-year-old man presents to the emergency department with worsening abdominal pain over the last few weeks. When questioned further he believes this pain has been present for many months. He also has felt queasy for some time, noting multiple episodes of vomiting for no apparent reason, which has been increasing in frequency of late which he believes to be due to chronic gastroenteritis. He has been taking over-the-counter antacids without any improvement in symptoms. Blood pressure is 120/80 mm Hg, heart rate 85 beats per minute (bpm). Labwork is unremarkable. Palpation of the abdomen reveals a pulsatile mid-epigastric mass with severe tenderness. Which of the following findings in this patient correlates with the impending risk of rupture?

A. Abdominal tenderness on palpation
B. Pulsatile abdominal mass
C. Nausea
D. Hemodynamic stability

79.6 A 62-year-old female presents to her primary care office for routine follow-up. Patient states she thinks she had an upper respiratory infection many months ago because her voice became hoarse in addition to a dry cough that has never improved with some blood noted in her sputum recently. She denies any infectious symptoms. She also notes vague chest and back pain over the same period of time and pain with swallowing. What is the **MOST LIKELY** diagnosis for this patient?

A. Tuberculosis
B. Gastroesophageal reflux
C. Recurrent upper respiratory tract infections
D. Thoracic aortic aneurysm (TAA)

79.7 A patient is diagnosed with a 4.5-cm AAA at age 65, currently being followed in the vascular surgery clinic. Which testing modality would be most appropriate for surveillance purposes?

A. Magnetic resonance imaging (MRI)
B. Duplex ultrasound
C. Computed tomography angiography (CTA)
D. None of the above

79.8 A 76-year-old female patient with a history of hypertension, chronic tobacco abuse, and known Crawford Type II AAA with a last documented diameter of 5.2 cm presents to the emergency department via emergency medical services (EMS) with acute onset bilateral flank pain approximately 30 minutes ago. Blood pressure is 92/45 mm Hg and heart rate 115 bpm. Emergent CT scan demonstrates a ruptured aneurysm with considerable blood accumulation in the retroperitoneal space. What is the expected risk of mortality of this patient within the next 24 hours?

A. 30%
B. 50%
C. 70%
D. 90%

79.9 An 81-year-old male with a history of coronary artery disease, hypertension, and hyperlipidemia presents to clinic 1 month after undergoing repair for a suprarenal AAA with endovascular aneurysm repair (EVAR) by vascular surgery. What is the most appropriate means of surveillance to be completed at this visit?

A. CT angiography
B. Duplex ultrasound
C. MRI
D. No surveillance imaging is required at this time.

79.10 An atherosclerotic lesion penetrating the internal elastic lamina into the media **BEST** characterizes this entity:

A. Aortic dissection
B. Penetrating aortic ulcer
C. Atheroma
D. Atherosclerosis

ANSWERS

79.1 The correct answer is D.
Rationale: Dissections involving the thoracic aorta distal to the left subclavian takeoff (type B) may extend along the length of the aorta, potentially compromising renal blood flow. They may result in aneurysm development and can potentially rupture leading to retroperitoneal bleeding. While dissections may result in thrombosis of the false lumen, the takeoff distal to the left subclavian artery would make an acute CVA very unlikely.

79.2 The correct answer is C.
Rationale: ECG abnormalities in patients with dissection are common; however, those mimicking acute occlusion of a coronary artery are not. Less than 10% of acute type A aortic dissections show evidence of new Q waves or ST elevations. A study of more than 1,500 patients with ST-segment elevation myocardial infarction (STEMI) determined that only 0.51% were secondary to aortic dissection.[1] In addition, in a

study of more than 400 patients with a presenting ECG concerning for STEMI, 11% had delayed door-to-balloon time because of a CT scan looking for stroke, PE, or aortic dissection. Only 4% of scans changed management by identifying stroke, while none found an aortic dissection.[2] While this patient's presentation may be concerning for dissection potentially involving the right coronary artery, the likelihood of this is low and should not delay the transfer of this patient to the cath lab for likely revascularization in this acute inferior STEMI.

79.3 The correct answer is C:
Rationale: This patient is presenting with an acute type B aortic dissection and should be immediately started on IV antihypertensive treatment with a first-line medication such as a beta-blocker with dual alpha- and beta-receptor blockade, nondihydropyridine calcium channel blockers, or vasodilators. Beta-blockers are ideal given their effect on blood pressure and heart rate, while vasodilator therapy initiation before heart rate control may result in reflex tachycardia and increased aortic shear stress (**Table 79.1**).

79.4 The correct answer is C:
Rationale: In the absence of genetically mediated disorders (Ehlers-Danlos syndrome, Turner syndrome, bicuspid aortic valve or familial TAA, and dissection) or Marfan syndrome, where elective repair should be performed at diameters from 4.0 to 5.0 cm, patients should be considered for surgical intervention for ascending or descending TAA or thoracoabdominal aneurysms greater than or equal to 5.5 cm. This patient has not reached a size requiring urgent repair; however, he should be referred to vascular or cardiothoracic surgery at the time of AAA or TAA discovery.

79.5 The correct answer is A:
Rationale: A pulsatile abdominal mass is consistent with AAA, and nausea and hydronephrosis may occur with compression of nearby structures such as the duodenum and ureters, respectively. Hemodynamic stability would be more associated with an unruptured AAA. Tenderness to palpation correlates best with impending risk of rupture.

79.6 The correct answer is D:
Rationale: The most common symptoms of TAA are vague pain in the chest, back, flank, or abdomen. Large TAAs can present with symptoms associated with compression of nearby structures. Hoarseness due to laryngeal nerve compression, chronic cough due to tracheal compression, dysphagia due to esophageal compression, and hemoptysis or hematemesis from erosion into the pulmonary structures of the esophagus can be seen. General symptoms of tuberculosis include weakness, fevers, weight loss, and night sweats. Neither gastroesophageal reflux nor recurrent upper respiratory tract infections would fit best with this constellation of symptoms.

79.7 The correct answer is B:
Rationale: The imaging modality of choice for both diagnosing and surveilling AAA (in the absence of repair) is the B-mode ultrasound, with sensitivity and specificity approaching 100%. However, for preoperative planning, multidetector computed tomography (MDCT) is superior in demonstrating more precise information regarding the sizing of grafts and locations of peripheral vessels. MRI can be considered

TABLE 79.1 Antihypertensive Agents for Aortic Dissection

	Drug	Initial IV Dose	Infusion Dose	Onset/Duration of Action	Side Effects	Considerations
Beta-adrenergic receptor blockers	Esmolol	250-500 µg/kg over 1 min	25-50 µg/kg/min, titrate up to max 300 µg/kg/min	1-2 min; 10-30 min	Nausea, flushing, bronchospasm, bradycardia, first-degree heart block	Nonhepatic, nonrenal clearance, avoid in acutely decompensated heart failure
	Labetalol	20 mg followed by 20-50 mg bolus every 10 min up to 300 mg	0.5-2 mg/min, titrate to max 10 mg/min	2-5 min; 2-6 h	Nausea, vomiting, paresthesias, bronchospasm, dizziness, bradycardia, first-degree heart block	Avoid in acutely decompensated heart failure; use with caution in obstructive airway disease.
Nondihydropyridine calcium channel blockers	Diltiazem	0.25-0.35 mg/kg	5-20 mg/h	1-3 min, 0.5-10 h	Nausea, bradycardia, first-degree heart block, dizziness	Avoid in acutely decompensated heart failure.
	Verapamil	5-10 mg, may repeat in 5-10 min		3-5 min; 0.5-6 h	Nausea, bradycardia, first-degree heart block, dizziness	Avoid in acutely decompensated heart failure.
Vasodilators	Nitroprusside		0.25-0.5 µg/kg/min, titrate to max 10 µg/kg/min	Immediate; 1-10 min	Elevated intracranial pressure, decreased cerebral blood flow, reduced coronary flow in coronary artery disease, cyanide and thiocyanate toxicity, nausea, vomiting, muscle spasm, flushing, sweating	To minimize cyanide toxicity, infusion duration should be as short as possible and ≤2 µg/kg/min. For patients with higher doses (ie, >500 µg/kg and >2 µg/kg/min) administer sodium thiosulfate infusion to avoid cyanide toxicity.

(continued)

TABLE 79.1 Antihypertensive Agents for Aortic Dissection (continued)

	Drug	Initial IV Dose	Infusion Dose	Onset/Duration of Action	Side Effects	Considerations
	Nicardipine		2.5-5 mg/h, titrate to max 15-30 mg/h	5-15 min; 0.5-8 min	Tachycardia, headache, dizziness, nausea, flushing, local phlebitis, edema	
	Clevidipine		1-2 mg/h, titrate up to 16 mg/h	2-4 min; 5-15 min	Atrial fibrillation, nausea, lipid allergy	Nonrenal, nonhepatic clearance
Second-line agents	Nitroglycerin		5-200 µg/min	2-5 min; 5-10 min	Hypoxemia, reflex sympathetic activation with tachycardia, headache, vomiting, flushing, methemoglobinemia, tolerance	Useful in patients with coronary ischemia or acute pulmonary edema
	Enalaprilat	1.25-5 mg IV every 6 h		15-30 min; 6 h	Precipitous fall in pressure with high-renin states; variable response, headache, dizziness	Slow onset, variable response, long duration of effect; avoid in acute myocardial infarction, renal impairment, or pregnancy

IV, intravenous.

Adapted from Black JH III, Burke CR. Management of acute type B aortic dissection. In: Collins KA, ed. *UpToDate.* 2024. Accessed December 13, 2022. https://www.uptodate.com/contents/management-of-acute-aortic-dissection; Hiratzka LF, Bakris GL, Beckman JA, et al. 2010 ACCF/AHA/AATS/ACR/ASA/SCA/SCAI/SIR/STS/SVM guidelines for the diagnosis and management of patients with thoracic aortic disease: a report of the American College of Cardiology Foundation/American Heart Association Task Force on Practice Guidelines, American Association for Thoracic Surgery, American College of Radiology, American Stroke Association, Society of Cardiovascular Anesthesiologists, Society for Cardiovascular Angiography and Interventions, Society of Interventional Radiology, Society of Thoracic Surgeons, and Society for Vascular Medicine. *Circulation.* 2010;121(13):e266-e369; Tsai TT, Nienaber CA, Eagle KA. Acute aortic syndromes. *Circulation.* 2005;112:3802-3813; Marik PE, Rivera R. Hypertensive emergencies: an update. *Curr Opin Crit Care.* 2011;17:569-580.

for diagnostic purposes but limitations include increased cost and study time, poorer spatial resolution, limited thrombus and calcium visualization, and interference from any metallic implants.

79.8 **The correct answer is D.**
Rationale: Mortality after aortic aneurysm rupture exceeds 90%. Aortic aneurysm rupture requires expedited management with priorities including rapid stabilization of the patient and preparation for definitive operative treatment, which may include emergent transfer to a higher level of care (**Figure 79.1**).

STEP 1
Identify patients at risk for acute AoD

Consider acute AoD in all patients presenting with:
- Chest, back, or abdominal pain
- Syncope
- Symptoms consistent with perfusion deficit (ie, CNS, mesenteric, myocardial, or limb ischemia)

STEP 2
Bedside risk assessment

Focused bedside pre-test risk assessment for acute AoD.

❶ High Risk Conditions
- Marfan Syndrome
- Connective tissue disease
- Family history aortic disease
- Known aortic valve disease
- Recent aortic manipulation
- Known thoracic aortic aneurysm

+

❷ High Risk Pain Features
Chest, back or abdominal pain described as the following:
- Abrupt at onset/severe in intensity
and
- Ripping/tearing/sharp or stabbing quality

+

❸ High Risk Features
- Evidence of perfusion deficit
- Pulse deficit
- Systolic BP differential
- Focal neurologic deficit (in conjunction with pain)
- Murmur of aortic insufficiency (new or not known to be old and in conjunction with pain)
- Hypotension or shock state

Determine pre-test risk by combination of risk conditions, history, and exam

STEP 3
Risk based diagnosis evaluation

Low Risk
No high risk features present

Proceed with diagnostic evaluation as clinically indicated by presentation

Intermediate Risk
Any single high risk feature present

ECG consistent with STEMI?

YES → Likely primary ACS. In absence of other perfusion deficits strongly consider immediate coronary re-perfusion therapy. If coronary angiography performed is culprit lesion identified?

High Risk
Two or more high risk features present

Immediate surgical consultation and arrange for expedited aortic imaging

520

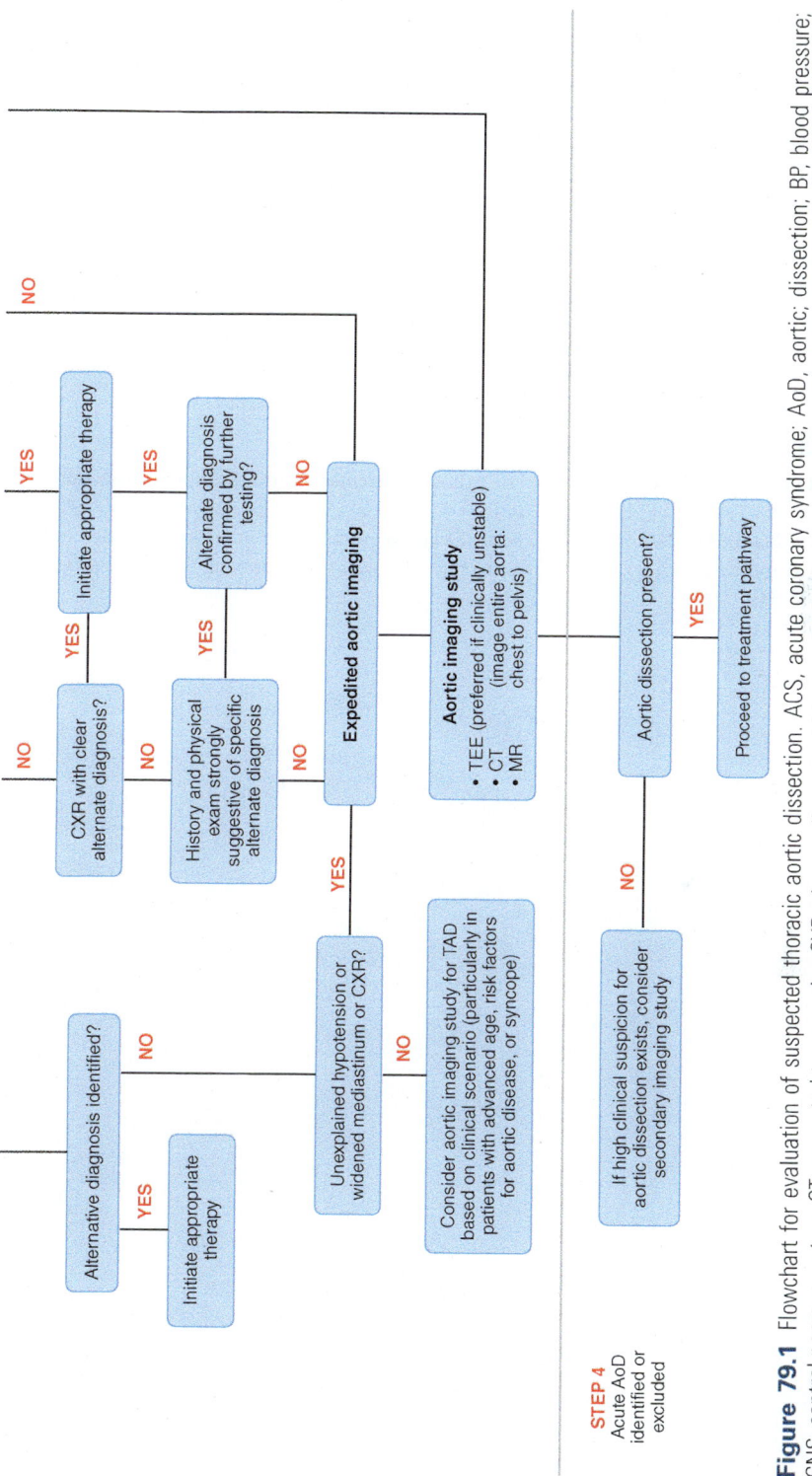

Figure 79.1 Flowchart for evaluation of suspected thoracic aortic dissection. ACS, acute coronary syndrome; AoD, aortic; dissection; BP, blood pressure; CNS, central nervous system; CT, computed tomography; CXR, chest radiograph; ECG, electrocardiogram; MR, magnetic resonance imaging; STEMI, ST-segment elevation myocardial infarction; TAD, thoracic aortic dissection; TEE, transesophageal echocardiography. (Reprinted with permission from Hiratzka LF, Bakris GL, Beckman JA, et al. 2010 ACCF/AHA/AATS/ACR/ASA/SCA/SCAI/SIR/STS/SVM guidelines for the diagnosis and management of patients with thoracic aortic disease: a report of the American College of Cardiology Foundation/American Heart Association Task Force on Practice Guidelines, American Association for Thoracic Surgery, American College of Radiology, American Stroke Association, Society of Cardiovascular Anesthesiologists, Society for Cardiovascular Angiography and Interventions, Society of Interventional Radiology, Society of Thoracic Surgeons, and Society for Vascular Medicine. *Circulation.* 2010;121(13):e266-e369.)

79.9 The correct answer is A:
Rationale: MDCT angiography would be performed at the 1-month follow-up visit following EVAR for AAA to assess for any endoleak around the device and aneurysm enlargement. In the absence of these features, ultrasound imaging can be performed at 6 and 12 months, and then annually. Neither Duplex ultrasound nor MRI are the preferred means of imaging at this time duration after surgical intervention. Failure to do surveillance imaging at this point is not appropriate management.

79.10 The correct answer is B:
Rationale: An ulcerating atherosclerotic lesion penetrating the internal elastic lamina into the media is a penetrating aortic ulcer. An uncomplicated atheroma and atherosclerosis do not involve penetration into the media.

REFERENCES

1. Zhu Q, Tai S, Tang L, et al. STEMI could be the primary presentation of acute aortic dissection. *Am J Emerg Med.* 2017;35(11):1713-1717.
2. Armstrong EJ, Kulkarni AR, Hoffmayer KS, et al. Delaying primary percutaneous coronary intervention for computed tomographic scans in the emergency department. *Am J Cardiol.* 2012;110(3):345-349.

PERIPHERAL ARTERY DISEASE
Brian Conway and Neil Yager

CHAPTER 80

QUESTIONS

80.1 A 56-year-old male with a history of coronary artery disease (CAD), diabetes mellitus and 30-pack-year smoking history, and recent revascularization for bilateral femoral artery disease presents for follow-up. Which of the following statements regarding peripheral artery disease and lipid management is **TRUE**?

   A. Levels of low-density lipoproteins (LDL) are higher in patients with established peripheral arterial disease (PAD).
   B. New-onset diabetes mellitus is strongly associated with the establishment of PAD.
   C. Older age and diabetes are associated with the development of tibial-level disease.
   D. Patients with PAD tend to have higher levels of high-density lipoprotein (HDL).

80.2 Which of the following findings is least likely to be present with regard to acute limb ischemia?

   A. Painful and pale limb below the level of the occlusion
   B. Diminished or absent pulses
   C. Easy fatigability of the affected limb
   D. Paralysis

80.3 Which of the following statements is **FALSE** regarding the Rutherford classification of acute limb ischemia?

   A. Class I is consistent with viable limb without any immediate threat.
   B. Mild sensory impairment is present in class I.
   C. Class III is consistent with irreversible damage.
   D. Sensory and motor impairment is present in class III.

80.4 A 64-year-old male with a history of abdominal aortic aneurysm (AAA), 4.5 cm in diameter, returns to clinic for continued surveillance. Recent imaging demonstrated a right iliac artery with focal dilatation of 1.8 cm, approximately 60% of the vessel's reference diameter. Which of the following statements is **INCORRECT** with regard to this patient's peripheral vascular disease?

Questions and Answers are based on Chapter 80: Peripheral Arterial Disease by Joseph J. Ingrassia, Matt Finn, and Sahil Parikh in Cardiovascular Medicine and Surgery, First Edition.

A. Aneurysmal disease is defined as a focal dilation that is 50% larger than the referenced diameter.
B. When the common iliac artery is greater than 1.6 cm, it should be followed independently from a concomitant AAA.
C. Repair would be indicated for symptomatic iliac aneurysms, those greater than 3 cm in diameter, expand greater than 6 mm in 6 months, or greater than 1 cm in a year.
D. When endovascular repair for AAAs is planned, iliac aneurysmal disease of stable dimensions can be left alone and monitored serially.

80.5 A 65-year-old female with a history of smoking and hypertension is scheduled to undergo ankle-brachial index (ABI) testing for worsening bilateral leg discomfort she has been noticing when going for her evening walk with her husband. Right upper extremity 130/90 mm Hg, left upper extremity 150/100 mm Hg, right lower extremity 120/80 mm Hg, and left lower extremity 110/70 mm Hg. Which of the following is **CORRECT** regarding the interpretation of this patient's ABI?

A. Right ABI = 120/130 = 0.92
B. Right ABI = 120/150 = 0.8
C. Left ABI = 110/130 = 0.84
D. Left ABI = 150/110 = 1.36

80.6 The patient in **Question 80.5** subsequently undergoes pulse volume recording (PVR) to help provide diagnostic information regarding the degree of arterial insufficiency long the lower extremities. Which of the following features would **MOST LIKELY** be found in the left lower extremity?

A. Preserved dicrotic notch
B. Quicker systolic upstroke
C. Loss of amplitude
D. Steeper appearance

80.7 A 70-year-old male with a history of chronic hypertension, hyperlipidemia, and who has smoked 1 to 2 cigars daily for the last 40 years recently underwent ABIs which resulted in 0.92 and 0.95 on the right and the left, respectively. Which of the following findings regarding exercise ABIs is **CORRECT**?

A. A post-exercise systolic blood pressure drop of 40 mm Hg would be a positive test for PAD.
B. A post-exercise systolic blood pressure drop of 10% is considered a positive test for PAD.
C. Exercise ABIs only provide a subjective assessment of exercise tolerance.
D. PVRs are recorded in an upright position.

80.8 A patient with suspected claudication undergoes ABI testing with borderline abnormal results (0.94). Clinical suspicion for claudication remains high given the patient's complaints of leg pain within 2 minutes of exertion, relieved with rest. Toe-brachial index (TBI) testing is subsequently performed yielding grossly abnormal results. What is the **BEST** next step?

A. Exercise therapy and risk factor modification
B. Revascularization
C. Imaging
D. Exercise ABI

80.9 Which of the following statements is **TRUE**?

A. The use of phosphodiesterase inhibitor cilostazol has been shown to improve walking distance in patients with claudication.
B. A 64-year-old male with a history of heart failure with mildly reduced ejection fraction and peripheral artery disease with claudication symptoms, already attending supervised exercise therapy (SET), should be started on cilostazol for optimization.
C. Blood pressure control in patients with peripheral artery disease should be optimized by using beta-blockers and calcium channel blockers.
D. A 74-year-old male with a history of CAD and PAD with claudication should be treated with high-intensity statin therapy ± ezetimibe or proprotein convertase subtilisin/kexin type 9 inhibitor (PCSK9i) to achieve goal LDL less than 70 mg/dL.

80.10 A 76-year-old female with diabetes with known aortoiliac artery disease presents to the clinic. She has had a long-standing history of diabetic foot ulcers which have required referral to podiatry in the past for debridement. She currently complains of skin ulceration which has been healing very slowly of late. She was diagnosed with chronic limb-threatening ischemia (CLTI) and has recently completed computed tomography angiography (CTA) and digital subtraction angiography (DSA) for further anatomic evaluation. Hemodynamically significant stenosis was noted in the aortoiliac vasculature; however, no occlusion was present. What would be the **BEST** treatment strategy for this patient at this time?

A. Optimize medical management, referral to a walking program, diabetes optimization, initiation/continuation of high-intensity statin, aspirin, and angiotensin-converting enzyme/angiotensin receptor blocker (ACE/ARB).
B. Schedule for bypass surgery for lower extremity revascularization.
C. Schedule for endovascular revascularization.
D. None of the above

ANSWERS

80.1 **The correct answer is C.**

Rationale: LDL interestingly tends to be lower in patients with established PAD compared to healthy controls. Long-standing or poorly controlled diabetes is associated with PAD, whereas new-onset diabetes is not as strongly associated. Patients with PAD tend to have lower levels of HDL, and the protective effect of HDL may be more important than the deleterious effects associated with elevated LDL.

80.2 The correct answer is C.
Rationale: The "six Ps" of acute limb ischemia are painful and pale limb distal to the **level** of the occlusion with diminished or absent pulses that can eventually progress to poikilothermia, paresthesia, and paralysis if left untreated. Easy fatigability is more common with chronic limb ischemia.

80.3 The correct answer is B.
Rationale: Class I is devoid of motor or sensory impairments whereas IIa is **associated** with a marginally threatened limb where sensory impairment may be minimal or none (**Table 80.1**).

TABLE 80.1 Rutherford Classification for Acute Limb Ischemia

Category	Sensory Impairment	Motor Impairment	Arterial Doppler Signal	Venous Doppler Signal
Class I Viable—no immediate threat	No	No	Audible	Audible
Class IIa Marginally threatened	Minimal or none	No	±	Audible
Class IIb Immediately threatened	Involves forefoot ± rest pain	Mild to moderate	Usually inaudible	Audible
Class III Irreversible	Anesthetic	Paralytic/rigor	Inaudible	Inaudible

Data from Rutherford RB, Baker JD, Ernst C, et al. Recommended standards for reports dealing with lower extremity ischemia: revised version. *J Vasc Surg.* 1997;26:517-538.

80.4 The correct answer is D.
Rationale: Whenever planning AAA repair with endovascular aneurysm repair (EVAR), any iliac artery aneurysm should also be included to ensure adequate seal.

80.5 The correct answer is B.
Rationale: ABIs are measured as the systolic ankle blood pressure for the respective limb divided by the largest of the upper extremity systolic blood pressures.

80.6 The correct answer is C.
Rationale: The normal contour of a PVR consists of a sharp systolic upstroke, a dicrotic notch in the downstroke, and a gradual descent back to the baseline. As the disease proximal to the measurement site increases, the waveform loses the dicrotic notch, shows a slower systolic upstroke, and demonstrates a loss of amplitude with a rounded appearance (**Figure 80.1**).

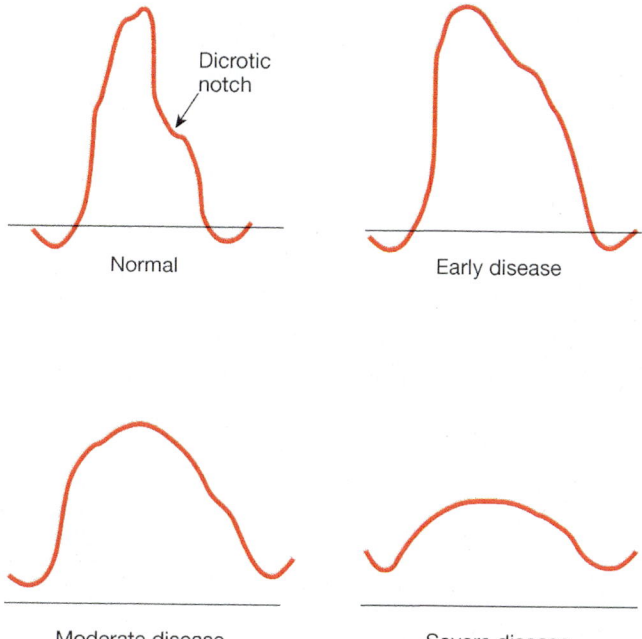

Figure 80.1 Segmental volume plethysmography in peripheral vascular disease. Variations in the contours of the pulse volume recording with segmental volume plethysmography reflect the severity of peripheral vascular disease. Mild disease is characterized by the absence of a dicrotic notch. With progressive obstruction, the upstroke and downstroke become equal, and with severe disease, the amplitude of the waveform is blunted. (Adapted with permission from Rajagopalan S, Dean SM, Mohler ER, Mukherjee D. *Manual of Vascular Diseases*. 2nd ed. Wolters Kluwer Health/Lippincott Williams & Wilkins; 2011. Figure 16.4.)

80.7 **The correct answer is A.**
Rationale: Exercise PVRs obtained with PVRs at rest are inconclusive. Supine blood pressures are taken before and after walking on a treadmill until claudication symptoms **cause** the cessation of exercise. Testing provides an objective assessment of a patient's walking tolerance. A positive test for PAD is when post-exercise systolic blood pressure (SBP) decreases greater than 30 mm Hg or post-ABI decreases greater than 20%.

80.8 **The correct answer is A.**
Rationale: When initial ABIs are borderline abnormal but there is high clinical suspicion for PAD, TBIs should be performed. If these are normal, the patient should subsequently undergo exercise ABI. If TBI is abnormal, risk factors modification and exercise therapy should be pursued.

80.9 **The correct answer is A.**
Rationale: Cilostazol is contraindicated with heart failure. Blood pressure optimization should **include** ACE/ARB medications. LDL goals for PAD are less than 70 mg/dL; however, goal LDL for PAD with concomitant CAD is less than 50 mg/dL.

80.10 The correct answer is A.

Rationale: Revascularization should not be performed proactively to prevent progression of **CLTI** and this patient should be medically optimized before consideration of invasive revascularization. For patients with claudication and aortoiliac involvement, an endovascular first approach is preferred. In femoropopliteal occluded segments, there is equipoise between endovascular and surgical options. However, in CLTI, the optimal revascularization strategy is unknown and currently is determined by factors such as referral center expertise and patient preference (**Table 80.2**).

TABLE 80.2 Antithrombotic Medical Regimens

PAD Category	Antithrombotic Treatment Strategy	Notes
PAD without prior revascularization	SAPT	Clopidogrel preferred over ASA Ticagrelor or ASA if contraindication to clopidogrel exists
PAD periprocedural revascularization	DAPT 1 mo; followed by ASA + rivaroxaban 2.5 mg orally twice daily	± PPI based on bleeding risk
PAD with remote prior revascularization	ASA Clopidogrel 75 mg daily ASA + rivaroxaban 2.5 mg orally bid	
PAD with stable CAD	ASA + rivaroxaban 2.5 mg orally bid	Independent of history of revascularization
PAD with CAD and recent ACS or PCI	DAPT for length of CAD indication followed by ASA + ticagrelor 60 mg orally bid OR ASA + rivaroxaban 2.5 mg orally bid	Factors favoring ticagrelor over rivaroxaban: complex coronary artery disease, bifurcation stents, multivessel PCI
PAD with indication for anticoagulation without prior revascularization	OAC + clopidogrel 75 mg daily OR OAC monotherapy	Addition of clopidogrel based upon bleeding risk
PAD with indication for anticoagulation with prior revascularization	OAC + clopidogrel 75 mg daily 1 mo post-revascularization followed by OAC ± clopidogrel	Maintenance of clopidogrel based upon bleeding risk
PAD, asymptomatic without history of revascularization or additional vascular disease	No antithrombotic treatment	

ACS, acute coronary syndrome; ASA, acetylsalicylic acid; CAD, coronary artery disease; DAPT, dual antiplatelet therapy; OAC, oral anticoagulation; PAD, peripheral arterial disease; PCI, percutaneous coronary intervention; PPI, proton pump inhibitor; SAPT, single antiplatelet therapy.

CEREBROVASCULAR DISEASE

Brian Conway and William Bachman

CHAPTER 81

QUESTIONS

81.1 A 64-year-old female with a history of hypertension, hyperlipidemia, and recently diagnosed breast cancer presents to the emergency department (ED) via emergency medical service (EMS) after the acute onset of left arm weakness, and left facial droop was noticed by her husband while she was in the kitchen making lunch. Her husband became most worried when he noticed her speech became slurred. What is the **MOST LIKELY** finding on computed tomography angiography (CTA) for this patient?
   A. Right M2 occlusion
   B. Right parietal hemorrhagic stroke
   C. Right A1 occlusion
   D. Right posterior cerebral artery (PCA) occlusion

81.2 A 46-year-old female with a history of epilepsy and hypertension, and taking oral contraceptives drives to the ED at the insistence of her supervisor. The patient works as a nurse at a dermatology clinic and has been noticing headaches, blurry vision, and slight weakness in her right arm since arriving at work. Which of the following characteristics favor her presentation **NOT** being related to an acute stroke?
   A. Right arm weakness
   B. Headaches
   C. Personal transportation rather than ambulance
   D. Blurry vision

81.3 A 76-year-old male presents to the ED after a fall at home while walking to the bathroom just after breakfast. Directly before attempting to ambulate to the bathroom, his wife states he had become extremely confused and developed garbled speech. She thinks she first noticed symptoms just over an hour ago. Patient has no contraindications for thrombolytics or mechanical thrombectomy. Which of the following statements is **CORRECT**?
   A. For thrombolytic therapy, goal for door-to-needle time is less than 90 minutes.
   B. For mechanical thrombectomy, goal for door-to-device time is less than 60 minutes.
   C. Blood sugar should be maintained greater than 140 mg/dL
   D. Blood pressure should be kept below 185/110 mm Hg

*Questions and Answers are based on Chapter 81: Cerebrovascular Disease by Steven R. Bailey in Cardiovascular Medicine and Surgery, First Edition.

81.4 A 72-year-old female who lives outside of Buffalo, NY, presents to her closest community hospital with stroke-like symptoms which began approximately 3 hours ago. Her presentation was unfortunately delayed due to a massive snowstorm. Emergent CTA is performed demonstrating an occlusion of a distal branch of the M2 segment of the middle cerebral artery (MCA). NIHSS (National Institutes of Health Stroke Scale) score is 20. She does **NOT** take any oral anticoagulation. Which of the following statements regarding emergent treatment are **CORRECT**?

A. Start intravenous (IV) heparin, and then transfer to the nearest level 1 stroke center for consideration of mechanical thrombectomy.
B. Start IV heparin and load with aspirin, and then transfer to the nearest level 1 stroke center for consideration of mechanical thrombectomy.
C. IV tissue plasminogen activator (tPA) should be administered.
D. Immediate transport to a level 1 stroke center for consideration of mechanical thrombectomy.

81.5 Which of the following is **NOT** an absolute contraindication for administering tPA for an acute thrombotic stroke?

A. Prior ischemic stroke 2 months ago
B. Preexisting dementia
C. Gastrointestinal (GI) bleed 2 weeks ago
D. History of intracranial hemorrhage

81.6 A 61-year-old female with a history of Crohn's disease on infliximab presents to her local community hospital ED via EMS after noticing acute onset left arm weakness, garbled speech, and left facial droop at home. Computed tomography (CT) demonstrates a large, right parietal ischemic infarct. Patient has had multiple colorectal surgeries in the past for bowel obstructions; however, denies any recent hematochezia. Labwork is unremarkable; notably, hemoglobin is 14.5, platelets are 300k and international normalized ratio (INR) is 1. Last known normal examination was 30 minutes ago. The nearest level 1 stroke center is 1 hour away. What is the most appropriate next step in this patient's management?

A. No absolute contraindications—give tPA.
B. Emergent transport to the nearest level 1 stroke center for consideration of mechanical thrombectomy.
C. Given her prior colorectal surgeries, tPA is contraindicated and she should be started on therapeutic IV heparin instead.
D. Emergent transport to the nearest level 1 stroke center for consideration of mechanical thrombectomy

81.7 A 70-year-old male with a history of coronary artery disease with stents, diabetes mellitus, atrial fibrillation, hypertension, and hyperlipidemia presents to the ED at a level 1 stroke center with concerns for an acute stroke. His last known normal examination was 8 hours ago. CTA demonstrates a proximal MCA occlusion. NIHSS is 8. What would be the **BEST** treatment option at this time?

A. tPA
B. Therapeutic heparin/Lovenox
C. Mechanical thrombectomy
D. Antiplatelet therapy

81.8 A 72-year-old female with a history of hypertension and hyperlipidemia is admitted with an acute ischemic stroke. She underwent uncomplicated thrombectomy after the discovery of a left internal carotid artery occlusion. Which of the following would be the most appropriate medication regimen at the time of discharge with respect to secondary prevention?

A. Discharge on clopidogrel 75 mg daily
B. Discharge on aspirin 81 mg daily
C. Discharge on aspirin 81 mg daily and atorvastatin 80 mg daily
D. Discharge on clopidogrel 75 mg daily and atorvastatin 20 mg daily

81.9 An 84-year-old male presents to his primary care clinic with worsening headaches and vision changes of increasing intensity over the last few hours. He recalls headaches prior to this episode approximately 1 week ago. CT head is negative; however, the patient continues to complain of a worsening headache and his vision has **NOT** improved. Which of the following strategies would be the least likely to provide beneficial information at this time?

A. Perform a lumbar puncture.
B. Repeat CT.
C. Magnetic resonance imaging (MRI) with fluid-attenuated inversion recovery (FLAIR) imaging
D. Angiography

81.10 A 62-year-old female is being followed in the neurosurgery clinic for surveillance of a 2-cm saccular aneurysm in the anterior segment of the circle of Willis. Which of the following statements regarding medical therapy for this patient is **CORRECT**?

A. Aspirin therapy should not be given to this patient as intracranial hemorrhage size would be worse if the aneurysm were to rupture in the future.
B. Aspirin therapy should be given to this patient as intracranial hemorrhage size would not be changed if the aneurysm were to rupture in future.
C. Anticoagulation should be given to reduce the risk of thrombosis.
D. Vasospasm risk is elevated post aneurysm rupture and should be treated with oral beta–blockers.

ANSWERS

81.1 The correct answer is A.
Rationale: Ischemic strokes account for over 70% of all strokes. The MCA is the most commonly affected vascular distribution. An MCA infarction typically results in contralateral hemiparesis, facial paralysis, and sensory loss of the face and upper extremity. Gaze preference to the side of the lesion may also be seen. The lower extremity is less commonly involved. Patients may also exhibit signs of dysarthria, aphasia, and hemispheric neglect with MCA infarcts. Parietal strokes may cause aphasia, loss of coordination, and difficulties with writing, proprioception, and executive functioning. Anterior cerebral artery strokes are rare accounting for only 3% of all cerebrovascular accidents (CVAs).

81.2 The correct answer is C.
Rationale: More than 30% of cases of patients presenting with stroke-like symptoms are due to other etiologies. Typical features suggesting nonstroke etiologies include younger age, mild symptoms, no history of vascular risk factors, and arrival to the ED by personal transportation.

81.3 The correct answer is D.
Rationale: The goal for door-to-needle time is less than 60 minutes, whereas the goal for door-to-device time is less than 90 minutes. Blood sugar should be maintained greater than 50 mg/dL and blood pressure less than 185/110 mm Hg (**Table 81.1**).

TABLE 81.1 Indications for Intravenous Tissue Plasminogen Activator Therapy

Current indications: Class I recommendations

Stroke symptom(s) onset within 3 h and the following are present:
- 18 y of age or older
- Severe stroke[a]
- Mild but disabling stroke[b]

Stroke symptom(s) onset 3-4.5 h ago and the following are present:
- 18-79 y of age
- Without a history of both diabetes mellitus and prior stroke
- NIHSS score ≤25
- Not taking oral anticoagulants
- Without imaging evidence of ischemic injury involving more than one-third of the middle cerebral artery territory
- Blood pressure can be lowered safely and maintained <185/110 mm Hg.
- Blood glucose >50 mg/dL
- Mild to moderate early ischemic changes on noncontrast CT scan
- With antiplatelet drug monotherapy or combination therapy
- With end-stage renal disease with normal aPTT

aPTT, activated partial thromboplastin time; CT, computed tomography.
[a]Severe stroke is defined as National Institutes of Health Stroke Scale (NIHSS) score of 21 or greater.
[b]**Mild but disabling** is a NIHSS score of 20 or less but with significant mental or physical disability.
Data from Powers WJ, Rabinstein AA, Ackerson T, et al. Guidelines for the early management of patients with acute ischemic stroke: 2019 update to the 2018 guidelines for the early management of acute ischemic stroke: a guideline for healthcare professionals from the American Heart Association/American Stroke Association. *Stroke.* 2019;50(12):e344-e418.

81.4 The correct answer is C.
Rationale: Patients 18 years or older who present within 3 hours of symptom onset having a mild but disabling stroke, or severe stroke without contraindications have a class I indication for IV-tPA administration. Patients presenting at 3 to 4.5 hours of symptom onset, from ages 18 to 79 without prior stroke or diabetes, and NIHSS score less than or equal to 25, not taking oral anticoagulants, and without imaging evidence of involvement of greater than one-third of the MCA territory are also considered class I for IV tPA administration. Notably, aspirin administration within 48 hours of ischemic stroke has been shown to decrease the risk of a second stroke (**Figure 81.1**).

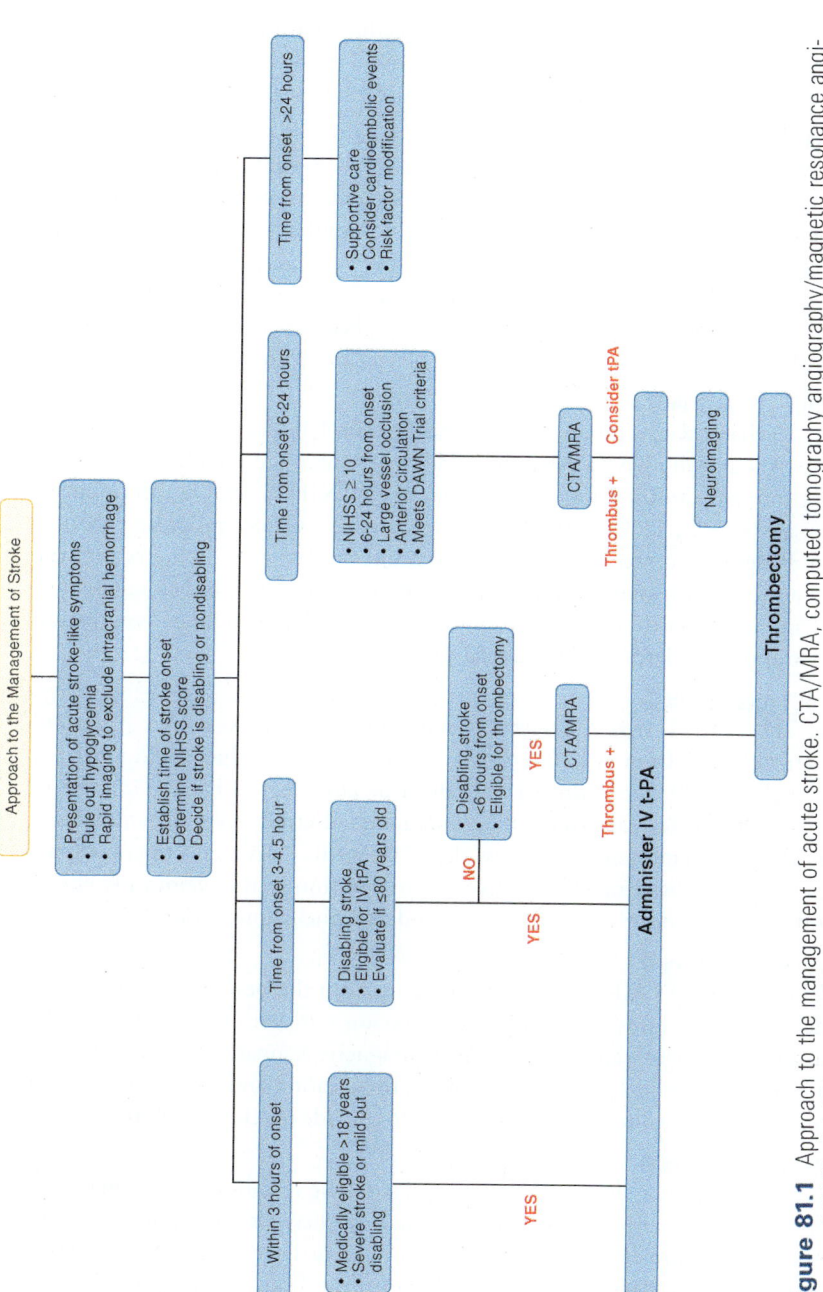

Figure 81.1 Approach to the management of acute stroke. CTA/MRA, computed tomography angiography/magnetic resonance angiography; DAWN trial, DWI or CTP Assessment With Clinical Mismatch in the Triage of Wake-Up and Late Presenting Strokes Undergoing Neurointervention With Trevo; NIHSS, National Institutes of Health Stroke Scale; tPA, tissue plasminogen activator; IV, intravenous. (Adapted from Powers WJ, Rabinstein AA, Ackerson T, et al. Guidelines for the early management of patients with acute ischemic stroke: 2019 update to the 2018 guidelines for the early management of acute ischemic stroke: a guideline for healthcare professionals American Heart Association/American Stroke Association. *Stroke.* 2019;50(12):e344-e418; From Nogueira RG, Jadhav AP, Haussen DC, et al. Thrombectomy 6 to 24 hours after stroke with a mismatch between deficit and infarct. *N Engl J Med.* 2018;378:11-21. Copyright © 2018 Massachusetts Medical Society. Reprinted with permission from Massachusetts Medical Society.)

81.5 The correct answer is B.
Rationale: Class III contraindications for tPA administration include acute intracranial hemorrhage, prior ischemic stroke or severe head trauma within 3 months, history of intracranial hemorrhage, structural GI bleeding within 21 days, and others. Preexisting dementia is one of many relative contraindications (Class of Recommendation [COR] IIb) that does not absolutely preclude the use of tPA.

81.6 The correct answer is B.
Rationale: While there are no absolute contraindications for thrombolytics mentioned for this patient (and prior colorectal surgery is not a contraindication, in the absence of recent bleeding), mechanical thrombectomy with stent thrombus retrievers carries a Class I-C-EO for patients presenting less than 6 hours after the onset of acute stroke and is largely considered first-line therapy for this population. Percutaneous stent management of stroke, except in the management of an acute complication of an endarterectomy or stent procedure, has limited utility in the setting of a patient with an acute stroke.

81.7 The correct answer is C.
Rationale: Mechanical thrombectomy also has a class I indication for individuals older than 18 years who have a prestroke modified Rankin score less than 1, occlusion of the internal carotid artery or proximal MCA, NIHSS score greater than or equal to 6, and ASPECTS (Alberta Stroke Program Early CT Score) greater than or equal to 6. Patients who present greater than 6 hours but less than 24 hours after the onset of symptoms with an occlusion of the internal carotid artery or M1 segment of the MCA and disproportionately severe clinical deficits relative to infarct volume on imaging are also candidates for mechanical thrombectomy.

81.8 The correct answer is C.
Rationale: The POINT trial (Platelet-Oriented Inhibition in New TIA [transient ischemic attack] and Minor Ischemic Stroke) demonstrated a reduction in recurrent ischemic strokes at 90 days with use of aspirin or clopidogrel. Early initiation of high-intensity statin decreases both fatal and nonfatal stroke with recommended target low-density lipoprotein (LDL) less than 70 mg/dL. This seems to encompass both the cholesterol-lowering effects of statins in addition to the pleiotropic effects of anti-inflammation, decreased thrombosis, and endothelial protection.

81.9 The correct answer is B.
Rationale: MRI with FLAIR or a lumbar puncture are the best tests to follow up an inconclusive noncontrast CT if clinical suspicion remains high for intracranial aneurysm rupture. Angiography (CTA, MRA [magnetic resonance angiography], or invasive) is another useful option in identifying the location and size of intracranial aneurysms. Repeat noncontrast CT is not likely to provide much meaningful benefit.

81.10 The correct answer is B.
Rationale: Medical therapy for hypertension and smoking cessation have been shown to decrease the risk of aneurysm rupture in small studies. Use of aspirin does not seem to increase the size of intracranial aneurysm hemorrhage, and in one randomized trial was found to decrease the risk of hemorrhage from an unruptured intracranial aneurysm. Conversely, anticoagulants seem to increase the risk and severity of intracranial aneurysm hemorrhage; however, these have been poorly studied. Vasospasm after aneurysm rupture is seen in 40% to 70% of patients and can lead to recurrent stroke. This should be managed with calcium channel blockers.

RENAL ARTERY STENOSIS*

Brian Conway and Neil Yager

CHAPTER 82

QUESTIONS

82.1 A 75-year-old male with a history of hypertension (HTN) on hydrochlorothiazide and losartan presents to the clinic for a routine follow-up. Blood pressures checked at home over the last 6 months have ranged from 155/95 to 190/130 mm Hg. His past medical history is only remarkable for chronic tobacco misuse for the last 40 years. Examination is consistent with a bruit noted over the abdomen. Laboratory values include creatinine 1.4 mg/dL, sodium 137 mEq/L, and potassium 3.4 mEq/L. What is the **MOST** LIKELY diagnosis for this patient?

A. Abdominal aortic aneurysm (AAA)
B. Descending thoracic aorta dissection
C. Renal artery stenosis
D. Essential HTN

82.2 A 27-year-old woman on two antihypertensive medications presents to the clinic for follow-up on HTN. She eats a vegetarian diet, exercises for 30 minutes 5 days a week, and has a body mass index (BMI) of 25. She is a nonsmoker and drinks alcohol very rarely. Blood pressure in clinic is 165/90 mm Hg. She states she is compliant with medications. On physical examination, an abdominal bruit is noted just to the left of the umbilicus. What is the **MOST** LIKELY diagnosis?

A. Fibromuscular dysplasia
B. Peripheral artery disease
C. Raynaud disease
D. Hyperaldosteronism

82.3 Epidemiologic studies have shown that the strongest predictor of developing atherosclerotic renal artery stenosis (ARAS) is a history of:

A. Essential HTN
B. Coronary artery disease
C. Peripheral vascular disease
D. Diabetes mellitus

82.4 Which of the following statements is **INCORRECT** regarding invasive management of ARAS?

*Questions and Answers are based on Chapter 82: Renal Artery Atherosclerosis by Jose D. Tafur and Christopher J. White in Cardiovascular Medicine and Surgery, First Edition.

A. Hemodynamically significant ARAS with a mean translesional gradient greater than 10 mm Hg and systolic gradient greater than 20 mm Hg should undergo either percutaneous stenting of the affected vessel or be referred for open surgical intervention.
B. Multiple randomized controlled trials regarding medical therapy alone versus medical therapy with percutaneous intervention for hemodynamically significant ARAS have demonstrated no difference with regard to blood pressure management and progression of chronic kidney disease.
C. Open surgical repair of the diseased segment of renal artery for patients with flow-limiting ARAS has been largely replaced by less invasive endovascular procedures due to a higher risk of complications with open surgery and overall similar benefits with regard to patency rates, blood pressure controls, and progression in renal dysfunction.
D. The complication rate for renal artery stenting is around 2%, with the most common complications arising from femoral access.

82.5 Favorable predictors of improvement in chronic ischemic nephropathy from ARAS with renal revascularization include all the following **EXCEPT**:

A. Reduction in glomerular filtration rate (GFR) during angiotensin-converting enzyme inhibitor (ACEI) or angiotensin receptor blocker (ARB) treatment
B. A recent gradual decrease in serum creatinine concentration
C. Absence of fibrosis in the glomerulus or interstitium on renal biopsy
D. Kidney pole-to-pole length greater than 8.0 cm

82.6 A 76-year-old male with a history of heart failure with preserved ejection fraction (HFpEF) and HTN on losartan, atenolol, and furosemide presents to the hospital with worsening shortness of breath over the last 3 weeks. He also notes a 15-pound weight gain and new lower extremity swelling. He was admitted for an acute exacerbation of heart failure and started on intravenous (IV) diuretics. Blood pressure on admission was elevated at 160/90 mm Hg. He underwent renal ultrasonography which was consistent with unilateral hemodynamically significant ARAS. After 3 days of hospitalization, the patient has been diuresed to his perceived dry weight. This was his third admission for heart failure exacerbation this year. What is the **BEST** next step in his management at this time?

A. Optimization of guideline-directed medical therapy for heart failure
B. Computed tomography (CT) abdomen/pelvis to help guide potential future intervention
C. Aggressive risk factor modification
D. Renal angiography with percutaneous stenting

82.7 Which statement regarding the pathogenesis of ARAS is **INCORRECT**?

A. Renal hypoperfusion leads to renin release and eventual pressure natriuresis of the unaffected kidney.
B. With bilateral renal artery stenosis, overactivation of the renin-angiotensin-aldosterone system (RAAS) occurs due to hypoperfusion to the affected kidneys and leads to vasoconstriction and pressure diuresis to prevent systemic volume overload.
C. Ischemic nephropathy can occur when lesions are greater than 70% stenosed, leading to excretory dysfunction.
D. Hemodynamically significant lesions may lead to atrophy of the affected kidney and interstitial fibrosis.

82.8 A 74-year-old male with a history of stage II chronic kidney disease and resistant HTN on four antihypertensives, including a diuretic, is admitted to the hospital for hypertensive urgency in the setting of medication noncompliance and dietary indiscretions. He was initially managed on IV antihypertensives but transitioned back to oral medications on day 2 of hospitalization. He was subsequently sent for renal angiography that demonstrated unilateral renal artery stenosis of 60% in the right renal artery and minimal atherosclerotic changes noted on the left. Hemodynamic evaluation reveals a hyperemic systolic gradient of 18 mm Hg and a mean gradient of 8 mm Hg. What should be the next step in treatment?

A. Proceed with renal artery stenting for an angiographically significant lesion of the right renal artery.
B. Refer to vascular surgery for consideration of open renal artery surgery.
C. Optimize oral antihypertensive therapy.
D. Refer for renal denervation.

82.9 A 78-year-old female with a history of HFpEF, stage IV chronic kidney disease secondary to long-standing uncontrolled HTN on hydralazine and amlodipine, presents to the hospital with profound, rapidly developing shortness of breath at rest over the last 12 to 24 hours and progressive anasarca. She is adamant that she has maintained medication compliance since receiving health insurance approximately 2 years ago. Blood pressure on admission was elevated at 170/90 and 165/80 mm Hg on the right and left upper extremities, respectively. Labs show a creatinine of 1.8 mg/dL, sodium of 129 mEq/L, and potassium of 4.7 mEq/L. Chest x-ray demonstrates diffuse bilateral Kerley B lines and peribronchial cuffing. Troponin is mildly elevated and there are no electrocardiogram (ECG) changes to suggest acute myocardial ischemia as the etiology for her decompensation. Patient requires bilevel positive airway pressure (Bi-pap) to maintain adequate oxygen saturation and is admitted to the step-down unit for decompensated heart failure. Computed tomography angiography (CTA) performed in the emergency department to rule out pulmonary embolism is extended to the abdomen and demonstrates a right kidney of 6 cm in length and left of 14 cm. After medical stabilization with diuresis and adequate blood pressure control on three antihypertensives, she undergoes renal angiography which demonstrates right ARAS of 70% with a translesional systolic gradient of 25 mm Hg. What is the most appropriate next step in this patient's management?

A. Proceed with renal artery stenting for an angiographically significant lesion of the right renal artery.
B. Refer to vascular surgery for consideration of open renal artery surgery.
C. Optimize oral antihypertensive therapy.
D. Refer for renal denervation.

82.10 A 72-year-old male presents to his outpatient cardiology office visit. 3 months ago, he was discharged from the hospital after an admission for hypertensive emergency. Over the course of his hospitalization, a renal artery ultrasound was performed demonstrating left renal atrophy with left renal artery narrowing. He subsequently underwent renal angiography demonstrating a flow-limiting lesion in the left renal artery for which a stent was placed. He has been appropriately maintained on dual antiplatelet therapy without complications. However, blood pressure remains elevated despite three oral antihypertensive medications which had been up-titrated in the outpatient setting. What is the **BEST** next step in management?

A. Continued escalation in antihypertensive therapy with goal blood pressure less than 120/80 mm Hg
B. Magnetic resonance imaging (MRI) to assess for in-stent restenosis (ISR)
C. Schedule for renal angiography with an assessment of the previously stented region.
D. Renal Doppler ultrasound

ANSWERS

82.1 The correct answer is C.
Rationale: HTN and bruit over the abdomen are most likely ARAS. AAA may present with abdominal discomfort or a notable pulsatile mass on examination, which is not present. Aortic dissections tend to present with tearing or ripping pain, acute in onset. While the patient has only been managed on a single antihypertensive agent, the finding of an abdominal bruit should raise suspicion for ARAS.

82.2 The correct answer is A.
Rationale: Fibromuscular dysplasia represents 10% to 30% of renal artery stenosis (RAS) patients and is what this patient is presenting with. Peripheral arterial disease would be more likely in older males with risk factors for atherosclerosis. Raynaud characteristic vasospastic features would not necessarily present with resistant HTN. Hyperaldosteronism would not explain an abdominal bruit.

82.3 The correct answer is C.
Rationale: While HTN, coronary artery disease, and diabetes are all risk factors for developing atherosclerotic disease, confirmed atherosclerotic peripheral vascular disease is the strongest predictor of ARAS.

82.4 The correct answer is A.
Rationale: Not all hemodynamically significant cases of ARAS should be referred for invasive intervention. Those asymptomatic patients with hemodynamically significant ARAS have not been shown to benefit from stenting when compared to medical therapy alone. Percutaneous intervention in this population has been deemed rarely appropriate by the SCAI (Society for Cardiovascular Angiography and Interventions) appropriate use criteria and carries a IIb/C recommendation from the American Heart Association/American College of Cardiology (AHA/ACC) recommendations. Randomized controlled trials have yet to demonstrate superiority in renal artery stenting compared to medical therapy for moderate or greater degrees of stenosis. Since the greatest procedural risk for renal artery stenting is related to femoral access, many operators are opting for a radial artery approach. The surgical complication rate for open repair ranges from 5% to 7% and the benefits following open surgery compared to percutaneous intervention have shown no significant differences. For these reasons, open surgery has largely been supplanted by less invasive renal artery stenting.

82.5 The correct answer is B.
Rationale: A recent acute/rapid increase in serum creatinine concentration predicts favorably improvement in renal dysfunction after revascularization.

82.6 The correct answer is D.
Rationale: Renal artery revascularization carries a IB recommendation from the AHA/ACC for patients with unilateral ARAS and recurrent heart failure. This does not require any further imaging to perform. Risk factor modification for atherosclerotic disease should always be addressed for these patients; however, addressing underlying ARAS is of paramount importance at this stage (**Table 82.1**).

TABLE 82.1 Current Appropriate Use Criteria From the Society for Cardiovascular Angiography and Interventions and American Heart Association/American College of Cardiology Guideline Recommendations

Hemodynamically Significant RAS[a] Scenario	SCAI Appropriate Use Criteria	AHA/ACC Recommendations	
		Class	Level of Evidence
Cardiac disturbance syndrome with hypertension • Flash pulmonary edema, NSTEMI • Unstable angina	Appropriate	I IIa	B
CKD stage IV with kidney size >7 cm • Bilateral ARAS	Appropriate	IIa	B
CKD stage IV without another explanation • Bilateral or unilateral with solitary kidney ARAS	Appropriate	IIb	B
Resistant hypertension (failing maximally tolerated doses of at least three agents including a diuretic) • Bilateral or unilateral with solitary kidney ARAS • Unilateral ARAS	Appropriate May be appropriate	IIa	B
Recurrent CHF with unilateral ARAS	May be appropriate	I	B
Asymptomatic	Rarely appropriate	IIb	C

ACC, American College of Cardiology; ACS, acute coronary syndrome; AHA, American Heart Association; ARAS, atherosclerotic renal artery stenosis; CHF, congestive heart failure; CKD, chronic kidney disease; NSTEMI, non-ST-elevation myocardial infarction; SCAI, Society for Cardiovascular Angiography and Interventions.

[a]Hemodynamically significant renal artery stenosis (RAS): (a) 50% to 70% (moderate) stenosis with resting/hyperemic translesional mean gradient greater than 10 mm Hg, and/or systolic gradient greater than 20 mm Hg; or renal fractional flow reserve (RFFR) less than or equal to 0.8 or (b) greater than 70% to 99% (severe) stenosis.

82.7 The correct answer is B.

Rationale: Stimulation of RAAS results in pressure natriuresis of the unaffected kidney which acts to prevent systemic volume overload. This, however, necessitates adequate perfusion to the unaffected kidney. Bilateral RAS (or solitary RAS with a single functioning kidney) results in a lack of natriuresis and leads to sodium and fluid retention, potentially precipitating heart failure.

82.8 The correct answer is C.

Rationale: Angiography demonstrates moderate stenosis (50%-70%), however, without resting/hyperemic systolic translesional gradients greater than 20 mm Hg or mean gradients greater than 10 mm Hg. This lesion is not hemodynamically significant, and he would be best treated with medication management/optimization. The patient does have chronic kidney disease; however, it has not progressed to stage IV or greater, which would have made percutaneous intervention appropriate if the lesion was hemodynamically significant (class IIb/LOE B [Level of Evidence B]). Also, if the lesion was hemodynamically significant, percutaneous intervention may be appropriate on the basis of resistant HTN alone for unilateral RAS (IIa/B). He should undergo medication optimization and likely workup for other potential secondary causes of HTN.

82.9 The correct answer is A.

Rationale: This patient is presenting with an acute decompensation of HFpEF with evidence of flash pulmonary edema and angiographically and hemodynamically significant right ARAS. He should undergo percutaneous intervention with stenting of the diseased segment based on ACC/AHA Guidelines (Class I/B) (see **Table 82.1**).

82.10 The correct answer is D.

Rationale: Escalating antihypertensive therapy in a patient with recent percutaneous intervention for flow-limiting renal artery stenosis should arouse suspicion for ISR. Continued escalation of oral antihypertensive therapy in light of this would not be appropriate. MRI would be affected by metal artifacts and not provide accurate intraluminal assessment. Further imaging should be performed before sending back for invasive assessment. Renal Doppler ultrasound is the first-line imaging modality to assess stent patency.

MESENTERIC ARTERIAL DISEASE*

Brian Conway and William Bachman

CHAPTER 83

QUESTIONS

83.1 All of the following characteristics are associated with acute mesenteric ischemia EXCEPT:

A. Increased age
B. Cardiac disease (arrhythmias, CHF [congestive heart failure], recent MI [myocardial infarction], valvular disease)
C. Male gender
D. Intra-abdominal tumors

83.2 Which of the following findings would NOT support a diagnosis of chronic mesenteric ischemia?

A. Epigastric pain 60 minutes after a meal
B. Significant weight loss
C. History of coronary artery disease
D. Difficult to localize, moderate to severe abdominal pain

83.3 A 52-year-old male with a history of tobacco abuse and recently diagnosed non–small cell lung cancer presents to the emergency department (ED) with nagging abdominal pain over the last week. What is the MOST LIKELY form of mesenteric ischemia in this patient?

A. Intestinal arterial thrombosis
B. Mesenteric venous thrombosis
C. Intestinal arterial thromboembolism
D. Nonocclusive mesenteric ischemia

83.4 An 84-year-old male with a history of hypertension, hyperlipidemia, tobacco abuse, and coronary artery bypass approximately 10 years ago presents to the clinic with worsening postprandial abdominal pain. He has had long-standing abdominal discomfort, especially after meals, but has been concerned over 30 pounds of weight loss over the last 6 months, and he believes the severity of pain has started to worsen. He has been taking proton pump inhibitors and calcium carbonate over-the-counter without any improvement in symptoms. What is the MOST LIKELY cause of this patient's weight loss?

A. Colorectal cancer
B. Acute pancreatitis
C. Chronic mesenteric ischemia
D. Diverticulitis

*Questions and Answers are based on Chapter 83: Mesenteric Arterial Disease by Stefanos Giannopoulos and Ehrin J. Armstrong in Cardiovascular Medicine and Surgery, First Edition.

83.5 A 64-year-old female presents to the hospital with acute onset intractable abdominal pain and nausea without vomiting. Plain abdominal radiograph demonstrates a dilated bowel but no evidence of volvulus or free intraperitoneal air. Labwork is otherwise unremarkable. The team is concerned about mesenteric ischemia. Which of the following imaging studies would be MOST appropriate at this time?

   A. Duplex ultrasound
   B. Computed tomography angiography (CTA)
   C. Magnetic resonance angiography (MRA)
   D. Arterial angiography

83.6 A 72-year-old female with a history of colorectal cancer presents to the ED with poorly defined abdominal pain which began earlier that day. Blood pressure on arrival is 85/40 mm Hg with heart rate 105 beats per minute (bpm). She is started on a 1-L bolus of IV fluids. There is guarding on the examination with rebound tenderness. CTA is performed which demonstrates a complete occlusion of the superior mesenteric artery. Which is the BEST next step in this patient's treatment?

   A. Immediate exploratory laparotomy
   B. Thrombolytics
   C. Endovascular therapy
   D. Medical management

83.7 An 82-year-old male with a history of coronary artery bypass grafting (CABG), hypertension, and hyperlipidemia presents to cardiology clinic for a routine follow-up. He complains of predictable abdominal discomfort 30 minutes after meals which has been present for the last month or more. He remains on guideline-directed medical therapy (GDMT) for his coronary artery disease. Which would be the first-line intervention for suspected chronic mesenteric ischemia?

   A. Continue GDMT.
   B. Open surgery
   C. Angioplasty with stenting
   D. Either B or C

83.8 Which of the following statements regarding intervention for mesenteric ischemia is NOT TRUE?

   A. Most periprocedural deaths following revascularization for acute mesenteric ischemia are due to progression of intestinal ischemia.
   B. Interventional treatment of acute or chronic mesenteric ischemia is complicated by death in up to 50% of cases.
   C. Percutaneous transluminal angioplasty is associated with lower target repeat revascularization rates during follow-up.
   D. Surgical repair has been associated with higher morbidity rates compared to interventional treatment.

83.9 Which of the following statements regarding follow-up after intervention for mesenteric ischemia is INCORRECT?

A. After surgical revascularization, additional laparotomy is rarely required to reevaluate intestinal blood flow.
B. Anticoagulant therapy should be given in cases of mesenteric embolism.
C. Antiplatelet agents and statins are recommended after acute thromboembolic arterial occlusion of an atherosclerotic mesenteric artery.
D. Nutritional needs should be addressed immediately postoperative and adjunctive parenteral nutrition should be started if necessary.

83.10 Which of the following statements regarding surveillance imaging after mesenteric revascularization is CORRECT?

A. Annual surveillance
B. 3-, 6-, 12-month intervals and annually thereafter
C. Every 6 months
D. No surveillance required. Reimage if symptoms redevelop.

ANSWERS

83.1 The correct answer is C.
Rationale: Females tend to have a higher incidence of acute mesenteric ischemia. Risk factors typically consistent with atherosclerosis (smoking, hypertension, hyperlipidemia, diabetes, metabolic syndrome, sedentary lifestyle) seem to portend a higher risk for chronic mesenteric ischemia. Embolic occlusions are the most common source for acute mesenteric ischemia (40%-50%). Several factors predisposing to thrombus formation or embolization include cardiac disease, hypovolemia, intra-abdominal tumors, increased age, and female gender.

83.2 The correct answer is D.
Rationale: Patients with chronic mesenteric ischemia tend to present with a long-standing history of progressive, worsening epigastric postprandial pain approximately 10 to 180 minutes after a meal. This leads to avoidance of meals and weight loss. Patients also tend to have a history of vascular disease. Acute mesenteric ischemia tends to present with pain out of proportion to the examination and is very often difficult to localize.

83.3 The correct answer is B.
Rationale: Mesenteric venous thrombosis usually affects the small intestines and younger patients with hypercoagulable states. Onset is insidious and pain is less severe compared to the other forms of acute mesenteric ischemia. Intestinal arterial thrombosis usually presents in patients with a history of chronic mesenteric ischemia with postprandial pain and may include a history of coronary or peripheral arterial disease. Due to the chronic nature of disease, collateral flow development, signs and symptoms are less severe compared to arterial embolization. Acute mesenteric ischemia due to nonocclusive arterial

or venous (older adults) disease usually develops symptoms of intestinal ischemia over several days and is typically present after a prodrome of intestinal irritation, discomfort, or malaise. Acute arterial embolization is the most rapid in the evolution of symptoms and is associated with the most painful and robust presentation.

83.4 The correct answer is C:
Rationale: The chronic nature of postprandial abdominal pain in this older male patient with known vascular disease makes mesenteric ischemia the most likely diagnosis. Note weight loss and nutritional deficiencies are very commonly associated with this diagnosis. Colorectal cancer, while also potentially resulting in rapid weight loss, likely would not present with postprandial pain and may be more likely to be accompanied by gastrointestinal (GI) bleeding. Acute pancreatitis would not likely follow such a prolonged time course and generally presents with epigastric pain and tenderness that may radiate to the back. Diverticulitis tends to present with sharp left lower quadrant pain with rebound tenderness and guarding on examination.

83.5 The correct answer is B:
Rationale: CTA has a sensitivity of 96% to 100% and specificity up to 94% for mesenteric ischemia. Ultrasound may have otherwise been a good alternative test; however, dilated loops of the bowel can limit its sensitivity, as can obesity and calcified vessels. In addition, it can only detect proximal arterial occlusions. MRA would be a reasonable alternative, especially given its lack of radiation, but it may overestimate the severity of disease and is timely and costly. Arterial angiography is mainly used for preoperative planning after the diagnosis of mesenteric ischemia is established.

83.6 The correct answer is A:
Rationale: Patients presenting with hemodynamic instability, signs of peritonitis, and advanced intestinal ischemia who are not at high risk for surgery should undergo immediate exploratory laparotomy. Stable patients can undergo endovascular therapy. Thrombolytics can be lifesaving in emergency cases of arterial occlusion; however, this would not be the first line. Medical therapy can be helpful in select patients; however, surgery should be pursued in this unstable patient who would otherwise be a good candidate for surgical revascularization (**Table 83.1**).

83.7 The correct answer is D:
Rationale: Surgery has traditionally been considered to have more durable results. Endovascular interventions have been increasingly utilized as first-line therapy. The decision about which to use is typically made by the operator, taking into account comorbidities, severity of disease, patient clinical status, and other risk factors. Bare-metal stents or covered grafts have been shown to have better patency rates and lower revascularization rates compared to balloon angioplasty alone (**Table 83.1**).

83.8 The correct answer is C:
Rationale: Angioplasty is associated with higher target repeat revascularization when compared to surgical revascularization.

TABLE 83.1 Treatment Modalities for Acute and Chronic Mesenteric Ischemia

A. Contemporary Endovascular Treatment Options for Mesenteric Ischemia

Endovascular Approach	Indications	Technique	Considerations	Recommended Surveillance Imaging
Thrombolysis	Acute arterial occlusion, distal lesions	Anticoagulation with heparin	• Within 8-10 h from symptoms onset • No signs of advanced ischemia consider vasodilation • Risk for bleeding	• CTA • Duplex ultrasound measuring hemodynamic variables;
Mechanical thrombectomy	Acute arterial occlusion	Aspiration, stent retriever, atherectomy, combined approach	• Within 8-10 h from symptom onset • No signs of advanced ischemia, if unsuccessful consider open conversion.	
Percutaneous transluminal angioplasty ± stenting	• Usually for acute or chronic mesenteric ischemia • Chronic mesenteric ischemia	Balloon angioplasty with bail-out stenting, primary stenting with bare-metal stents or covered grafts	• Risk for dissection • Plain balloon angioplasty has higher restenosis rates than stenting. • Consider antithrombotic therapy, especially when stents or covered grafts are deployed.	• Adjust follow-up imaging according to patient's risk factors for disease recurrence. • Timely reintervention

(continued)

TABLE 83.1 Treatment Modalities for Acute and Chronic Mesenteric Ischemia (continued)

B. Contemporary Surgical Treatment Options for Mesenteric Ischemia

Surgical Approach	Indications	Technique	Considerations	Recommended Surveillance Imaging
Exploratory laparotomy	• Severe intestinal ischemia • Advanced disease with signs of peritonitis	Abdominal exploration to identify: ischemic intestinal segments and perforations, bleeding sites	• Nonviable intestinal segments should be resected. • If intestinal viability is questionable, consider revascularization and reassessment.	• Consider a second exploratory laparotomy. • CTA Imaging studies at 3, 6, 12 mo, and every year thereafter
Revascularization	• Patients who are hemodynamically unstable • Advanced intestinal ischemia • Radiologic findings of necrotic intestines	• Embolectomy and full intestinal inspection • Mesenteric bypass • Endarterectomy • Translocation of superior mesenteric artery	• Endarterectomy and translocation of the superior mesenteric artery should be avoided in acute arterial occlusion. • Autologous grafts should be preferred for mesenteric bypass, especially when perforation and peritonitis have occurred. • Reevaluate intestinal blood flow after revascularization. • Leave abdominal wall open if a second laparotomy is planned.	

CTA, computed tomography angiography.

83.9 The correct answer is A.
Rationale: Frequently after surgical revascularization for mesenteric ischemia, additional laparotomy is needed within 24 to 48 hours after the indexed procedure to assess intestinal blood flow. Anticoagulants are indicated in cases of mesenteric embolism.

83.10 The correct answer is B.
Rationale: 3-, 6-, and 12-month intervals are recommended for surveillance imaging following mesenteric revascularization and annually thereafter. Most restenosis occurs within the first 6 months following revascularization, and restenosis is higher in the endovascular subset of patients (5%-15%). There is no specific recommendation regarding the optimal imaging modality.

VENOUS THROMBOEMBOLISM*

Hamza Oglat and Robert D. Millar

CHAPTER 84

QUESTIONS

84.1 A 63-year-old male with a history of obesity and osteoarthritis underwent right hip replacement surgery. There were no complications. He had pain for several days after the surgery limiting his mobility. A week after the surgery, he presented to the emergency department (ED) with right lower extremity swelling and calf pain. He was diagnosed with deep vein thrombosis (DVT). For how long should he be treated with anticoagulation?

   A. 3 months
   B. 6 months
   C. 12 months
   D. Indefinitely

84.2 Which of the following is a provoking risk factor for DVT?

   A. Hormone replacement therapy
   B. Malignancy
   C. Pregnancy
   D. All of the above

84.3 Which of the following patients with DVT would benefit the most from invasive strategies such as catheter-directed thrombolysis (CDT) or thrombectomy?

   A. A 59-year-old patient with DVT involving the popliteal vein
   B. A 59-year-old patient with DVT involving the peroneal vein
   C. A 59-year-old patient with DVT involving the common femoral vein
   D. A 59-year-old patient with DVT involving the posterior tibial vein

84.4 In which of the following situations is a negative D-dimer assay adequate to rule out DVT?

   A. A 73-year-old male with metastatic colon cancer who is bedridden and is presenting with swelling of his entire right leg
   B. A 57-year-old female with diabetes mellitus and peripheral neuropathy who is presenting with erythema and swelling of her left lower leg
   C. A 59-year-old male status post recent knee replacement surgery presenting with calf swelling and tenderness
   D. A 67-year-old male who has been hospitalized for the past week due to multiple fractures following a motor vehicle collision who has developed swelling of his left leg

---

*Questions and Answers are based on Chapter 84: Venous Thromboembolism by Stephanie M. Madonis and J. Stephen Jenkins in Cardiovascular Medicine and Surgery, First Edition.

84.5 A 43-year-old female with metastatic breast cancer is presenting with 1 day of right lower extremity swelling and pain. Right calf swelling and tenderness were noted on her physical examination. What is the **BEST** next step in the management of this patient?

   A. Venous ultrasound of the right lower extremity
   B. D-dimer assay
   C. Start anticoagulation.
   D. Clinical observation

84.6 A 55-year-old female with a history of hypertension and diabetes mellitus presented to the ED with left lower extremity swelling and pain after a long trip. A venous ultrasound was performed, and she was found to have a thrombus in the popliteal vein. Her medical team decided to start a direct oral anticoagulant (DOAC). Which of the following DOACs require pretreatment with a parenteral anticoagulant before their initiation for the treatment of DVT?

   A. Apixaban and rivaroxaban
   B. Apixaban and edoxaban
   C. Rivaroxaban and dabigatran
   D. Edoxaban and dabigatran

84.7 A 52-year-old female with breast cancer was found to have DVT in the left common femoral vein. Which of the following anticoagulants is the preferred agent for the treatment of this patient?

   A. Warfarin
   B. Enoxaparin
   C. Apixaban
   D. Rivaroxaban

84.8 A 33-year-old female who is pregnant at 10 weeks of gestation developed DVT in the right common femoral vein. Which of the following anticoagulants is the preferred agent for the treatment of this patient?

   A. Dabigatran
   B. Rivaroxaban
   C. Enoxaparin
   D. Warfarin

84.9 A 75-year-old male was admitted to the hospital with an intracerebral hemorrhage. He was noted to have swelling in his left leg. A venous ultrasound was performed and revealed a thrombus in the left common femoral vein. Which of the following is the **BEST** next step in the management of DVT in this patient?

   A. Start anticoagulation with unfractionated heparin.
   B. Start anticoagulation with low-molecular-weight heparin.
   C. Start anticoagulation with a DOAC.
   D. Inferior vena cava (IVC) filter placement.

84.10 A 52-year-old female who is obese with a history of varicose veins presents to the ED with redness and warmth along the medial aspect of her right leg. The area is tender on examination. A venous ultrasound was performed and revealed thrombus in the greater saphenous vein to within 3 cm of the saphenofemoral junction. What is the most appropriate next step in the management of this patient?

A. Start apixaban.
B. Start ibuprofen.
C. Start local compression and heat application.
D. All of the above

ANSWERS

84.1 The correct answer is A.
Rationale: The patient had a provoked DVT, and guidelines recommend at least 3 months of anticoagulation. The provoking risk factor in his case was hip replacement surgery. Patients with unprovoked DVT are at high risk of recurrence, and thus it is recommended that they be treated with long-term anticoagulation (**Figure 84.1**).

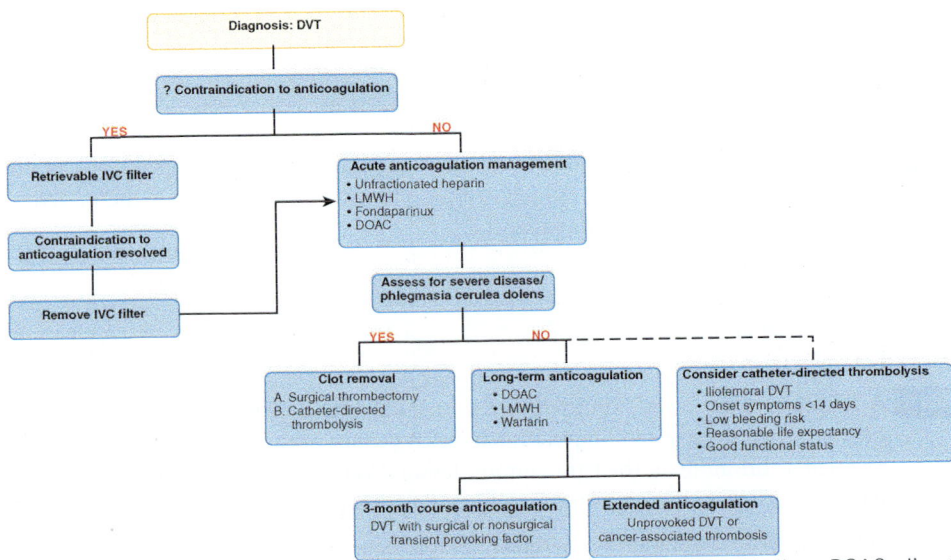

Figure 84.1 Approach to the management of acute deep vein thromboembolism. DOAC, direct oral anticoagulant; DVT, deep vein thrombosis; IVC, inferior vena cava; LMWH, low-molecular-weight heparin. (Adapted with permission from Liu D, Peterson E, Dooner J, et al. Diagnosis and management of iliofemoral deep vein thrombosis: clinical practice guideline. *CMAJ*. 2015;187[17]:1288-1296.)

84.2 The correct answer is D.

Rationale: Identification of provoking risk factors is an important part of the evaluation of patients with DVT due to management and prognostic implications. Hormone replacement therapy, malignancy, and pregnancy are all provoking risk factors for DVT.

Current guidelines advocate for at least 3 months of anticoagulation for provoked DVTs, whereas long-term anticoagulation is recommended for patients with unprovoked events because of a high risk of recurrence. Provoking risk factors can be further subdivided into transient or persistent. Transient risk factors are those that resolve after they have "provoked" a DVT and include events such as recent trauma, surgery, confinement to bed or prolonged immobilization, use of oral contraceptives or hormone replacement therapy, and pregnancy.

Potential permanent or persistent risk factors include malignancy, hereditary thrombophilia, inflammatory bowel disease, collagen vascular disease, chronic renal disease, congestive heart failure, obesity, and tobacco use disorder. It is approximated that 25% to 50% of DVT cases have no identifiable predisposing risk factor or trigger and are therefore classified as being "unprovoked."

84.3 The correct answer is C.

Rationale: Patients with DVTs involving the common femoral or iliac veins have worse prognoses and have a higher risk for adverse outcomes compared to patients with DVTs that do not involve the common femoral or iliac veins. Randomized controlled trials showed improved iliofemoral patency and a lower incidence of post-thrombotic syndrome in patients with DVTs involving the common femoral or iliac veins who were treated with CDT with or without thrombectomy compared to those patients treated with anticoagulation alone. The use of thrombectomy is being further evaluated in several ongoing clinical trials.

84.4 The correct answer is B.

Rationale: Based on the use of the Wells Scoring System for DVT, all of the patients mentioned in options of **Question 84.4** have a high pretest probability for DVT except for patient B. An alternative diagnosis (cellulitis) is more likely in patient B. A negative D-dimer assay has a high negative predictive value in patients with a low or intermediate pretest probability for DVT (**Table 84.1**).

TABLE 84.1 Pretest Probability of Deep Vein Thrombosis (Wells Score)

Clinical Finding	Points
• Paralysis, paresis, or recent orthopedic casting of lower extremity	1
• Recently bedridden for more than 3 d or major surgery within 4 wk	1
• Localized tenderness along distribution of deep venous system	1
• Swelling of entire leg	1
• Calf swelling by more than 3 cm when compared to the asymptomatic leg (measured 10 cm below tibial tuberosity)	1

(continued)

TABLE 84.1 Pretest Probability of Deep Vein Thrombosis (Wells Score) (continued)

Clinical Finding	Points
• Pitting edema (greater in the symptomatic leg)	1
• Collateral superficial veins (non-varicose vein)	1
• Active cancer or cancer treated within previous 6 mo	1
• Alternative diagnosis more likely than that of DVT (eg, Baker cyst, cellulitis, superficial vein thrombosis, postphlebitic syndrome, inguinal lymphadenopathy)	−2
Risk Score Interpretation	**Points**
• High probability of DVT	3-8
• Moderate probability	1-2
• Low probability	−2 to 0

Wells Scoring System for DVT: −2 to 0 points: low probability; 1-2 points: moderate probability; 3-8 points: high probability.

Modified from Wells PS, Anderson DR, Bormanis J, et al. Value of assessment of pretest probability of deep-vein thrombosis in clinical management. *Lancet.* 1997;350(9094):1795-1798. Copyright © 1997 Elsevier, with permission.

84.5 The correct answer is C.
Rationale: When the clinical suspicion for DVT is high, treatment with anticoagulation should be started while the workup is being performed to confirm the diagnosis.

84.6 The correct answer is D.
Rationale: Edoxaban and dabigatran require pretreatment with a parenteral anticoagulant for at least 5 days before their initiation. On the other hand, apixaban and rivaroxaban provide their effects immediately, and no pretreatment with a parenteral anticoagulant is required. Of note, a higher dose of apixaban and rivaroxaban is used in the initial period of therapy followed by a dose reduction.

84.7 The correct answer is B.
Rationale: Low-molecular-weight heparins are the preferred anticoagulants in patients with malignancy. Warfarin is not recommended in patients with malignancy unless the patient cannot be on a low-molecular-weight heparin or a DOAC.

84.8 The correct answer is C.
Rationale: The incidence of DVT in pregnant women is about 6 times the incidence in nonpregnant women. Warfarin should be avoided in the treatment of acute DVT due to adverse effects on the fetus. Vitamin K antagonists cross the placenta readily and are associated with adverse pregnancy outcomes. The preferred anticoagulants are low-molecular-weight heparin or unfractionated heparin because they do not cross the placenta. The use of DOACs is contraindicated in pregnancy as they have not been sufficiently tested.

84.9 The correct answer is D.
Rationale: The patient was admitted with an intracerebral hemorrhage which is an absolute contraindication to anticoagulation. An IVC filter can be placed in patients with DVT and an absolute contraindication to anticoagulation to decrease the risk of thrombus migration from the lower extremities to the pulmonary arteries, reducing the risk of pulmonary embolism.

84.10 The correct answer is D.
Rationale: This patient was diagnosed with superficial vein thrombosis. The majority of patients with this condition are treated conservatively with local compression, heat application, and the use of nonsteroidal anti-inflammatory drugs with no need for anticoagulation. However, patients with superficial vein thrombosis within 3 to 5 cm of the saphenofemoral or saphenopopliteal junctions are treated with anticoagulation as they are considered to be equivalent in risk for developing DVT.

PULMONARY EMBOLISM

Hamza Oglat and Robert D. Millar

CHAPTER 85

QUESTIONS

85.1 A 68-year-old male presents to the emergency department (ED) with shortness of breath and pleuritic chest pain. Computed tomographic pulmonary angiography (CTPA) reveals a pulmonary embolus (PE). What is the **MOST LIKELY** site of thrombus formation in this patient?

   A. Proximal lower extremity veins
   B. Distal lower extremity veins
   C. Upper extremity veins
   D. Right ventricle (RV)

85.2 A 71-year-old male with a history of diabetes mellitus and hypertension and recent right knee replacement surgery presents to the ED with shortness of breath following a car trip from Florida to New York. Workup in the ED reveals PE. Which of the following is the strongest predisposing factor for developing PE in this patient?

   A. Diabetes mellitus
   B. Hypertension
   C. Recent knee replacement surgery
   D. Prolonged car travel

85.3 Which of the following patients presenting to the ED with shortness of breath and tachycardia (heart rate [HR] >100 beats per minute [bpm]) on examination have the highest probability of having PE?

   A. A 66-year-old male with left leg swelling and pain 10 days after left hip replacement surgery
   B. A 59-year-old smoker with hemoptysis
   C. A 71-year-old male with metastatic lung cancer
   D. A 55-year-old female with a history of deep vein thrombosis (DVT)

85.4 A 76-year-old male with metastatic colon cancer is presenting to the ED with shortness of breath. His HR is 115 bpm. Physical examination reveals left leg swelling and tenderness. Which of the following is the **BEST** next step in establishing the diagnosis in this patient?

   A. D-dimer assay
   B. Ventilation/perfusion ($\dot{V}/\dot{Q}$) lung scintigraphy
   C. CTPA
   D. Invasive pulmonary angiography

---

*Questions and Answers are based on Chapter 85: Pulmonary Embolism by Debabrata Mukherjee and Richard A. Lange in Cardiovascular Medicine and Surgery, First Edition.

85.5 A 43-year-old female presents to the ED with pleuritic chest pain following a long flight from Australia to New York. Her HR is 68 bpm. Her oxygen saturation is 99% on room air. Physical examination is unremarkable. Performing which of the following tests would be most appropriate to rule out PE?

A. Electrocardiogram (ECG)
B. Chest radiograph
C. D-dimer assay
D. CTPA

85.6 A 58-year-old female with breast cancer is presenting to the ED with shortness of breath. Her HR is 105 bpm. A D-dimer assay was performed and came back elevated. Which of the following is the **BEST** next step in the management of this patient?

A. V̇/Q̇ lung scintigraphy
B. CTPA
C. Invasive pulmonary angiography
D. No further testing is indicated.

85.7 The use of thrombolytic therapy in patients with PE and RV dysfunction is associated with increased risk of which of the following?

A. Major bleeding
B. Intracranial hemorrhage
C. All-cause mortality
D. Both A and B

85.8 A 69-year-old male presents to the ED after a syncopal event. He is complaining of shortness of breath. His blood pressure is 80/50 mm Hg. His HR is 130 bpm, and his oxygen saturation is 85%. An ECG reveals sinus tachycardia with no other abnormalities. A bedside echocardiogram reveals depressed RV contractility. A troponin comes back elevated. The patient was resuscitated with intravenous (IV) fluids with slight improvement in his blood pressure. CTPA shows a saddle PE. Which of the following is the **BEST** next step in the management of this patient?

A. Apixaban
B. Warfarin
C. Low-molecular-weight heparin
D. Thrombolytic therapy

85.9 A 60-year-old female with a history of breast cancer is presenting to the ED with shortness of breath and pleuritic chest pain. Her blood pressure is 115/70 mm Hg, her HR is 110 bpm, and her oxygen saturation is 93%. An ECG shows sinus tachycardia with no other abnormalities. A troponin level is mildly elevated. CTPA shows PE and RV dilation. Which of the following is the **BEST** next step in this patient?

A. Low-molecular-weight heparin
B. Systemic thrombolysis
C. Catheter-directed thrombolysis
D. Surgical pulmonary embolectomy

85.10 A 67-year-old female underwent left knee replacement surgery with no complications. 12 days later she presents to the ED with shortness of breath. Her HR is 104 bpm, her blood pressure is 132/78 mm Hg, and her oxygen saturation is 95% on room air. CTPA shows PE. Which anticoagulant is preferred for this patient?

A. Unfractionated heparin
B. Low-molecular-weight heparin
C. Warfarin
D. Rivaroxaban

ANSWERS

85.1 The correct answer is A.
Rationale: The most common sites of thrombus formation in patients with PE are the proximal lower extremity veins which include the iliac, femoral, and popliteal veins.

85.2 The correct answer is C.
Rationale: Diabetes mellitus, hypertension, and prolonged car travel are all considered weak predisposing risk factors for PE. Knee replacement surgery is a strong risk factor for PE.
Predisposing factors for venous thromboembolism and PE have been categorized into strong, moderate, or weak risk factors. Strong risk factors include lower-limb fracture, hospitalization for heart failure or atrial fibrillation/flutter (within the previous 3 months), hip or knee replacement, major trauma, myocardial infarction (within the previous 3 months), any previous venous thromboembolism or PE, and spinal cord injury.

Moderate risk factors include arthroscopic knee surgery, autoimmune diseases, blood transfusions, central venous lines, IV catheters and leads, oral contraceptive therapy, postpartum period, infection (specifically pneumonia, urinary tract infection [UTI], and HIV), inflammatory bowel disease, malignancy, paralytic stroke, and thrombophilia.

Relatively weak risk factors include bed rest for more than 3 days, diabetes mellitus, systemic hypertension, immobility owing to sitting (ie, prolonged car or air travel), increasing age, laparoscopic surgery, obesity, pregnancy, and presence of varicose veins. Estrogen-containing oral contraceptive agents are associated with elevated thromboembolism risk, and their use is the most frequent risk factor for thromboembolism and PE in women of reproductive age.

85.3 The correct answer is A.
Rationale: The most frequently used prediction rules are the revised Geneva rule (see **Table 85.1**) and the Wells rule to assess the probability of PE.

For the Wells score, 3.0 points are assigned to the clinical symptoms of DVT, 3 points if PE is the most likely diagnosis, 1.5 points for HR greater than 100 bpm, 1.5 points for immobilization or surgery within 4 weeks, 1.5 points for previous DVT or PE, 1 point for hemoptysis, and 1 point for malignancy.

Patient A has the highest Wells score, 9.0 (3 + 3 + 1.5 + 1.5).

85.4 The correct answer is C.

Rationale: CTPA is the diagnostic modality of choice in patients with a high clinical probability of PE. The D-dimer assay is used in patients with a low or intermediate clinical probability of PE due to its high negative predictive value. V/Q lung scintigraphy is preferred in certain clinical scenarios when performing CTPA could lead to harm such as in patients with advanced kidney disease. Invasive pulmonary angiography is not the preferred diagnostic modality in patients with PE because CTPA offers similar diagnostic accuracy with lower procedural risk.

85.5 The correct answer is C.

Rationale: This patient has a low probability of PE. The D-dimer assay is used to rule out PE in patients with low or intermediate clinical probability due to its high negative predictive value. Both the ECG and the chest radiograph are nonsensitive and nonspecific for PE. CTPA is the diagnostic modality of choice in patients with a high clinical probability of PE.

85.6 The correct answer is B.

Rationale: This patient with an intermediate probability of PE has an elevated D-dimer level. The D-dimer assay has a low positive predictive value and thus does not confirm PE. Further testing is needed to establish the diagnosis of PE. In this case, CTPA is the diagnostic modality of choice. V/Q lung scintigraphy is done in certain clinical scenarios when CTPA is not preferred such as in patients with advanced kidney disease. Invasive pulmonary angiography is not preferred over CTPA as CTPA is less invasive and offers similar diagnostic accuracy with lower procedural risk.

85.7 The correct answer is D.

Rationale: A meta-analysis of 16 thrombolysis trials in patients with PE and RV dysfunction showed that the use of thrombolysis was associated with increased risks of major bleeding and intracranial hemorrhage. The all-cause mortality rate was lower in patients who received thrombolysis.

85.8 The correct answer is D.

Rationale: This patient has a high-risk PE with evidence of RV dysfunction, an elevated troponin level, and hemodynamic instability. Thrombolytic therapy is the treatment of choice in patients with high-risk PE and hemodynamic instability (**Table 85.2**).

85.9 The correct answer is A.

Rationale: This patient has an intermediate-risk PE with evidence of RV dysfunction and an elevated troponin level. Studies have shown no improved short- or long-term clinical or functional outcomes with the use of either catheter-directed thrombolysis or embolectomy in patients with intermediate-risk PE. The ASH (American Society of Hematology) guidelines suggest anticoagulation alone over the routine use of thrombolysis in patients with intermediate-risk PE.

85.10 The correct answer is D.

Rationale: Novel oral anticoagulants (NOACs) such as rivaroxaban are preferred for the treatment of patients with PE without hemodynamic instability.

TABLE 85.1 The Revised Geneva Clinical Prediction Rule for Pulmonary Embolism

Items	Clinical Decision Rule Points	
	Original Version[9]	Simplified Version[10]
Previous PE or DVT	3	1
Heart rate		
75-94 bpm	3	1
≥95 bpm	5	2
Surgery or fracture within the past month	2	1
Hemoptysis	2	1
Active cancer	2	1
Unilateral lower-limb pain	3	1
Pain on lower-limb deep venous palpation and unilateral edema	4	1
Age >65 y	1	1
Clinical probability		
Three-level score		
Low	0-3	0-1
Intermediate	4-10	2-4
High	≥11	≥5
Two-level score		
PE unlikely	0-5	0-2
PE likely	≥6	≥3

bpm, beats per minute; DVT, deep vein thrombosis; PE, pulmonary embolism.
From Konstantinides SV, Meyer G, Becattini C, et al; ESC Scientific Document Group. 2019 ESC Guidelines for the diagnosis and management of acute pulmonary embolism developed in collaboration with the European Respiratory Society (ERS). *Eur Heart J.* 2020;41(4):543-603. Reproduced by permission of The European Society of Cardiology.

TABLE 85.2 Classification of Pulmonary Embolism Severity and the Risk of Early (In-Hospital or 30-Day) Death

Early Mortality Risk		Indicators of Risk			
		Hemodynamic Instability[a]	Clinical Parameters of PE Severity and/or Comorbidity PESI Class III-V or sPESI dI	RV Dysfunction on TTE or CTPA[b]	Elevated Cardiac Troponin Levels[c]
High		+	(+)[d]	+	(+)
Intermediate	Intermediate-high	−	+[e]	+	+
	Intermediate-low	−	+[e]	One (or none) positive	
Low		−	−	−	Assessment optional: if assessed, negative

CTPA, computed tomography pulmonary angiography; PE, pulmonary embolism; PESI, Pulmonary Embolism Severity Index; RV, right ventricular; sPESI, simplified Pulmonary Embolism Severity Index; TTE, transthoracic echocardiogram.
[a]One of the following clinical presentations: cardiac arrest, obstructive shock (systolic blood pressure [BP] <90 mm Hg or vasopressors required to achieve a BP ≥90 mm Hg despite an adequate filling status, in combination with end-organ hypoperfusion), or persistent hypotension (systolic BP <90 mm Hg or a systolic BP drop ≥40 mm Hg for >15 minutes, not caused by new-onset arrhythmia, hypovolemia, or sepsis).
[b]Prognostically relevant imaging (echocardiography or CTPA) findings in patients with acute PE.
[c]Elevation of further laboratory biomarkers, such as plasma N-terminal pro-B-type natriuretic peptide 600 ng/L or more, plasma heart-type fatty acid-binding protein 6 ng/mL or more, or copeptin 24 pmol/L or more, may provide additional prognostic information.
[d]Hemodynamic instability, combined with PE confirmation on CTPA and/or evidence of RV dysfunction on TTE, is sufficient to classify a patient into the high-risk PE category. In these cases, neither calculation of the PESI nor measurement of troponins or other cardiac biomarkers is necessary.
[e]Signs of RV dysfunction on TTE (or CTPA) or elevated cardiac biomarker levels may be present despite a calculated PESI of I-II or an sPESI of 0. Until the implications of such discrepancies for the management of PE are fully understood, these patients should be classified into the intermediate-risk category.
From Konstantinides SV, Meyer G, Becattini C, et al. 2019 ESC guidelines for the diagnosis and management of acute pulmonary embolism developed in collaboration with the European Respiratory Society (ERS): the Task Force for the diagnosis and management of acute pulmonary embolism of the European Society of Cardiology (ESC). *Eur Heart J.* 2020;41(4):543-603. Reproduced by permission of The European Society of Cardiology.

SECTION 7 CARDIOVASCULAR SURGERY

CORONARY ARTERY BYPASS SURGERY*
Mohammad El-Hajjar and Samuel Kim

CHAPTER 86

QUESTIONS

86.1 Which of the following scenarios is coronary artery bypass grafting (CABG) **NOT** indicated for survival benefit?

A. Significant stenosis (>70% diameter) in two major coronary arteries that include one being proximal left anterior descending (LAD) artery

B. In survivors of sudden cardiac arrest with presumed ischemia-mediated ventricular tachycardia caused by significant (>70% diameter) stenosis in a major coronary artery

C. An asymptomatic individual with noted left main coronary artery of greater than 50% stenosis

D. None of the above. All presented scenarios have indications for CABG for survival benefit.

86.2 Which of the following scenarios would emergent CABG **NOT** be indicated in?

A. A patient presenting with acute myocardial infarction with subsequent failed percutaneous intervention and ongoing chest pain

B. A patient presenting with ST–segment elevation myocardial infarction (STEMI) with known multivessel disease but amendable to percutaneous coronary intervention (PCI)

C. A patient presenting with acute myocardial infarction and noted ventricular septal rupture with hemodynamic instability

D. To preserve left ventricular (LV) function in a patient who presented for elective PCI procedure with subsequent development of acute coronary occlusion with ongoing ischemia and inability to restore vessel patency percutaneously

86.3 Which of the following statements regarding conduits for coronary bypass graft is **TRUE**?

A. There is no significant difference in patency rate between the usage of saphenous venous graft and arterial graft.

B. Late graft disease (>12 months) of venous grafts is due to intimal hyperplasia at the anastomosis site.

C. The radial artery graft is the preferred conduit to any vessel in CABG.

D. The radial artery is prone to more spasms as compared to internal mammary artery (IMA) graft.

Questions and Answers are based on Chapter 86: Coronary Artery Bypass Grafting by Michael E. Jessen in Cardiovascular Medicine and Surgery, First Edition.

86.4 A 53-year-old male with a past medical history of known coronary artery disease and hypertension presents to the emergency department with anginal symptoms. His current regimen includes aspirin 81 mg and amlodipine 10 mg once daily. His high-sensitivity troponin was mildly elevated on admission. He underwent cardiac catheterization with demonstration of two-vessel disease with significant stenosis (>70%) in the left circumflex and proximal LAD arteries. What factors will assist in the decision regarding candidacy for coronary artery bypass surgery?

   A. Hemoglobin A1c
   B. LV ejection fraction
   C. Patient risk profile assessment
   D. All of the above

86.5 A 65-year-old female with a previous medical history of hypertension, diabetes mellitus type 2, and dyslipidemia presented to the hospital with complaints of chest discomfort and noted to have an elevated troponin with electrocardiogram demonstrating lateral T-wave inversions. She underwent cardiac catheterization and noted to have multivessel disease with mid-LAD artery, proximal right coronary artery, and mid-left circumflex involvement. What further intervention would you recommend at this time?

   A. PCI with multiple drug-eluting stent placements
   B. PCI with multiple bare-metal stent placements
   C. Coronary artery bypass surgery
   D. Medical therapy only

86.6 A 49-year-old gentlemen underwent coronary artery bypass surgery after initially presenting for acute coronary syndrome (ACS) and found to have multivessel coronary artery disease. No post-procedural complications were noted and he remained hemodynamically stable without pressor or mechanical support device requirements with an average blood pressure of 145/95 mm Hg. Which of the following antiplatelet should be added to aspirin 81 mg at this time?

   A. Clopidogrel
   B. Dipyridamole
   C. Rivaroxaban
   D. None of the above

86.7 In the patient in **Question 86.6**, an echocardiogram was obtained and noted significant LV systolic dysfunction with an estimated ejection fraction of 30%. What further management strategy would be considered at this time?

   A. Beta-blocker
   B. Implantable cardioverter-defibrillator implantation
   C. Amlodipine
   D. None of the above

86.8 A 53-year-old female underwent coronary artery bypass surgery for two-vessel coronary artery disease and LV systolic dysfunction after presenting with myocardial infarction. In addition to antiplatelet strategy, you have recommended the addition of beta-blocker for the following reason(s):

A. To prevent postoperative atrial fibrillation
B. Improve survival in the setting of myocardial infarction
C. Survival benefit given LV dysfunction
D. All of the above

86.9 A 73-year-old female presents to the cardiology clinic for a post-discharge follow-up after receiving coronary artery bypass surgery. She has an additional medical history of hypertension and dyslipidemia, and she is currently on aspirin, clopidogrel, metoprolol, lisinopril, and pravastatin 40 mg. You discuss with the patient her cholesterol management and plan to obtain a lipid panel. What medication changes would you recommend at this time?

A. Increase pravastatin dose to 80 mg.
B. Change statin to rosuvastatin 20 mg once daily.
C. Add ezetimibe 10 mg once daily.
D. Change statin to atorvastatin 20 mg once daily.

86.10 A 55-year-old male with a past medical history, COPD, hypertension, and active tobacco use presented to the hospital with complaints of chest pain. He underwent cardiac catheterization with demonstration of proximal LAD artery and left circumflex artery stenosis. Patient was evaluated and deemed to be an appropriate surgical candidate. What is the optimal method for revascularization for coronary artery bypass surgery?

A. Left internal mammary artery (LIMA) and radial artery graft
B. Radial artery and saphenous vein grafts
C. Hybrid procedure with IMA and PCI
D. LIMA and vein graft

ANSWERS

86.1 **The correct answer is D.**
Rationale: CABG has been demonstrated to result in improved survival in patients with greater than 50% stenosis of the left main coronary artery, greater than 70% stenosis in three major coronary arteries, and greater than 70% stenosis in two major coronary arteries when one is affecting the proximal LAD artery. The survival benefit is more apparent when associated with impaired LV function.

CABG or PCI is recommended to improve survival in those who survived presumed ischemia-mediated ventricular tachycardic sudden cardiac arrest due to suspected significant coronary artery stenosis.

CABG is recommended to improve survival in those with greater than 50% stenosis of the left main coronary artery, regardless of presence or lack of anginal symptoms.

86.2 **The correct answer is B.**
Rationale: Most patients who present with and are diagnosed with STEMI undergo percutaneous coronary angiography with intervention, and subsequently a small portion of this group will be found to have unsuitable coronary anatomy for PCI

or coronary occlusions that cannot be opened. In these scenarios, emergency CABG may be indicated, especially if they have suitable anatomy for bypass, persistent ischemia of significant area of myocardium, and/or hemodynamic instability refractory to nonsurgical therapy.

Emergency CABG is recommended in patients undergoing surgical repair of postinfarction mechanical complications. Such examples include ventricular septal rupture, free wall rupture, and papillary muscle infarction/rupture with resulting mitral valve insufficiency.

Emergency CABG should be considered in patients who develop acute coronary occlusion while undergoing elective PCI to preserve LV function, as long as the risk profile is not prohibitive.

86.3 The correct answer is D.
Rationale: The radial artery is morphologically different as compared to the IMA and is more prone to spasms after grafting.

It has been noted that up to 15% of saphenous vein grafts occluded by 1 year and angiographic studies demonstrated a 40% to 50% occlusion rate at 10 years. The radial artery was associated with a lower incidence of adverse cardiac events, rate of graft occlusion, incidence of myocardial infarction, and need for revascularization as compared to saphenous venous grafts in a combined analysis of several studies at a 5-year follow-up.

Early (<1 month) graft occlusion is a result of thrombosis from either technical imperfection in the construction of the graft, poor runoff in the target vessel, or vein graft endothelial injury during harvesting. Intermediate (1-12 month) graft stenosis is generally due to intimal hyperplasia near the anastomotic site. Late graft disease (>12 months) results from the development of atherosclerotic disease.

The LIMA is the preferred conduit for use in CABG and is the standard of care, especially as the conduit for the LAD. It is associated with the highest 10-year patency rate (>90%), survival and freedom from cardiac events when compared to other vascular conduits.

86.4 The correct answer is D.
Rationale: Coronary artery bypass surgery has a class I recommendation for improvements in patients with significant (>70%) stenosis of proximal LAD plus one additional major coronary artery and is an especially preferred revascularization option in patients with diabetes.

CABG offers survival benefits in many patients with complex coronary arteries, as mentioned earlier, and the magnitude of the benefit tends to be greater in patients with LV systolic dysfunction up to a certain degree of severity. In patients with extreme LV dysfunction (eg, LVEF <20%), especially when accompanied with LV remodeling, the risk versus benefit ratio may guide decisions away from CABG. In these scenarios, myocardial viability may provide useful additional information, particularly in patients without anginal symptoms.

To better accurately inform patients of their risk of mortality and/or development of complications following CABG, several risk models have been established. The most commonly used tools are the Society of Thoracic Surgeons (STS), the Adult Cardiac Surgery Database Predictive Risk of Mortality (PROM), and the European System for Cardiac Operative Risk Evaluation (EuroSCORE II).

86.5 The correct answer is C.

Rationale: CABG has a class I recommendation to improve survival in significant stenosis in three major coronary arteries, especially in patients with LV systolic dysfunction.

STITCH (Surgical Treatment for Ischemic Heart Failure) trial is one of the largest trials that investigated the survival benefit of CABG with guideline-directed medical therapy versus medical therapy alone in patients between July 2002 and May 2007. It recruited 1,212 patients with LV ejection fraction of 35% or less with coronary artery disease and demonstrated significant survival benefit with CABG at 10 years compared to medical therapy alone.

A large meta-analysis of pertinent randomized trials demonstrated survival benefit of CABG as compared to PCI in those with multivessel disease as well. One such included study was the SYNTAX (Synergy Between Percutaneous Coronary Intervention With Taxus and Cardiac Surgery) trial that compared CABG versus PCI. At the 5-year follow-up, CABG was demonstrated to be superior in patients with intermediate to high SYNTAX scores. At the 10-year follow-up, no reported differences were noted between CABG and PCI, but a survival benefit was seen for CABG in those with three-vessel disease.

86.6 The correct answer is A.

Rationale: A systematic review and meta-analysis that included 20 randomized trials investigated aspirin with ticagrelor or aspirin and clopidogrel and noted its effectiveness in reducing saphenous vein graft failure as compared to aspirin monotherapy with no significant difference in major adverse outcomes (major bleeding, myocardial infarction, or death). As such, many surgical teams initiate this strategy in the early postoperative period and continue it for 12 months. The usage of aspirin in combination with P2Y12 inhibitor has a class IIb recommendation. An additional indication for dual antiplatelet initiation in this patient is the presentation of ACS and thereby providing further support for the addition of clopidogrel. Furthermore, it remains a Class 1 indication to prescribe clopidogrel with aspirin (DAPT [dual antiplatelet therapy]) after ACS irrespective of treatment modality, that is, medical therapy, PCI, or CABG.

Early studies had demonstrated the combination of aspirin and dipyridamole improved vein graft patency but subsequently the benefits were concluded to be minimal. As a result, guidelines do not recommend the addition of dipyridamole to aspirin.

One large trial did not demonstrate reduction of saphenous vein graft failure by the combination of rivaroxaban to aspirin. Overall, data regarding the benefit of oral anticoagulant are limited.

86.7 The correct answer is A.

Rationale: Patients who have undergone coronary artery bypass surgery commonly have associated cardiovascular risk factors, such as hypertension in our patient, and appropriate treatment of these conditions improve their long-term outcomes. As the patient has evidence of LV dysfunction, management with beta-blocker and/or angiotensin-converting enzyme inhibitors would be the ideal choice. Patients with severely depressed LV function (<35%) should have their LV function reassessed 3 months following CABG. If the LV dysfunction severity continues to persist, an implantable cardioverter-defibrillator should be considered.

86.8 The correct answer is D:
Rationale: Beta-blockers are recommended in nearly all patients who have undergone CABG for several different reasons. It is an effective agent for preventing postoperative atrial fibrillations and has been shown to improve survival following myocardial infarction and in those with LV systolic dysfunction.

86.9 The correct answer is B:
Rationale: It is recommended that following CABG, all patients should undergo intensive lipid management as current evidence supports reduction of progression of atherosclerosis not only in the native coronary circulation but in the bypass grafts as well. As such, current guidelines recommend high-intensity statin therapy (atorvastatin 40-80 mg or rosuvastatin 20-40 mg) as the preferred pharmacologic approach and have a goal of low-density lipoprotein cholesterol of less than 100 mg/dL.

86.10 The correct answer is A:
Rationale: The LIMA is undoubtedly the preferred conduit for use in CABG, especially when grafting to the LAD artery. This construct is associated with the highest 10-year patency rate as well as freedom from cardiac events as opposed to any other conduit. Due to this finding, there have been consideration of bilateral IMA grafting but is currently controversial. The multicenter prospective randomized arterial revascularization trial (ART) trial randomized patients to single or bilateral IMA grafting and unfortunately no significant differences were noted between the two groups in terms of mortality or rate of adverse cardiovascular events with 10 years of follow-up. The bilateral IMA group, however, did have a significant increased rate of sternal wound complications. The interpretation of this trial was complicated, however, by a high rate of crossover (14% allocated to bilateral IMA received single IMA with radial artery). Further studies are required.

A meta-analysis that combined six randomized controlled trials investigated and compared radial artery grafts versus saphenous vein grafts. With a mean 5-year follow-up, it was revealed that the radial artery graft arm had a significantly lower incidence rate of adverse cardiac events and a significantly lower rate of graft occlusion, myocardial infarction, and need for repeat revascularization. These data suggest that the usage of radial artery graft is beneficial as compared to the saphenous vein graft and is the preferred second conduit of choice in CABG.

There have been many randomized controlled trials that compared radial artery grafts versus saphenous vein grafts (with both groups receiving single IMA grafts as well).

Minimally invasive approaches for coronary artery bypass surgery have emerged with some procedures performed through a small anterolateral minithoracotomy incision. This, however, limits the operation to anastomosis of the LIMA to the LAD and a few other vessels. Some centers have developed a hybrid revascularization for the treatment of multivessel coronary artery disease with surgical revascularization of the LAD that is followed by PCI to the other vessels. Data on this procedure on the short and intermediate outcomes are limited and further investigations are required.

AORTIC VALVE SURGERY

Hamza Oglat and William Bachman

QUESTIONS

87.1 How is aortic valve stenosis most commonly detected?
   A. Transthoracic echocardiogram
   B. Physical examination
   C. Cardiac-gated computed tomography
   D. Cardiac magnetic resonance imaging

87.2 A 78-year-old male presented to the cardiology clinic for evaluation of progressive exertional dyspnea. On physical examination, he was noted to have a harsh, late peaking, crescendo-decrescendo systolic ejection murmur. A transthoracic echocardiogram was performed and showed aortic valve peak flow velocity of 4.5 m/s, mean gradient of 48 mm Hg and aortic valve area of 0.9 cm^2. Left ventricular ejection fraction is preserved. Based on his transthoracic echocardiogram, which stage of aortic valve stenosis does this patient have?
   A. Stage D1
   B. Stage D2
   C. Stage D3
   D. Stage D4

87.3 Which of the following patients with aortic valve stenosis **DOES NOT** have a class I recommendation for aortic valve replacement?
   A. A 73-year-old female with symptomatic, severe, high-gradient aortic valve stenosis
   B. A 75-year-old male with asymptomatic, severe, aortic valve stenosis, and left ventricular ejection fraction of 45%
   C. A 78-year-old male with asymptomatic, severe, aortic valve stenosis, and left ventricular ejection fraction of 60%
   D. A 65-year-old male with severe, aortic stenosis undergoing coronary artery bypass surgery

87.4 Which of the following patients with aortic valve stenosis who meet indications for aortic valve replacement is **BEST** treated with transcatheter aortic valve replacement (TAVR) rather than surgical aortic valve replacement (SAVR) based on the Society of Thoracic Surgeons (STS) risk score?
   A. Patient with low surgical risk
   B. Patient with intermediate surgical risk
   C. Patient with high surgical risk
   D. Patient with prohibitive surgical risk

*Questions and Answers are based on Chapter 87: Aortic Valve Surgery by Andres Samayoa Mendez and Amy E. Hackmann in Cardiovascular Medicine and Surgery, First Edition.

875 Which of the following patients with aortic valve regurgitation have a class IIa recommendation for aortic valve replacement?
A. A 55-year-old male with symptomatic severe aortic valve regurgitation
B. A 55-year-old male with severe aortic valve regurgitation undergoing coronary artery bypass surgery
C. A 55-year-old male with asymptomatic severe aortic valve regurgitation, left ventricular ejection fraction of 56%, and left ventricular end-systolic dimension (LVESD) of 54 mm
D. A 55-year-old male with asymptomatic severe aortic valve regurgitation and left ventricular ejection fraction of 45%

876 A 33-year-old female with a history of intravenous (IV) drug use presents to the emergency department (ED) with 1 week of fevers, difficulty breathing, orthopnea, and paroxysmal nocturnal dyspnea. Her heart rate is 130 bpm and blood pressure is 89/40 mm Hg. Examination is significant for cool extremities and crackles on lung auscultation. Transthoracic echocardiogram was performed and shows mobile vegetation on the aortic valve and severe aortic valve regurgitation. What is the **BEST** approach and timing for aortic valve replacement in this patient?
A. Early SAVR
B. Early TAVR
C. Delayed SAVR
D. Delayed TAVR

877 A 49-year-old male is presenting for evaluation of progressive dyspnea on exertion. He is an avid rock climber and noticed decreased exercise tolerance. Examination is significant for a harsh crescendo-decrescendo systolic ejection murmur. Transthoracic echocardiogram reveals severe aortic valve stenosis. He would like to be treated, so he can continue rock climbing. Which of the following interventions is most appropriate for this patient?
A. SAVR with mechanical valve
B. SAVR with bioprosthetic valve
C. TAVR
D. Percutaneous aortic balloon dilation

878 Which of the following is a risk factor for porcelain aorta?
A. Systemic inflammatory disease
B. Radiation-induced heart disease
C. Chronic kidney disease
D. All of the above

879 Compared to aortic valve replacement alone, aortic root enlargement followed by aortic valve replacement is associated with which of the following?
A. Higher mortality rate
B. Increased rate of permanent pacemaker implantation
C. Higher stroke rate
D. Longer cardiopulmonary bypass and cross-clamp times

87.10 Cardiac surgery in patients with extensive aortic calcifications is associated with increased risk of:
- A. Stroke
- B. Death
- C. A and B
- D. None of the above

ANSWERS

87.1 The Correct answer is B.
Rationale: Aortic valve stenosis is most commonly detected by physical examination which is further evaluated with a transthoracic echocardiogram. Cardiac-gated computed tomography and cardiac magnetic resonance imaging are adjunctive diagnostic modalities that may be used to further assess aortic valve disease.

87.2 The correct answer is A.
Rationale: This patient has symptomatic, severe, high-gradient aortic valve stenosis. This is stage D1. Stage D2 is symptomatic, severe, low-flow, low-gradient aortic valve stenosis with reduced left ventricular ejection fraction. Stage D3 is symptomatic, severe, paradoxical low-flow, low-gradient aortic valve stenosis with normal left ventricular ejection fraction. There is no stage D4.

87.3 The correct answer is C.
Rationale: Class I recommendations for aortic valve replacement include patients with stage D1 aortic valve stenosis (choice A), patients with asymptomatic severe aortic valve stenosis and left ventricular ejection fraction of less than 50% (choice B), and patients with severe aortic stenosis undergoing other cardiac surgery (choice D). Asymptomatic severe aortic valve stenosis in patients with left ventricular ejection fraction greater than 50% is not a class I recommendation for aortic valve replacement (choice C) (**Table 87.1**).

87.4 The correct answer is D.
Rationale: STS risk score predicts the risk of mortality and is a tool that is used by the Heart Valve Team to help determine the approach for aortic valve replacement. SAVR is recommended in patients with low or intermediate surgical risk. Either TAVR or high-risk SAVR can be recommended in patients with high surgical risk based on Heart Valve Team evaluation. TAVR is recommended in patients with prohibitive surgical risk.

87.5 The correct answer is C.
Rationale: All of the patients mentioned in the options of **Question 87.5** have a class I recommendation for aortic valve replacement except the patient in choice C. Patients with asymptomatic severe aortic valve regurgitation, left ventricular ejection fraction greater than or equal to 50%, and LVESD of greater than 50 mm have a class IIa recommendation for aortic valve replacement. Patients with symptomatic

TABLE 87.1 Indications for Aortic Valve Replacement

	Class of Recommendation	Recommendations
Aortic stenosis	Class I (should)	Stage D1 AS
		Asymptomatic severe AS and LVEF <50%
		Severe AS undergoing other cardiac surgery
	Class IIa (reasonable)	Asymptomatic critical AS (MG ≥60 mm Hg and V_{max} ≥5 m/s) and low surgical risk
		Asymptomatic severe AS with decreased exercise tolerance or decreased blood pressure during exercise
		Stage D2 with V_{max} ≥4 m/s or MG ≥40 mm Hg on low-dose dobutamine stress test
		Stage D3, normotensive, LVEF >50% with AS as the most likely cause of symptoms
		Moderate AS undergoing other cardiac surgery
	Class IIb (may be considered)	Asymptomatic severe AS, rapid disease progression, and low surgical risk
Aortic regurgitation (chronic)	Class I (should)	Symptomatic severe AR
		Asymptomatic severe AR and LVEF <50%
		Severe AR undergoing other cardiac surgery
	Class IIa (reasonable)	Asymptomatic severe AR, LVEF ≥50%, and severe LV dilation (LVESD >50 mm)
		Moderate AR undergoing other cardiac surgeries
	Class IIb (may be considered)	Asymptomatic severe AR, LVEF <50%, and progressive severe LV dilation (LVEDD >65 mm)

AR, aortic regurgitation; AS, aortic stenosis; LV, left ventricle; LVEDD, left ventricular end-diastolic dimension; LVEF, left ventricular ejection fraction; LVESD, left ventricular end-systolic ejection fraction; MG, mean gradient; V_{max}, maximum aortic velocity.

severe aortic valve regurgitation (choice A), patients with severe aortic valve regurgitation undergoing other cardiac surgery (choice B), and patients with asymptomatic severe aortic valve regurgitation and left ventricular ejection fraction of less than 50% (choice D) have a class I recommendation for aortic valve replacement.

876 The correct answer is A.

Rationale: This patient has infective endocarditis and acute severe aortic valve regurgitation. She is hypotensive and has signs of systemic hypoperfusion. Acute aortic valve regurgitation is a surgical emergency and better outcomes are seen with early aortic valve replacement. SAVR is the treatment for aortic valve regurgitation, both acute and chronic.

87.7 The correct answer is B.
Rationale: Mechanical valves are generally preferred in patients younger than 50 years old because of the deterioration that may happen with bioprosthetic valves. However, this patient's hobby puts him at high risk of bleeding if he takes anticoagulation, and thus a bioprosthetic valve would be preferred in this case. SAVR and not TAVR is recommended in patients with low or intermediate surgical risk. Percutaneous aortic balloon dilation is performed as a bridge to aortic valve replacement in patients with severe aortic valve stenosis who need delay in aortic valve replacement or are severely symptomatic.

87.8 The correct answer is D.
Rationale: The risk for porcelain aorta is increased in patients with systemic inflammatory disease, radiation-induced heart disease, and chronic kidney disease.

87.9 The correct answer is D.
Rationale: Longer cardiopulmonary bypass and cross-clamp times were observed with aortic root enlargement followed by aortic valve replacement compared to aortic valve replacement alone. There is no difference in mortality, permanent pacemaker implantation, or stroke rates with aortic root enlargement followed by aortic valve replacement compared to aortic valve replacement alone.

87.10 The correct answer is C.
Rationale: Patients with extensive aortic calcifications undergoing cardiac surgery are at increased risk of stroke and death.

MITRAL VALVE SURGERY

Hamza Oglat and William Bachman

CHAPTER 88

QUESTIONS

88.1 Which of the following is **NOT** a class I recommendation for mitral valve (MV) surgery?
  A. Symptomatic severe primary MV regurgitation
  B. Asymptomatic severe primary MV regurgitation with left ventricular ejection fraction (LVEF) of 55%
  C. Asymptomatic severe primary MV regurgitation with end-systolic dimension (ESD) of 45 mm
  D. Asymptomatic severe primary MV regurgitation with ESD of 37 mm

88.2 A 63-year-old male presented to the cardiology clinic with exertional shortness of breath and orthopnea. His echocardiogram revealed severe MV regurgitation with focal degenerative changes involving less than half of the posterior MV leaflet. His LVEF is 65%, and ESD is 35 mm. Which of the following is the most appropriate intervention for this patient?
  A. MV replacement
  B. MV repair
  C. Transcatheter edge-to-edge repair (TEER)
  D. Routine surveillance echocardiogram in 6 months

88.3 A 59-year-old female with known severe primary MV regurgitation is presenting for a follow-up visit. She continues to be active and has no exertional symptoms. Her LVEF is 65%, and ESD is 34 mm. She would like to know if undergoing MV surgery is reasonable. Which of the following statements is **CORRECT**?
  A. It is reasonable to undergo MV repair if expected surgical mortality is less than 1% with greater than 95% likelihood of successful and durable repair.
  B. It is reasonable to undergo MV repair if expected surgical mortality is less than 5% with greater than 95% likelihood of successful and durable repair.
  C. It is reasonable to undergo MV repair if expected surgical mortality is less than 1% with greater than 85% likelihood of successful and durable repair.
  D. It is not reasonable to undergo MV repair regardless of expected surgical mortality or the likelihood of successful and durable repair.

88.4 What is the first step in managing patients with symptomatic severe secondary MV regurgitation?

*Questions and Answers are based on Chapter 88: Mitral Valve Surgery: A Pathoanatomic Approach by Vinay Badhwar, Jahnavi Kakuturu, and Chris C. Cook in Cardiovascular Medicine and Surgery, First Edition

A. TEER
B. MV repair
C. MV replacement
D. Guideline-directed medical therapy (GDMT) optimization

88.5 Mitral regurgitation due to MV leaflet prolapse falls under which Carpentier classification?

A. Type 1
B. Type 2
C. Type 3A
D. Type 3B

88.6 Which of the following is a predictor of potential failure of MV repair?

A. Prior MV repair
B. Mitral annular calcification involving the base of the leaflet
C. Tissue destruction from endocarditis
D. All of the above

88.7 All of the following are determinants of successful MV repair **EXCEPT**:

A. Stabilization of the MV annulus
B. Achieving a coaptation depth of less than 5 mm
C. Restoration of normal leaflet motion
D. Immediate post repair transesophageal echocardiogram showing no more than trace to mild mitral regurgitation

88.8 Which of the following is a chordal preserving technique used in patients undergoing chord-sparing MV replacement?

A. Using artificial chords of polytetrafluoroethylene
B. Maintaining posterior leaflet chordal attachments only
C. Dividing the anterior leaflet and incorporating its chords in the posterior annular suture line
D. All of the above

88.9 Which of the following is **NOT** a risk factor for development of systolic anterior motion after MV repair?

A. Thick basal interventricular septum (>15 mm)
B. Decreased distance between the coaptation point and interventricular septum (<25 mm)
C. Increased left ventricular end-diastolic volume
D. Bilateral MV leaflet prolapse

88.10 Which of the following statements about the anatomy of the MV is **CORRECT**?

A. Anterior leaflet constitutes two-thirds of the valve orifice area.
B. Posterior leaflet constitutes one-half of the valve orifice area.
C. Anterior leaflet constitutes two-thirds of the annular circumference.
D. Posterior leaflet constitutes one-third of the annular circumference.

ANSWERS

88.1 The correct answer is D.

Rationale: Class I recommendation for MV surgery in severe primary MV regurgitation includes symptomatic patients and those who are asymptomatic with either LVEF of less than or equal to 60% or ESD of 40 mm or greater (**Figure 88.1**).

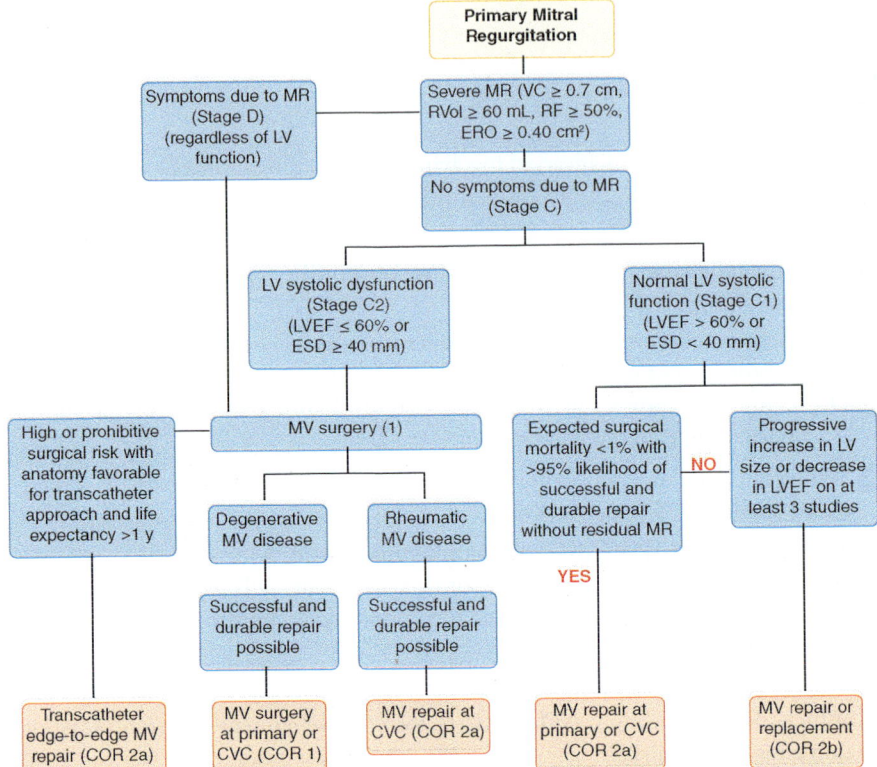

Figure 88.1 Guidelines for the management of primary mitral regurgitation. COR, class of recommendation; CVC, cardiovascular center; ERO, effective regurgitant orifice area; ESD, end-systolic volume; LV, left ventricular; LVEF, left ventricular ejection fraction; MR, mitral regurgitation; MV, mitral valve; RF, regurgitant fraction; RVol, regurgitant volume; VC, vena contracta; y, year. (Reprinted from Otto CM, Nishimura RA, Bonow RO, et al. 2020 ACC/AHA Guideline for the management of patients with valvular heart disease: a Report of the American College of Cardiology/American Heart Association Joint Committee on clinical practice guidelines. *Circulation.* 2021;143(5):e35-e71. Copyright © 2021 by the American College of Cardiology Foundation and the American Heart Association, Inc., with permission.)

88.2 The correct answer is B.

Rationale: The patient has symptomatic severe primary MV regurgitation and intervention is indicated instead of routine surveillance. MV replacement is considered a class III recommendation (harmful) in patients with focal degenerative changes involving less than half of the posterior MV leaflet. Those patients should undergo

MV repair (class I recommendation). TEER is considered in patients with high or prohibitive risk for MV surgery.

88.3 The correct answer is A.

Rationale: In patients with asymptomatic severe primary MV regurgitation with LVEF greater than 60% and ESD less than 40 mm, it is reasonable (class IIa recommendation) to undergo MV repair if expected surgical mortality is less than 1% with greater than 95% likelihood of successful and durable repair.

88.4 The correct answer is D.

Rationale: All patients with symptomatic severe secondary MV regurgitation should be on optimal GDMT, preferably supervised by a heart failure specialist. If they continue to be symptomatic despite optimal GDMT, then MV interventions can be considered (**Figure 88.2**).

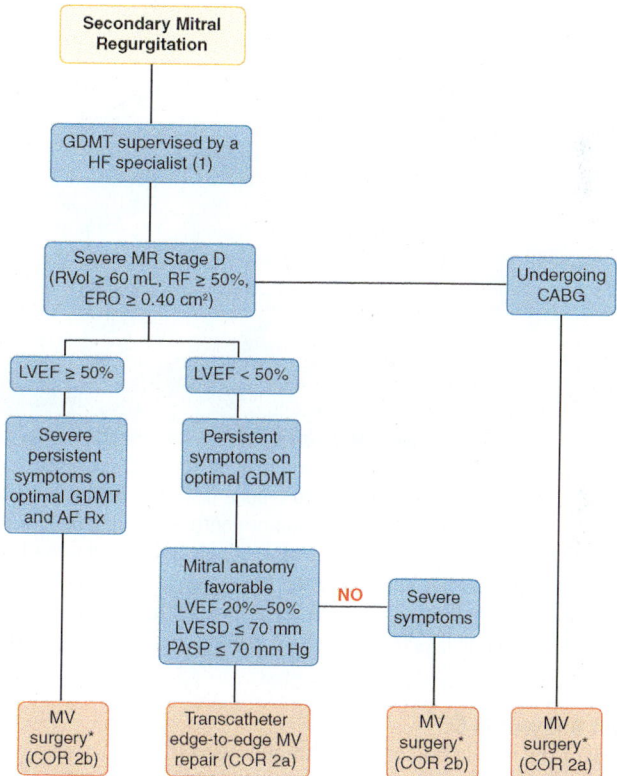

Figure 88.2 Guidelines for the management of secondary mitral regurgitation. *Chordal-sparing MV replacement may be reasonable to choose over downsized annuloplasty repair. AF, atrial fibrillation; CABG, coronary artery bypass grafting; COR, class of recommendation; ERO, effective regurgitant orifice area; GDMT, guideline-directed medical therapy; HF, heart failure; LVEF, left ventricular ejection fraction; LVESD, left ventricular end-systolic volume; MR, mitral regurgitation; MV, mitral valve; PASP, pulmonary artery systolic pressure; RF, regurgitant fraction; RVol, regurgitant volume; Rx, treatment. (Reprinted from Otto CM, Nishimura RA, Bonow RO, et al. 2020 ACC/AHA Guideline for the management of patients with valvular heart disease: a Report of the American College of Cardiology/American Heart Association Joint Committee on clinical practice guidelines. *Circulation*. 2021;143(5):e35-e71. Copyright © 2021 by the American College of Cardiology Foundation and the American Heart Association, Inc., with permission.)

88.5 The correct answer is B.

Rationale: The Carpentier classification is used to define MV leaflet motion in MV regurgitation. Type 1 is normal leaflet motion, type 2 is excessive leaflet motion (such as with primary degenerative prolapse or chordal rupture causing a flail leaflet), type 3A is restricted leaflet motion in systole and diastole (such as with rheumatic disease or radiation), and type 3B is restricted leaflet motion in systole only.

88.6 The correct answer is D.

Rationale: Prior MV repair, mitral annular calcification involving the base of the leaflet and tissue destruction from endocarditis are predictors of potential failure of MV repair. In addition, leaflet calcium or restriction is also a predictor of potential failure.

88.7 The correct answer is D.

Rationale: Achieving a coaptation depth of greater than, rather than less than, 5 mm is a determinant of successful MV repair. The other choices are all determinants of successful MV repair (**Figure 88.3**).

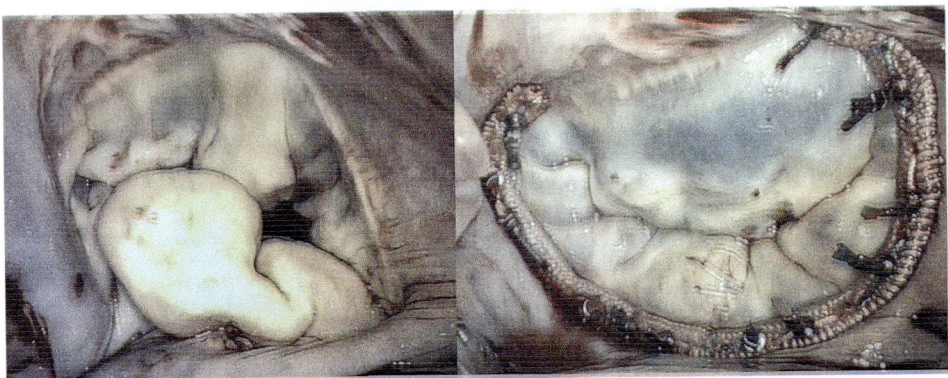

Figure 88.3 Repair of diffuse posterior leaflet prolapse or flail. Diffuse multi scallop involvement of the posterior leaflet (left) often requires efforts to reduce posterior leaflet height while preserving leaflet motion. This may be accomplished by resection or nonresection supportive techniques. In this case, both were applied by a central focal resection and a single polytetrafluoroethylene (PTFE) suture that both repaired the resected leaflet and supported the repair to the papillary muscle at the same time (right). (From Roberts HG, Rankin JS, Wei LM, et al. Respectful resection to enhance the armamentarium of mitral valve repair: is less really more? *J Thorac Cardiovasc Surg.* 2018;156:1854-1855.)

88.8 The correct answer is D.

Rationale: All of the listed choices are techniques used in chord-sparing MV replacement.

88.9 The correct answer is C.

Rationale: All of the choices listed in **Question 88.9** are risk factors for development of systolic anterior motion after MV repair except for choice C. A small hyperdynamic left ventricle with reduced end-diastolic volume is a risk factor for development of systolic anterior motion after MV repair.

88.10 The correct answer is A.

Rationale: The anterior leaflet constitutes two-thirds of the valve orifice area and one-third of the annular circumference. The posterior leaflet constitutes one-third of the valve orifice area and two-thirds of the annular circumference.

THORACIC AORTIC SURGERY

Andrew J. Castellano

CHAPTER 89

QUESTIONS

89.1 A 50-year-old male with a past medical history significant for hypertension and heavy tobacco use presents to the emergency department at 2 AM with sudden onset back pain that awoke him from sleep 2 hours before presentation. On arrival, he was noted to have a blood pressure of 200/90 mm Hg. On examination, he appeared pale and diaphoretic and had a 4/6 early diastolic decrescendo murmur. Laboratory data revealed a hemoglobin of 13.0 g/dL, a high-sensitivity troponin of 89 ng/L, and a creatinine of 1.8 μmol/L. What is the next **BEST** test to order?

- A. Transesophageal echocardiogram
- B. Transthoracic echocardiogram
- C. Computed tomography (CT) chest with contrast
- D. CT chest/abdomen/pelvis with contrast

89.2 A patient is referred to your office after a 4.3-cm thoracic aortic aneurysm was identified incidentally on a chest CT. One year later, a repeat chest CT notes the aneurysm is now measuring 4.9 cm. What is the next **BEST** step?

- A. Repeat chest CT in 3 months.
- B. Repeat chest CT in 6 months.
- C. Repeat chest CT in 1 year.
- D. Referral to cardiothoracic surgery

89.3 A 40-year-old male with a past medical history of hypertension and Marfan syndrome presents to establish care. He has a strong family history of Marfan syndrome and states his father died at an early age from an aortic dissection. As part of your screening, an echocardiogram is performed which reveals a thin tricuspid aortic valve and a 5.1-cm aortic root. You start him on losartan for a blood pressure of 140/80 mm Hg. What is the next **BEST** step in the management of this patient?

- A. Perform a transesophageal echocardiogram.
- B. Repeat transthoracic echocardiogram in 6 months.
- C. Refer for surgery.
- D. Follow up in 1 year.

89.4 A 42-year-old male with a past medical history significant for hypertension and hyperlipidemia on valsartan 80 mg daily and atorvastatin 20 mg nightly presents to your office for follow-up. He appears nervous at today's visit, and he informs you that his father was just recently hospitalized for an aortic dissection. What is the next **BEST** step in the management of this patient?

*Questions and Answers are based on Chapter 89: Thoracic Aortic Surgery by Yuki Ikeno, Akiko Tanaka, and Anthony L. Estrera in Cardiovascular Medicine and Surgery, First Edition.

A. Reassurance
B. Echocardiography
C. Genetic testing
D. Magnetic resonance imaging (MRI) of the chest

89.5 A patient is being discharged from the hospital after a thoracic endovascular aortic repair (TEVAR) was performed for an ascending aortic aneurysm of 5.6 cm. He feels well and has no complaints. He has a blood pressure of 118/76 mm Hg well managed on losartan and carvedilol. Heart rate is 80 beats per minute (bpm). When should follow-up imaging be performed?

A. 1 month
B. 6 months
C. 12 months
D. Only if symptoms arise

89.6 A 46-year-old male with a history of Marfan syndrome, hypertension, dyslipidemia, and a 4.2-cm thoracic aortic aneurysm is seen in the office for follow-up. He has been feeling quite well and has no complaints. He has a blood pressure of 136/82 mm Hg, a heart rate of 52 bpm, and a respiratory rate of 12 breaths/min. He is on carvedilol 25 mg bid, omeprazole 40 mg daily, and rosuvastatin 10 mg at bed time. What is the next **BEST** step in the management of this patient's care?

A. Follow up in 6 months without additional changes.
B. Start losartan 50 mg daily
C. Decrease carvedilol to 12.5 mg bid.
D. Start hydrochlorothiazide 12.5 mg daily.

89.7 A 70-year-old Asian female with a past medical history of poorly controlled diabetes, peripheral vascular disease, hypertension, dyslipidemia, and chronic obstructive pulmonary disease (COPD) presents to the emergency department with complaints of chest and back pain that occurred abruptly approximately 2 hours before her presentation. On arrival, she was noted to have a blood pressure of 142/78 mm Hg, a heart rate of 87 bpm, and a respiratory rate of 18 breaths/min. She has a CT of her chest performed that demonstrates a crescent-shaped thickening of the aortic wall measuring 8 mm absent of blood flow. There is no evidence of a false lumen. What is the **MOST LIKELY** diagnosis?

A. Aortic dissection
B. Penetrating arteriosclerotic ulcer
C. Intramural hematoma
D. Pseudoaneurysm

89.8 During an aortic root replacement, you measure the annulus to be 27 mm. What size Dacron graft should be used?

A. 27 mm
B. 28 mm
C. 30 mm
D. 32 mm

89.9 A 45-year-old female who is morbidly obese with a past medical history significant for coronary artery disease, hypertension, dyslipidemia, and a 30-pack-year tobacco history presents to the emergency department with complaints of sudden onset back pain. A CT chest/abdomen/pelvis with contrast is performed that reveals a dissection of the aortic root extending proximal to the innominate artery. How would you classify this particular type of dissection?

A. Stanford Type A, DeBakey Type I
B. Stanford Type A, DeBakey Type II
C. Stanford Type B, DeBakey Type IIIa
D. Stanford Type B, DeBakey Type IIIb

89.10 A 52-year-old male with a past medical history significant for hypertension, dyslipidemia, and obesity presents to the emergency department with complaints of diffuse chest, back, and abdominal pain. Vital signs are significant for a respiratory rate of 18 breaths/min, a heart rate of 92 bpm, and a blood pressure of 142/90 mm Hg. An emergent CT scan is performed which shows acute aortic dissection of the aorta distal to the left subclavian extending past the celiac artery. He is given 2 mg of intravenous (IV) morphine that helps improve his pain. What is the next appropriate step in the management of this patient?

A. IV esmolol 25 μg/kg/min
B. IV nicardipine 5 mg/h
C. IV dobutamine 2 μg/kg/min
D. Oral metoprolol tartrate 25 mg every 6 hours

ANSWERS

89.1 The correct answer is D.
Rationale: This patient is presenting with signs and symptoms concerning for acute aortic dissection. Abrupt onset of chest/back pain is the most frequent symptom of acute aortic dissection. This patient had an early diastolic decrescendo murmur suggestive of aortic regurgitation that can be a complication of aortic dissection. CT chest/abdomen/pelvis with contrast is the next best step to order to obtain a diagnosis without delay. A CT chest would not evaluate the abdominal aorta and in a patient with a presumably new kidney injury, renal artery involvement must be a consideration. Although the potential risk of kidney injury associated with contrast exists, the logistical considerations of a transesophageal echocardiogram, especially overnight, will likely delay the time to diagnosis.

KEY POINTS

✓ The prompt diagnosis of acute aortic dissection is critical in increasing the chance of survival given the significantly high mortality rate associated with this condition. CT chest/abdomen/pelvis with contrast allows for a timely diagnosis with complete evaluation of the aortic tree.

89.2 The correct answer is D.

Rationale: Referral to cardiac surgery is the best next step in the management. This patient experienced a 0.6-cm expansion of their thoracic aortic aneurysm. According to the 2022 AHA/ACC (American Heart Association/American College of Cardiology) Guidelines for the Diagnosis and Management of Aortic Disease, it is a class 2a recommendation for aortic repair if the diameter is less than 5.5 cm with an associated increased risk of rupture. One feature associated with an increased risk of thoracic aortic aneurysm rupture is rapid growth which is defined as 0.5 cm/y or more. Since this patient's aorta grew 0.6 cm in 1 year, referral to cardiothoracic surgery is appropriate. Repeat imaging of any duration would delay the time to treatment.

KEY POINTS

- For thoracic aortic aneurysms with a diameter less than 5.5 cm, referral for surgery should be considered when associated with an increased risk of rupture. These features include rapid growth (confirmed increase in diameter of ≥0.5 cm/y), symptomatic aneurysm, significant change in aneurysm appearing, saccular aneurysm or presence of penetrating atherosclerotic ulcers.

89.3 The correct answer is C.

Rationale: In patients with Marfan syndrome and other connective tissue diseases, the management of aortic disease is more stringent compared to those without. According to the 2022 AHA/ACC Guidelines for the Diagnosis and Management of Aortic Disease, in patients with Marfan syndrome and an aortic root diameter of 5.0 cm or more, surgery to replace the aortic root and ascending aorta is a class 1A recommendation. It is even a class 2A recommendation for surgery if a patient with Marfan syndrome has an aortic root diameter of 4.5 cm or more and features associated with an increased risk of aortic dissection. A repeat transthoracic echocardiogram and a follow-up in 1 year would delay the time to treatment. A transesophageal echocardiogram might be beneficial if aortic valve features are unclear on transthoracic echocardiogram but in this case the aortic valve was well visualized.

KEY POINTS

- Close attention must be paid in patients with connective tissues disorders such as Marfan syndrome with the associated aortic disease as the timing of intervention differs from those without.

89.4 The correct answer is B.

Rationale: Thoracic aortic imaging is recommended for first-degree relatives of all individuals with thoracic aortic disease. Therefore, an echocardiogram is the next best step in the management of this patient whose father was just diagnosed with an aortic dissection to screen for an asymptotic aneurysm. An MRI of the chest is costly and time consuming. If an echocardiogram was unsuccessful at visualizing the aorta, then an MRI might be an appropriate next step. Genetic testing would be an appropriate next step if this patient were found to have an aortic aneurysm.

KEY POINTS

✓ Thoracic aortic imaging is recommended for first-degree relatives of all individuals with thoracic aortic disease.

89.5 The correct answer is A.
Rationale: For patients who undergo TEVAR or aortic surgery, aortic imaging should be performed after 1 month to rule out early complications. Additional imagining should then be performed after 6 months, 12 months, and then yearly thereafter. In situations when no progression of disease occurs, it is reasonable to increase monitoring to every 2 years. Waiting to repeat imaging only if symptoms arise would be inappropriate.

KEY POINTS

✓ For patients who undergo TEVAR or aortic surgery, routine surveillance should be performed to rule out asymptomatic disease progression.

89.6 The correct answer is B.
Rationale: In patients with thoracic aortic aneurysms, medical management is mainly focused on blood pressure control and surveillance imaging. In general, beta-blockers are the most common antihypertensive prescribed. In patients with Marfan syndrome, treatment with beta-blockers or angiotensin receptor blockers (ARBs) at maximally tolerated doses is recommended. In this patient, his blood pressure is inadequately controlled despite being on a higher dose of beta-blocker, and therefore an additional agent is warranted. Losartan, an ARB, would be an appropriate addition. Given the fact that the patient is asymptotic, decreasing carvedilol would be unnecessary and would likely cause the blood pressure to rise even more.

89.7 The correct answer is C.
Rationale: An intramural hematoma forms when blood is present within the medial layer of the aorta without an obvious tear or patent false lumen. This differs from an aortic dissection that involves an intimal tear through which blood enters and rapidly separates the media, thereby forming a false lumen. A penetrating arteriosclerotic ulcer penetrates the internal elastic lamina of the aortic wall. In some situations, the blood entering the aortic media through these ulcers may be confined after atherosclerotic scarring takes place, thereby forming a pseudoaneurysm.

KEY POINTS

✓ It is important to be able to understand the anatomy and pathophysiology of the various types of thoracic aortic disease as the management of each one may vary significantly.

89.8 The correct answer is C.

Rationale: A 30-mm Dacron graft would be the proper size to use when the annulus measures 27 mm. The size of the Dacron graft is determined by adding 3 mm to the size of the annulus. All of the other answer choices would be improperly sized.

KEY POINTS

- During an aortic root replacement, the size of the Dacron graft is determined by adding 3 mm to the size of the annulus.

89.9 The correct answer is B.

Rationale: This patient's aortic dissection involves only her ascending aorta, which extends from the sinotubular junction to the innominate artery. Stanford Type A dissections involve the ascending aorta with or without involvement of the descending aorta. Stanford Type B dissections only involve the descending aorta. DeBakey Type I dissections involve the ascending aorta, aortic arch, and descending aorta. DeBakey Type II dissections involve the ascending aorta only. DeBakey Type IIIa dissections involve only the descending aorta proximal to the celiac artery compared to a Type IIIb, which involves the entire descending aorta extending distal to the celiac artery.

KEY POINTS

- Understanding the correct classifications of aortic dissections is important to properly identify and manage patients appropriately.

89.10 The correct answer is A.

Rationale: Esmolol would be the correct first-line agent given to this patient who is presenting with an acute Type B aortic dissection. Anti-impulse therapy is critical in the management of acute aortic dissection with a target heart rate less than 60 bpm and a systolic blood pressure less than 120 mm Hg. IV esmolol is a fast-acting selective beta-1 blocker that will provide both a decrease in heart rate and blood pressure. If target blood pressure is not achieved, IV nicardipine would be an appropriate second-line agent to assist in further reduction of blood pressure. Inotropic agents should be avoided in acute aortic dissection as they increase the left ventricular contractility (dP/dt) and can worsen the shear stress. Due to the delayed onset and inability for rapid titration, initial use of oral medications is not recommended.

KEY POINTS

- Rapid initiation of anti-impulse therapy with reduction in both heart rate and blood pressure with beta-blockade is crucial after the diagnosis of an acute aortic dissection.

PERIPHERAL ARTERIAL SURGERY

Samuel Kim and Neil Yager

CHAPTER 90

QUESTIONS

90.1 A 45-year-old male with a past medical history of coronary artery disease, dyslipidemia, chronic kidney disease, and tobacco use presents to your clinic for regular follow-up. The patient states that his mother recently underwent femoral bypass surgery for peripheral arterial disease (PAD) and thus is concerned he may need it as well. You explain most patients with peripheral vascular disease have:

A. Asymptomatic disease
B. Critical limb-threatening ischemia
C. Intermittent claudication
D. Both B and C

90.2 A 63-year-old gentleman presents to your clinic with complaints of leg pain while walking. His medical history includes diabetes mellitus type 2 and hypertension. In addition to a history and physical examination, what screening test would assist in diagnosing PAD?

A. Computed tomography angiography (CTA)
B. Pulse volume recording
C. Ankle-brachial index (ABI)
D. Magnetic resonance angiography (MRA)

90.3 Which of the following examinations would **NOT** be used to aid with the localization of the level of disease?

A. ABI
B. Pulse volume recording/segmental pressure
C. History and physical examination
D. CTA/MRA

90.4 A 75-year-old male presents to your clinic after completing ABI testing due to concerns about PAD. He had initially reported symptoms of right leg pain with walking that has progressively worsened. You review the results and note the ABI ratio of the right lower extremity is 0.3 and the left lower extremity is 0.85. How do you interpret this data?

A. Right: moderate PAD, left: no PAD
B. Right: severe PAD, left: mild PAD
C. Right: severe PAD, left: no PAD
D. Right: moderate PAD, left: moderate PAD

Questions and Answers are based on Chapter 90: Peripheral Arterial Surgery by Michael C. Siah, Gerardo Gonzalez-Guardiola, Khalil Chamseddin, James A. Walker, and Melissa L. Kirkwood in Cardiovascular Medicine and Surgery, First Edition.

90.5 A 72-year-old female with a medical history of hypertension, dyslipidemia, active tobacco use, heart failure, and diabetes mellitus type 2 presents to your clinic for follow-up of leg pain after completion of ABI with findings compatible with moderate PAD. Her current medication includes lisinopril 20 mg, metoprolol succinate 50 mg, pravastatin 40 mg, and metformin. Her blood pressure at her outpatient follow-up appointment is 145/84 mm Hg and recent bloodwork includes a total cholesterol level of 183 mg/dL, triglyceride of 81 mg/dL, high-density lipoprotein (HDL) of 53 mg/dL, and low-density lipoprotein (LDL) of 113 mg/dL with a most recent hemoglobin A1c (HgbA1c) of 6.8%. Along with intensifying medical therapy, what additional workup and/or treatment would be recommended for her newly diagnosed PAD?

- A. CTA/MRA
- B. Referral to vascular specialist for revascularization
- C. Supervised exercise program
- D. No further evaluation or treatment changes indicated at this time

90.6 In the patient from **Question 90.5**, what additional management would be suggested at this time?

- A. Change pravastatin to atorvastatin 80 mg.
- B. Intensify blood pressure regimen for stricter control.
- C. Lifestyle modification
- D. All of the above

90.7 At the 3-month follow-up, the patient from **Question 90.5** reports no significant improvement in her claudication symptoms. An updated echocardiogram did note moderate left ventricular dysfunction in the interim. What additional medication or treatment would you recommend at this time to manage her PAD?

- A. Cilostazol
- B. Pentoxifylline
- C. Ranolazine
- D. Morphine

90.8 A 73-year-old male with a medical history consisting of dyslipidemia, diabetes mellitus, PAD presents to your clinic for follow-up and states that his intermittent claudication has remained unchanged and is affecting his quality of life. He has been compliant with his supervised exercise program and with his medications that includes cilostazol. He was seen by a vascular specialist and deemed to be a suitable candidate for revascularization and is awaiting CTA images. Which of the following factors would determine the treatment modality for this patient?

- A. Trans-Atlantic Inter-Society Consensus (TASC) classification
- B. Anatomic location of occlusive lesion
- C. Comorbidities
- D. All of the above

90.9 The patient in **Question 90.8** underwent revascularization with arterial bypass of the femoral lesion with no significant procedural complications and was discharged. He presents to your clinic and reports significant symptomatic improvement but is concerned regarding the risk of restenosis and requests the **BEST** method for monitoring its recurrence. What would you suggest for long-term surveillance?

A. Monitoring for recurrence of symptoms
B. Routine ABI
C. Routine duplex ultrasound
D. Routine CTA

90.10 Which of the following statements is **NOT TRUE** regarding revascularization?

A. Asymptomatic PAD patients should be considered for open surgical reconstruction for occlusive disease due to risk of progression.
B. Patients with critical limb-threatening ischemia generally are affected by various levels (aortoiliac, femoral-popliteal, and/or infrageniculate) and all require reconstruction for adequate perfusion for limb salvage.
C. All patients with critical limb-threatening ischemia undergo revascularization with open surgical reconstruction.
D. Patients with PAD require multiple interventions in their lifetime.

ANSWERS

90.1 The correct answer is A.

Rationale: PAD is divided into three distinct categories: asymptomatic disease, intermittent claudication, and critical limb-threatening ischemia. Most patients with PAD have asymptomatic disease with the combination of intermittent claudication and critical limb-threatening ischemia being significantly less common. However, the combination of intermittent claudication and critical limb-threatening ischemia is the primary indication for referral to vascular providers.

90.2 The correct answer is C.

Rationale: Noninvasive vascular studies assist in providing objective data regarding the presence and severity of PAD in addition to the history and physical examination. ABI is recommended as the first-line test to screen for and diagnose patients with PAD if signs, symptoms, and risk factors are present (Class Ia recommendation per Society for Vascular Surgery [SVS] 2017 guidelines). It has a sensitivity of 79% to 95% and a specificity of greater than 95%.

Pulse volume recordings and further advanced images (CTA/MRA) are recommended in symptomatic patients who are considered for revascularization (**Table 90.1**).

90.3 The correct answer is A.

Rationale: ABI is the first-line test to diagnose PAD. Other evaluation and/or testing are used to assist with the localization and planning for patients who are suitable candidates for revascularization.

Pulse volume recordings/segmental pressures are recommended in symptomatic patients who are considered for revascularization to quantify and localize the level of the arterial disease (Class IIc recommendation per SVS 2017 guidelines). It may, however, be falsely elevated in those with extensive collaterals and limitation exists in those with multivessel disease and provides no assessment of profunda femoris or nonaxial vessels. A decrease of 20 mm Hg across any level is suggestive of significant disease with segmental pressure measurements.

TABLE 90.1 Diagnostic Studies for PAD

Diagnostic Modality	Sensitivity/ Specificity	Limitations/ Drawbacks	Guideline Recommendation SVS 2017
Ankle-brachial index (ABI)	Sensitivity 79%-95% Specificity >95%	Falsely elevated with tibial calcification, not used for localization, screening tool	**Class IA:** first-line test to diagnose PAD in patients with consistent signs, symptoms, and risk factors. For ABI >0.9 and symptoms of claudication, exercise ABI recommended.
Duplex ultrasonography	Detect >50% stenosis aortoiliac: sensitivity 86%, specificity 97% Fem-pop: sensitivity 80%, specificity 96% Infragenicular: sensitivity 83%; specificity 84%	Operator dependent, body habitus	**Class IB:** recommended in symptomatic patients being considered for revascularization
Segmental pressures/ pulse volume recordings	No data	Falsely elevated with extensive collaterals, no assessment of profunda femoris or nonaxial vessels, limited with multilevel disease	**Class IIC:** recommended in symptomatic patients being considered for revascularization to quantify arterial disease and localize level of disease
CTA/MRA	CTA: sensitivity 93%, specificity 95% MRA: sensitivity 95%, specificity 95%	Limited evaluation of small-caliber vessels, extensive calcification, radiation exposure, nephrotoxicity, no assessment of hemodynamics	**Class IB:** recommended in symptomatic patients being considered for revascularization
Catheter angiography	Sensitivity 100%	Invasive, motion artifact, two-dimensional, access site complications, nephrotoxic	

CTA, computed tomography angiography; fem-pop, femoropopliteal; MRA, magnetic resonance angiogram; PAD, peripheral arterial disease; SVS, Society of Vascular Surgery 2017.

The physical examination, in addition to a well-documented history, is the initial approach in patients with PAD with a focus on the presence and quality of peripheral perfusion and could provide clues on the localization. For example, the constellation of thigh/buttock claudication, impotence, and physical examination of absent femoral pulses would suggest aortoiliac occlusive disease and is known as Leriche syndrome.

CTA is recommended in symptomatic patients being considered for revascularization (Class Ib recommendation per SVS 2017 guidelines) with a sensitivity of 93% and a specificity of 95%. Both CTA and MRA have largely replaced catheter angiography for the accurate assessment of disease distribution. Limited evaluation for those with small-caliber vessels, extensive calcification, radiation exposure, and nephrotoxicity. In addition, it does not provide any hemodynamic assessments.

90.4 The correct answer is B.

Rationale: ABI is a calculated ratio using the highest ankle systolic pressure divided by the highest brachial artery systolic pressure. The ratio is interpreted as follows:

Normal: 1.0 to 1.4
Mild to moderate PAD: 0.4 to 0.9
Severe PAD: less than 0.4

For patients with ABI between 0.9 and 1.4 with symptoms consistent with PAD, exercise ABI testing is recommended. It is performed by obtaining a resting ABI followed by a patient exercising on a treadmill (⨯2 mph at a 12° incline for 20 minutes or until forced to stop due to symptoms) and concludes with a postexercise ABI. The following would indicate PAD: 20% decrease in ABI from baseline, 30 mm Hg drop in ankle systolic pressure, or greater than 3 minutes to recovery of baseline ankle systolic pressure.

In patients with an abnormal ABI (<0.90) with lifestyle-limiting symptoms despite guideline-directed medical therapy, further diagnostic imaging is indicated and evaluation for revascularization would be appropriate.

ABI greater than 1.4 suggests calcified vessels due to increased cuff pressures required to occlude the vessels and is more common in diabetic and renal failure patients. As a result, AHA (American Heart Association)/ACA (American College of Cardiology) guidelines recommend toe-brachial index as the next diagnostic step with a value of less than 0.7 suggestive of PAD (see **Table 90.1**).

90.5 The correct answer is C.

Rationale: In addition to risk factor modification, a supervised exercise program is the first-line therapy in intermittent claudication and has the highest level of recommendation per the AHA/ACC 2016 guidelines. It allows for the development of collaterals and angiogenesis, augmentation of skeletal muscle efficiency, and improvement in the microcirculation sensitivity to nitric oxide vasodilation. According to a 2012 Cochran Review, a supervised exercise program led to an increased maximal walking time and pain-free walking distance with exercise when compared to placebo. The regimen involves having the patient walk greater than 30 minutes at least 3 times per week for at least 12 weeks with patients instructed to walk until maximum pain is experienced followed by a brief rest period to allow for symptom resolution and the continuation of walking again. At 3 months follow-up, the presence/degree of symptoms are reevaluated to determine if further treatment/intervention is required.

This patient does not exhibit signs/symptoms suggestive of critical limb ischemia nor has conservative medical management been initiated and thus this should be performed before revascularization. CTA/MRA are obtained once consideration for revascularization has been decided.

90.6 The correct answer is D.
Rationale: All patients with symptomatic PAD should have risk factor management with both pharmacologic and lifestyle modifications as it has been shown to benefit this patient population. SVS guidelines provide Class Ia with evidence for smoking cessation with demonstration of a significant reduction of risk for limb loss in this patient population. Antihypertensive regimen with goal blood pressure of less than 140/90 mm Hg and a goal of less than 130/80 mm Hg for those with diabetes or chronic kidney disease should be implemented with first-line therapy with angiotensin-converting enzyme inhibitors (AHA/ACC Class IIa recommendation). Management of hyperlipidemia includes moderate to high-intensity statin therapy to maintain LDL less than 100 and less than 70 mg/dL in higher-risk individuals. For diabetes mellitus, the HgbA1c goal should aim for less than 7.0%. Additional guideline therapy includes the usage of long-term antiplatelet therapy with a single agent of aspirin with clopidogrel as an acceptable alternative.

90.7 The correct answer is B.
Rationale: In patients with no symptomatic improvement or worsening in symptoms after conservative management with a supervised exercise program, pharmacologic agents can be considered as an adjunctive therapy. U.S. FDA (Food and Drug Administration)-approved drugs for patients with intermittent claudication include cilostazol and pentoxifylline. In a randomized control trial, cilostazol was demonstrated to yield more benefit in terms of increased maximal walking distance when compared to pentoxifylline with a 6-month treatment. In the 2015 SVS guideline, cilostazol 100 mg bid is recommended for claudication without evidence of heart failure with a Class IIa recommendation. If patients are not candidates for this medication, pentoxifylline 400 mg tid is recommended with a Class IIb recommendation.

Cilostazol is a phosphodiesterase inhibitor that is prescribed at a dosage of 100 mg twice daily with ACC/AHA Class Ia recommendation and SVS Class IIa recommendation for intermittent claudication. It is contraindicated in patients with any level of heart failure.

Ranolazine is an antianginal medication that is not indicated at this time given no complaints of chest discomfort (**Table 90.2**).

90.8 The correct answer is D.
Rationale: There are several revascularization modalities for patients requiring PAD revascularization. It includes endovascular techniques with the usage of drug-coated balloon angioplasty and/or drug-eluting stent placements, endarterectomy, and surgical arterial bypass. Therapy selection is determined based on the specific needs for the patient with consideration of a variety of factors that include but are not limited to anatomic location and extent of occlusive disease, extent of tissue loss, patient's comorbidities, history of previous intervention, and overall risk of anesthesia. The TASC guidelines were created to assist in the decision for treatment modality. For example, TASC A lesions should be treated with endovascular techniques for both aortoiliac and infrainguinal occlusive disease with TASC D treated with surgery.

TABLE 90.2 Medications Used for Peripheral Arterial Disease

Drugs	Dosage	Side Effects	Recommendation
Aspirin	75-325 mg daily	Rash, abdominal pain, tinnitus, bleeding, nausea	SVS Class IA AHA/ACC Class IA
Clopidogrel	75 mg daily	Bleeding, acute liver failure, aplastic anemia, agranulocytosis	SVS Class IB AHA/ACC Class IA
ACE inhibitor (ramipril)	10 mg daily	Dry cough, hyperkalemia, kidney failure, angioedema, pancreatitis	AHA/ACC Class IIA
Statin	Atorvastatin 40-80 mg daily (high intensity) Rosuvastatin 20-40 mg daily (high intensity)	Myopathy, new-onset diabetes, liver failure	SVS Class IA AHA/ACC Class IA
Cilostazol	100 mg bid	Fluid retention, headaches, abdominal pain, palpitations	SVS Class IIA AHA/ACC Class IA
Pentoxifylline	400 mg tid, titrated to 1,800 mg daily	Nausea, headache, anxiety, insomnia	SVS Class IB

ACC, American College of Cardiology; ACE, angiotensin-converting enzyme; AHA, American Heart Association; SVS, Society of Vascular Surgery.

90.9 The correct answer is C.

Rationale: The main causes of restenosis following any of the revascularization procedures are technical defects, intimal hyperplasia, and recurrence of atherosclerosis. Preemptive identification of narrowing can benefit the primary patency rate of the primary intervention and thus should be routinely monitored.

Duplex ultrasonography can identify threatened open or endovascular revascularizations and allows for early intervention and repair of the narrowed segments. This is suggested with findings of (a) focal peak systolic velocity greater than 300 cm/s in any segment/bypass graft and (b) low velocities of less than 40 to 45 cm/s throughout the segment/bypass graft.

Recurrent leg symptoms and a significant decrease of ABI of 0.15 or more have poor sensitivity to detect recurrence. It has been reported that it can detect only 50% of the cases.

90.10 The correct answer is A.

Rationale: For patients who are asymptomatic with PAD, open surgical reconstruction for occlusive disease is not indicated.

In general, intermittent claudication has a single level of disease whereas critical limb-threatening ischemic patients have multiple levels. Revascularization can be performed with an endovascular approach with drug-coated balloons and drug-eluting stents or via a surgical approach with endarterectomy and arterial bypass. TASC guidelines and classifications assist in assisting the preferred approach in patients affected by intermittent claudication and critical limb-threatening ischemia. Post-intervention, all patients should be monitored to identify threatened open or endovascular revascularizations as it may help preserve the primary patency.

CAROTID ENDARTERECTOMY*

Meet Patel

CHAPTER 91

QUESTIONS

91.1 A 67-year-old female presents to the clinic with a history of recurrent episodes of transient neurologic symptoms. She describes experiencing sudden onset weakness and numbness on her left side that typically resolves within a few minutes. The patient reports these episodes have occurred multiple times over the past week. She denies any associated speech difficulties, visual changes, or loss of consciousness. The patient has a significant smoking history and hypertension. The physician performs an ultrasound of the extracranial arteries to evaluate for carotid artery disease. Physician discusses transcarotid artery revascularization (TCAR) for further management of patient carotid artery disease. Which of the following findings is **NOT** a contraindication to TCAR?

A. Distance between the access site (at common carotid artery [CCA] above clavicle) and the lesion less than 5 cm
B. Diameter of CCA less than 6 mm
C. CCA access and carotid occlusion sites are not free of significant disease (ie, no thrombus/calcification within 1 cm of either site)
D. Lesions extending above the level of the second cervical vertebra

91.2 A 65-year-old male with a history of hypertension and smoking presents with transient ischemic attacks (TIAs). A carotid ultrasound is ordered to evaluate for carotid artery disease. The examination includes grayscale imaging, color Doppler imaging, and spectral Doppler velocity measurements. The ultrasound findings reveal a noncalcified plaque in the internal carotid artery (ICA) with a peak systolic velocity (PSV) of 250 cm/s and an internal carotid artery to common carotid artery peak systolic velocity ratio (ICA/CCA PSV) of 3.5. What is the most appropriate management for this patient based on the ultrasound findings?

A. Medical management with antiplatelet therapy and aggressive risk factor modification
B. Carotid endarterectomy (CEA)
C. Carotid artery stenting (CAS)
D. Further imaging with computed tomography angiography (CTA)

---

*Questions and Answers are based on Chapter 91: Carotid Artery Revascularization by Fatemeh Malekpour, Gerardo Gonzalez-Guardiola, Sooyeon Kim, and Melissa L. Kirkwood in Cardiovascular Medicine and Surgery, First Edition.

91.3 A 65-year-old male with a history of hypertension, diabetes mellitus, and dyslipidemia presents to the clinic for routine follow-up. Patient has a significant smoking history of 1 pack per day for the last 30 years. He denies any episodes of weakness, numbness, syncope, headache, or neck pain. His current medications include lisinopril, metformin, and atorvastatin. On physical examination, his blood pressure is 145/90 mm Hg, heart rate is regular at 80 beats per minute (bpm), and a carotid bruit is noted. The neurologic examination was normal. Which imaging modality would be the most appropriate next step in the management of this patient?

A. Ultrasound
B. Computed tomography (CT)
C. Magnetic resonance imaging (MRI)
D. Echocardiogram

91.4 A 60-year-old man with a history of hypertension, hyperlipidemia, and tobacco use presents with transient right-sided weakness that resolved within 10 minutes. Imaging revealed a left middle cerebral artery infarct. Carotid Doppler ultrasound showed severe carotid artery stenosis. The patient is started on medical management for extracranial carotid disease. Which of the following is **NOT** recommended for secondary prevention of ischemic stroke in this patient?

A. Aspirin 81 mg daily
B. Clopidogrel 75 mg daily
C. Dual antiplatelet therapy (DAPT) with aspirin and clopidogrel for 3 months
D. Oral anticoagulation with warfarin

91.5 A 60-year-old male presents to his primary care physician for a routine physical examination. His medical history is significant for hypertension and hyperlipidemia, for which he is taking amlodipine and atorvastatin. His blood pressure is 140/90 mm Hg, and his body mass imaging (BMI) is 30 kg/m². Carotid ultrasound reveals the presence of a plaque in his left ICA, with a stenosis of 45%. What is the most appropriate management for this patient?

A. Observation and repeat ultrasound in 1 year
B. Referral for CEA
C. Optimization of blood pressure and lipid levels
D. Referral for CAS

91.6 A 78-year-old male patient with a past medical history (PMH) of hypertension, dyslipidemia, and obesity presents with a history of recurrent TIAs and a 45% stenosis of the right ICA. The patient has no history of coronary artery disease or atrial fibrillation. What is the **BEST** management option for this patient?

A. Optimal medical management
B. CEA
C. CAS
D. Observation and close follow-up

91.7 A 65-year-old male patient presents with a recent onset of left-sided weakness, slurred speech, and difficulty in walking. A CT scan of the brain without contrast is unremarkable for acute pathology. A carotid Doppler ultrasound shows an 80% stenosis of the left ICA. The patient is scheduled for carotid revascularization, and the options of CEA and CAS are discussed with the patient. Which of the following is the most appropriate treatment option for this patient?
   A. CEA
   B. CAS
   C. Either CEA or CAS is appropriate.
   D. Medical management without revascularization

91.8 A 65-year-old male with a history of laryngeal cancer presents to the hospital with a TIA involving his right side. The patient reports that he has been experiencing episodes of weakness and numbness in his right arm and leg for the past week. He underwent a laryngectomy and tracheostomy 5 years ago and has been receiving radiation therapy for head and neck cancer. A carotid Doppler ultrasound shows an 80% stenosis of the right ICA. Which of the following is the most appropriate management for this patient?
   A. CEA
   B. CAS
   C. Antiplatelet therapy alone
   D. Conservative management

91.9 A 65-year-old male with a history of hypertension, diabetes mellitus, and dyslipidemia presents to the emergency department (ED) with complaints of right-sided weakness and numbness that started 3 hours ago. He had similar episodes last week that lasted for a few minutes and resolved spontaneously. The patient went to his primary care physician yesterday and was noted to have left-sided carotid bruit. He denies any episodes of weakness, numbness, syncope, headache, or neck pain. Patient is currently taking lisinopril, metformin, and atorvastatin. On physical examination, his blood pressure is 145/90 mm Hg, heart rate is regular at 80 bpm, and left-sided carotid bruits were noted. The neurologic examination showed strength of 2/5 in the right upper and lower extremity. Which imaging modality would be the most appropriate next step in the management of this patient?
   A. Carotid duplex ultrasound
   B. MRI head without intravenous (IV) contrast
   C. CT head without contrast
   D. Magnetic resonance angiography (MRA) head without IV contrast

91.10 A 65-year-old male presents to the clinic with a history of recent TIA. He reports episodes of sudden weakness and numbness on his left side that resolve within a few minutes. The patient has a significant smoking history, hypertension, and recent myocardial infarction (MI). On physical examination, vitals were within normal limits, and no focal neurologic deficits were noted. A carotid ultrasound was performed, which revealed 85% stenosis in the right external carotid artery. The physician recommended intervention for further management and provided different treatment options to the patient. Which of the following is a disadvantage of CAS compared to CEA?

A. Higher risk of periprocedural MI
B. Higher risk of periprocedural stroke
C. Worse outcomes in patients with difficult surgical neck anatomy
D. Higher risk of facial neuropathy

ANSWERS

91.1 The correct answer is D.
Rationale: The options provided represent potential contraindications to TCAR, except for option D, which is not a contraindication. Lesion extending above the level of the second cervical vertebrae is a contraindication for CEA and an indication for doing TCAR or CAS. To achieve proximal control of the CCA during the procedure, an incision is made at the base of the neck. Subsequently, percutaneous access of the common femoral vein (CFV) is obtained in either groin. A specially designed short sheath is then carefully inserted into the proximal CCA, ensuring caution to avoid manipulation of the carotid bulb and ICA. The next step involves connecting the CCA and CFV using a flow reversal system equipped with a built-in filter. This flow reversal system takes advantage of the temporary pressure gradient created by linking the carotid artery and femoral vein. It establishes a retrograde flow from the ICA toward the CFV. As a result, the diminished antegrade flow toward the ICA significantly reduces the risk of distal embolization during the procedure. For the successful and safe insertion of the arterial sheath in TCAR, specific anatomic criteria must be fulfilled. These criteria include:
- The distance between the access site (located at the CCA above the clavicle) and the lesion should be greater than 5 cm. The diameter of the CCA should be larger than 6 mm.
- Both the access site in the CCA and the carotid occlusion site should be free from significant disease, such as thrombus or calcification, within a 1-cm radius of either location.

91.2 The correct answer is B.
Rationale: The ultrasound findings indicate the presence of a noncalcified plaque in the ICA with a PSV of 250 cm/s and an ICA/CCA PSV of 3.5. These are both indicators of a significant carotid artery stenosis. ICA PSV is a primary parameter for identifying carotid artery stenosis while ICA/CCA PSV is an additional parameter. ICA PSV greater than 230 indicates more than 70% stenosis while an ICA/CCA PSV between 2 and 4 indicates stenosis between 50% and 69%. A stenosis 50% or more is considered significant in symptomatic patients for evaluation for surgery, and this patient is symptomatic with TIAs. Therefore, the most appropriate management for this patient based on the ultrasound findings is CEA. Primary and additional parameters for assessing the degree of stenosis are shown in **Table 91.1**. Medical management with antiplatelet therapy and aggressive risk factor modification is also important in the management of carotid artery disease, but surgical intervention is warranted in this case. CAS is the preferred approach over CEA for

patients who have challenging surgical neck anatomy, including conditions like tracheostomy, contralateral nerve palsy, previous neck radiation, or lesions located near the clavicle or above the level of the C2 vertebral body. This patient does not have these risk factors and thus, CEA remains the preferred intervention. Further imaging with CTA would not change the management of this patient.

TABLE 91.1 Society of Radiologists in Ultrasound Consensus Criteria

Degree of Stenosis (%)	Primary Parameters		Additional Parameters	
	ICA PSV (cm/s)	Plaque Estimate (%)	ICA/CCA PSV Ratio	ICA EDV (cm/s)
Normal	<125	None	<2.0	<40
<50	<125	<50	<2.0	<40
50-69	125-230	≥50	2.0-4.0	40-100
≥70 but less than near occlusion	>230	≥50	>4.0	>100
Near occlusion	High, low, or undetectable	Visible	Variable	Variable
Total occlusion	Undetectable	Visible, no detectable lumen	Not applicable	Not applicable

From Rasmussen TE, Clouse WD, Tonnessen BH. *Handbook of Patient Care in Vascular Diseases*. 6th ed. Philadelphia, PA: Wolters Kluwer; 2018. Table 12.1.

91.3 The correct answer is A.

Rationale: In this scenario, the most appropriate imaging modality for the evaluation of carotid artery disease would be ultrasound. The 2016 American College of Radiology (ACR) Appropriateness Criteria states that imaging is recommended for asymptomatic patients who have significant risk factors for cerebrovascular events or exhibit a carotid bruit during physical examination. This patient has a history of hypertension, diabetes mellitus, and dyslipidemia and has the presence of carotid bruit on physical examination which warrants further imaging workup. Ultrasound is the preferred initial test in asymptomatic patients as it is noninvasive, cost-effective, and widely available. The ACR, American Institute of Ultrasound in Medicine (AIUM), Society for Pediatric Radiology (SPR), and Society of Radiologists in Ultrasound (SRU) gave joint recommendations for the technique of performing an ultrasound of the extracranial arteries. The examination should include grayscale imaging (B-mode), color Doppler imaging, and spectral Doppler velocity measurements. Ultrasound can also help in the evaluation of the internal carotid artery end-diastolic velocity (ICA EDV), PSV, and ICA/CCA PSV, which are useful adjuncts to quantify the severity of the disease. The study should aim to examine the complete pathway of the common carotid arteries, carotid bulbs, internal carotid arteries, vertebral arteries, and origins of the ECA (external carotid arteries). The description should encompass plaque morphology, including composition and intima-media thickness. In addition, the study should accurately document the precise location of plaques in areas where there is increased velocity resulting in stenosis, accompanied by post-stenotic turbulence. CT and MRI can also be used in the evaluation of carotid artery disease, especially in symptomatic patients. However, they are not the initial imaging modalities of choice in asymptomatic patients. CT has the disadvantage of exposing the patient to ionizing radiation, and MRI is time-consuming and expensive. CT and MRI may be useful in detecting anatomic variants, incidental comorbidities, or further characterizing lesions such as dissection, intramural hematoma, or ulcerated plaques. Vessel wall imaging MRI is particularly valuable in patients with vasculitis. Therefore, in this scenario, the most appropriate imaging modality for the evaluation of carotid artery disease would be ultrasound.

91.4 The correct answer is D.
Rationale: Medical management is the cornerstone of all treatments of extracranial carotid disease. All patients should begin medical optimization of their comorbidities. In cases of noncardioembolic ischemic stroke or TIA, the preferred approach for reducing the risk of recurrent ischemic stroke and other cardiovascular events, while minimizing the risk of bleeding, is antiplatelet therapy rather than oral anticoagulation. For patients with noncardioembolic ischemic stroke or TIA, the following options are indicated for secondary prevention of ischemic stroke: aspirin at a daily dose of 50 to 325 mg, clopidogrel at 75 mg, or a combination of aspirin at 25 mg and extended-release dipyridamole at 200 mg taken bid. In patients with recent minor noncardioembolic ischemic stroke (National Institute of Health Stroke Scale [NIHSS] score ≤3) or high-risk TIA (age, blood pressure, clinical feature, duration and diabetes [ABCD2] score ≥4), DAPT with aspirin and clopidogrel should be initiated promptly (preferably within 12-24 hours of symptom onset and within 7 days at the latest) and continued for a period of 21 to 90 days. After the DAPT phase, single antiplatelet therapy (SAPT) should be continued to further reduce the risk of recurrent ischemic stroke. However, individuals who are already receiving oral anticoagulation for conditions like atrial fibrillation or prosthetic heart valves may not derive significant additional benefits from the addition of an antiplatelet agent, except in select cases involving unstable angina or coronary artery stenting. Recent studies suggest that newer oral anticoagulants, such as dabigatran, may carry a lower risk of intracranial hemorrhage compared to warfarin, making them a more favorable choice for many patients. As a result, for individuals with extracranial carotid disease, it is not recommended to use warfarin as oral anticoagulation for secondary prevention of ischemic stroke.

91.5 The correct answer is C.
Rationale: This patient's carotid plaque is less than 50% stenosis, which is considered mild. However, it is important to note that plaque progression from less than 50% stenosis to more than 50% stenosis has been associated with increased odds of cerebrovascular accident (CVA), especially if it progresses to more than 70% stenosis. Therefore, the primary goal of management in this patient is to prevent plaque progression and the development of more severe stenosis. Medical optimization of his hypertension and hyperlipidemia is the most appropriate management for this patient, as larger plaques have been shown to be less fibrotic, more

lipid-laden, and contain more inflammatory cells and intraplaque hemorrhage. Optimization of blood pressure and lipid levels may prevent plaque progression and reduce the risk of major adverse cardiovascular events (MACE), stroke, and cardiovascular deaths. Observation and repeat ultrasound in 1 year may be appropriate if there is no significant change in the degree of stenosis. Referral for CEA or stenting is not indicated at this time, as the patient's stenosis is mild and the patient is asymptomatic. Intervention may be considered in symptomatic patients with stenosis greater than 50% especially if stenosis is greater than 70% in symptomatic patients.

91.6 The correct answer is A.

Rationale: Common medications used in the medical management of extracranial carotid arteries include status, antiplatelets, and anticoagulation medications. Appropriate medication should be chosen for management based on the patient's condition. For patients who have experienced a TIA or non-disabling ischemic stroke within the past 6 months, along with severe (70%-99%) carotid artery stenosis on the same side, CEA is recommended as a means to reduce the risk of future strokes. However, this recommendation is valid only if the estimated risk of perioperative complications and mortality is less than 6%. In cases where the TIA or ischemic stroke is recent, but the degree of stenosis is less than 50%, revascularization with CEA or CAS is not recommended for reducing the risk of future strokes. A comprehensive analysis conducted by Rothwell et al revealed no significant benefit from CEA in patients with less than 50% ICA stenosis. In patients who have recently experienced a TIA or ischemic stroke and have moderate (50%-69%) carotid stenosis on the same side, as confirmed by catheter-based or noninvasive imaging, CEA is recommended to reduce the risk of future strokes. However, the decision to proceed with CEA should consider individual patient-specific factors such as age, sex, comorbidities, and an estimated perioperative morbidity and mortality risk of less than 6%.

91.7 The correct answer is A.

Rationale: In symptomatic patients, outcomes following CEA are more favorable compared to CAS, especially when performed within the first week of symptoms. This patient is symptomatic with an 80% stenosis, and therefore, carotid revascularization is recommended. The patient does not have any difficult surgical neck anatomy such as the presence of tracheostomy, contralateral nerve palsy, prior neck radiation, or lesions close to the clavicle or above the level of C2 vertebral body. Therefore, CEA is the most appropriate treatment option for this patient. Several studies have shown similar stroke risks in patients with difficult surgical neck anatomy after CEA or CAS, but a higher incidence of cranial nerve injury after CEA. In addition, CAS may be associated with a higher risk of in-stent restenosis and thromboembolic events. Both the North American Symptomatic Carotid Endarterectomy Trial (NASCET) and European Carotid Surgery Trial (ECST) included individuals with symptomatic carotid disease and found a noteworthy rise in the risk of major stroke or death in the medical treatment groups compared to the intervention groups. NASCET revealed that patients with symptomatic carotid stenosis more than 70% experienced advantages from CEA, with a 29% decrease in relative risk of stroke or death over a span of 5 years. Thus, medical management without revascularization is not recommended for these patients.

91.8 The correct answer is B.
Rationale: CEA tends to yield more favorable outcomes than CAS in symptomatic patients, particularly when conducted within the initial week of symptoms. However, the patient described in the vignette has difficult surgical neck anatomy due to tracheostomy and prior neck radiation, which makes CEA challenging and increases the risk of complications such as cranial nerve injury.

CAS is the preferred approach over CEA for patients with challenging surgical neck anatomy, such as those with tracheostomy, contralateral nerve palsy, previous neck radiation, or lesions located near the clavicle or above the C2 vertebral body level. Multiple studies have demonstrated comparable stroke risks between CEA and CAS in this patient population. However, CEA is associated with a higher occurrence of cranial nerve injury. Therefore, the most appropriate intervention for this patient would be CAS. The patient is symptomatic and requires treatment to prevent further stroke, hence option antiplatelet therapy alone and conservative management are not appropriate choices. Medical management is usually considered appropriate for asymptomatic patients with less than 70% stenosis and symptomatic patients with less than 50% stenosis. Intervention is necessary for this patient who is symptomatic with stenosis exceeding 70%.

91.9 The correct answer is C.
Rationale: As per the 2016 American College of Radiology (ACR) Appropriateness Criteria, imaging is recommended for asymptomatic individuals presenting with notable cerebrovascular risk factors or the presence of a carotid bruit during physical examination. In such cases, initial evaluation may involve ultrasound, CT, or MRI. However, for symptomatic patients, cross-sectional imaging techniques such as CT scan or MRI are preferred. CT head without contrast is the ideal test of choice in patients with new focal neurologic defects that are fixed or worsening and started less than 6 hours ago as CT without contrast is necessary to exclude hemorrhage as a cause of the deficit. It is a highly effective diagnostic tool for distinguishing between ischemic and hemorrhagic stroke. In the management of eligible patients with acute ischemic stroke, the primary treatment approach is IV thrombolysis. This therapy is considered first line and should be administered within 4.5 hours of symptom onset or the last known time the patient was neurologically stable. MRI head without IV contrast should be obtained if there is a new focal neurologic defect, fixed or worsening which started more than 6 hours ago. MRI is more sensitive than CT for acute infarct. MRA head without IV contrast is the ideal screening study of choice in patients who have the risk of unruptured aneurysm, including patients with polycystic kidney disease, patients who have at least two first-degree relatives with a history of subarachnoid hemorrhage (SAH), and those with previously ruptured and treated aneurysms. Carotid duplex ultrasound is the preferred initial test in asymptomatic patients as it is noninvasive, cost-effective, and widely available. However, a patient who has ongoing symptoms of stroke needs urgent CT head without contrast for further evaluation. CTA of the head and neck with CT perfusion, or MRA with diffusion-weighted imaging (DWI), with or without MR perfusion-weighted imaging (PWI) is useful for evaluating patients who may be eligible for mechanical thrombectomy.

91.10 The correct answer is B.

Rationale: CAS is associated with a higher risk of periprocedural stroke compared to CEA. An analysis of multiple randomized controlled trials revealed that CAS was associated with a higher risk of stroke or death within 30 days compared to CEA. This finding was further supported by a large observational study and a multicenter randomized controlled trial, both of which demonstrated a greater incidence of periprocedural stroke with CAS when compared to CEA within 30 days. Four trials reported the rate of periprocedural MI, with a weighted average incidence of 2.6% (95% CI, 0.4-6.3) for CEA and 0.9% (0.05%-2.9%) for CAS. The risk of MI was significantly higher in the CEA group (odds ratio: 2.69, 95% CI, 1.06-6.79; $P = .036$; $I2 = 0\%$; $P = .700$). In six studies that assessed periprocedural cranial facial neuropathy, one study reported no occurrences of this complication. The average weighted event rate for CEA was found to be 7.5% (95% CI, 5.8-9.4), whereas for CAS, it was 0.45% (0.01%-1.0%). The analysis demonstrated a higher risk of cranial facial neuropathy in the CEA group (odds ratio: 10.25, 95% CI, 4.02-26.13; $P < .001$; $I2 = 0\%$; $P = .754$). CAS is the preferred approach over CEA for patients with challenging surgical neck anatomy, such as those with tracheostomy, contralateral nerve palsy, previous neck radiation, or lesions located near the clavicle or above the C2 vertebral body level. In conclusion, CAS has a better periprocedural risk of MI, facial neuropathy, and better outcomes in patients with difficult surgical neck anatomic but was associated with a significantly higher risk of periprocedural stroke compared to CEA.

SUGGESTED READINGS

Mukherjee D, Lange RA, eds. *Cardiovascular Medicine and Surgery*. 1st ed. LWW; 2022.

Benjamin EJ, Blaha MJ, Chiuve SE, et al. Heart disease and stroke statistics-2017 update: a report from the American Heart Association. *Circulation*. 2017;135(10):e146-e603.

Mukherjee D, Lange RA, eds. *Cardiovascular Medicine and Surgery*. 1st ed. LWW; 2022.

Barnett HJM, Taylor DW, Haynes RB, et al. Beneficial effect of carotid endarterectomy in symptomatic patients with high-grade carotid stenosis. *N Engl J Med*. 1991;325(7):445-453.

Mukherjee D, Lange RA, eds. *Cardiovascular Medicine and Surgery*. 1st ed. LWW; 2022.

https://www.ncbi.nlm.nih.gov/pmc/articles/PMC4495083/

Rothwell PM, Eliasziw M, Gutnikov SA, et al. Analysis of pooled data from the randomised controlled trials of endarterectomy for symptomatic carotid stenosis. *Lancet*. 2003;361(9352):107-116.

Rothwell PM, Eliasziw M, Gutnikov SA, Warlow CP, Barnett HJM. Endarterectomy for symptomatic carotid stenosis in relation to clinical subgroups and timing of surgery. *Lancet*. 2004;363(9413):915-924.

Rothwell PM, Gibson R, Warlow CP. Interrelation between plaque surface morphology and degree of stenosis on carotid angiograms and the risk of ischemic stroke in patients with symptomatic carotid stenosis. *Stroke*. 2000;31(3):615-621.

Rothwell PM, Warlow CP. Low risk of ischemic stroke in patients with reduced internal carotid artery lumen diameter distal to severe symptomatic carotid stenosis: cerebral protection due to low poststenotic flow? *Stroke*. 2000;31(3):622-630

TRANSPLANTATION AND LONG-TERM IMPLANTABLE MECHANICAL CIRCULATORY SUPPORT*

Phillip Olsen and Dmitri Belov

CHAPTER 92

QUESTIONS

92.1 Which of the following patients **DOES NOT** require referral to an advanced heart failure program as per ACC (American College of Cardiology)/AHA (American Heart Association) guidelines?

A. A 58-year-old man with ischemic cardiomyopathy who required reduction in doses of spironolactone and sacubitril-valsartan due to recurrent presyncopal symptoms and hypotension at home

B. A 63-year-old woman with a history of nonischemic cardiomyopathy who presents for her fourth hospitalization in the past year for dyspnea related to her heart failure (HF). She takes dapagliflozin, bisoprolol, spironolactone, and sacubitril-valsartan at home.

C. A 67-year-old man with STEMI (ST-segment elevation myocardial infarction) 3 days ago who has an ejection fraction of 20% to 25% on echocardiogram weaned off intra-aortic balloon pump on hospital day 2

D. A 60-year-old woman with a history of ischemic cardiomyopathy and cardiac resynchronization therapy-defibrillator (CRT-D) who is hospitalized with recurrent ventricular tachycardia and appropriate defibrillator shocks

92.2 Which of the following patients is most appropriate for referral for a heart transplant?

A. An 82-year-old man with ischemic cardiomyopathy with left ventricular ejection fraction (LVEF) less than 10% and New York Heart Association (NYHA) Class III symptoms

B. A 58-year-old woman with a history of myocardial infarction and severe secondary mitral regurgitation with recurrent HF hospitalizations

C. A 48-year-old woman with persistent NYHA Class IV symptoms after myocarditis who is on full guideline-directed medical therapy and has received CRT-D

D. A 62-year-old man with ischemic cardiomyopathy with LVEF less than 25%, NYHA Class III symptoms, and left bundle branch block on ECG

92.3 Which of the following patients is **MOST LIKELY** to be ventricular assist device (VAD) eligible?

Questions and Answers are based on Chapter 92: Transplantation and Long-Term Implantable Mechanical Circulatory Support by Ryan J. Vela and Matthias Peltz in Cardiovascular Medicine and Surgery, First Edition.

A. A 60-year-old man with ischemic cardiomyopathy with LVEF less than 25% with peripheral artery disease (PAD) and prior complete lower extremity bypass
B. A 57-year-old woman with end-stage renal disease (ESRD) on hemodialysis for 2 years and nonischemic cardiomyopathy with LVEF less than 25%
C. A 38-year-old man with a history of intracranial bleed and spontaneous retroperitoneal bleeding with fulminant myocarditis
D. A 55-year-old man with ischemic cardiomyopathy with LVEF less than 25%, extensive tobacco use, and porcelain aorta noted on a computed tomography (CT) scan

92.4 Which of the following patients are likely to have symptom improvement with left ventricular assist device (LVAD) implantation?

A. A 60-year-old man with cardiogenic shock unable to be weaned from intra-aortic balloon pump and vasopressors
B. A 55-year-old woman maintained on home milrinone whose last hospitalization was 6 months ago
C. A 57-year-old man with NYHA 3B HF who is symptomatic with minimal activity and is homebound
D. All of the above

92.5 A 63-year-old man with unknown medical history is found down by Emergency Medical Services (EMS) and brought to the hospital. He is found to be in shock with rapidly escalating vasopressor requirements. Point-of-care ultrasound shows a severely reduced LVEF and hypokinetic right ventricle. What is the most appropriate next step?

A. Temporary mechanical circulatory support
B. Durable LVAD implantation
C. Cardiac transplantation
D. Palliative care and withdrawal of support

92.6 All the following are **TRUE** regarding the bicaval technique for orthotopic heart transplant as compared to the biatrial technique **EXCEPT**:

A. Fewer arrhythmias after transplantation
B. Decreased implantation time
C. Decreased need for pacemaker insertion
D. Slightly increased perioperative and long-term survival

92.7 Which of the following valvular conditions requires surgical correction at the time of LVAD insertion?

A. Moderate tricuspid regurgitation
B. Moderate mitral regurgitation
C. Presence of a mechanical aortic valve
D. Mild aortic regurgitation

92.8 Which of the following surgical management options for the failing heart has the greatest 5-year survival?

A. LVAD
B. Total artificial heart
C. Heart-lung transplant
D. Orthotopic heart transplant

92.9 Which of the following statements **BEST** describes VAD outcomes?
- A. LVAD outcomes display equal long-term results to heart transplantation.
- B. Short- and intermediate-term outcomes of LVAD therapies are approaching those of orthotopic heart transplantation.
- C. Short-term LVAD outcomes show significantly higher mortality as compared to orthotopic heart transplantation with improvement at intermediate follow-up.
- D. Orthotopic heart transplantation displays significantly higher short mortality as compared to LVADs but ultimately has improved long-term survival.

92.10 Which of the following statements is **FALSE** regarding complications of VAD therapy?
- A. One- and 2-year survival after LVAD implantation is nearing that heart transplantation but serious complications remain prevalent.
- B. Major complications of LVAD therapy include device (driveline) infection and gastrointestinal (GI) bleeding.
- C. Complications are highest in the first year after LVAD implantation and event rate during the first year is predictive of subsequent event rate.
- D. Device thrombosis is the most common serious complication associated with LVAD therapy.

ANSWERS

92.1 The correct answer is C.
Rationale: The patient with recent STEMI without a known history of severely reduced ejection fraction and not currently on guideline-directed medical therapy does not obligate advanced HF referral. It is well established that appropriate utilization of guideline-directed therapy can lead to significant improvement in ejection fraction and symptoms of HF, a low ejection fraction alone does not warrant referral. The remaining cases all exhibit evidence of symptomatic and progressive HF and would thus be appropriate for advanced HF referral.

92.2 The correct answer is C.
Rationale: The 48-year-old woman with a history of myocarditis and persistent severe HF symptoms would likely be most appropriate for a heart transplant listing. Many factors are considered when listing for transplant, including a thorough medical comorbidity evaluation as well as an assessment of social and financial support to ensure an long-term success. The patient in A has an advanced age that would likely preclude listing for transplant. The 58-year-old woman with secondary mitral regurgitation should first be considered for transcutaneous mitral valve repair before transplantation. The 62-year-old man with a widened QRS and left bundle branch block with HF symptoms and severely reduced ejection fraction should first be considered for CRT before consideration of transplant listing.

92.3 The correct answer is A.
Rationale: Of these patients, the patient with peripheral arterial disease as their primary comorbidity is most likely to be eligible for VAD implantation. Patients with ESRD have poor outcomes with VADs and are generally not candidates for VAD. Severe central vascular calcifications can be problematic for the surgical approach and prohibit VAD implantation. A history of multiple life-threatening bleeds would preclude anticoagulation and thus make a patient ineligible for LVAD implantation which typically requires chronic anticoagulation and an international normalized ratio (INR) of 2 to 3.

92.4 The correct answer is D.
Rationale: All these patients are likely to have symptomatic improvement with LVAD implantation as per the Risk Assessment and Comparative Effectiveness of Left Ventricular Assist Device and Medical Management (ROADMAP) study. The patients described by answers A and B are described by (Interagency Registry for Mechanically Assisted Circulatory Support) INTERMACS class 1 and 3, respectively, and have clear benefits with device implantation. Answer C describes an INTERMACS Class 5 patient, who is likely to have *symptomatic* improvement as per the ROADMAP study, but with increased complications and no increase in survival benefit (**Table 92.1**).

92.5 The correct answer is A.
Rationale: The most appropriate next step is the use of temporary mechanical support and monitoring for clinical improvement. The patient has unknown medical comorbidities and the acuity of his cardiac dysfunction is unknown, so transplantation or implantation of durable mechanical circulatory support would be inappropriate. Palliative care and withdrawal of support would be premature at this point; however, they may later be appropriate if complications develop while on temporary mechanical circulatory support (**Figure 92.1**).

92.6 The correct answer is B.
Rationale: The bicaval technique is favored in the United States and slightly increases implantation time as anastomoses are required to be formed between the inferior and superior vena cava in addition to left atrial, pulmonary artery, and aortic anastomoses. This technique generally results in fewer arrhythmias, reduced tricuspid regurgitation, reduced need for pacemakers, and a slight increase in perioperative and long-term survival. In comparison, the biatrial technique involves retaining sizable left and right atrial cuffs, followed by aortic and pulmonary artery anastomoses. The biatrial technique is considered a relatively simple approach with the advantages of shorter ischemic times and reduced risk of venous anastomotic complications.

92.7 The correct answer is C.
Rationale: The presence of a mechanical aortic valve at the time of LVAD implantation requires either patch oversewing of the aortic valve or replacement with a bioprosthetic valve. Mechanical valves are at increased risk of thrombosis with reduced blood flow through the valve given the significant flow through the LVAD. Aortic regurgitation greater than mild requires correction due to the risk of ineffective cardiac output with increased regurgitant volumes through the aortic valve. There is no current consensus on the need to intervene in tricuspid or mitral regurgitation.

TABLE 92.1 INTERMACS Classification

NYHA Class	Heart Failure Stage	INTERMACS Profile	INTERMACS Profile Description
4	D	1	Critical cardiogenic shock—"crash and burn" patient characterized by hypotension requiring escalating vasoactive infusion requirement, organ malperfusion, lactic acidosis
4	D	2	Progressive decline on inotropic support as demonstrated by increasing dose requirements, refractory volume overload, malnutrition, and worsening end-organ perfusion
4	D	3	Inotrope dependent—patient either hospitalized or at home with stable end-organ perfusion and volume status
4	D	4	Resting symptoms—describes a patient with heart failure symptoms at rest and with activities of daily living that increase even with minimal activity. Patients typically are congested with difficulty in managing volume status and are often intolerant of GDMT.
3b	C	5	Exertion intolerant—patients are comfortable at rest and with activities of daily living around the house but become symptomatic with minimal increases in activity and are mostly homebound.
3b	C	6	Exertion limited—patients who are comfortable at home and with basic activities outside the house. Patients may have experienced recent deteriorations and are intolerant of minor exertions such as grocery shopping.
3	C	7	Stable patient who can perform typical daily activities both within and outside the home environment with no recent decompensations but develops symptoms with moderate increases in activity.

GDMT, guideline-directed heart failure medical therapy; INTERMACS, Interagency Registry for Mechanically Assisted Circulatory Support; NYHA, New York Heart Association.
TCS—Temporary Circulatory Support—modifier applies to hospitalized patients with profiles 1 to 3 that are maintained on a temporary mechanical circulatory support device, such as intra-aortic balloon pump, percutaneous or surgical ventricular assist device, or extracorporeal membrane oxygenation.
A—Arrhythmia—can apply to any INTERMACS profile for patients with frequent, symptomatic arrhythmias affecting the patient's clinical course, including frequent implantable cardiodefibrillator shocks needed for cardioversion.
FF—Frequent Flyer—this modifier includes patients with frequent heart failure exacerbation admissions (two within 3 months or three in 6 months) and applies to nonhospitalized profile 3 and profiles 4 to 6 patients.

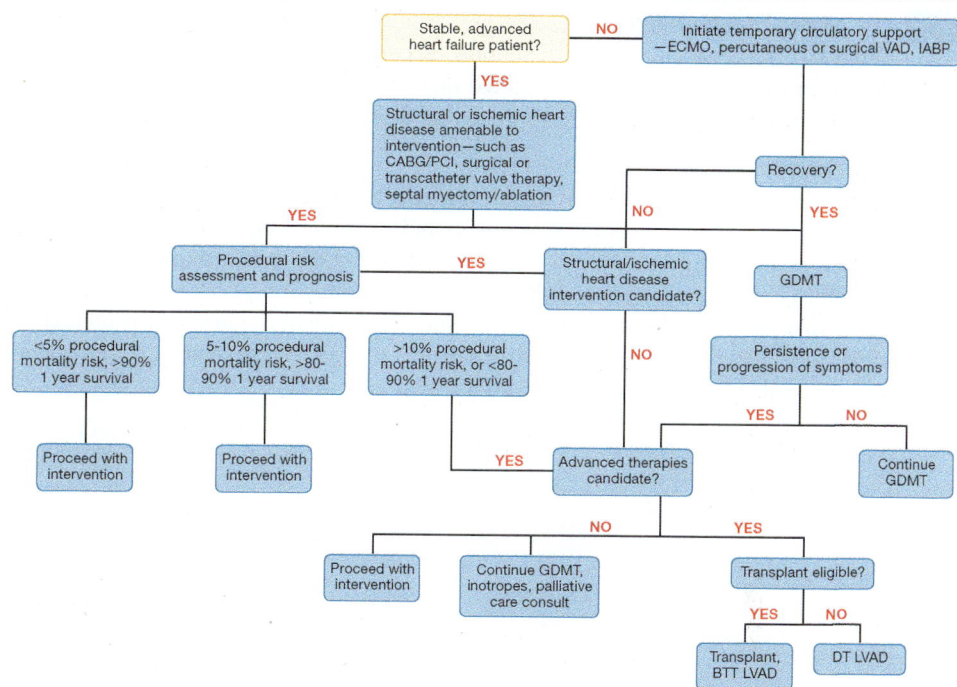

Figure 92.1 Surgical decision-making in patients with advanced heart failure. Patient stability on presentation is the most immediate concern when evaluating a candidate for advanced heart failure therapies or other interventions. Patients classified as INTERMACS class 1 and 2 are usually too unstable to be considered for high-risk coronary artery bypass grafting, valve surgery, or transcatheter interventions. These patients often benefit from temporary circulatory support to stabilize them and reassess their candidacy. Patients classified as INTERMACS class 3 to 7 are, by definition, hemodynamically stable and can be evaluated for various treatment options. Decision-making for candidates with underlying coronary or structural heart disease is often based on the anticipated perioperative risk and subsequent outcomes. Patients with a procedural risk and expected 1-year survival better or similar to transplantation or LVAD placement should undergo these procedures preferentially. Transplantation or LVAD implantation may be preferable for high-risk cases if the patient is otherwise deemed a candidate and agrees to move forward. Patients who are not deemed suitable candidates for advanced therapies should be offered high-risk surgery or transcatheter therapies. BTT, bridge to transplantation; CABG, coronary artery bypass grafting; DT, destination therapy; ECMO, extracorporeal membrane oxygenation; GDMT, guideline-directed medical therapy; IABP, intra-aortic balloon pump; LVAD, left ventricular assist device; PCI, percutaneous coronary intervention; VAD, ventricular assist device.

92.8 The correct answer is D.

Rationale: Orthotopic heart transplant has the most favorable short- and long-term survival outcomes reported, with an estimated 5-year survival at 72% as compared to the other listed options. Total artificial hearts are usually used as a bridge to transplant and generally kept hospitalized but have 4-year survival outcomes reported at 18.2%. LVAD 5-year survival is estimated at 42.7% and combined heart-lung transplant survival is estimated at 54.5%. Donor organ availability continues to be the primary impediment to heart transplants.

92.9 The correct answer is B.
Rationale: As ventricular assist technologies continue to develop along with further improvements in guideline-directed medical therapy for HF, LVAD short- and intermediate-term outcomes are approaching those of heart transplantation.

92.10 The correct answer is D.
Rationale: Device thrombosis is an uncommon but serious complication of LVAD therapy. More prevalent complications include GI bleeding and device infection. With continued improvement in device technology, short- and intermediate-survival outcomes now approach those of heart transplantation. Complication risk is highest in the first year after device implantation and event rate in the first year is predictive of the likelihood of future events, with a rate of up to 40% per year in patients who suffered multiple adverse events during the first year.

SURGICAL APPROACH FOR CONGENITAL HEART DISEASE*

Robert L. Carhart and Anderson C. Anuforo

CHAPTER 93

QUESTIONS

93.1 A baby is born at term to a relatively healthy 28-year-old G2P'2 woman. APGAR (Appearance [skin color], Pulse [heart rate, HR], Grimace [reflex irritability], Activity [muscle tone], and Respiration [breathing rate and effort]) scores were 7 in 1 minute and 9 in 5 minutes, baby weighs 6 lbs (2.72 kg). The pregnancy history and delivery course were essentially uneventful. Auscultation at birth reveals no significant systolic murmurs and vitals are within normal limits for a newborn except for pulse oximetry on the right hand, which is 85% on ambient air. On day 2 of life, the baby is noted to be tachycardic at 160 beats per minute (bpm). Physical examination reveals poorly perfused extremities with cyanosis and weak pulses. Chest x-ray reveals an enlarged cardiac silhouette with pulmonary edema. A stat echocardiogram is ordered and reveals a dilated right ventricle and atrium and a small left ventricle on a four-chamber view. Other views reveal dysfunctional left-sided valves and small ascending aorta and arch.

What is the **MOST LIKELY** diagnosis?

A. Hypoplastic left heart syndrome (HLHS) with patent ductus arteriosus (PDA) dependence
B. Ventricular septal defect (VSD)
C. Tetralogy of Fallot (TOF)
D. Transposition of the great arteries (TGA)

93.2 A 34-year-old male presented to the emergency department with a 1-month history of worsening shortness of breath especially with moderate to strenuous activities. He reports a history of a "hole in the heart" diagnosed in early childhood. Vital signs show a respiratory rate (RR) of 20/min, HR 90 bpm, T 37.4 °C, and blood pressure (BP) 116/78 mm Hg; cardiac auscultation reveals a moderate intensity pansystolic murmur and loudest in the left lower sternal border, which increases in intensity with the hand grip maneuver. Chest x-ray shows an enlarged cardiac silhouette and mild pulmonary edema, and electrocardiogram (ECG) shows normal sinus rhythm with right axis deviation, incomplete right bundle branch block, and right ventricular hypertrophy.

---

*Questions and Answers are based on Chapter 93: Surgical Approaches for Common Congenital Heart Diseases by Timothy J. Pirolli, Ryan R. Davies, Camille L. Hancock Friesen, and Robert D. B. Jaquiss in Cardiovascular Medicine and Surgery, First Edition.

Which imaging modality would be ideal in calculating the ratio of pulmonic to systemic blood flow (Qp:Qs)?
A. Transthoracic echocardiogram
B. Transesophageal echocardiogram
C. Cardiac catheterization
D. Chest arterial computed tomography (CT) angiography

93.3 A 3-year-old male child is hospitalized for a 1-month history of worsening exertional dyspnea. He immigrated to the United States and has never had a well-child visit till today. His mother reports that since infancy, he has had increased respiratory effort during meals with resultant poor feeding and weight gain. Vital signs show a RR 24/min, HR 120 bpm, BP 95/30 mm Hg, T 37.4 °C, and Spo_2 94% on ambient air; cardiac auscultation reveals a harsh pansystolic murmur and loudest in the left lower sternal border, which is associated with a diastolic decrescendo murmur and widened pulse pressure. Chest x-ray shows an enlarged cardiac silhouette and mild pulmonary edema, and ECG shows increased voltage in leads II, III, aVF, V5, and V6. An echocardiogram confirms the presence of a perimembranous VSD.

Which echocardiographic finding would be a contraindication to VSD closure?
A. Worsening aortic insufficiency
B. Suprasystemic severe pulmonary hypertension
C. Development of a double-chambered right ventricle
D. Pulmonary artery pressure is greater than half of the systolic blood pressure (SBP)

93.4 A 24-year-old female patient presents for a routine follow-up with her cardiologist. She has a history of a VSD diagnosed at birth for which she has been routinely followed up at regular intervals. She had a transthoracic echo done a few hours before her appointment that showed persistence of left-to-right shunt. Doppler echocardiography is used to obtain further parameters. Pulmonary vascular resistance (PVR) is estimated at 300 dynes/s/cm^5 using the tricuspid regurgitation velocity (TRV) and the time velocity integral (TVI) and systemic vascular resistance is estimated at 800 dynes/s/cm^5 using the ratio of the peak mitral regurgitant velocity (MRV) and left ventricular outflow (LVOT) TVI. Similar values are obtained on invasive hemodynamic evaluation, and pulmonary artery systolic pressure (PASP) is about 55% of systemic pressure.

What is the **BEST** next step in the management of this patient?
A. Surgical closure
B. Device closure
C. Consult with Allegheny County Health Department (ACHD) and Public Health (PH) experts.
D. Initiate combination therapy with Bosentan and phosphodiesterase (PDE)-5 inhibitors.

CHAPTER 93 | Surgical Approach for Congenital Heart Disease

93.5 A 6-month-old infant with no past significant medical history born at full term to a 26-year-old woman was transported to a tertiary care pediatric facility in respiratory failure. A 911 call was made due to worsening shortness of breath, and the child required intubation by the Emergency Medical Services (EMS) en route. The parents report poor weight gain, excessive sweating, and fast breathing during feeds but denied any upper respiratory symptoms, associated fever, vomiting, or diarrhea. They also deny any history of trauma or ingestion before presentation. They also report that intermittent episodes of agitation are usually associated with bluish discoloration of lips and extremities, which typically improves with folding the legs to the chest. Embryologically, the patient's disease is believed to arise from the underdevelopment of the conus due to defective migration of neural crest cells.

Which of the following is **NOT** a potential treatment modality for this patient?
A. Modified Blalock-Taussig-Thomas (BTT) shunt in a staged manner
B. Valve-sparing pulmonary arterioplasty with VSD repair in a few months
C. Emergency stenting of the PDA
D. Fontan repair

93.6 A 17-year-old male is admitted for a 6-week history of anorexia, easy satiety, abdominal distension, lower extremity swelling, and worsening dyspnea. He had a Fontan procedure completed 11 years ago for HLHS. His past medical history is significant for a neo-aorta created via a Norwood procedure and a right-modified BTT shunt created on the fourth day of life, a hemi-Fontan (superior cavopulmonary anastomosis) at the sixth month of life at which time the BTT shunt was closed, and at 6 years of age the Fontan, that is, total cavopulmonary connection (TCPC) circulation was completed with a lateral tunnel. He reports optimal growth, development, respiratory and functional status in relation to exertion since the Fontan until his most recent review by his pediatric cardiologist 6-weeks ago when pedal edema and exertional dyspnea were elicited. During the visit, ECG showed sinus rhythm without abnormal Q waves or ST/T wave abnormalities. A transthoracic echocardiogram reveals optimal systolic and diastolic function of the systemic ventricle without atrioventricular (AV) valve dysfunction, intracardiac clots, or TCPC obstruction, and a bubble contrast study was positive for a L-R interatrial shunt but negative for pulmonary arteriovenous malformations. Lasix 40 mg daily was prescribed in addition to his ongoing antiplatelet therapy at that visit; however, he presented today due to worsening of symptoms.

Vitals showed BP 90/50 mm Hg, HR 80 bpm, RR 22/min, SpO_2 94% on ambient air and temperature of 37 °C. Physical examination revealed a young man in mild respiratory distress with generalized pitting edema of the lower extremities and abdominal wall. The chest examination exposed a midline zipper scar and clear auscultation findings. The abdominal examination was positive for fluid thrill and hepatomegaly.

Admission laboratory results:

Na (sodium)—138 mmol/L

K (potassium)—4.4 mmol/L

Cl (chlorine)—100 mmol/L

HCO_3 (bicarbonate)—24 mmol/L

BUN (blood urea nitrogen)—15 mmol/L

Creatinine—0.6 mg/dL

Glucose—105 mg/dL

Ca (calcium)—7.8 mg/dL

Albumin—2.1 mg/dL

Total protein—4.2 mg/dL

AST (aspartate aminotransferase)—65 U/L

ALT (alanine aminotransferase)—60 U/L

ALP (alkaline phosphatase)—55 U/L

T (total) bilirubin—1.5 mg/dL

D (direct) bilirubin—0.2 mg/dL

INR (international normalized ratio)—1.05

Urinalysis is negative for proteins, ketones, or glucose, and the chest x-ray showed no overt anomalies. Urine protein-creatinine ratio is within normal limits at 120 mg/g. CT of the abdomen and pelvis was most significant for hepatomegaly and moderately severe ascites. Lasix was converted to the IV route and the dose was doubled without improvement in fluid overloaded status. Cardiac catheterization and angiography were performed and did not show a step up to suggest a new shunt.

Which of the following is the **MOST LIKELY** etiology of this patient's clinical change?
A. Protein-losing enteropathy (PLE)
B. Ischemic hepatic injury
C. Nephrotic range proteinuria from membranous nephropathy
D. Obstruction of the cavopulmonary circulation system

93.7 A 2-month-old male infant is evaluated for poor feeding, increased respiratory effort, and poor weight gain. He has been hospitalized thrice since birth. On physical examination, a thrill is noted along the left sternal border. A grade 4/6 holosystolic murmur is heard at the left sternal border obscuring the S2. The remainder of the physical examination is unremarkable. Echocardiograms show enlarged left atrium and left ventricle, along with a perimembranous VSD. The patient is referred to surgery for further evaluation.

What is the optimal technique in this patient to avoid heart block during a perimembranous VSD repair?
A. Taking shallow suture bites (3-5 mm) through the endocardium on the right ventricle
B. Taking large suture bites (5-10 mm) through the endocardium on the right ventricle
C. Taking large suture bites through the endocardium in the left ventricle
D. Taking shallow suture bites through the endocardium on the right atrium

93.8 A 64-year-old man undergoes a preoperative evaluation before repair of a torn anterior cruciate ligament. His cardiovascular history includes repaired TOF. He has no symptoms.

On physical examination, vital signs are normal. Jugular venous distension and a prominent wave are noted. A right ventricular heave is present. A single S2 is heard, as is a grade 4/6 diastolic murmur best heard in the left second and third intercostal spaces. The diastolic murmur increases with inspiration. Echocardiography shows impaired right ventricular systolic function.

Which of the following is the most appropriate next step in management?
A. Transcatheter aortic valve replacement (TAVR)
B. Pulmonary valve replacement
C. Mitral valve replacement
D. Closure of the VSD

93.9 A newborn is diagnosed with HLHS. Which of the following interventions is the initial management strategy for stabilizing the patient's condition and improving systemic perfusion?
A. Immediate surgical repair of the hypoplastic left heart
B. Administration of prostaglandin E1 (PGE1) infusion
C. Initiation of inotropic support with dobutamine
D. Placement of a systemic-to-pulmonary artery shunt

93.10 A 2-year-old child presents with cyanosis, a harsh systolic murmur, and clubbing of the fingers. He has no known medical conditions. His vitals in clinic include BP of 100/50 mm Hg, HR of 120 bpm, and RR of 30/min. An echocardiogram reveals a large VSD, pulmonary stenosis, overriding aorta, and right ventricular hypertrophy. Which of the following **BEST** describes the pathophysiologic basis of these findings in TOF?
A. Left-to-right shunting at the VSD leading to pulmonary congestion
B. Decreased pulmonary blood flow due to severe pulmonary valve stenosis
C. Right-to-left shunting at the VSD causing systemic hypoxemia
D. Left ventricular hypertrophy secondary to increased afterload

ANSWERS

93.1 The correct answer is A.
Rationale: The patient's presentation with the rapid development of profound cyanosis and hemodynamic compromise (shock) following PDA closure in 24 to 48 hours after birth suggests a PDA-dependent congenital heart disease. The SpO_2 of 85% suggests some mixing of arterial and venous blood but the echo findings strongly suggest HLHS. The continuous murmur of a PDA is not unexpected in a newborn as opposed to an isolated systolic murmur. The absence of systolic murmurs makes a VSD of TOF less likely. A VSD would likely have a pansystolic murmur loudest in the left lower sternal border unless it is very large. A TOF would likely have the pulmonic systolic ejection murmur and/or the pansystolic murmur of the VSD. TGA tends to present with moderate-to-severe cyanosis at birth, a significantly lower oxygen saturation, that is unresponsive to supplemental O_2, and the murmur of a septal defect. TGA would also be dependent on the PDA, but the echo findings described suggest a HLHS diagnosis.

93.2 The correct answer is C.

Rationale: This patient has VSD based on clinical findings. The degree of shunting could be calculated by cardiac catheterization or cardiac magnetic resonance imaging (MRI) as the ratio of Qp:Qs. Transthoracic or transesophageal echocardiography can estimate the degree of shunting by measuring the pressure gradient across the VSD, but they do not give a precise Qp:Qs. An arterial chest CT angiography would be indicated in evaluating for an aortic dissection or aneurysm but not to estimate Qp:Qs. Most VSDs have Qp:Qs less than 1.5:1. VSDs with a moderate shunt (Qp:Qs of 1.5-2.3:1) typically result in mild-moderately increased right ventricular and pulmonary arterial pressures, as well as signs and symptoms of congestive heart failure. Large defects (Qp:Qs >2.3:1) have unrestrictive shunts with minimal pressure gradient between the two ventricles. This equalization (or near-equalization) of ventricular pressures can lead to left ventricular dilation and increased end-diastolic pressures, resulting in increased left atrial pressures, pulmonary venous pressures, and progressive symptoms of heart failure.

93.3 The correct answer is B.

Rationale: The American Heart Association (AHA)/American College of Cardiology (ACC) released an evidence-based, expert consensus guideline algorithm for surgical closure of VSDs in adults. VSD closure is contraindicated in patients with suprasystemic pulmonary hypertension, often in patients with unrepaired VSDs who survive until adulthood as the pulmonary vascular disease may develop leading to right-to-left shunting (Eisenmenger syndrome) and cyanosis due to chronic elevations of pressure and flow across the VSD. These patients are typically inoperable.

Patients with estimated pulmonary artery pressures greater than half-systemic or continued enlargement of left-sided cardiac structures likely warrant surgical closure of their VSD. Patients with smaller VSDs who are asymptomatic may be monitored for spontaneous closure. The presence of associated congenital defects, development of a double-chambered right ventricle, or worsening aortic insufficiency may also be indications for surgery.

93.4 The correct answer is C.

Rationale: If the patient has a VSD with L-R shunt, with hemodynamic assessment showing PVR greater than 1/3 systemic and PASP greater than 50% of systemic pressure, the best next step is a consultation with an adult congenital heart disease specialist and pulmonary hypertension expert. However, if the patient has a VSD with L-R shunt with echo finding of LV enlargement and hemodynamic findings of Qp:Qs $1.5 \geq 1$, PVR less than 1/3 systemic and PASP less than 50% of systemic, would be an indication for surgical or device closure. In the event of a VSD with R-L shunt, combination therapy would be an option but this would need to be guided by the results of invasive monitoring that would also confirm the diagnosis of pulmonary artery hypertension (PAH). Further details are described in **Figure 93.1**.

93.5 The correct answer is D.

Rationale: The Fontan procedure is a procedure required in the definitive management of the univentricular heart, for example, tricuspid atresia or HLHS via the creation of a TCPC. It is not indicated for treatment of TOF.

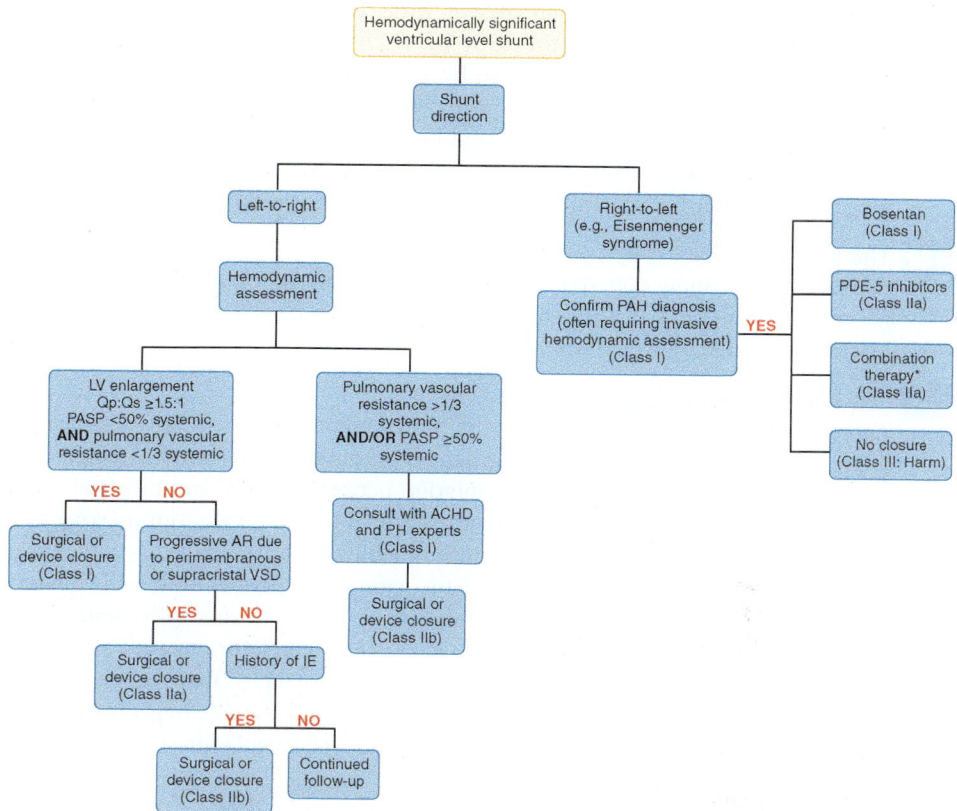

Figure 93.1 Management for hemodynamically significant VSD in adults. Critical decisions are based on echocardiography and cardiac catheterization. ACHD, adult congenital heart disease; AR, aortic regurgitation; IE, infective endocarditis; LV, left ventricle; PAH, pulmonary artery hypertension; PASP, pulmonary artery systolic pressure; PDE, phosphodiesterase; PH, pulmonary hypertension; Qp:Qs, pulmonary to systemic blood flow; VSD, ventricular septal defect.

As a result of the wide range of pathophysiology, intervention may be required urgently or emergently in the neonatal or infancy period or may be scheduled electively at 4 to 6 months of age like any other VSD. Management modalities include neonatal complete repair in the neonatal period or emergency stenting of the PDA, modified BTT shunt in a staged repair, and valve-sparing pulmonary arterioplasty with VSD repair in the older infant.

93.6 The correct answer is A.

Rationale: PLE is a known complication of Fontan circulation. This patient is hypoalbuminemic, hypoproteinemic, and hypocalcemic with mildly elevated liver enzymes and normal INR, which is suggestive of PLE and unlikely to be due to ischemic hepatic injury. The specific mechanism for PLE is not fully understood, but it often presents with ascites, hypoproteinemia, and diuretic-resistant edema. Fecal alpha-1-antitrypsin is elevated in PLE and is a measure of gastrointestinal protein loss.

Ischemic hepatic injury would present with transaminitis in the high 100s to 1,000s but would usually be preceded by an ischemic insult. Nephrotic range proteinuria would usually be indicated by a positive urinalysis (if the protein was albumin) and would usually be supported by a urine protein-creatinine ratio of 3 mg/g or more. Obstruction of the cavopulmonary circulation system must be ruled out before focusing on PLE and neither the echocardiogram nor hemodynamics suggests this. A cardiac MRI would not be ideal to confirm this.

93.7 The correct answer is A.
Rationale: The conduction system follows a course along the inferior margin of a perimembranous or inlet VSD, thus superficial bites (or bites 3-5 mm away from the margin of the defect) are critical to prevent heart block.

93.8 The correct answer is B.
Rationale: Pulmonary regurgitation is the most common postoperative sequela of TOF repair. Pulmonary valve replacement is a common intervention required in adults with repaired TOF. Close collaboration between surgical and catheterization laboratory/intervention teams provides the optimal forum for decision-making and support for intervention. Guidelines recommend either percutaneous or surgical pulmonary valve replacement indicated for patients with symptoms with moderate or worse pulmonary regurgitation and asymptomatic patients with moderate or worse pulmonary regurgitation with ventricular enlargement or impaired right ventricular systolic function. The timing of pulmonary valve replacement can be decided by an ACHD multidisciplinary team, and the patient may be able to get his anterior cruciate ligament (ACL) repaired before pulmonary valve replacement.

93.9 The correct answer is B.
Rationale: In patients with HLHS, PGE1 is critical to maintain ductal patency and improve systemic perfusion. PGE1 helps keep the ductus arteriosus open, allowing for shunting of blood from the systemic circulation to the pulmonary circulation, which helps improve oxygenation and systemic perfusion, minimize the risk of shock and myocardial ischemia. This is a crucial step in the management of HLHS before more definitive surgical interventions can be planned.

93.10 The correct answer is B.
Rationale: The four cardinal anatomic features of TOF are VSD, right ventricular outflow tract (RVOT) obstruction, right ventricular hypertrophy, and aortic override. These arise from the underdevelopment of the conus (also called the infundibulum), which is the muscle in which the pulmonary valve sits. Thus the hypoplasia of the conus causes RVOT obstruction and decreased pulmonary blood flow. In addition, with underdevelopment of the conus—a muscle that normally grows large enough to contribute a portion of the interventricular septum—there is a canal VSD that forms. The VSD is unrestrictive and thus increases pressures in the right ventricle resulting in right ventricular hypertrophy. The underdeveloped conus fails to "push" the aorta back into normal anatomic location over the left ventricle resulting in aortic override of the interventricular septum.

CHEST WALL INFECTIONS FOLLOWING OPEN HEART SURGERY*

CHAPTER 94

Robert L. Carhart, Monique Monita, and Hiba Zafar

QUESTIONS

94.1 A 63-year-old male is 6 days post-op after receiving a coronary artery bypass grafting (CABG) procedure. The patient did receive two units of packed red blood cells during the operation. During his hospitalization, the patient's blood glucose levels have fluctuated between 202 and 285 mg/dL. Today, the patient reports chills and overnight he had a fever of 38.3 °C. On physical examination, there is redness at the incision site with mild purulent drainage. Blood work and cultures were obtained this morning. What microorganism is most commonly associated with superficial and deep sternal wound infections of the chest wall following open heart surgery?

A. *Streptococcus pyogenes*
B. *Staphylococcus aureus*
C. *Corynebacterium diphtheria*
D. *Bacteroides fragilis*

94.2 A 68-year-old woman with a history of chronic kidney disease (CKD) stage 2, type 2 diabetes on oral antihyperglycemic medications, and a body mass index (BMI) of 32 is being prepped for her CABG procedure with planned single internal thoracic artery grafting. She has **NOT** been hospitalized previously, lives at home with her partner, and denies any history of previous infections. The patient has several nonmodifiable risk factors that increase the risk of surgical site infection. Which intravenous (IV) antibiotic medication is recommended for prophylaxis?

A. Ampicillin
B. Zosyn
C. Cefazolin
D. Vancomycin

94.3 A 72-year-old male is 6 days post-op from a CABG procedure and is taken back to the operating room (OR) for surgical site wound exploration. He was noted to have a fever of 38.5 °C overnight with leukocytosis at 14,000/μL. Physical examination findings included swelling, tenderness, and redness to the lower 1/3 of the incision site. Upon superficial debridement of the infected sternotomy incision, a sternal wire becomes exposed. After further evaluation, there is no separation of tissue layers. What complication has occurred in this patient?

A. Deep sternal wound infection
B. Deep incisional surgical site infection
C. Partial wound dehiscence
D. Medical adhesive-related skin injury

*Questions and Answers are based on Chapter 94: Chest Wall Infections Following Open Heart Surgery by Michael A. Wait in Cardiovascular Medicine and Surgery, First Edition.

Section 7: Cardiovascular Surgery

94.4 Proper surgical technique and postoperative management are crucial to reducing the incidence of chest wall infections in patients receiving open heart surgery. Which of the following should be avoided as it contributes toward surgical wound infections?
   A. Negative pressure wound therapy
   B. Limited electrocautery
   C. Intranasal mupirocin
   D. Bone wax marrow

94.5 A 57-year-old woman with a recent history of CABG with grafting of both right and left internal thoracic arteries is being evaluated for flap placement for wound dehiscence. The lower third of the median sternotomy has separated and an intercostal artery-supported vertical rectus myocutaneous flap is being considered for wound closure. In this procedure, what two vessels are ligated?
   A. Deep and superficial inferior epigastric artery and vein
   B. Superior phrenic and mediastinal artery and vein
   C. Axillary and lateral thoracic artery and vein
   D. Anterior intercostal and pericardiacophrenic artery and vein

94.6 A 74-year-old female is 22 days post-op from a CABG procedure complicated by a deep sternal wound infection. The patient received debridement of infected tissue, antibiotics, and negative pressure wound therapy has been applied. The incisional wound shows granulation tissue without purulent drainage. The patient's BMI is 20 and there is limited pectoralis muscle available. What surgical approach can be used for closure in such a scenario?
   A. Transverse upper gracilis flap
   B. Right rectus abdominis flap with left pectoralis myoplasty flap
   C. Intercostal artery-supported vertical rectus myocutaneous flap
   D. Omentoplasty with chest wall fasciocutaneous flap

94.7 A 49-yo male presents to the emergency department (ED) after undergoing CABG for significant left main disease on cardiac catheterization, with 80% stenosis of the left anterior descending (LAD) and left circumflex (LCx) arteries. He notes pain and swelling around his median sternotomy incision, with purulent drainage from the site. Last night, the patient reported having fevers to 38.3 °C thus had his wife drive him to the ED for further evaluation. Which of the following organisms is **MOST LIKELY** to be isolated from his mediastinal fluid?
   A. B. fragilis
   B. S. aureus
   C. Staphylococcus epidermidis
   D. Pseudomonas aeruginosa

94.8 A 53-yo female presents to the ED after undergoing surgical aortic valve replacement, with fevers, erythema, and active purulent drainage from the surgical incision. She is started on broad-spectrum antibiotics and taken to the OR for surgical debridement and reconstruction. Which of the following measures is indicated as surgical prophylaxis in this patient?

A. Nasal application of mupirocin
B. Application of vancomycin paste to sternal edges
C. Use of topical skin disinfectant such as chlorhexidine or isopropyl alcohol
D. Use of gentamicin-collagen sponges

94.9 A 60-yo male with a prior medical history of type 2 diabetes mellitus, hypertension, hyperlipidemia, metabolic syndrome, and obesity is admitted to the hospital post-CABG for concerns for deep sternal wound infection. He is taken to the OR where cultures of the purulent drainage are sent for microbiologic evaluation and undergoes debridement of the wound. A phlegmon is found requiring further sharp excisional debridement. The patient has notable multiple chest wall incisions, with a similar history of deep sternal wound infection in the past. Discussions between the cardiovascular surgeon and plastic reconstructive surgeon are underway to determine the appropriate management of this patient's complex poststernotomy wound. Which of the following reconstructive techniques have been shown to have the **BEST** mortality benefits in these patients?

A. Transdiaphragmatic omentoplasty
B. Latissimus dorsi myoplasty
C. Pectoralis myoplasty

94.10 A 59-yo male presents to the ED for evaluation after recent bypass surgery with median sternotomy incision. He reports chest wall pain around his site of incision, with fevers to 37.7 °C, and states he tried taking Tylenol which helped with the fever but has **NOT** touched his pain. He denies any active drainage from his surgical site. States he called his cardiologist who advised him to come to the ED. On examination, he is febrile to 38.5 °C, with the remainder of his vital signs normal. After evaluation by the cardiovascular surgery team, the patient is admitted to the hospital and taken to the OR for concerns for sternal wound infection.

Upon further conversation with the patient after surgical debridement, he tells you he had a prolonged hospital stay of over 1 week and a half post-surgery due to complications with blood counts, and management of his blood sugars. Which of the following has **NOT** been observed with increased infection risk post median sternotomy?

A. Antibiotic prophylaxis more than 60 minutes before incision
B. Multiple blood transfusions post-surgery
C. Postoperative hyperglycemia
D. Statin therapy

ANSWERS

94.1 The correct answer is B.
Rationale: The patient in this vignette has several factors that contributed to development of his chest wall infection including inadequate blood glucose control and receiving blood transfusions. The infection rate increases with the increased use of packed red blood cell units. In addition, as the patient has redness at the incision site and purulent drainage, this suggests a superficial wound infection. *S. aureus* is the most common microorganism isolated from both superficial and deep sternal wound infections from heart surgery. Other common organisms include *S. epidermidis* and alpha-hemolytic streptococcus.

94.2 The correct answer is C.
Rationale: According to STS (Society of Thoracic Surgeons) guideline recommendations, IV cefazolin or cefuroxime can be administered for antibiotic prophylaxis to prevent the occurrence of wound infection as the likely organism is *S. aureus* or *S. epidermidis*.

94.3 The correct answer is A.
Rationale: The patient has a chest wall infection following open heart surgery. Superficial wound infections are those limited to the epidermis, dermis, and superficial subcutaneous adipose. In addition, the patient has symptoms supporting this type of infection including swelling, tenderness, and redness at the incision site. However, as a sternal wire was exposed during debridement, the chest wall infection is now classified as deep sternal wound infection.

94.4 The correct answer is D.
Rationale: Bone marrow max is a topical hemostatic agent and impairs normal wound healing by promoting inflammation, fibrosis, and a foreign body reaction. The use of bone marrow wax is associated with deep sternal wound infection and sternal dehiscence. Negative pressure wound therapy provides many advantages including decreased wound swelling and exudate, enhanced blood flow, and decreased time to wound closure. Limited electrocautery is recommended as it improves blood supply to incision edges. Intranasal mupirocin is one form of antibiotic prophylaxis.

94.5 The correct answer is A.
Rationale: By ligating the deep and superficial inferior epigastric artery and vein, the segmental intercostal vessels mature and eventually dilate, allowing for collaterals to form with the lower remnants of the internal thoracic arteries and inferior epigastric artery.

94.6 The correct answer is D.
Rationale: In patients with deep sternal wound infection, treatment includes limited radical debridement, antibiotics tailored to the cultured organism, and the use of wound vacuum tissue. Following these steps, nonrigid reconstruction using pectoralis muscle is often employed as local muscles can be accessed through the same incision site as the surgery. In those patients with limited muscle mass, packing of tissue from the greater omentum of the stomach is a useful surgical procedure as this

tissue is rich in vascular endothelial growth factor and promotes wound healing as it is a well-vascularized tissue. Following mobilization and placement of the omentum, skin coverage is required and can be achieved from chest wall fasciocutaneous skin advancement or split-thickness skin graft.

94.7 The correct answer is B.
Rationale: S. aureus is the most common organism (~80%) isolated from superficial and deep sternal wound infections. *Staphylococcus* species including *S. aureus*, *S. epidermidis*, and alpha-hemolytic streptococcus continue to predominate as the leading bacterial organisms isolated from deep sternal wound infections.

94.8 The correct answer is C.
Rationale: Use of topical skin disinfectants such as chlorhexidine or isopropyl alcohol is a mainstay of surgical prophylaxis of deep sternal wound infection (DSWI). Studies involving prophylactic intranasal mupirocin in comparison with placebo showed no reduction in overall surgical site infections by *S. aureus*. Likewise, use of gentamicin-collagen sponges or vancomycin paste in patients undergoing cardiac operations was not associated with a reduced risk of DSWI.

94.9 The correct answer is C.
Rationale: Comparisons between pectoralis, latissimus, or rectus myoplasty and omentoplasty have been conducted. Nonrandomized, single-center reports have reported the superiority of pectoralis myoplasty techniques more than omentoplasty in terms of overall mortality benefit in these patients, in the absence of sternal bone necrosis.

94.10 The correct answer is D.
Rationale: While not specific to deep sternal wound infections, studies have demonstrated that preoperative administration of statins has reduced the incidence of all infections. Blood transfusion post cardiac surgery along with elevated hemoglobin A1c (HbA1c) and hyperglycemia are also associated with increased infection risk. While antibiotic prophylaxis is proven to prevent surgical site infections, administration of antibiotics more than 60 minutes before incision or greater than 30 minutes after incision has been associated with deep sternal wound infections.

SECTION 8 PREVENTIVE CARDIOLOGY

CHAPTER 95
PREVENTIVE CARDIOLOGY/ PATHOPHYSIOLOGY OF ATHEROSCLEROSIS*

Robert L. Carhart, Anojan Pathmanathan, and Niranjan Ojha

QUESTIONS

95.1 A 41-year-old smoker male presents to cardiology office for establishing care. He has a strong family history of premature coronary heart disease. His father died of heart attack at the age of 47 years. His blood pressure at the office was 119/75 mm Hg. The lipid panel and diabetes screening tests were sent to laboratory. The patient wants to know about the effect of smoking on coronary heart disease.

- A. Smoking has no effect on atherosclerosis.
- B. Smoking is considered as one of the factors in the initiation of atherosclerosis.
- C. There is no benefit to quitting smoking now since atherosclerosis might have already started.
- D. The morbidity and mortality caused by smoking are not preventable.

95.2 A 52-year-old male underwent cardiac catheterization for activity limiting stable angina. He has a critical disease in his right coronary artery and underwent angioplasty and stenting. He also has some plaque deposit in his left anterior descending artery, which was **NOT** flow limiting based on intravascular ultrasound (IVUS) and physiologic studies. Virtual histology IVUS showed fibrocalcific plaque. Which of the following feature is **NOT** considered a feature of a stable plaque?

- A. Thick fibrous cap
- B. Small necrotic core
- C. Microcalcifications
- D. Increased collagen content

95.3 A 74-year-old male with a history of diabetes mellitus type 2 and hyperlipidemia presented with acute onset chest pain that began 4 hours ago. His home medications include metformin ER 1,000 mg daily, empagliflozin 10 mg daily, and atorvastatin 20 mg nightly. His electrocardiogram (ECG) showed some nonspecific T-wave changes in the inferior leads. He has high-sensitivity troponin drawn, which was elevated above the 99th percentile of normal range. He subsequently underwent cardiac catheterization and he got a stent in the mid-right coronary artery. What is the **MOST LIKELY** reason for his non–ST-segment-elevation myocardial infarction (NSTEMI)?

- A. Plaque rupture
- B. Plaque erosion
- C. Embolic event
- D. Coronary vasospasm

*Questions and Answers are based on Chapter 95: Pathophysiology of Atherosclerosis by Marcio Sommer Bittencourt, Giuliano Generoso, and Raul D. Santos in Cardiovascular Medicine and Surgery, First Edition.

95.4 Heart disease is the leading cause of death in the United States, and the risk of heart disease death differs by race and ethnicity. Which of the following statements is **TRUE** regarding the epidemiology of heart disease?

   A. From 1999 through 2017, death rates for heart disease decreased for all racial and ethnic groups.
   B. Non-Hispanic Black persons were more than twice as likely as non-Hispanic Asian or Pacific Islander persons to die of heart disease from 1999 to 2017.
   C. Non-Hispanic Black adults aged 20 and over were most likely to have hypertension.
   D. Asian Indian men, Filipino men, and Filipino women have a high risk of coronary artery disease and heart attack compared with White people.
   E. All of the above are correct.

95.5 A 37-year-old female is recently diagnosed with type 2 diabetes mellitus. Her lipid panel showed isolated hypertriglyceridemia for which she was referred to a cardiologist. Patient wants to the implication of her triglyceride level. Which of the following is **NOT CORRECT** regarding triglyceride levels in the blood?

   A. The level of triglyceride fluctuates with fasting and postprandial states.
   B. The triglycerides have no role in atherogenesis and atherosclerotic heart disease.
   C. Triglyceride-rich lipoproteins have been associated with an increased risk of atherosclerosis.
   D. In studies, the reduction of triglycerides led to a reduction in cardiovascular events.

95.6 Diabetes mellitus is considered a major risk factor for atherosclerosis. Which of the following mechanisms explains atherosclerosis in a patient with diabetes?

   A. Production of reactive oxygen species
   B. Formation of advanced glycation end products with activation of their receptor axis
   C. Vascular damage by polyol (ie, sorbitol) pathway metabolites
   D. All of the above

95.7 A 65-year-old White male with a history of diabetes mellitus type 2 and hypertension is in a cardiologist's office for follow-up on his hypertension. His home medications include lisinopril 40 mg nightly, metformin 1,000 mg tid, and empagliflozin 10 mg daily. His blood pressure today in the office was 129/83 mm Hg, heart rate was 72 beats per minute. His lipid profile showed low-density lipoprotein (LDL) cholesterol of 101 mg/dL and total cholesterol of 180 mg/dL. He is encouraged to participate in strength and cardio exercises and the booklet was provided about healthy eating habits and diet. What would be the appropriate next step in management?

   A. Moderate-intensity statin
   B. High-intensity statin
   C. Inclisiran
   D. Lipid-lowering treatment is not indicated at this time.

95.8 A 40-year-old male with a family history of premature coronary artery disease in his father presented to discuss his coronary artery calcium (CAC) score. He doesn't have any symptoms. His CAC score was 150. What is the most appropriate management strategy?

A. Lifestyle modification: exercise and healthy eating habit
B. Risk factor modification: weight loss and smoking cessation
C. Patient should be started on statin.
D. A and B
E. A, B, and C

95.9 A 52-year-old male with a history of coronary artery disease with a recent angioplasty and stenting presented for hospital discharge follow-up. He was discharged on aspirin, Plavix, metoprolol, and atorvastatin. His lab drawn at the time of discharge showed elevated lipoprotein at a level of 20 mg/dL. What is the significance of lipoprotein a (Lp(a)) level?

A. Lp(a) has elevated cholesterol content.
B. Lp(a) has proinflammatory and prothrombotic effects.
C. Lp(a) serum level is dependent on heredity.
D. A and B
E. A, B, and C

95.10 Which of the following is **TRUE** about vulnerable plaque?

A. It is a result of continuous inflammatory insult associated with development of lipid core that may increase the risk of plaque rupture.
B. It has a thick fibrous cap.
C. The plaque has well-structured calcifications.
D. Statin therapy increases the plaque vulnerability.

ANSWERS

95.1 The correct answer is B.

Rationale: Atherosclerosis is the primary etiology for a broad spectrum of clinical manifestations of cardiovascular diseases (CVDs) that comprises ischemic heart disease, cerebrovascular disease, and peripheral artery disease. Smoking is considered one of the factors in the initiation of atherosclerosis. The chemicals you inhale when you smoke cause damage to the heart and blood vessels. Any amount of smoking, even occasional smoking, can cause damage to the heart and blood vessels. Quitting smoking will prevent further damage to the heart and blood vessels, and it is the main preventable cause of death and illness in the United States.

95.2 The correct answer is C.

Rationale: In atheroma progression, the process of clearing dead cells and associated cellular debris (called efferocytosis) becomes dysfunctional, thereby accumulation of cellular debris and deposition of cholesterol crystals contribute to the formation of the necrotic core. Smooth muscle cell migration and proliferation continue, building additional cell layers that result in a thick fibrous cap that covers the necrotic core. This cover protects the plaque against rupture and its consequent core exposure to prothrombotic factors. Vascular calcifications is another factor in plaque stabilization. Although microcalcifications in the fibrous cap may generate instability and predispose to plaque rupture initially, the evolution to extensive organized, structured calcifications may lead to a lower risk of thrombotic events because of biomechanical stability.

95.3 The correct answer is B.
Rationale: In patients taking lipid-lowering therapies, plaque erosion, and ulceration rather than plaque rupture is more common. In advanced stages of atherosclerosis, apoptosis and consequent desquamation of endothelial cells occur, configuring areas of plaque erosion that, in contrast with plaque ruptures, contain few inflammatory cells, abundant extracellular matrix, and neutrophil extracellular traps. The result is the organization of a less occlusive "white" thrombus with plaque erosion, which is more likely to be associated with the clinical presentation of a NSTEMI. Coronary artery emboli is a less common yet important cause of nonatherosclerotic STEMI. Coronary vasospasms usually appear normal in coronary angiography.

95.4 The correct answer is E.
Rationale: Although there has been a reduction in CVD deaths for all ethnicities, the incidence in African Americans is still higher than in non-Hispanic Whites and twice as high as in Hispanics. There are recent reports suggesting Asian Indian men, Filipino men, and Filipino women have a higher risk of coronary artery disease and heart attack compared to White people. The economic burden of heart disease is also significant. In the United States, heart disease has an economic impact of $218 billion annually. By 2035, direct costs of all CVD may exceed $750 billion, with more than half in hospital spending and $350 billion in productivity losses.

95.5 The correct answer is B.
Rationale: The role of triglycerides in atherosclerosis is not clear but triglyceride-rich lipoproteins have been associated with an increased risk of atherosclerosis. Triglyceride-depleted remnants of chylomicrons and very low-density lipoprotein (VLDL) may induce atherosclerosis by their relatively elevated cholesterol content rather than triglyceride content per se. However, the addition of triglycerides in those particles may increase oxidative stress and inflammation and play a role in atherogenesis. Excess triglycerides in lipoproteins also reduce the antiatherogenic properties of high-density lipoprotein (HDL) particles and lead to the formation of small dense LDL particles that are more prone to oxidation. In some studies such as REDUCE-IT (Reduction of Cardiovascular Events With Icosapent Ethyl–Intervention Trial), the reduction of triglycerides led to a reduction in cardiovascular events.

95.6 The correct answer is D.
Rationale: Diabetes mellitus is characterized as a chronic disease with high blood glucose levels and insulin resistance. Diabetes contributes to micro- and macrovascular structural changes that double the risk of ischemic heart disease, stroke, and peripheral arterial disease. The main mechanisms associated with hyperglycemia that participate in atherogenesis are production of reactive oxygen species, formation of advanced glycation end products with activation of their receptor axis, vascular damage caused by polyol (ie, sorbitol) pathway metabolites, activation of the diacylglycerol-protein kinase C pathway, which regulates endothelial permeability, extracellular matrix synthesis/turnover, cell growth, angiogenesis, cytokine activation, and leukocyte adhesion; and chronic vascular inflammation.

95.7 The correct answer is B.

Rationale: Different clinical risk scores or calculators can be used to stratify the cardiovascular risk in an asymptomatic patient. The atherosclerotic cardiovascular disease (ASCVD) risk calculator is one of them. Based on the information, this patient's ASCVD risk score would be 28.6%. High-intensity statin is recommended because of known diabetes and the 10-year risk is 7.5% or more.

95.8 The correct answer is E.

Rationale: The CAC score measured by a noncontrast cardiac computed tomography scan is a useful risk stratification tool. The CAC score may improve risk prediction and help shared decision-making on the need for pharmacologic interventions to reduce risk. Those who have no coronary calcium (CAC 0) show an extremely low incidence of cardiovascular outcomes and would have limited benefit from pharmacologic treatment. Conversely, a more extensive calcification (CAC >100 Agatston units) supports statin initiation even in individuals considered to be at low risk based on clinical factors.

95.9 The correct answer is E.

Rationale: Lp(a) is an LDL-modified low-density atherogenic particle that contains apolipoprotein(a) in its structure and its serum levels are highly dependent on heredity. It has elevated cholesterol content and has proinflammatory and prothrombotic effects. Elevated level of Lp(a) has strong independent association with coronary heart disease and stroke as well as calcific degenerative aortic stenosis. There are ongoing trials on therapies to decrease Lp(a) level.

95.10 The correct answer is A.

Rationale: Vulnerable plaques are a result of continuous inflammatory insult associated with development of lipid core that may increase the risk of plaque rupture, and it may develop in different stages of plaque progression. Different inflammatory processes and expansion of necrotic lipid core lead to thinning of the fibrous cap. Statin therapy reduces the plaque vulnerability and stabilizes the fibrous cap and slows plaque progression.

CARDIOVASCULAR DISEASE RISK ASSESSMENT IN CLINICAL PRACTICE

Jacqueline S. Coppola, Joshua Schulman-Marcus, and Sulagna Mookherjee

CHAPTER 96

QUESTIONS

96.1 In the United States, routine risk estimation for primary prevention is recommended between which ages?
- A. 20 to 30
- B. Men older than 40, women older than 50
- C. 40 to 75
- D. 35 to 50

96.2 According to primary prevention atherosclerotic cardiovascular disease (ASCVD) risk scores, a 45-year-old male patient without diabetes is presenting to your clinic to initiate care. You calculate his 10-year ASCVD risk score to be 15%, with a significant family history of ASCVD. What is the next **BEST** step?
- A. Emphasize healthy lifestyle to reduce risk factors.
- B. Start aspirin 81 mg daily.
- C. Routine 6-month follow-up in clinic.
- D. Start atorvastatin 20 mg.

96.3 A 60-year-old male presents to primary care clinic for a routine follow-up appointment. He has no history of diabetes but has a persistently elevated low-density lipoprotein (LDL) of 150 mg/dL despite diet and lifestyle modifications. His ASCVD risk is calculated and found to be 10%, but the patient is undecided about starting statin therapy because he has heard about negative side effects including liver problems and myositis. Based on 2018/2019 ACC/AHA (American College of Cardiology/American Heart Association) guidelines, what is the next **BEST** step to discuss with patient?
- A. Obtain coronary artery calcium (CAC) screening to help guide decision-making.
- B. Start moderate-intensity statin regardless of concerns.
- C. Only emphasize diet and lifestyle modifications.
- D. Start Zetia as first-line option.

96.4 Which of the following is **NOT** a tool for calculating risk stratification for ASCVD?
- A. Pooled Cohort Equation (PCE)
- B. Systemic Coronary Risk Evaluation (SCORE)
- C. Quantification of Risk Assessment Tool 3 (QRISK3)
- D. quick Sequential Organ Failure Assessment (qSOFA)

*Questions and Answers are based on Chapter 96: Cardiovascular Disease Risk Assessment in Clinical Practice by Miguel Cainzos-Achirica, Karan Kapoor, Tanuja Rajan, and Roger S. Blumenthal in Cardiovascular Medicine and Surgery, First Edition.

96.5 Which test helped to establish the prognostic value of a CAC score of zero?

A. QRISK3
B. Multiethnic Study of Atherosclerosis Risk Score (MESA)
C. SCORE
D. PCE

96.6 A 55-year-old White male with no history of smoking, significant cardiac family history, or diabetes is found to have a 10-year ASCVD risk score of 6.5%. The decision is made to have a CAC score, which subsequently comes back at 150. What is the next **BEST** step at today's visit?

A. Start atorvastatin 20 mg daily along with baby aspirin.
B. Start aspirin daily only.
C. Dietary changes only
D. Recommend 5 times per week cardiovascular exercise alone with no medical therapy.

96.7 Which of the following is **NOT** an appropriate modality for noninvasive ASCVD risk stratification by 2019 ESC (European Society of Cardiology) guidelines?

A. Femoral arterial plaque burden
B. Carotid intima-media thickness (CIMT)
C. Transthoracic echocardiogram (TTE)
D. CAC score

96.8 Which of the following modalities for risk stratification should **NOT** be done on asymptomatic individuals solely for the purpose of risk assessment?

A. CAC score
B. Cardiac computed tomographic angiography (CCTA)
C. PCE
D. SCORE

96.9 Which of the following subgroups is **NOT** considered a special population that may require additional screening or testing for ASCVD risk assessment?

A. Women
B. Under 40 years of age
C. Low socioeconomic status
D. Over 70 years of age

96.10 Which of the following is **NOT** a risk-enhancing factor for the 2019 ACC/AHA guidelines for primary prevention of ASCVD?

A. Metabolic syndrome
B. History of preeclampsia in previous pregnancy
C. High-sensitivity C-reaction protein (CRP) greater than 1.5
D. Ankle-brachial index (ABI) less than 0.9

ANSWERS

96.1 The correct answer is C.
Rationale: In the United States, routine risk estimation for primary prevention is recommended between ages 40 and 75. In Europe, risk factor screening for ASCVD risk stratification is recommended for men older than 40, and women older than 50, or who are postmenopausal. Traditional ASCVD risk factor evaluation is recommended every 4 to 6 years starting at age 20 years; 30-year risk estimate can be calculated up to age 59 years old.

96.2 The correct answer is D.
Rationale: In patients aged 40 to 75 without diabetes and an ASCVD risk score between 7.5% and less than 20%, moderate-intensity statin (eg, atorvastatin 20 mg) to reduce LDL-C by 30% to 49% should be implemented. If ambiguity persists, consider a CAC screening score. Statin therapy should be considered if levels are between 1 and 99, and statin therapy is initiated for CAC greater than 100. Diet and lifestyle modification should always be encouraged with medical therapy.

96.3 The correct answer is A.
Rationale: Guidelines currently would favor starting statin therapy for primary prevention in patients between 40 and 75 years of age with an elevated LDL and ASCVD risk score greater than 7.5%. However, given this patient does not have diabetes, and/or if the risk decision is uncertain, it would be appropriate to consider CAC scoring. If the coronary artery disease (CAD) is 0, statin therapy is not mandated, unless smoking or family history is a factor. A CAC of 1 to 99 favors statin especially in patients greater than age 55. For those who have a CAC greater than 100, statin therapy should be implemented regardless of age or other factors.

96.4 The correct answer is D.
Rationale: The PCE has been recommended by ACC/AHA since 2013 to predict 10-year atherosclerotic events. The SCORE has been recommended for use by ESC/EAS (European Atherosclerosis Society) to predict an individual's 10-year risk of fatal ASCVD events. QRISK3 is typically used in the United Kingdom, which uses the health information of 4 million British men and women; there may be an advantage to this given that it is using data specific to a specific region. qSOFA is a tool used to quickly identify sepsis-related organ failure and is not a tool to be used in the risk stratification of ASCVD.

96.5 The correct answer is B.
Rationale: MESA is a multiethnic prospective cohort study of U.S. adults free of cardiovascular disease (CVD) where all the participants initially underwent CAC scoring. Baseline CAC burden was independently associated with incident events after more than 10 years of follow-up. CAC also demonstrated incremental prognostic value beyond previous traditional risk factors at predicting future outcomes.

96.6 The correct answer is A.

Rationale: Given the patient's borderline risk score, the appropriate decision was made to obtain a CAC score. Patients with CAC of 0 and no additional risk factors likely do not need to start statin therapy. Those with scores of 1 to 99 should be considered for statin therapy, and those with scores over 100 should be started on at least moderate-intensity statin. While diet and exercise are extremely important, this degree of CAC would benefit from statin therapy for additional risk reduction of ASCVD events. Starting baby aspirin without starting statin therapy would not be the best choice (**Figure 96.1**).

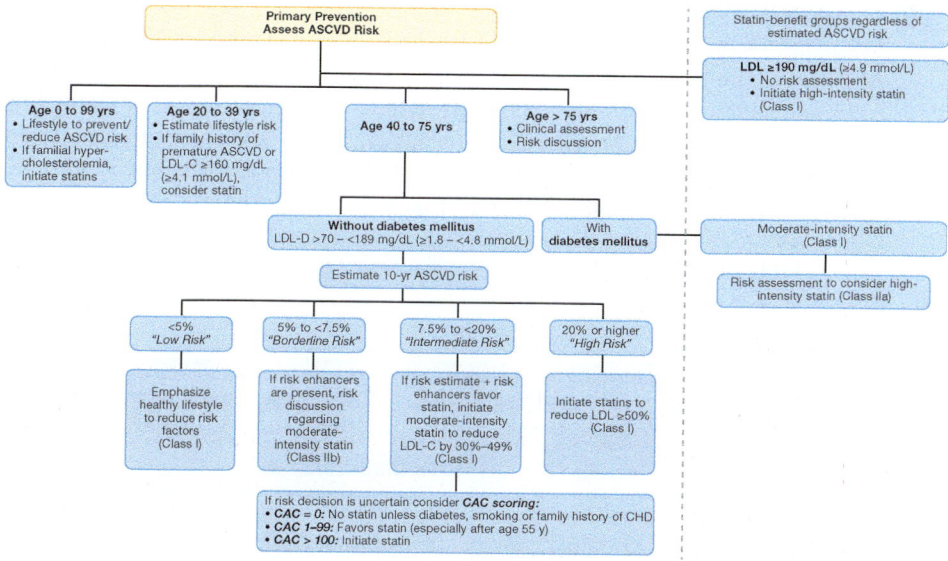

Figure 96.1 Risk assessment algorithm recommended in 2018/2019 ACC/AHA Guidelines. ASCVD, atherosclerotic cardiovascular disease; CAC, coronary artery calcium; LDL, low-density lipoprotein. (Reprinted with permission from Grundy SM, Stone NJ, Bailey AL, et al. 2018 AHA/ACC/AACVPR/AAPA/ABC/ACPM/ADA/AGS/APhA/ASPC/NLA/PCNA guideline on the management of blood cholesterol: a report of the American College of Cardiology/American Heart Association Task Force on Clinical Practice Guidelines. *Circulation.* 2018;139(25):e1082-e1143. ©2018 American Heart Association, Inc.)

96.7 The correct answer is C.

Rationale: Femoral arterial plaque burden, CIMT, and CAC scores are all appropriate noninvasive modalities for ASCVD risk stratification. CIMT demonstrated a 9% increase in future ASCVD for each 0.1-mm increase in CIMT thickness. There is a Class IIa, LOE B (Level of Evidence B) for the assessment of arterial plaque (carotid and/or femoral) as a potential modifier in individuals at low or intermediate risk. The net reclassification significantly improved with either carotid plaque burden (0.23) or CAC (0.25), with major adverse cardiovascular events (MACE) rates increasing in the setting of higher carotid plaque burden and higher CAC.

96.8 The correct answer is B.

Rationale: The ability of CCTA to detect noncalcified plaque makes it an attractive test for potential ASCVD risk assessment. However, studies on the added prognostic value of CCTA beyond traditional risk factors for risk assessment are scarce. No societal body recommends using CCTA in *asymptomatic* individuals for risk assessment alone.

96.9 The correct answer is D.

Rationale: Risk assessment in special populations needs to be monitored closely as they have specific characteristics that may be associated with increased ASCVD risk for fatal and nonfatal cardiac events. These groups include women with a history of premature menopause, and women in the job market with increased levels of stress and workplace conflicts. Other groups include patients less than 40 years old, patients greater than 75 years of age, as well as patients with low socioeconomic status which makes them particularly vulnerable to ASCVD.

96.10 The correct answer is C.

Rationale: Demographic and clinical features associated with a higher average ASCVD risk (at the group level) are labeled "risk-enhancing factors," by the ACC/AHA guidelines, and "risk modifiers" by the ESC/EAS. These include a family history of coronary heart disease (CHD)/ASCVD, South Asian ancestry, increased levels of circulating lipoprotein [a], chronic kidney disease, metabolic syndrome, history of preeclampsia, and ABI less than 0.9, among others. High-sensitivity C-reactive protein of greater than or equal to 2.0 is also listed as a risk-enhancing factor (**Table 96.1**).

TABLE 96.1 Risk-Enhancing Factors and Risk Modifiers Included in Relevant 2018/2019 ACC/AHA and the 2019 ESC/EAS Guidelines

Risk-Enhancing Factors	Risk Modifiers
2018 Multi-Society Guideline on the Management of Cholesterol and 2019 ACC/AHA Guideline on the Primary Prevention of ASCVD	2019 ESC/EAS Guidelines for the Management of Dyslipidaemias
Family history of premature ASCVD	Family history of premature CVD
Primary hypercholesterolemia (LDL-C ≥160 mg/dL)	
Metabolic syndrome	
	Obesity and central obesity
Chronic kidney disease	Chronic kidney disease
Chronic inflammatory conditions (rheumatoid arthritis, advanced psoriasis, systemic lupus erythematosus, HIV infection)	Chronic immune-mediated inflammatory disorders; treatment for HIV infection
History of premature menopause and history of pregnancy-associated conditions that increase later ASCVD risk such as preeclampsia	
High-risk race/ethnicity (eg, South Asian ancestry, Native American)	
Persistently elevated primary hypertriglyceridemia (≥175 mg/dL, nonfasting)	Increased triglycerides
High-sensitivity C-reactive protein ≥2.0 mg/L	Increased high-sensitivity C-reactive protein

TABLE 96.1 Risk-Enhancing Factors and Risk Modifiers Included in Relevant 2018/2019 ACC/AHA and the 2019 ESC/EAS Guidelines *(continued)*

Risk-Enhancing Factors	Risk Modifiers
Lp(a) ≥50 mg/dL or ≥125 nmol/L	Extreme Lp(a) elevation; Lp(a) should be considered in selected patients with a family history of premature CVD and for reclassification in people who are borderline between moderate and high risk.
ApoB ≥130 mg/dL	Increased ApoB
Ankle-brachial index <0.9	Ankle-brachial index <0.9 or >1.4
	Presence of albuminuria
CAC score not listed as a risk-enhancing factor	CAC score >100
	Presence of carotid or femoral plaque
	Social deprivation
	Physical inactivity
	Psychosocial stress including vital exhaustion
	Major psychiatric disorders
	Atrial fibrillation
	Left ventricular hypertrophy
	Obstructive sleep apnea
	Nonalcoholic fatty liver disease

ACC, American College of Cardiology; AHA, American Heart Association; ApoB, apolipoprotein B; ASCVD, atherosclerotic cardiovascular disease events; CAC, coronary artery calcium; CVD, cardiovascular disease; EAS, European Atherosclerosis Society; ESC, European Society of Cardiology; HIV, human immunodeficiency virus; LDL-C, low-density lipoprotein cholesterol; Lp(a), lipoprotein a.

LIFESTYLE IMPLEMENTATION FOR CARDIOVASCULAR DISEASE PREVENTION: A FOCUS ON SMOKING CESSATION, DIET, AND PHYSICAL ACTIVITY*

Jacqueline S. Coppola, Joshua Schulman-Marcus, and Sulagna Mookherjee

CHAPTER 97

QUESTIONS

97.1 According to "Life's Simple 7," optimum health is defined as the presence of ideal values for all the following **EXCEPT**:
   A. Smoking cessation for more than 6 months
   B. Heart-healthy diet
   C. Body mass index (BMI) less than 25 kg/m^2
   D. Total cholesterol less than 200 mg/dL

97.2 Smoking leads to which of the following?
   A. Hemophilia states
   B. Decreased inflammation
   C. Endothelial dysfunction and injury
   D. Reduced risk of thrombosis

97.3 In 2019, what percentage of the U.S. adult population continued to smoke cigarettes?
   A. 6%
   B. 14%
   C. 27%
   D. 39%

97.4 When discussing smoking cessation advice and treatment, which of these accurately describes the 5 A method?
   A. Approach/Accept/Access/Accuse/Action
   B. Adapt/Address/Advice/Agree/Aim
   C. Ask/Advise/Assess/Assist/Arrange
   D. Allow/Alter/Analyze/Announce/Answer

97.5 Which of the following foods and recommended consumption is **CORRECT**?
   A. Sodium—moderation
   B. Legumes—caution
   C. Lean meat—high
   D. Coffee—moderation

97.6 Which of the following diets is associated with significantly lower cardiovascular disease (CVD) incidence and CVD/all-cause mortality?

---

*Questions and Answers are based on Chapter 97: Lifestyle Implementation for Cardiovascular Disease Prevention: A Focus on Smoking Cessation, Diet, and Physical Activity by Oluwaseun E. Fashanu, Gowtham R. Grandhi, and Erin D. Michos in Cardiovascular Medicine and Surgery, First Edition.

A. Vegetarian diet
B. Mediterranean diet
C. Ketogenic diet
D. Dietary approaches to stop hypertension (DASH) diet

97.7 Which of the following is **NOT TRUE** regarding physical activity and fitness?
A. About half of the U.S. population does not achieve recommended activity.
B. Physical activity has reduced the risk of some cancer types.
C. It would increase the economic burden of CVD.
D. It affects various aspects of health including mental health.

97.8 Which of the following accurately matches the type of exercise, metabolic equivalents (METs) achieved, and intensity level of the exercise?
A. Recreational swimming—3.0 to 5.9—moderate
B. Driving—1.6 to 2.9—sedentary
C. Jogging—3.0 to 5.9—vigorous
D. Walking briskly—less than 1.5—light

97.9 Special considerations are made for children and adolescents. How much physical activity is recommended by the 2018 Physical Activity Guideline for children and adolescents?
A. 30 minutes of moderate activity 5 times per week
B. 90 minutes of vigorous activity 3 times per week
C. 45 minutes of moderate to vigorous activity on weekdays

97.10 Which of the following is **NOT** a form of nicotine replacement therapy (NRT) for patients interested in smoking cessation?
A. Lozenge
B. Emollient cream
C. Nasal spray
D. Oral inhalers

ANSWERS

97.1 The correct answer is A.
Rationale: All are correct answer choices except A. To achieve their 2020 impact goal, the American Heart Association (AHA) developed the concept of "Life's Simple 7," which defined seven modifiable risk factors that contribute to cardiovascular (CV) health. Optimal CV health is defined by at least 5 of 7 metrics: not smoking or smoking cessation for more than 12 months, heart-healthy diet, BMI less than 25 kg/m^2, total cholesterol less than 200 mg/dL, optimal physical activity levels, blood pressure (BP) less than 120/80 mm Hg, glucose less than 100 mg/dL, and absence of clinical atherosclerotic cardiovascular disease (ASCVD). Based on recent data, none of the U.S. adult population met ideal levels of all seven metrics, with only 5% meeting six ideal metrics, and approximately 41% having two or less.

972. The correct answer is C.
Rationale: Smoking leads to oxidative stress, increased sympathetic activation, endothelial dysfunction/injury, inflammation, and hypercoagulable states, leading to increased atherogenesis and increased thrombosis risk with resultant CVD. Smoking cessation reduces the risk of CVD morbidity and mortality as well as all-cause mortality.

973. The correct answer is B.
Rationale: There has been a decline in the proportion of U.S. adults who smoke in recent years. Nevertheless, in 2019, about 34.1 million representing 14% of the U.S. adult population continued to smoke cigarettes. Cigarette smoking remains the leading cause of preventable disease and mortality in the United States according to the 2020 U.S. Surgeon General report and has been the focus of public health interventions in recent times.

974. The correct answer is C.
Rationale: As outlined in the 2019 ACC (American College of Cardiology)/AHA Guideline for primary prevention, tobacco use should be addressed at every visit and individuals who smoke should be counseled to quit. One approach that has been shown to be effective is the Five As method, which consists of Ask, Advise, Assess, Assist, and Arrange. All patients should be asked about tobacco use. Readiness to quit should be assessed at every visit; counseling, pharmacotherapy, and referrals to assist with quitting should be offered. Follow-up for patients who were willing to quit should be clearly outlined. Quitting smoking should be readdressed at every visit for patients who are unwilling to quit (**Table 97.1**).

975. The correct answer is D.
Rationale: According to the table listed, the components of a heart-healthy diet consist of a high intake of leafy vegetables, fruits, whole grains, and legumes. Vegetable oils, nuts, seeds, seafood, low-fat dairy, lean meat, and coffee should all be consumed in moderation. One should exercise caution when consuming animal fat, refined grains, fruit juices, and tinned fruits. Those following a heart-healthy diet should restrict sodium, added sugars, processed red meats, and saturated and trans fats (**Table 97.2**).

TABLE 97.1 Five As Approach to Counseling Against Tobacco Use

Ask	All patients should be **asked** about tobacco use.
Advise	Tobacco users should be **advised** to quit.
Assess	Readiness to quit should be **assessed** at every visit.
Assist	Provide counseling, pharmacotherapy, and referrals to **assist** with quitting.
Arrange	**Arrange** follow-up contacts for those willing to quit and readdress quitting at follow-up for those unwilling to quit.

TABLE 97.2 Components of Heart-Healthy Diet

High	Moderation	Caution	Restrict
Leafy vegetables, fruits, whole grains, legumes	Vegetable oils, nuts, seeds, seafood, low-fat dairy, lean meat, coffee	Animal fat, refined grains, fruit juices, tinned fruits	Sodium, added sugar, processed and red meat, saturated and *trans* fats

97.6 The correct answer is B.

Rationale: Fewer CVD-related deaths are found in Mediterranean countries (eg, Greece, Spain, and Italy), when compared to the United States and northern Europe. This has kindled interest in their dietary habits. The Mediterranean diet, which is typically rich in vegetables, whole grains, fruits, nuts/seeds, legumes, and olive oil, along with moderate consumption of seafood, poultry, and low-fat dairy, is associated with significantly lower CVD incidence and CVD/all-cause mortality. Benefits of this diet were noted in 1999 in the Lyon Diet Heart Study, which explored the effect of the Mediterranean diet among individuals with myocardial infarction (MI) on secondary CVD prevention. The study reported a significant reduction in major adverse cardiac events: 54% and 72% reduction in all-cause mortality and nonfatal MI/cardiac mortality, respectively. For primary prevention, The PREDIMED (Prevention with Mediterranean Diet) randomized control trial demonstrated a 31% lower risk of MI, stroke, and CVD mortality among those assigned to the Mediterranean diet plus extra-virgin olive oil, and a 28% lower risk for the Mediterranean diet plus nuts, when compared to a low-fat diet. This study complements a prior study that demonstrated a 33% and 25% reduction in coronary heart disease (CHD) and all-cause mortality, respectively, among those who consume a Mediterranean diet.

97.7 The correct answer is C.

Rationale: According to the 2018 Physical Activity Guidelines Advisory Committee Report, about half of the U.S. population remains inactive or do not achieve the recommended levels of physical activity. Physical activity has been shown to affect various aspects of human health including, but not limited to, mental health, reduced risk of a variety of cancers, as well as improved CV health. Thus, increasing physical activity has been identified as a low-cost intervention that can reduce the burden of CVD, premature mortality, and the economic burden of CVD globally.

97.8 The correct answer is A.

Rationale: Sedentary activities are less than 1.5 METs, and examples include sitting, watching television (TV), lying, and driving. Light activity has a MET equivalent of 1.6 to 2.9 and examples include leisure walking (at <2 mph), light household chores, and cooking. Moderate activity level is when an MET level of 3.0 to 5.9 is achieved and includes walking briskly (3-4 mph), vacuuming, recreational swimming, and doubles tennis. Vigorous activity is greater than or equal to 6 METs and includes jogging, running, swimming laps, singles tennis, heavy gardening, mowing grass, and shoveling snow (**Table 97.3**).

TABLE 97.3 Intensities of Physical Activity

Intensity	Sedentary Behavior	Light	Moderate	Vigorous
METs	≤1.5	1.6-2.9	3.0-5.9	≥6
Examples	Sitting, watching TV, lying, driving	Leisure walking (≤2 mph), light household chores, cooking	Walking briskly (3-4 mph), vacuuming, recreational swimming, tennis (doubles)	Jogging, running, swimming laps, tennis (single), heavy gardening, mowing grass, snow shoveling

METs, metabolic equivalents; mph, miles per hour; TV, television.

97.9 The correct answer is D.

Rationale: The 2018 Physical Activity Guideline recommends that children and adolescents perform at least 60 minutes of moderate to vigorous activity daily, including muscle and bone strengthening physical activity. Based on 2017 data, only about 46.5% of students report having 60 minutes or more of physical activity for at least 5 days per week.

97.10 The correct answer is B.

Rationale: NRT comes in many different forms to suit the needs of patients. This includes gum, lozenges, nasal sprays, oral inhalers, and patches. Emollient cream is not one of the NRTs available for patients. A combination of both counseling and pharmacotherapy is recommended to maximize the success of quitting in nonpregnant individuals. Data on the safety of NRT in pregnant or breastfeeding mothers are limited, so NRT should be used with caution. Two non-nicotine oral medications have also been used for smoking cessation including sustained-release bupropion and varenicline (**Table 97.4**).

TABLE 97.4 U.S. Food and Drug Administration–Approved Pharmacotherapies for Smoking Cessation

Nicotine replacement therapies (NRTs)	Gum	No more than 24 gums or 20 lozenges daily
	Lozenge	If smoking occurs ≤30 min after waking start with 4 mg, otherwise use 2 mg.
	Nasal spray	No more than 40 sprays daily
	Oral inhaler	No more than 16 cartridges daily (10 mg per cartridge)
	Patch	7, 14, or 21 mg. Use 21-mg patch if smokes ≥10 cigarettes daily.
Non-nicotine oral medications	Sustained-release bupropion	150 mg titrated up to 300 mg daily. May be used in combination with other NRTs
	Varenicline	0.5 mg titrated up to 1 mg daily

DIABETES AND CARDIOMETABOLIC MEDICINE*

CHAPTER 98

Jacqueline S. Coppola, Joseph D. Sacco, and Sulagna Mookherjee

QUESTIONS

98.1 In the United States, what percentage of the population will develop type 2 diabetes mellitus (T2DM) over the course of their lifetime?

A. 15%
B. 33%
C. 25%
D. 50%

98.2 Which of the following is a characteristic of type 1 diabetes mellitus (T1DM)?

A. Associated with poor lifestyle
B. Low ketoacidosis incidence
C. Human leukocyte antigen (HLA) association
D. Obese weight

98.3 Which of the following is **NOT** a direct effect of adipose tissue on the pathogenesis in T2DM?

A. Increased free fatty acids
B. Decreased adiponectin
C. Increased cytokines and other proteins
D. Increased glucose production

98.4 Which of the following is a common symptom of diabetes mellitus (DM)?

A. Acanthosis nigricans
B. Increased energy
C. Decreased urinary output
D. Improved wound healing

98.5 Which of the following laboratory values confirms the diagnosis of DM?

A. Hemoglobin A1c (HbA1c) of 6.0%
B. Symptoms with random plasma glucose of 175 mg/dL
C. Fasting plasma glucose of 135 mg/dL
D. 2-hour plasma glucose after oral glucose test of 180 mg/dL

---

*Questions and Answers are based on Chapter 98: Diabetes and Cardiometabolic Medicine by Cara Reiter-Brennan, Omar Dzaye, and Michael J. Blaha in Cardiovascular Medicine and Surgery, First Edition.

98.6 A 65-year-old male with a past medical history of heart failure and myocardial infarction is presenting to your clinic today for an annual physical examination. After reviewing his routine labs for this appointment, you notice his A1c has increased from 6.4% to 7.3%. According to the 2019 American Diabetes Association/European Association for the Study of Diabetes (ADA/EASD) Standards of Medical Care, which of the following medications should be started as a first-line agent?

   A. Metformin
   B. Linagliptin
   C. Pioglitazone
   D. Empagliflozin

98.7 Which medication is **CORRECTLY** paired with its appropriate side effect?

   A. Glucagon-like peptide 1 receptor agonist GLP1-RA—medullary thyroid tumors
   B. Dipeptidyl peptidase 4 inhibitors (DPP-4 inhibitors)—bladder cancer
   C. Metformin—weight gain
   D. Sodium-glucose cotransporter-2 (SGLT2) inhibitors—pancreatitis

98.8 Drugs that lower cardiovascular disease (CVD) risk including all the following **EXCEPT:**

   A. GLP1-RAs
   B. Metformin
   C. DPP-4 inhibitors
   D. SGLT2 inhibitors

98.9 By how much can insulin reduce HbA1c levels in patients with T2DM?

   A. Up to 4.9%
   B. Up to 2.3%
   C. Up to 6.7%
   D. Up to 1.5%

98.10 What is the leading cause of morbidity and mortality in patients with type 1 diabetes?

   A. Peripheral vascular disease
   B. Diabetic kidney disease
   C. Atherosclerotic cardiovascular disease (ASCVD)
   D. Neuropathy

98.11 Stress-induced hyperglycemia affects up to what percentage of post-cardiac surgery patients?

   A. 10%
   B. 25%
   C. 40%
   D. 75%

ANSWERS

98.1 **The correct answer is B.**
Rationale: Over the course of their lifetime, about 33% or 1/3 of the population will develop T2DM. DM is one of the leading causes of death worldwide (30%) and CVD-related deaths account for 70% of all deaths among patient with DM. T2DM is the most common form of DM (>90%), whereas T1DM makes up about 5% of all patients with DM.

98.2 **The correct answer is C.**
Rationale: T1DM makes up 5% of all diabetic cases. Research suggests that T1DM is caused by an autoimmune response, often triggered by a viral infection. The most common antibodies found in patients with T1DM are anti-glutamic acid decarboxylase (anti-GAD) antibodies, which target GAD, an enzyme found in the pancreatic cell. These promote the destruction of insulin-producing beta-cells in the pancreas, ultimately resulting in absolute insulin deficiency. The age of onset of T1DM is usually during childhood and adolescence. T1DM is not typically associated with a poor lifestyle. Most patients with T1DM are thin or normal weight. The incidence of ketoacidosis in patients with T1DM is high. Therapy requires insulin in all cases. All other choices are characteristics of T2DM (**Table 98.1**).

TABLE 98.1   Differential Diagnosis of Type 1 and Type 2 Diabetes Mellitus

	Type 1 Diabetes Mellitus	Type 2 Diabetes Mellitus
Proportion of all diabetic cases (%)	5	95
Pathogenesis	Absolute insulin deficiency	Relative insulin deficiency and insulin resistance
Genetics	Human leukocyte antigen (HLA) association	No HLA association, but strong genetic disposition
Age of onset	Primarily childhood and adolescence	Predominantly >40 y of age, but rising incidence among youths <20 y of age (4.8% per year increase among individuals <20 y)
Associated with poor lifestyle	No	Yes
Weight	Thin or normal weight	Obese
Ketoacidosis incidence	High	Low
Therapy	Insulin required	Lifestyle, antidiabetic medication—insulin

98.3 The correct answer is D.

Rationale: Expanded visceral mass leads to an increase in free fatty acids and other cytokines and proteins that inhibit insulin action, as well as a decrease in factors that enhance insulin signaling, such as adiponectin. These changes result in blocking the action of insulin in the liver and skeletal muscle at the level of the insulin receptor and at postreceptor signaling sites. This results in a failure of insulin to suppress hepatic glucose production and to promote glucose uptake into the muscle. The resulting hyperglycemia normally increases insulin secretion by pancreatic beta-cells. In patients with T2DM, the combination of resistance to insulin action and a genetically determined impairment of the beta-cell response to elevated glucose levels results in hyperglycemia and subsequent T2DM (**Figure 98.1**).

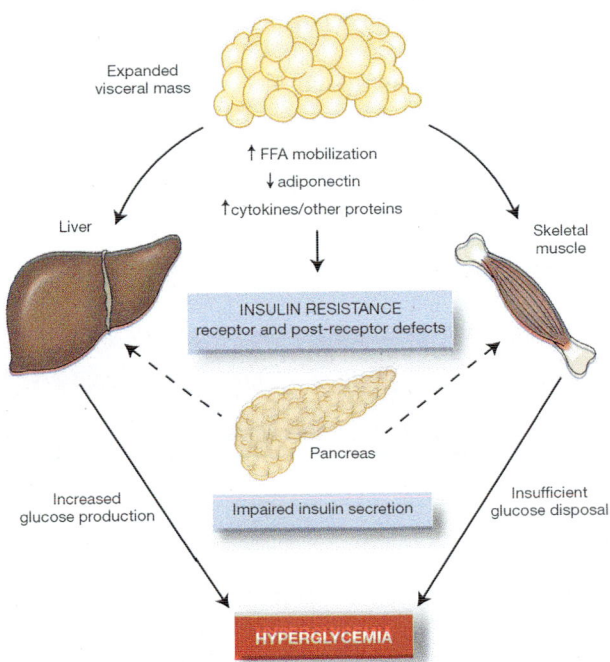

Figure 98.1 Pathogenesis of type 2 diabetes mellitus (T2DM). Pathogenesis of obesity-related T2DM. The expanded visceral fat mass in upper body obesity elaborates several factors that contribute to tissue insulin resistance. These include an increase in circulating free (nonesterified) fatty acids (FFAs) and other cytokines and proteins that inhibit insulin action, as well as a decrease in factors that enhance insulin signaling, such as adiponectin. These changes result in a block to insulin action in the liver and skeletal muscle at the level of the insulin receptor and at postreceptor signaling sites, resulting in a failure of insulin to suppress hepatic glucose production and to promote glucose uptake into muscle. The resulting hyperglycemia is normally countered by increased insulin secretion by pancreatic beta-cells. In persons with T2DM, the combination of resistance to insulin action and a genetically determined impairment of the beta-cell response to hyperglycemia results in hyperglycemia, and T2DM ensues. (Reprinted with permission from Rubin R, Strayer DS, Rubin E. *Rubin's Pathology: Clinicopathologic Foundations of Medicine*. 6th ed. Wolters Kluwer Health/Lippincott Williams & Wilkins; 2011, Figure 22.5.)

98.4 The correct answer is A.
Rationale: The other choices are typical symptoms of DM including polyuria, polydipsia, polyphagia, fatigue, calf cramps, visual impairment, disturbed wound healing, and pruritus. Weight loss is commonly seen in T1DM. Benign acanthosis nigricans is commonly seen in T2DM.

98.5 The correct answer is C.
Rationale: The diagnosis of DM includes typical symptoms of hyperglycemia and random plasma glucose greater than or equal to 200 mg/dL, HbA1c greater than or equal to 6.5%, fasting plasma glucose greater than or equal to 126 mg/dL, or a 2-hour plasma glucose after oral glucose tolerance testing greater than or equal to 200 mg/dL.

98.6 The correct answer is D.
Rationale: The 2019 ADA/EASD Standards of Medical Care recommends an individualized approach to pharmacologic therapy of DM in which cardiovascular comorbidities, body weight, side effects, risk of hypoglycemia, cost, and patient preference should all be considered. In this patient, with new onset T2DM and a history of heart failure, SGLT2 inhibitors, or empagliflozin, should be the preferred first-line agent to treat DM. In 2019, the European Society of Cardiology (ESC) guidelines recommended SGLT2 inhibitors or GLP1-RA monotherapy to metformin naïve patients with ASCVD or high-CVD risk.

98.7 The correct answer is A.
Rationale: GLP1-RAs have an U.S. Food and Drug Administration (FDA) Black Box warning of causing medullary thyroid c-cell tumors. Thiazolidinediones, specifically pioglitazone, are associated with bladder cancer. Metformin has a known association with lactic acidosis and gastrointestinal (GI) side effects. SLGT2 inhibitors may cause genital yeast and urinary tract infections.

98.8 The correct answer is C.
Rationale: Medications that lower CVD risk include metformin, SGLT2 inhibitors, and GLP1-RAs. Metformin can also promote weight reduction (2%-3%), has no harmful effects on the cardiovascular system, and may benefit patients with heart failure. SGLT2 inhibitors have demonstrated the reduction of heart failure-related end points and progression of kidney disease in patients with T2DM. GLP1-RAs have demonstrated high efficacy in reducing hyperglycemia as well as cardiovascular benefits, are associated with marked weight loss, and show few severe side effects. DPP-4 inhibitors have only moderate glycemic reduction without any consistent cardiac risk reduction.

98.9 The correct answer is A.
Rationale: Insulin can reduce HbA1c levels up to 4.9% in patients with T2DM. Therapy intensification through the addition of insulin to oral regimens offers many benefits including a reduction in HbA1c levels; one study reviewed that those on a combination of insulin and metformin insulin and metformin had fewer incidences of hypoglycemia along with less weight gain.

98.10 The correct answer is C.
Rationale: ASCVD is the leading cause of morbidity and mortality in patients with DM. In addition, individuals with DM are at risk of suffering from heart failure, and evidence has suggested that rates for hospitalization from heart failure are 2-fold higher in patients with DM.

98.11 The correct answer is C.
Rationale: Stress-induced hyperglycemia affects up to 40% of patients after cardiac surgery, irrespective of diabetic status, and is associated with higher in-hospital mortality and morbidity. Interestingly, moderate glycemic control is sufficient to improve outcomes as tight glycemic control (<140 mg/dL) during cardiac surgery was associated with increased complications. A perioperative blood glucose level of more than 150 and less than 180 mg/dL sustained through a continuous intravenous (IV) infusion pump for cardiac surgery patients with DM is recommended. During the Intensive Care Unit (ICU) stay, a blood glucose level between 150 and 180 mg/dL should be maintained for patients with and without DM.

LIPID DISORDERS

Jacqueline S. Coppola, Joseph D. Sacco, and Sulagna Mookherjee

CHAPTER 99

QUESTIONS

99.1 What percentage of the U.S. population has total cholesterol levels greater than 240 mg/dL?

   A. 7%
   B. 12%
   C. 26%
   D. 43%
   E. 55%

99.2 Which of the following is **NOT** identified as a secondary cause of dyslipidemia?

   A. Pregnancy
   B. Preeclampsia
   C. Early onset menopause
   D. HIV
   E. Hypothyroidism

99.3 What is the purpose of the endogenous pathway of lipid metabolism that occurs in the liver?

   A. Where fatty acids are absorbed and repackaged into apoB-48-containing TG (triglyceride)-rich chylomicrons
   B. Location where chylomicrons are broken down by lipoprotein lipase
   C. Production of triacylglycerol (TAG)-rich very low-density lipoprotein (VLDL) that transport TG and cholesterol to target tissues
   D. Extracellular lipoprotein lipase degrades TAG in VLDL.
   E. Apo C-II and ape E are returned to high-density lipoprotein (HDL).

99.4 In which of the following scenarios should lipid-lowering therapy be initiated?

   A. 45-year-old healthy male with apolipoprotein B (apoB) levels less than 1.5 g/L and TG levels less than 1.5 mmol/L
   B. 26-year-old female who is obese and currently pregnant
   C. 47-year-old male with no significant past medical history and low-density lipoprotein C (LDL-C) of 145 mg/dL
   D. 50-year-old female with coronary artery calcium (CAC) score of 110 Agatston units
   E. 60-year-old male with CAC of 0, and atherosclerotic cardiovascular disease (ASCVD) risk of 5%

*Questions and Answers are based on Chapter 99: Lipid Disorders by Bibin Varghese, Renato Quispe, and Seth S. Martin in Cardiovascular Medicine and Surgery, First Edition.

99.5 A 55-year-old male with a past medical history of myocardial infarction (MI) status-post left anterior descending (LAD) stent, type 2 diabetes mellitus, and obesity is presenting for follow-up after hospitalization 3 months later. His medications include atorvastatin 80 mg, dual-antiplatelet therapy, low-dose beta-blocker, and metformin. He has been adhering to diet and lifestyle modifications since his event and has lost 10 pounds since his admission. Labs are obtained prior to his visit, and it is noted that on his lipid panel that his LDL-C is 86 mg/dL. What is the next step at this visit?

    A. Continue diet and lifestyle modifications only.
    B. Add alirocumab 75 mg SQ (subcutaneous) every 2 weeks to his regimen.
    C. Add ezetimibe 10 mg once daily.
    D. Add cholestyramine 3,750 mg once daily.
    E. Add niacin 1,000 mg once daily.

99.6 A 70-year-old female with history of hypertriglyceridemia was started on a new medication about 3 months ago and is presenting to the emergency department with complaints of right-sided abdominal pain. Ultrasound of her abdomen reveals cholelithiasis. She cannot remember the names of her medications. Which medication was likely started 3 months ago, given her current presentation to the emergency department?

    A. Cholestyramine
    B. Icosapent ethyl
    C. Niacin
    D. Ezetimibe
    E. Fenofibrate

99.7 An 80-year-old male with a past medical history of hyperlipidemia and obesity has been following recently with a new geriatrician. You received a call from his doctor with concerns of polypharmacy, and he is requesting to discontinue some of his medications, specifically his atorvastatin 40 mg. His most recent LDL-C is 95 mg/dL. Patient has never had adverse effects from the medication. He has no history of peripheral vascular disease (PVD), MI, or cardiovascular accident (CVA). What is your recommendation to the geriatrician?

    A. Stop atorvastatin.
    B. Decrease dose to 20 mg.
    C. Decrease dose to 10 mg.
    D. Continue atorvastatin at current dose.
    E. Add ezetimibe.

99.8 A 55-year-old female with elevated CAC, 1,000 Agatston units, was recently started on atorvastatin 80 mg daily about 1 month ago. She presents to your office with complaints of myalgias and would like to discuss the side-effect profile of this medication with you. In addition to discussion and education with the patient, what is your next **BEST** step?

    A. Check creatinine kinase (CK) level.
    B. Decrease to atorvastatin 40 mg.
    C. Change to rosuvastatin 20 mg.
    D. Stop all lipid-lowering therapies.
    E. Send patient home with follow-up in 2 weeks.

99.9 A 60-year-old female with a past medical history of type 2 diabetes mellitus, unspecified hyperlipidemia, and hypertension has recently transferred to your office to establish ongoing outpatient care. Her current medications include metformin 1,000 mg daily, atorvastatin 80 mg, and lisinopril 10 mg. Her vital signs are all stable today with a heart rate of 78 beats per minute (bpm), blood pressure 119/76 mm Hg, and normal respiratory rate and temperature. She reports during the visit that she has **NOT** been regularly followed by any physician and does **NOT** recall the last time she had routine labs drawn. You order a lipid panel, HgbA1c, complete blood count, and comprehensive metabolic panel. Her total cholesterol is 148 mg/dL, HDL is 56 mg/dL, and her TGs are 375 mg/dL. What is your next recommendation to the patient?

A. Continue current medication regimen.
B. Change atorvastatin 80 mg to rosuvastatin 40 mg.
C. Stop statin therapy.
D. Discuss with patient addition of proprotein convertase subtilisin/kexin type 9 (PCSK9) inhibitors.
E. Start *n*-3 long-chain fatty acid, icosapent ethyl

99.10 Which of the following is an absolute contraindication for initiation of PCSK9 inhibitors?

A. Active malignancy
B. Atrial fibrillation
C. Declining medication by patient
D. Gout
E. All of the above

ANSWERS

99.1 **The correct answer is B.**
Rationale: More than 12% of the U.S. population, about 29 million people, have total cholesterol levels greater than 240 mg/dL. 7% of U.S. adolescents, ages 6 to 19, have high cholesterol. Only 55% of the patients eligible for lipid-lowering therapy are currently taking it.

99.2 **The correct answer is A.**
Rationale: All of the following including diabetes mellitus, hypothyroidism, medications, chronic kidney disease, nephrotic syndrome, cirrhosis, inflammatory diseases (rheumatoid arthritis, psoriasis, HIV), premature menopause, and preeclampsia should be considered in the right clinical context as contributors to dyslipidemia. Nonmodifiable risk factors such as age, sex, family history, and ethnicity should also be considered.

99.3 **The correct answer is C.**
Rationale: The endogenous pathway occurs in the liver and is responsible for the production of TAG-rich VLDL that transport TG and cholesterol to target tissues. A and B are both part of the endogenous pathway, where lipid metabolism begins, occurring in the intestines. D occurs in tissues (adipose), and E occurs in circulation as byproducts of the breakdown of intermediate-density lipoprotein (IDL) (**Figure 99.1**).

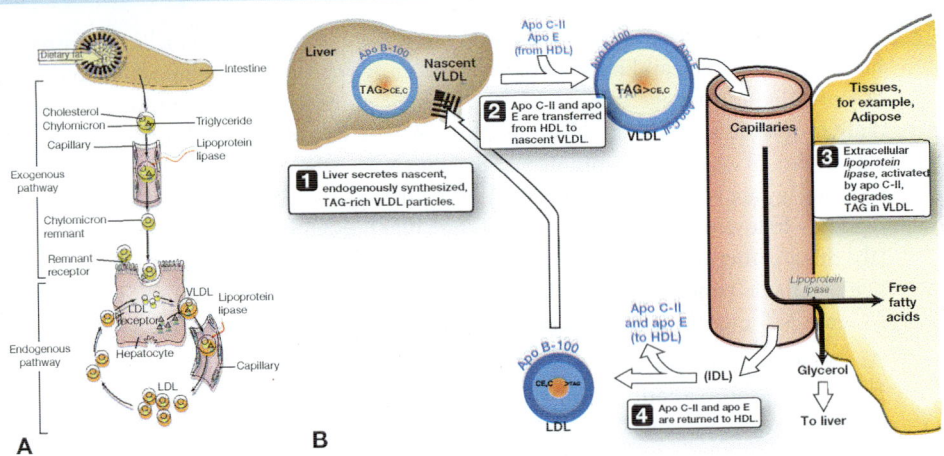

Figure 99.1 Lipid metabolism begins with exogenous dietary intake of triglycerides (TGs) and cholesterol-rich foods that are metabolized, absorbed, and repackaged into chylomicrons in intestinal epithelial cells. These particles are secreted into the lymphatic system and enter the circulation. The liver also produces endogenous triacylglycerol (TAG-rich) very low-density lipoprotein (VLDL) particles that transport TG and cholesterol to target tissues. Lipoprotein lipase (LPL) found on endothelial cells breaks down TG from chylomicrons and VLDL. Once the TGs are processed, lipid and apolipoprotein exchanges occur with high-density lipoprotein (HDL), which results in the formation of remnant particles. Remnant chylomicron particles are taken up by the liver. After TG breakdown and HDL exchanges, VLDL remnant particles are called intermediate-density lipoprotein (IDL). The IDL particles are either taken up by the liver or undergo reaction with hepatic lipase and further lipid exchanges with HDL to form LDL. (**A**: Adapted with permission from Rubin E, Farber JL. *Pathology*. 3rd ed. Lippincott Williams & Wilkins; 1999, Figure 10.18; **B**: Adapted with permission from Harvey RA, Ferrier DR. *Lippincott Illustrated Reviews: Biochemistry*. 5th ed. Wolters Kluwer Health/Lippincott Williams & Wilkins; 2010, Figure 18.17.)

99.4 The correct answer is D.

Rationale: Reasons to consider initiation of lipid-lowering therapies include patients with LDL-C greater than 190 mg/dL, or age 40 to 75 years old with diabetes and LDL-C greater than or equal to 70 mg/dL, and CAC scores greater than 99 Agatston units. Special consideration, such as cigarette smoking, secondary causes of dislipoproteinemias, and familial lipid disorders—such as familial hypercholesterolemia (FH) or type III hyperlipidemia, should also be considered before deferring therapies.

99.5 The correct answer is C.

Rationale: While diet and lifestyle modification should be commended and absolutely continued, his LDL-C is still not at goal (≤70 mg/dL) after his event. Adjunct therapy is needed. Ezetimibe is an add-on therapy to statins for patients at high risk who do not meet their LDL-C goal. Ezetimibe typically lowers LDL-C 15% to 20% and would likely bring his LDL-C below 70 mg/dL. PCSK9 inhibitors and bile acid sequestrants are third- and fourth-line agents, respectively (added to statin + ezetimibe), to achieve LDL goal. Niacin is usually no longer recommended due to side-effect profile and lack of benefit.

99.6 The correct answer is E.

Rationale: Side-effect profile of fibrates, including fenofibrate and gemfibrozil, includes muscle injury and cholelithiasis. Side effects of cholestyramine include constipation and gastrointestinal (GI) upset, and icosapent ethyl causes diarrhea; however, only fibrates have been known to cause cholelithiasis. Fibrates decrease the synthesis and excretion of bile acid, therefore making it easier for cholesterol to precipitate and thereby increasing the risk of gallstones (**Table 99.1**).

99.7 The correct answer is D.

Rationale: For patients older than 75 years of age, there is established evidence of beneficial effects of statin therapy for secondary prevention but less so for primary prevention. However, guidelines recommend continuing high-intensity statin therapy for patients older than 75 years if there is no intolerance to the drug. This patient is tolerating this medication well, so therefore stopping the medication or reduction to a low- or moderate-intensity statin should not be recommended. There is no indication for addition of ezetimibe, as patient is not high risk, and his goal LDL is less than or equal to 100 mg/dL.

99.8 The correct answer is A.

Rationale: Myalgias are the most commonly reported side effect of statin therapy, but causality is often unclear. If there are concerns about statin-induced myalgias, as in this case, a plasma CK level should be checked. If normal, dose adjustments to the statin should be attempted. If the patient cannot tolerate the lowest possible dose, an alternative statin should be trialed. If the patient remains intolerant, a detailed history of all medications and conditions should occur. If no alternative explanation exists, then statin should be discontinued. A plan to rechallenge statin therapy should be considered and trialed again in the future. If CK levels are elevated on the initial screen, statin should be discontinued immediately.

99.9 The correct answer is E.

Rationale: n-3 long-chain fatty acid should be used in patients on statin therapy with TG levels 150 to 500 mg/dL. The REDUCE-IT (Reduction of Cardiovascular Events with Icosapent Ethyl-Intervention Trial) showed that the relative risk of cardiovascular events decreased by about 25% in patients on statin therapy at goal LDL-C levels with the addition of icosapent ethyl for persistent hypertriglyceridemia.

99.10 The correct answer is C.

Rationale: PCSK9 inhibitors are monoclonal antibodies injected subcutaneously every other week and are generally well tolerated with no major side effects, aside from injection site reactions. There are no absolute contraindications to starting this medication aside from a patient who does not want to take the medication. A "risk versus benefits" discussion may be helpful in this situation.

TABLE 99.1 Lipid Medications

Medication (Class)	Dosage (Orally, Unless Otherwise Indicate)	Therapeutic Use	LDL-C or TG Lowering	Clinical Benefit (Studies)	Side Effects
Statins	High-intensity statin therapy: Atorvastatin 40-80 mg once daily Rosuvastatin 20-40 mg once daily	First-line agent for primary or secondary ASCVD prevention	>50% ↓ LDL-C	↓ Risk (22%) for CV events ↓ 10% all-cause mortality	Myalgias, myopathy, liver injury, increased risk of diabetes
	Moderate-intensity statin therapy: Atorvastatin 10-20 mg once daily Rosuvastatin 5-10 mg once daily Fluvastatin 20-80 mg once daily Lovastatin 20-80 mg once daily Pravastatin 20-40 mg once daily		20%-55% ↓ LDL-C		
Inhibitors of cholesterol absorption	Ezetimibe 10 mg once daily	Add-on therapy to statins for patients at high risk who do not meet LDL-C goal (LDL-C <70 mg/dL) and patients with statin intolerance.	15%-20% ↓ LDL-C	↓ Relative risk (6%) for recurrent CV events in patients with ASCVD No large double-blind trial of ezetimibe monotherapy.	Gastrointestinal discomfort including diarrhea

PCSK9 inhibitors	Alirocumab 75-150 mg subcutaneously every 2 wk or 300 mg every 4 wk	Third-line agent after statins and ezetimibe to achieve LDL-C goal (LDL-C <70 mg/dL) in patients with ASCVD or hypercholesterolemia.	40%-65% ↓ LDL-C when added to statin ± ezetimibe	↓ Risk (~15%) for CV events in patients with stable atherosclerotic disease and those with clinical ASCVD. No clear mortality benefit	Injection site reactions
	Evolocumab 140 mg subcutaneously every 2 wk or 420 mg every 4 wk				
n-3 long-chain fatty acids	Icosapent ethyl (Vascepa) 4 g once daily	Possible use in patients at high risk on statin therapy with TG 150-500 mg/dL.	No LDL-C lowering; 20%-30% TG ↓	↓ Relative risk (25%) for CV events in patients on statin therapy at goal LDL-C levels.	Diarrhea, sore throat, joint pain
Bile acid sequestrants	Colesevelam 3,750 mg once daily or 1,875 mg bid Cholestyramine 3,750 mg once daily or 1,875 mg bid Colestipol 3,750 mg once daily or 1,875 mg bid	Fourth-line agent if not achieving LDL-C goal despite maximally tolerated lipid-lowering therapy	15%-20% LDL-C ↓	Possible ↓ risk (5%) for CV events No trial evaluating benefit as add-on to statin therapy	Constipation, GI upset, possible increase in TG levels
Fibrates	Fenofibrate 50-160 mg once daily Gemfibrozil 600 mg bid	Third-line agent if TG > 500 mg/dL despite maximally tolerated TG-lowering therapies	40%-50% TG ↓	Possible ↓ risk (16%) for CV events No clear mortality benefit	Muscle injury, cholelithiasis
Niacin	Niacin 500-2,000 mg once daily	Usually not recommended because of lack of benefit, side-effect profile, and more beneficial alternative therapies	15%-25% TG ↓ 10%-20% LDL-C ↓	No reduction in mortality or CV events	Flushing, nausea, pruritus, transaminitis, gout, hyperglycemia

ASCVD, atherosclerotic cardiovascular disease; CV, cardiovascular; GI, gastrointestinal; LDL-C, low-density lipoprotein cholesterol; PCSK9, proprotein convertase subtilisin/kexin type 9; TG, triglyceride.

HYPERTENSION

Robert L. Carhart, Sean Byrnes, Shweta Paulraj, and Subash Nepal

CHAPTER 100

QUESTIONS

100.1 A 66-year-old male with a history of smoking and hyperlipidemia is referred to your office by his primary care physician (PCP) for hypertension (HTN) management. He takes no medications for his HTN. His blood pressure (BP) in the PCP office last week was 145/82 mm Hg. His BP in the office today is 140/78 mm Hg. What is your recommendation, based on the ACC/AHA (American College of Cardiology/American Heart Association) guidelines?

   A. Advise diet and exercise and check back in 3 months.
   B. Start the patient on lisinopril 10 mg immediately.
   C. Send the patient home with ambulatory BP monitoring.
   D. His BP is well controlled so no therapy is required.

100.2 A 42-year-old female with a diagnosis of HTN comes to your office for a general follow-up. She is taking losartan 25 mg daily. Her BP in the office is 132/82 mm Hg, heart rate (HR) 75 bpm. Her atherosclerotic cardiovascular disease (ASCVD) risk is calculated at 6.2%. She advises you that she just found out she is pregnant. What is your recommendation today?

   A. Stop her losartan and start her on labetalol.
   B. Continue her current medication as she meets the ACC/AHA guidelines.
   C. Increase her losartan to 50 mg daily as she is above 130/80 mm Hg.
   D. Switch her to lisinopril 10 mg daily.

100.3 A 25-year-old male is referred by his PCP for HTN. His BP in the office today is 138/85. On history taking, you discover that he drinks about three beers a day, drinks two cups of coffee a day, and takes about 800 mg of ibuprofen daily due to a recent injury, and sleeps 10 hours a day. In this patient's case, all of the following have been shown to cause HTN **EXCEPT** what?

   A. Caffeine use
   B. Alcohol use
   C. Use of nonsteroidal anti-inflammatory drug (NSAIDs)
   D. Sleeping more than 8 hours

100.4 A 22-year-old male is referred to your clinic for HTN. His BP in the clinic today is 138/82. On physical examination, you notice a systolic murmur at the left paravertebral interscapular area and a continuous murmur over his upper back. What should be your next step to support your diagnosis?

Questions and Answers are based on Chapter 100: Hypertension by Amal Abdellatif, Mohamed B. Elshazly, Parag H. Joshi, and John W. McEvoy in Cardiovascular Medicine and Surgery, First Edition.

A. Check the electrocardiogram (ECG).
B. Order a computed tomography of the thorax.
C. Check BP on the leg.
D. Order echocardiogram.

100.5 A 72-year-old male with a history of HTN, coronary artery disease with a stent in the left main coronary artery 5 years ago, and systolic heart failure (ejection fracture 30%) comes to your office for a follow-up. His BP today is 150/93 mm Hg and HR is 70 beats per minute (bpm). His antihypertensives include lisinopril 20 mg once daily, metoprolol succinate 50 mg once daily, and spironolactone 50 mg once daily. All of the following are recommended choices in this patient **EXCEPT** what?

A. Add amlodipine.
B. Increase lisinopril.
C. Switch metoprolol succinate to carvedilol.
D. Increase Aldactone.

100.6 A 65-year-old female presents to the office for a routine annual check. Her HR is 72/min and BP in the office is 126/86 mm Hg. Her BP 1 year ago was 128/84 mm Hg. based on the current ACC/AHA guidelines, which of the following is **CORRECT**?

A. Given her systolic blood pressure (SBP) less than 130 mm Hg, she is considered to be normotensive.
B. Given her diastolic BP greater than 80 mm Hg, she has stage 1 HTN.
C. Given her SBP greater than 120 mm Hg, she is considered to have elevated BP.
D. Given her borderline BP, suspect masked HTN.

100.7 Which of the following patients can be classified as having drug-resistant HTN?

A. A 52-yo male with a BP of 144/78 mm Hg on carvedilol 3.125 mg bid, lisinopril 20 mg daily, and amlodipine 5 mg daily
B. A 73-yo male with a BP of 150/75 mm Hg on lisinopril 40 mg daily, carvedilol 25 mg bid, and indapamide 5 mg daily
C. A 61-yo female with a BP of 148/72 mm Hg on valsartan 320 mg daily, chlorthalidone 50 mg daily, metoprolol tartrate 100 mg bid, and amlodipine 5 mg daily
D. Both options B and C are correct.

100.8 Which of the following patients require initiation of antihypertensives at their initial office visit?

A. A 58-yo male with a BP of 138/84 mm Hg and no comorbidities
B. A 69-yo female with a BP of 145/82 mm Hg and no comorbidities
C. A 46-yo female with chronic kidney disease (CKD) and a BP of 126/70 mm Hg
D. A 62-yo male with a BP of 132/80 mm Hg and an estimated 10-year ASCVD score of 8%

100.9 A 49-yo-African American male presents for a routine health checkup. He is found to have a BP of 162/89 mm Hg. Which of the following medications represents the **BEST** regimen for his HTN?

A. Chlorthalidone 25 mg daily + lisinopril 5 mg daily
B. Carvedilol 12.5 mg twice daily
C. Hydralazine 25 mg tid + isosorbide dinitrate 20 mg tid
D. Amlodipine 2.5 mg daily

100.10 What is the most common cause of secondary HTN in terms of prevalence in the general population?

A. Primary hyperaldosteronism
B. Drug/alcohol induced
C. Obstructive sleep apnea
D. Hypothyroidism

ANSWERS

100.1 The correct answer is A.
Rationale: The first step in evaluating BP is to advise lifestyle modifications and repeat the BP in 3 months. If it is still elevated at about 130/80, then home BP monitoring or ambulatory BP monitoring is recommended. If still elevated about 130/80, then starting therapy at the subsequent visit is recommended if the ASCVD is greater than 10%, the patient has diabetes or CKD, or the patient is over 65.

100.2 The correct answer is A.
Rationale: Angiotensin-converting enzyme (ACE) and angiotensin receptor blocker (ARB) should be avoided in pregnancy as they have been found to be teratogenic. Since her BP is between 130 and 139/80 and 89 and her ASCVD less than 10%, there is no indication at this visit to increase her medication. While not the first line for HTN, alpha-methyldopa, labetalol, and nifedipine have been used for HTN in pregnancy.

100.3 The correct answer is D.
Rationale: Alcohol, caffeine, NSAIDs, decongestants, atypical antipsychotics, steroids, and antidepressants have been shown to induce HTN. While sleep restriction has been shown to increase BP, an increase in sleep has not.

100.4 The correct answer is C.
Rationale: Any young patient below 30 years of age with HTN and a systolic murmur at the left paravertebral interscapular area and continuous murmur over the chest/back should raise suspicion for aortic coarctation. The systolic murmur at the left paravertebral interscapular area is due to flow across the narrow coarctation area and continuous murmurs may be caused by flow through large collateral vessels. Coarctation may manifest as absent femoral pulses, BP discrepancy between the upper and lower extremities, and a systolic murmur at the left paravertebral interscapular area and continuous murmur on the back, chest, or abdominal bruit. While an echocardiogram is indicated, the quickest and next best step to support the diagnosis would be BP in the lower extremities.

100.5 The correct answer is A.
Rationale: Calcium channel blockers (CCBs) are a known negative inotrope, especially when combined with beta-blockers, and so their use should be avoided in patients with heart failure with reduced ejection function. All the other options are reasonable.

100.6 The correct answer is B.
Rationale: She has stage 1 HTN based on her diastolic BP. The recommendation is to assign the higher stage when SBP and diastolic BP are discordant.

100.7 The correct answer is D.
Rationale: Drug-resistant HTN is typically defined as SBP greater than or equal to 140 mm Hg despite adherence to at least three maximally tolerated doses of antihypertensives from complementary classes, including a diuretic at an appropriate dose, or when four or more medications are required to control SBP.

100.8 The correct answer is B.
Rationale: A 69-yo female with a BP of 145/82 mm Hg and no comorbidities. The 2017 Hypertension Clinical Practice guidelines recommended the initiation or intensification of antihypertensive treatment among patients with stage 1 HTN who belong to one of five high-risk categories: age 65 years or more, diabetes, CKD, clinical ASCVD, or a 10-year Pooled Cohort Equation (PCE) estimated ASCVD risk greater than or equal to 10%.

100.9 The correct answer is A.
Rationale: Initial combination therapy candidates include (1) patients with stage 2 HTN, and (2) patients whose BP is more than 20/10 mm Hg above treatment goal. Specific ethnic and age groups tend to demonstrate better responses to certain drug classes. For example, Black patients and older adults (ie, ≥60 years) may respond better to thiazide diuretics or CCBs, and therefore are recommended to start monotherapy with one of these classes should they bear no special indications otherwise for other drug classes. On the other hand, younger patients (ie, <50 years) tend to respond better to ACE inhibitors or ARBs and beta-blockers (although the latter group is only recommended in the presence of a special indication).

100.10 The correct answer is C.
Rationale: Obstructive sleep apnea has a prevalence of 25% to 50% and is a common cause of secondary HTN. These patients can have a loss of normal nocturnal BP fall. Screening and evaluation for the same is paramount in patients with obesity and Mallampati airway class III to IV.

CARDIAC REHABILITATION

Robert L. Carhart, Ronald Russo, Philip Chebaya, and Muhammad Malik

CHAPTER 101

QUESTIONS

101.1 A 60-year-old male with a history of type 2 diabetes mellitus (T2DM), hypertension, and stable coronary artery disease (CAD) presents to your clinic with complaints of intermittent bilateral lower extremity that is worse with activity. When asked regarding alleviating factors, the patients stated that his symptoms improve with rest. The physical examination was significant for faint dorsalis pedis pulses bilaterally with no skin changes or signs of peripheral ischemia. Patient's vitals were unremarkable. Based on the patient's presentation, she is sent for ankle-brachial index (ABI) testing and is diagnosed with bilateral peripheral artery disease with ABIs of 0.7 on the left and 0.65 on the right.

Which of the following is the next **BEST** step in the management of this patient?

A. Supervised exercise program (SEP)
B. Lower extremity surgical revascularization
C. Hyperbaric therapy
D. Start direct oral anticoagulant (DOAC).
E. Advise patients to avoid activity and remain sedentary until symptoms improve.

101.2 A 55-year-old obese female with a history of T2DM, hypertension, and stable CAD presents to your clinic stating she is frustrated with her cardiovascular health and wants to improve her exercise tolerance and lose weight to improve her quality of life. Patient states she spoke to a friend who was in a comparable situation and mentioned she was started in a cardiac rehab program and her quality of life had improved. Patient denies any known aortic stenosis, pulmonary hypertension, or any other acute health issues that would prevent her from exercising safely. After discussion, you agree patients would benefit most from an intensive cardiac rehab program.

Which of the variables mentioned earlier has shown significantly greater improvement in an intensive cardiac rehab program versus a traditional one?

A. Increase adipose tissue loss.
B. Blood pressure
C. Glucose control
D. Patient compliance

---

*Questions and Answers are based on Chapter 101: Cardiac Rehabilitation by Tamara Beth Horwich, Amir Behzad Rabbani, James S. Lee, and Arash B. Nayeri in Cardiovascular Medicine and Surgery, First Edition.

101.3 Socioeconomic disparities and lack of access to care have posed a challenge to participation and completion of cardiac rehab programs. In addition to the issues described earlier, the contact restrictions brought by the COVID-19 pandemic, home-based cardiac rehab has become an increasingly valuable tool. A recent review has shown similar outcomes between home-based and traditional cardiac rehab regarding quality of life, 1-year mortality, and need for revascularization.

What are some of the potential disadvantages associated with the use of home-based cardiac rehab?

A. Increase in waitlist times for programs
B. Less patient accountability
C. Overcoming logistical barriers
D. Concern for the safety of patients at high risk
E. B and D

101.4 A 65-year-old male who is morbidly obese with a history of poorly controlled T2DM, hypertension, and stable CAD reports to your office requesting to enroll in a cardiac rehab program as he states "He wants to get his life back on track." Patients' labs were significant for a hemoglobin (Hgb) of 11 and HbA1c of 9.5. Vitals during the visit were significant for a blood pressure of 182/118 at rest, which was reproducible when repeated manually. Patient denied any symptoms.

Which of the findings is considered a contraindication for the patient starting cardiac rehab?

A. Patient's HbA1c greater than 8
B. Hgb less than 12
C. Patient's diastolic blood pressure greater than 110
D. Patient's systolic pressure greater than 200
E. C and D

ANSWERS

101.1 The correct Answer is A.
Rationale: Based on the patients' medical history, presentation, and ABI testing results, it is clear that this patient has peripheral vascular (artery) disease. The patient is currently experiencing intermittent claudication with no obvious signs of terminal ischemia requiring urgent surgical intervention. As shown in the claudication: exercise versus endoluminal revascularization (CLEVER) and endovascular revascularization and supervised exercise (ERASE) trials, a supervised exercise program (SEP) has been shown to improve outcomes in patients with peripheral arterial disease (PAD) compared to medical therapy. SEP is also preferred to immediate revascularization therapy as the first line as it is minimally invasive. However, if patients' symptoms do not improve with a SEP and surgical revascularization is required, improved outcomes are seen when SEP is continued following the procedure.

Hyperbaric chamber has not shown efficacy in improving outcomes for patients experiencing intermittent claudication secondary to peripheral vascular disease.

DOACs are not considered first-line therapy for PAD due to limited evidence and benefits currently available.

KEY POINTS

- ✓ Patients with PAD experiencing intermittent claudication with no obvious signs of limb ischemia will benefit from SEP for first-line therapy.

101.2 The correct Answer is A.

Rationale: Intensive cardiac rehab programs have become increasingly prevalent in cardiology, due to their efficacy, efficiency, and growing insurance approval. Recent meta-analysis has shown a significant increase in the loss of adipose tissue in comparison to a traditional program.

Blood pressure and glucose control have shown improvement in intensive programs versus traditional cardiac rehab; however, none have shown significant differences.

KEY POINTS

- ✓ Intensive cardiac rehab programs are becoming increasingly popular and have been shown to significantly decrease adipose tissue greater than traditional programs.

101.3 The correct Answer is E.

Rationale: Home-based cardiology rehab programs are a suitable alternative to hospital-based cardiac rehab for those with difficulty accessing health care and socioeconomic disparities. However, the nature of home-based management can lead to unique challenges such as less supervision for patients at high risk and decreased compliance due to lack of accountability.

Weight times would be decreased due to increased availability for participation. In addition, not requiring transportation would decrease logistical barriers seen for many patients with socioeconomic disparities.

KEY POINTS

- ✓ Home-based cardiac rehab is a great alternative to hospital-based programs for those with difficulty accessing health care and socioeconomic disparities. However, continued research needs to be performed to evaluate its efficacy and outcomes.

101.4 The correct Answer is E.

Rationale: Contraindications for participation in cardiac rehab include diastolic blood pressure greater than 110 at rest or systolic blood pressure greater than 200 at rest. Other contraindications include but are not limited to severe symptomatic mitral regurgitation (MR), aortic stenosis (AS), pulmonary hypertension, and New York Heart Association (NYHA) class IV heart failure.

Elevated HbA1c and mild asymptomatic anemia are not contraindications for patients participating in cardiac rehab.

KEY POINTS

- Uncontrolled hypertension (>200/>110) at rest poses an increased risk for patients participating in cardiac rehab and therefore not recommended as the risks outweigh the benefits.

SECTION 9 ADULT CONGENITAL HEART DISEASE

ANATOMIC AND PHYSIOLOGIC CLASSIFICATION OF CONGENITAL HEART DISEASE*

CHAPTER 102

Robert L. Carhart and Harneet Bhatti

QUESTIONS

102.1 A 19-year-old female patient presents to the emergency department with shortness of breath. Vitals on presentation are blood pressure (BP) 120/88 mm Hg, heart rate (HR) 112 beats per minute (bpm). She is saturating at 97% on room air. Lungs are clear to auscultation. Electrocardiogram (ECG) demonstrates sinus tachycardia. Chest x-ray (CXR) demonstrates right isomerism. Which of the following is this condition generally associated with?

A. Asplenia
B. Polysplenia
C. Cyanosis
D. Ventricular septal defect

102.2 A 47-year-old male presents for an annual health screening. He has no past medical history and reports he runs 3 miles 3 times each week. Vitals include BP 124/70 and HR 87 bpm. On examination, lungs are clear to auscultation, and a decrescendo, diastolic murmur is heard along the left sternal border in the third intercostal space. A transthoracic echocardiogram is ordered that demonstrates mild aortic regurgitation and a dilated coronary sinus. What congenital abnormality does this patient likely have?

A. Ventricular septal defect
B. Persistent left superior caval vein
C. Atrial septal defect
D. Common arterial trunk

102.3 A 42-year-old male presents to the emergency department with complaints of worsening shortness of breath on exertion and palpitations. Vitals on presentation are BP 145/89 mm Hg, HR 97 bpm. He is saturating at 87% on room air. On physical examinations, lungs are clear to auscultation. There is a systolic murmur at the third intercostal space along the right sternal border and digital clubbing is noted in bilateral lower extremities. What is the next **BEST** step to help determine the diagnosis?

A. Computed tomography angiography (CTA) thorax
B. Transthoracic echocardiogram
C. Transesophageal echocardiogram
D. Ventilation/perfusion (V/Q) lung scan

*Questions and Answers are based on Chapter 102: Anatomic and Physiologic Classification of Congenital Heart Disease by David S. Majdalany and Francois Marcotte in Cardiovascular Medicine and Surgery, First Edition.

Section 9: Adult Congenital Heart Disease

102.4 A 36-year-old male presents to the clinic for an annual visit. He has **NOT** seen a physician since he was a child. On examination, a systolic murmur is heard at the second left intercostal space. Transthoracic echocardiogram demonstrates moderate pulmonic stenosis. Which of the following is the patient **MOST LIKELY** at risk for?

A. Cyanosis
B. Eisenmenger syndrome
C. Pulmonary embolism
D. None of the above

102.5 A 24-year-old male presents to the clinic with complaints of exertional shortness of breath and orthopnea. Vitals demonstrate BP 124/78 and HR of 88 bpm. He is saturating well on room air. Physical examination is significant for bilateral rales and lung bases, abdominal distension, and 2+ pitting edema in bilateral lower extremities. ECG demonstrates sinus rhythm. Transthoracic echocardiogram demonstrates a mid-left atrial (LA) membrane. What is the diagnosis?

A. Parachute mitral valve
B. Congenital aortic stenosis
C. Cor triatriatum
D. Double-inlet ventricle

102.6 A 32-year-old female with a known history of asthma presents to the emergency department with complaints of wheezing and shortness of breath. Vitals on presentation include BP 120/82 mm Hg and HR 89 bpm. She is saturating at 87% on room air. On physical examination, wheezing is noted bilaterally. The rest of the physical examination is unremarkable. Computed tomography (CT) thorax reveals atrioventricular (AV) discordance and ventriculoarterial (VA) discordance. What congenital abnormality does this patient likely have?

A. Ventricular septal defect
B. Atrial septal defect
C. Transposition of the great arteries (TGA)
D. Congenitally corrected transposition of the great arteries (CCTGA)

ANSWERS

102.1 The correct answer is A.
Rationale: Patients with situs ambiguous can have associated polysplenia or asplenia syndromes along with disordered arrangement of abdominal organs. Right isomerism is generally associated with asplenia whereas left isomerism is associated with polysplenia.

102.2 The correct answer is B.
Rationale: A persistent left superior caval vein is a pre-tricuspid shunt that can return venous blood to the right atrium (RA) through the coronary sinus, resulting in a dilated coronary sinus. It is usually a benign condition that does not cause any degree of cyanosis.

102.3 The correct answer is B.

Rationale: This patient likely has a patent ductus arteriosus (PDA) that led to the development of Eisenmenger syndrome given evidence of chronic hypoxia. A transthoracic echocardiogram will be the next best test to help determine this diagnosis. Gibson in 1900 described PDA continuous systolic and diastolic murmur, that is, machinery murmur. With Eisenmenger syndrome, elevated pulmonary pressures cause a reversal of the shunt to right-to-left, resulting in loss of the diastolic murmur and a presentation that can mimic primary pulmonary hypertension.

102.4 The correct answer is D.

Rationale: Pulmonic stenosis is an obstructive right heart lesion that on its own usually does not cause cyanosis. The significant obstructive prevents increased pulmonary artery pressures preventing Eisenmenger syndrome and hypoxia.

102.5 The correct answer is C.

Rationale: Cor triatriatum is a congenital anatomic defect that results from insufficient posterior LA wall resorption during the fusion of the pulmonary venous buds to the primitive LA. This can result in the formation of two separate sections of the LA that can lead to obstruction and heart failure (mitral stenosis physiology).

102.6 The correct answer is D.

Rationale: This patient likely has CCTGA. CT thorax demonstrates AV discordance along with VA discordance so that the left ventricle (LV) connected to the RA is delivering blood to the pulmonary artery (PA) and the LA connected to the right ventricle (RV) is delivering oxygenated blood to the aorta. CCTGA prevents cyanosis, unlike TGA.

EVALUATION OF SUSPECTED AND KNOWN ADULT CONGENITAL HEART DISEASE

Kellsey Peterson

QUESTIONS

103.1 Which of the following epidemiologic statements is **TRUE**?
  A. Congenital heart disease (CHD) is the second most common birth defect.
  B. The prevalence of CHD is 6 per 1,000 in the adult population.
  C. Shunt lesions such as atrial septal defect (ASD), ventricular septal defect (VSD), patent ductus arteriosus (PDA), or atrioventricular (AV) septal defects have been found to be more common in men.
  D. The number of adults living with CHD is expected to decrease.

103.2 Which of the following maternal risk factors are associated with CHD?
  A. Preeclampsia, hypertension, hyperlipidemia, methotrexate use
  B. Hyperlipidemia, HIV, tobacco use
  C. Maternal CHD, tobacco use, lithium use, methotrexate use
  D. Diabetes, acetaminophen use, hypertension, rheumatoid arthritis

103.3 Which of the following genetic syndromes is associated with the **CORRECT** congenital heart defects?
  A. Down syndrome: AV septal defects, VSD, ASD
  B. DiGeorge syndrome: coarctation of the aorta and bicuspid aortic valve
  C. Noonan syndrome: tetralogy of Fallot (ToF), interrupted aortic arch type B, truncus arteriosus, conoventricular VSDs, and other aortic arch abnormalities
  D. Turner syndrome: pulmonary valve stenosis, AV septal defect, aortic coarctation, and hypertrophic cardiomyopathy

103.4 A 29-year-old male is evaluated in your clinic for progressively worsening dyspnea on exertion. He has no known past medical history and does **NOT** take any medications. On examination, his blood pressure is 110/80 mm Hg, heart rate 75 beats per minute (bpm), and oxygen saturation 98% on room air. Cardiac examination reveals an S2 that does **NOT** vary with respiration and a prominent P2. An echocardiogram is performed that is notable for a mildly dilated right ventricle with reduced systolic function and pulmonary artery (PA) systolic pressure estimated at 56 mm Hg. Which of the following is the most appropriate next step in management?
  A. Repeat echo with bubble study.
  B. Right heart catheterization with shunt run
  C. Computed tomography angiogram (CTA)
  D. Cardiac magnetic resonance (CMR) imaging

*Questions and Answers are based on Chapter 103: Evaluation of Suspected and Known Adult Congenital Heart Disease by Andrew R. Pistner and Anitra W. Romfh in Cardiovascular Medicine and Surgery, First Edition.

CHAPTER 103 | Evaluation of Suspected and Known Adult Congenital Heart Disease

103.5 A 45-year-old female presents to your clinic for the evaluation of hypertension. She takes losartan 50 mg, amlodipine 10 mg, and hydrochlorothiazide 50 mg with excellent compliance. She is 4 feet 9 inches tall and weighs 125 lbs. Her blood pressure is 160/95 mm Hg from the right arm, heart rate 82 bpm, oxygen saturation 99% on room air. She is noted to have a wide, short neck without jugular venous distension. Cardiac examination reveals a regular rhythm with an early systolic ejection click followed by an ejection murmur at the left sternal border. Which of the following would you expect to find upon further evaluation?

A. A heavily calcified tricuspid aortic valve on echo with a peak velocity of 4.2 m/s
B. Blood pressure readings are as follows: 155/90 mm Hg left arm, 160/95 mm Hg right arm, 115/70 mm Hg left leg.
C. Upper extremity defects consisting of a hypoplastic or absent thumb
D. Chromosomal abnormality trisomy 21

103.6 A 46-year-old female is referred to your clinic for exertional shortness of breath and occasional palpitations. She has been told that she has had a murmur since childhood but denies any past medical or surgical history. Her blood pressure is 138/50 mm Hg, heart rate is 90 bpm, and oxygen saturation is 98% on room air. Cardiac examination is notable for a harsh, holosystolic murmur and soft, high-pitched, early diastolic decrescendo murmur at the left lower sternal border. Her echocardiogram reveals severe aortic regurgitation. Which of the following congenital cardiac abnormalities could explain this patient's findings?

A. Supracristal VSD
B. Muscular VSD
C. ToF
D. Ebstein anomaly

103.7 The chest x-ray shown in **Figure 103.1** is characteristic of what CHD?

A. Pulmonary stenosis
B. Congenitally corrected transposition of the great arteries
C. Partial anomalous pulmonary venous return (PAPVR) of the right pulmonary veins via the inferior vena cava (IVC)
D. Aortic coarctation

103.8 Which of the following congenital diagnoses is associated with the **CORRECT** electrocardiogram (ECG) findings?

A. Surgically repaired ToF: right axis deviation (RAD), right atrial enlargement (RAE), dominant R wave in V1
B. Ebstein anomaly: right bundle branch block (RBBB), increased QRS duration, increased QT duration
C. Secundum ASD: first-degree atrioventricular block (AVB), RAD, RAE, "crochetage pattern"
D. Pulmonary stenosis: first-degree AVB, RAE with Himalayan P waves, Wolff-Parkinson White (WPW) pattern

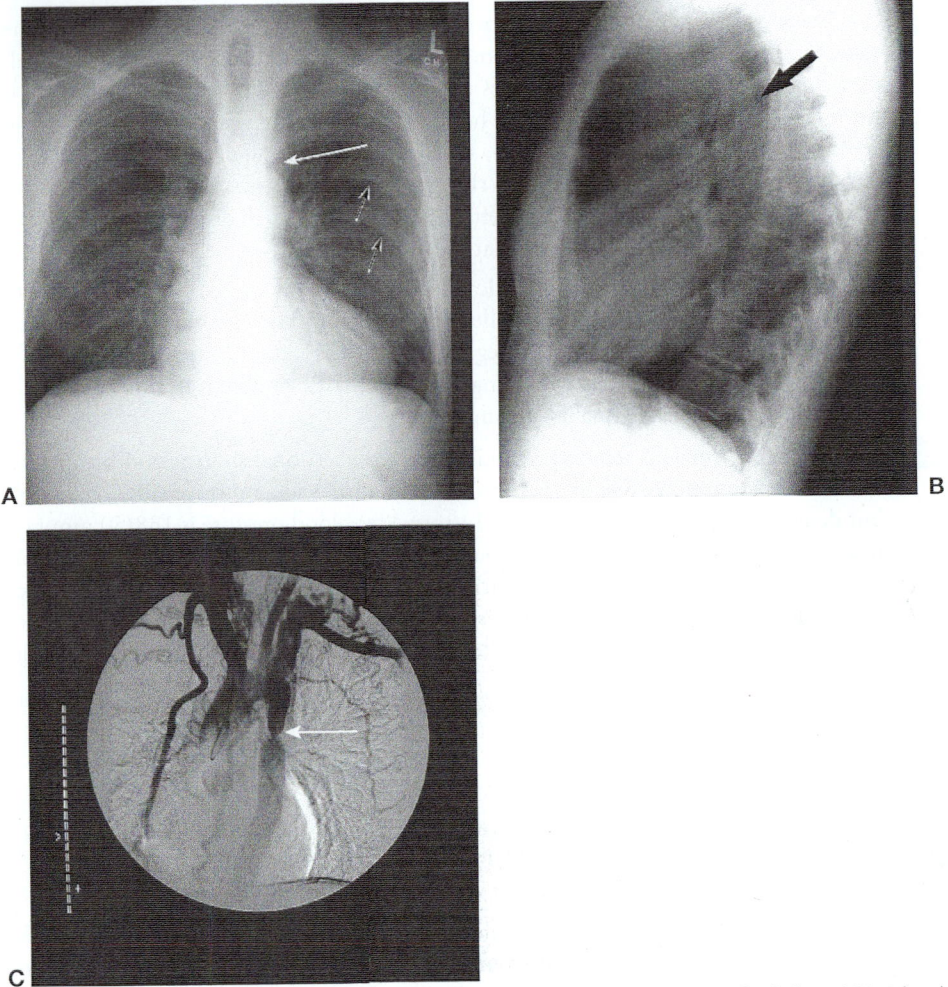

Figure 103.1 From Thompson BH, Erkonen WE. Chest. In: Smith WL, ed. *Radiology 101*. 4th ed. Wolters Kluwer; 2014:25-79, Figure 3.31.

103.9 You are meeting a 65-year-old female in your clinic for the first time to establish care after she just moved to the area. She has a history of "some heart or blood vessel problem" that was repaired when she was a child. She does **NOT** have any prior medical records on hand and does **NOT** know any details about her surgery. Her physical examination is notable for a scar beneath her left breast to mid-axilla. There is a notable delay when comparing the upstroke of the right radial pulse to the right femoral pulse. She also has drooping of the left eyelid as well as left pupil constriction. The patient underwent which of the following surgeries?

- A. Atrial septectomy
- B. Aortic valve surgery
- C. Central shunt
- D. Repair of coarctation of the aorta

103.10 A 76-year-old male is referred to your clinic for the evaluation of syncope. His history is notable for ToF status post transannular patch repair when he was 8 years old. He reports that he was washing dishes at the sink when he suddenly passed out and woke up on the floor. His medications include a baby aspirin, atorvastatin 10 mg, and a multivitamin. His blood pressure is 125/78 mm Hg, pulse is 85 bpm, and oxygen saturation is 99% on room air. His cardiac examination is notable for a widely split S2 and soft 2/6, an early diastolic decrescendo murmur heard **BEST** at the left sternal border. His ECG reveals normal sinus rhythm with rare premature ventricular contractions (PVCs) and a QRS duration of 195 milliseconds. What is the **MOST LIKELY** etiology of his syncope?

A. Ventricular arrhythmia
B. Transient complete heart block
C. Vasovagal syncope
D. WPW syndrome

ANSWERS

103.1 The correct answer is B.
Rationale: CHD is the most common (not second most) birth defect. The prevalence of CHD varies between 4 and 10 cases per 100 births and eventually 6 per 1,000 in the adult population. Studies have shown that shunt lesions are more common in women, while transposition of the great arteries and aortic coarctation are more commonly found in men. The number of adults living with CHD is expected to *increase* with the increasing success of surgery and modern medical treatment.

103.2 The correct answer is C.
Rationale: Maternal CHD is associated with an increased risk of CHD in their offspring estimated at 4% to 5%. Women who smoke tobacco in their first trimester or during the periconceptual period have an increased risk of having children with right-sided obstructive cardiac defects as well as both ASDs and VSDs. Maternal use of lithium has been associated with Ebstein anomaly in the fetus and folic acid antagonists, such as methotrexate, are associated with a 2-fold increase in CHD. Maternal diabetes and pregestational diabetes are associated with the risk of CHD but not maternal preeclampsia, hypertension, or hyperlipidemia. Certain maternal infections such as rubella have been associated with CHD; however, HIV has not. Maternal use of acetaminophen has proven safe.

103.3 The correct answer is A.
Rationale: Down syndrome is the most common chromosomal abnormality associated with CHD (prevalence of 40%-50%). Coarctation of the aorta and bicuspid aortic valve are associated with Turner syndrome which is caused by complete or partial absence of one of the X chromosomes. The defects listed in choice C are associated with DiGeorge syndrome which is a result of a microdeletion of chromosome 22. The defects listed in choice D are associated with Noonan syndrome owing to mutations in the PTPN11 gene.

103.4 The correct answer is D.

Rationale: This patient has evidence of right ventricular dysfunction and pulmonary hypertension with a key physical examination finding of fixed splitting of S2 which is observed in ASD. The interval between A2 and P2 normally increases with inspiration related to the prolonged right ventricular ejection owing to increased venous return and right-sided volumes, which is referred to as "physiologic splitting." In ASD, the A2-P2 interval does not vary with respiration. Furthermore, the loud or prominent P2 is suggestive of pulmonary hypertension. Given the echo and physical examination findings, the clinician should be suspicious of an ASD. This would be best evaluated further by CMR which allows you to identify anatomy and physiology (ie, assessment for shunt). An echo with a bubble study will help to identify a right-to-left shunt at the atrial level (ie, patent foramen ovale) but is not the next best step to identify a left-to-right shunt as would be expected with ASD leading to right heart enlargement and pulmonary hypertension as seen in this patient. A right heart catheterization would be an appropriate next step after identifying the anatomy to determine the hemodynamic significance. While a pulmonary embolism as assessed by CTA may be associated with pulmonary hypertension, it would not present in this fashion and be associated with fixed splitting of S2.

103.5 The correct answer is B.

Rationale: This patient has findings that are consistent with Turner syndrome including short stature and webbed neck. Furthermore, she has poorly controlled blood pressure which can be attributed to coarctation of the aorta. Her cardiac examination describes a bicuspid aortic valve. Lower extremity blood pressure should be greater than upper extremity blood pressure owing to pulse wave amplification. If the lower extremity blood pressure is less than the upper extremity by 20 mm Hg or more than the clinician should be suspicious of aortic coarctation. Answer choice A describes severe calcific/senile aortic stenosis that can be observed in anatomically correct tricuspid aortic valves in the older adults. Answer choice C describes Holt-Oram syndrome, which is an autosomal dominant genetic syndrome associated with cardiac defects including ASD and VSD. Answer choice D describes Down syndrome.

103.6 The correct answer is A.

Rationale: Keeping in mind "the company it keeps," concomitant aortic regurgitation can be seen in supracristal VSDs due to aortic valve cusp prolapse. The physical examination identifies a systolic murmur characteristic of a pressure-restrictive VSD as flow goes from a high- to a low-pressure chamber. The diastolic murmur is characteristic of aortic regurgitation. None of the other answers are appropriate choices.

103.7 The correct answer is D.

Rationale: The "3-sign" on this chest x-ray in **Figure 103.1** represents the classical radiographic appearance of aortic coarctation demonstrating the dilation of the aortic arch and left subclavian artery, indentation at the coarctation site, and post-stenotic dilation of the descending aorta. The indentation at the lateral aspect of the proximal descending aorta can be observed on the PA radiograph (large arrow, A) and posterior indentation involving the posterior aspect of the proximal descending aorta on the lateral radiograph (arrow, B). This can be better visualized in the aortic angiogram seen in image C. Rib notching of the underside of the ribs can also be observed resulting from chronic collateral blood flow via the intercostal arteries (small arrows, A). In pulmonary stenosis, a prominent and enlarged PA can be observed due to post-stenotic dilation. Congenitally corrected transposition of the great arteries demonstrates a narrow vascular pedicle with an "absent" aortic knob owing to the anterior-posterior relationship of the great vessels. PAVR of the right pulmonary veins via the IVC is referred to as the Scimitar syndrome given the curvilinear opacity of the anomalous veins seen on frontal radiographs.

103.8 The correct answer is C.
Rationale: Surgically repaired ToF is associated with RBBB and increased duration of the QRS interval (>180 milliseconds), which is associated with an increased risk of arrhythmia and sudden cardiac death. Ebstein anomaly is associated with first-degree AVB, "Himalayan P waves" that describe tall, peaked P waves characteristic of RAE, and increased risk of an accessory pathway leading to WPW syndrome. Pulmonary stenosis is associated with right heart enlargement and pulmonary hypertension, which causes RAE, RAD, and findings of right ventricular hypertrophy (dominant R wave in V1). Heller et al. described the crochetage pattern of the R wave in inferior limb leads as being frequent in patients with ASD, correlating with shunt severity and being independent of the RBBB pattern. Crochetage sign, resembling the work of crochet needle, is characterized by the presence of a notch near the apex of the R wave in inferior lead and is highly specific for the diagnosis of ostium secundum ASD.

103.9 The correct answer is D.
Rationale: This patient's physical examination findings are consistent with the repair of aortic coarctation via a left thoracotomy approach. Careful neurologic examination reveals Horner syndrome which can be seen in coarctation repaired by subclavian flap with ipsilateral findings. Furthermore, she has evidence of radio-femoral delay which is concerning for restenosis following her remote repair. Atrial septectomy is usually via a right thoracotomy. Aortic valve surgery and central shunt are performed via median sternotomy. Refer to **Figure 103.1**.

103.10 The correct answer is A.
Rationale: This patient's physical examination findings are consistent with pulmonary regurgitation which is often seen as a residual sequela of patients with repair of ToF. Increased duration of the QRS interval (>180 milliseconds) is associated with an increased risk of ventricular arrhythmia and sudden cardiac death. Complete heart block is seen in congenitally corrected transposition of the great arteries (2% annual incidence). This vignette is not characteristic of vasovagal syncope. WPW syndrome is seen in the Ebstein anomaly.

SUGGESTED READINGS

Heller J, Hagège AA, Besse B, et al. "Crochetage" (notch) on R wave in inferior limb leads: a new independent electrocardiographic sign of atrial septal defect. J Am Coll Cardiol. 1996; 27(4): 877–882.

PREGNANCY AND REPRODUCTIVE HEALTH IN ADULT CONGENITAL HEART DISEASE

Jacqueline S. Coppola, Joshua Schulman-Marcus, and Sulagna Mookherjee

CHAPTER 104

QUESTIONS

104.1 Which of the following is **NOT** a hemodynamic change associated with normal pregnancy?
- A. An increase in plasma volume that begins by 6 weeks gestation
- B. An increase in systemic vascular resistance
- C. A 20% increase in heart rate
- D. Increased left ventricular end-diastolic (LVED) volume with preserved left ventricular (LV) function

104.2 Pregnancy is a relative contraindication for which of the following studies?
- A. Echocardiography
- B. Exercise stress testing
- C. Computed tomography (CT) of the chest
- D. Gadolinium contrast magnetic resonance imaging (MRI)

104.3 Which of the following is **NOT** a characteristic shared between CARPREG II (Cardiac Disease in Pregnancy Study II) and ZAHARA (Zofenopril in the Management of Hypertension Associated With Pregnancy: A Randomized Clinical Trial) studies for predictors of pregnancy risk?
- A. High-risk aortopathy
- B. Prior arrhythmias
- C. Mechanical valve
- D. Cyanotic heart disease

104.4 Which of the following maternal cardiovascular risk is **CORRECTLY** paired with the modified WHO classification, associated risk, and lesion?
- A. WHO Class I—small increased risk of maternal mortality—unoperated atrial septal defect (ASD)
- B. WHO Class II—significantly increased risk of maternal mortality—mechanical valve
- C. WHO Class IV—extremely high risk of maternal mortality/pregnancy contraindicated—severe mitral stenosis
- D. WHO Class III—may fall into higher or lower risk class depending on patient factors—repaired ASD

*Questions and Answers are based on Chapter 104: Pregnancy and Reproductive Health in Adult Congenital Heart Disease by Evan F. Shalen and Abigail D. Khan in Cardiovascular Medicine and Surgery, First Edition.

CHAPTER 104 | Pregnancy and Reproductive Health in Adult Congenital Heart Disease

104.5 What is the baseline assessment recommendation for women who become pregnant and who have repaired tetralogy of Fallot (TOF)?

- A. Termination of pregnancy
- B. 39-week cesarean section
- C. Cardiac catheterization
- D. Echocardiography

104.6 What is the risk of offspring inheritance for congenital aortic stenosis if the mother is affected, but the father is unaffected?

- A. 3% to 4%
- B. 8% to 18%
- C. 25% to 30%
- D. No associated inheritance risk

104.7 A 26-year-old female Chinese immigrant with a past medical history of moderate mitral stenosis secondary to rheumatic disease without repair and normal LV function presents to your office at 8 weeks gestation and is currently asymptomatic. What is the most appropriate recommendation for this patient?

- A. Close monitoring with echocardiography, and start beta-blocker.
- B. Terminate pregnancy.
- C. Exercise stress testing.
- D. Start angiotensin-converting enzyme (ACE) inhibitor to reduce afterload.

104.8 A 37-year-old female with a past medical history of nonischemic cardiomyopathy with ejection fraction (EF) of less than 25% (identified on echocardiogram 1 month ago) on guideline-directed medical therapy including beta-blocker, angiotensin receptor/neprilysin (ARNI), sodium-glucose cotransporter 2 inhibitors (SGLT2i), aldosterone receptor antagonists (mineralocorticoid receptor antagonist [MRAs]), and Lasix is presenting to the clinic today for a routine follow-up appointment. She reports to you that she has recently been married and is interested in starting a biologic family. What is the most appropriate recommendation for her today?

- A. Change her medications to hydralazine and labetalol in preparation for pregnancy.
- B. Encourage her to start trying to conceive.
- C. Strongly advise against pregnancy and refer to heart failure/transplant specialist.
- D. Send for exercise stress testing.

104.9 The patient from **Question 104.8** returns to your clinic to discuss options regarding nonpermanent contraceptive methods. Which of the following would you recommend for this patient?

- A. Estrogen-containing intrauterine device (IUD)
- B. Oral contraceptive pills
- C. Condoms with spermicide
- D. Copper IUD

104.10 A 30-year-old female with a past medical history of Fontan procedure and 26 weeks gestation is presenting to the emergency department with complaints of shortness of breath and palpitations for the last 30 minutes. She is immediately connected to telemetry and vital signs are obtained. She is found to be supraventricular tachycardia (SVT) with a rate of 180, and low systolic blood pressure of 86. She now reports lightheadedness, and her repeat blood pressure is 75/40. What is the next **BEST** step?

A. Adenosine
B. Direct-current cardioversion (DCCV)
C. Intravenous metoprolol
D. Digoxin

ANSWERS

104.1 The correct answer is B.
Rationale: An understanding of the hemodynamic changes of pregnancy is critical to the management of pregnant adults with congenital heart disease (ACHD). The major cardiovascular changes associated with normal pregnancy include an increase in circulating plasma that begins at 6 weeks gestation and peaks at 50% of baseline by 32 weeks, a decrease in systemic vascular resistance and blood pressure, an approximately 20% increase in heart rate, ventricular remodeling, leading to increased LVED volume with preserved LV function, increase in cardiac output by about 50% to 60%, and a decreased preload with the performance of the Valsalva maneuver.

104.2 The correct answer is D.
Rationale: All of the following studies including echocardiography, exercise stress testing, and CT are considered safe in pregnancy. CT in pregnancy should be discussed with a radiologist; however, typical fetal radiation dose from maternal chest imaging is allowed, although there is known association between in utero radiation exposure and childhood malignancy. However, use of gadolinium in MRI is generally avoided as this has been defined as a category C (Animal reproduction studies have shown an adverse effect on the fetus, and there are no adequate and well-controlled studies in humans.) by the U.S. Food and Drug Administration (FDA).

104.3 The correct answer is A.
Rationale: Prior cardiac events or arrhythmias, higher NYHA (New York Heart Association) class (>2 for ZAHARA, and baseline III-IV for CARPREG II), cyanotic heart disease, mechanical valve, or high-risk left-sided valve disease with left ventricular outflow tract (LVOT) obstruction (CARPREG III aortic valve area <1.5 cm^2, subaortic gradient >30 mm Hg, mitral valve area <2 cm^2, or moderate-to-severe mitral regurgitation [MR], ZAHARA: peak aortic gradient >50 mm Hg or aortic valve area <1.0 cm^2) are all characteristics shared between the studies according to **Table 104.1**. However, CARPREG III incorporates ventricular dysfunction, pulmonary hypertension, coronary artery disease, high-risk aortopathy, and late pregnancy assessment. ZAHARA adds cardiac medications before pregnancy, moderate or more atrioventricular (AV) valve regurgitation, and moderate or greater pulmonary valve regurgitation.

TABLE 104.1 Predictors of Pregnancy Risk in the CARPREG II and ZAHARA Studies

CARPREG II	ZAHARA
Prior cardiac events or arrhythmias Higher NYHA class[a] or cyanosis Mechanical valve High-risk left-sided valve disease/LVOT obstruction[b]	
Ventricular dysfunction[c]	Cardiac medications before pregnancy
Pulmonary hypertension[d]	≥Moderate systemic atrioventricular valve regurgitation
Coronary artery disease	≥Moderate pulmonary valve regurgitation
High-risk aortopathy[e]	—
No prior cardiac intervention	—
Late pregnancy assessment[f]	—

Note: Merged cells indicate risk factors that are common to both scores.
LVOT, left ventricular outflow tract obstruction; NYHA, New York Heart Association.
[a]CARPREG II: Baseline NYHA III-IV status, ZAHARA = NYHA before pregnancy more than II.
[b]CARPREG II: aortic valve area less than 1.5 cm^2, subaortic gradient greater than 30 mm Hg, mitral valve area less than 2 cm^2, or moderate-to-severe mitral regurgitation, ZAHARA: Peak aortic gradient greater than 50 mm Hg or aortic valve area less than 1.0 cm^2.
[c]Left ventricular ejection fraction less than 55%.
[d]Right ventricular systolic pressure 50 mm Hg or more in the absence of right ventricular outflow obstruction.
[e]Marfan syndrome, bicuspid aortic valve with aortic diameter greater than 45 mm, Loeys-Dietz syndrome, vascular Ehlers-Danlos syndrome, or prior aortic dissection or pseudoaneurysm.
[f]First antenatal visit after 20 weeks' gestation.
Adapted from Silversides CK, Grewal J, Mason J, et al. Pregnancy outcomes in women with heart disease: the CARPREG II study. *J Am Coll Cardiol.* 2018;71:2419-2430; Drenthen W, Boersma E, Balci A, et al. Predictors of pregnancy complications in women with congenital heart disease. *Eur Heart J.* 2010;31:2124-2132.

104.4 The correct answer is C.

Rationale: Answer choice C correctly pairs all three—WHO Class IV: extremely high risk of maternal mortality or severe morbidity; pregnancy contraindicated. These lesions include pulmonary arterial hypertension, severe systemic ventricular dysfunction, peripartum cardiomyopathy with residual LV dysfunction, severe mitral stenosis, severe symptomatic aortic stenosis, Marfan syndrome with aorta greater than 45 mm, bicuspid aortopathy with aortic diameter greater than 50 mm, and severe native aortic coarctation (**Table 104.2**).

104.5 The correct answer is D.

Rationale: Most women with repaired TOF tolerate pregnancy well, with a reported maternal cardiac event rate of 7% or less. Heart failure and arrhythmias occur more frequently in women with right ventricular (RV) dysfunction and/or moderate-to-severe pulmonary regurgitation. Overall complication rates are low, even in those with significant pulmonary stenosis or regurgitation. Baseline assessment of pregnant women with repaired TOF includes echocardiogram, primarily to evaluate the RV

TABLE 104.2 Modified WHO Classification of Maternal Cardiovascular Risk

WHO Class	Associated Risk	Lesion
I	No detectable increased risk of maternal mortality and no/mild increase in morbidity	**Uncomplicated, small, or mild:** Pulmonary stenosis PDA Mitral valve prolapse **Repaired simple lesions** ASD or VSD PDA Anomalous pulmonary venous drainage **Isolated ectopic beats**
II	Small increased risk of maternal mortality or moderate increase in morbidity	Unoperated ASD or VSD Repaired tetralogy of Fallot Most arrhythmias
II or III	May fall into higher or lower risk classification based on additional patient factors	Mild left ventricular impairment Hypertrophic cardiomyopathy Native or tissue valvular heart disease not considered Class I or IV Marfan syndrome without aortic dilation Bicuspid aortic valve aortopathy with aorta diameter <45 mm Repaired coarctation
III	Significantly increased risk of maternal mortality or severe morbidity	Mechanical valve Systemic right ventricle Fontan circulation Unrepaired cyanotic heart disease Other complex CHD Marfan syndrome with aortic diameter 40-45 mm Bicuspid aortopathy with aortic diameter 45-50 mm
IV	Extremely high risk of maternal mortality or severe morbidity; pregnancy contraindicated	Pulmonary arterial hypertension Severe systemic ventricular dysfunction Peripartum cardiomyopathy with any residual left ventricular dysfunction Severe mitral stenosis Severe symptomatic aortic stenosis Marfan syndrome with aortic diameter >45 mm Bicuspid aortopathy with aortic diameter >50 mm Severe native aortic coarctation

ASD, atrial septal defect; CHD, congenital heart disease; PDA, patent ductus arteriosus; VSD, ventricular septal defect.
Data from Regitz-Zagrosek V, Blomstrom Lundqvist C, Borghi C, et al. ESC Guidelines on the management of cardiovascular diseases during pregnancy: the task force on the management of cardiovascular diseases during pregnancy of the European Society of Cardiology (ESC). *Eur Heart J.* 2011;32(24):3147-3197; Jastrow N, Meyer P, Khairy P, et al. Prediction of complications in pregnant women with cardiac diseases referred to a tertiary center. *Int J Cardiol.* 2011;151(2):209-213.

and the degree of pulmonary regurgitation. Clinical follow-up every trimester is recommended, and a third-trimester echocardiogram is useful, especially in settings where the clinical presentation has changed. Pulmonary valve replacement should be considered in symptomatic patients with RV enlargement and severe pulmonary regurgitation.

104.6 The correct answer is B.
Rationale: If the mother is affected with aortic stenosis, the risk of offspring inheritance of this lesion is 8% to 18%. However, if the father was the affected parent, the offspring has a 3% to 4% chance of inheritance of aortic stenosis (**Table 104.3**).

TABLE 104.3 Risk of Offspring Inheritance by Congenital Heart Disease (CHD) Lesion

CHD Lesion	Father Affected (%)	Mother Affected (%)
Atrial septal defect	1.5-3.5	4-6
Atrioventricular septal defect	1-4.5	11.5-14
Ventricular septal defect	2-3.5	6-10
Aortic stenosis	3-4	8-18
Pulmonic stenosis	2-3.5	4-6.5
Tetralogy of Fallot	1.5	2-2.5
Aortic coarctation	2-3	4-6.5
Patent ductus arteriosus	2-2.5	3.5-4
Hypoplastic left heart syndrome	21	
D-transposition of the great arteries	2	
L-transposition of the great arteries	3-5	
Ebstein anomaly	Unknown	6

Merged cells indicate offspring risk irrespective of parental gender. Reprinted from Cowan JR, Ware SM. Genetics and genetic testing in congenital heart disease. *Clin Perinatol*. 2015;42(2):373-393. Copyright © 2015 Elsevier, with permission.

104.7 The correct answer is A.
Rationale: Moderate and severe mitral stenosis are associated with a significant risk in pregnancy and should be monitored very closely. Echocardiographic gradients increase in pregnancy owing to increased cardiac output, and stenosis severity should be graded by pressure half-time and/or direct planimetry. Starting the patient on beta-blocker in pregnancy to maximize diastolic filling time is reasonable, as well as anticoagulation if the patient is at high risk for thromboembolism, including greater than or equal to moderate stenosis, left atrial spontaneous echocardiographic contrast, left atrial area greater than or equal to 40 mL/m^2, or with known atrial fibrillation. MR is better tolerated in pregnancy than mitral stenosis because the decreased afterload of the pregnant state decreases the regurgitant volume.

104.8 The correct answer is C.
Rationale: Pregnancy is contraindicated in those with left ventricular ejection fraction (LVEF) of less than 30%, as this is a WHO Class IV disease. The risk of pregnancy, including an irreversible decline in ventricular function, should be discussed. Patients at high risk, including those with Class III to IV symptoms, should have a preconception assessment by a heart failure/transplant specialist. In those at lower risk, medications should be reviewed for fetotoxicity before conception. ACE inhibitors, angiotensin receptor blockers, and aldosterone antagonists need to be stopped, ideally with monitoring for decompensation before pregnancy. Most beta-blockers, diuretics, hydralazine, and isosorbide dinitrate can be used during pregnancy.

104.9 The correct answer is D.
Rationale: Highly effective, long-acting, non–estrogen-containing IUDs (copper) are the preferred form of nonpermanent contraception for most women with high-risk cardiac conditions. Endocarditis after IUD placement, once considered to be a risk in some patients, is unlikely, and antibiotic prophylaxis is not required. A vagal response to IUD placement can occur and may be problematic in patients with severe pulmonary hypertension or Fontan physiology. These patients are not candidates for IUD placement in the office setting.

104.10 The correct answer is B.
Rationale: This patient is presenting with unstable SVT; the next most appropriate step is DCCV. Unstable arrhythmias are treated with DCCV, which is considered safe in pregnancy as current exposure to the fetus is minimal. Fetal monitoring is recommended post procedure. If the patient were stable, adenosine may be used and is not known to be associated with fetal adverse events. Intravenous metoprolol can also be used in appropriate cases. Calcium channel blockers and digoxin are considered relatively safe in the appropriate setting, although they do remain listed as pregnancy category C.

PHARMACOLOGIC THERAPY FOR ADULT CONGENITAL HEART DISEASE

Harneet Bhatti and Robert L. Carhart

CHAPTER 105

QUESTIONS

105.1 A 29-year-old female presents to the emergency department with complaints of palpitations that started 8 hours ago. She has never had such symptoms before. Vitals on presentation include blood pressure (BP) 119/84 mm Hg and heart rate 154 beats per minute (bpm). She is saturating well on room air. Electrocardiogram (ECG) demonstrates atrial flutter with rapid ventricular response (RVR). After a medication is given, the heart rate slows down to 87 bpm and repeat ECG shows a shortened PR interval and the presence of a delta wave. Which drug is appropriate to use in this patient?

A. Calcium channel blocker
B. Beta-blocker
C. Adenosine
D. Procainamide

105.2 A 18-year-old female with a known ventricular septal defect (VSD) presents to the clinic with complaints of "her heart racing" at random times of the day. She is given a 14-day event monitor that captures multiple episodes of supraventricular tachycardia (SVT) with the longest lasting 32 minutes. Her symptoms correlate with the captured events. Transthoracic echocardiogram demonstrated a small VSD and normal left ventricular function. Which of the following drugs should be prescribed?

A. Amiodarone
B. Sotalol
C. Flecainide
D. None of the above

105.3 An 18-year-old male presents to the emergency department with palpitations that have been persistent for the past many hours. Vitals on arrival include BP 127/78 mm Hg and heart rate 188 bpm. Physical examination is unremarkable **EXCEPT** for tachycardia on cardiac auscultation. ECG demonstrates SVT. Of note, the patient has a known history of transposition of the great arteries with repair. Which of the following medications should be given?

A. Amiodarone
B. Flecainide
C. Propafenone
D. Diltiazem

---

*Questions and Answers are based on Chapter 105: Pharmacologic Therapy for Adult Congenital Heart Disease by Dan G. Halpern, Rebecca Pinnelas, and Frank Cecchin in Cardiovascular Medicine and Surgery, First Edition.

Section 9: Adult Congenital Heart Disease

105.4 A 26-year-old male presents to the clinic with complaints of palpitations that are usually associated with exertion. He denies having any chest pain. He has a known history of hypoplastic left heart with repair with the Fontan procedure. Which of the following tachyarrhythmias is most commonly seen in such patients?

A. Atrial fibrillation
B. Intra-atrial reentrant tachycardia
C. Atrioventricular (AV) nodal reentry tachycardia
D. Ventricular tachycardia

105.5 A 23-year-old female presents for a new patient visit with a new cardiologist. She reports that she has a history of an atretic tricuspid valve requiring a Fontan procedure at 1 year of age. She also has history of a pulmonary embolism at the age of 18. She reports that she has been doing fine and denies any current complaints. She takes no medications. Vitals include BP 118/80 mm Hg and heart rate 76 bpm. ECG demonstrates sinus rhythm. Which medication should this patient be prescribed?

A. Procainamide
B. Diltiazem
C. Warfarin
D. Apixaban

105.6 A 24-year-old male presents to the clinic for follow-up. He reports that in the last year, he has had worsening shortness of breath. He has a known history of a VSD. Vitals include BP 130/82 mm Hg and heart rate 89 bpm, and he is saturating at 88% on room air. Physical examination reveals digital clubbing. Lungs are clear on auscultation. A soft holosystolic murmur is heard. He only takes aspirin 81 mg daily. What recommendations should be made about continued aspirin use?

A. Continue aspirin indefinitely.
B. Stop aspirin immediately.
C. Continue aspirin for the next 6 months.
D. Start clopidogrel along with aspirin.

105.7 A 36-year-old male presents to the clinic for follow-up. He has a known large atrial septal defect (ASD) with right-to-left shunting. Vitals in the clinic demonstrate BP 158/98 mm Hg and heart rate 76 bpm. He checks his BP at home and reports it has been similar. Physical examination reveals digital clubbing. What should be the next **BEST** step in management?

A. Prescribe lisinopril.
B. Prescribe losartan.
C. Prescribe diltiazem.
D. Cardiac catheterization for assessment of pulmonary vascular resistance (PVR)

105.8 A 34-year-old female presents to the clinic for follow-up. She has a known small VSD. She reports that she has been feeling well and denies any symptoms. She has an upcoming root canal treatment scheduled. She has never had dental work done in the past. Which of the following is the **BEST** recommendation for this patient?

A. Prescribe prophylactic antibiotic therapy before any dental procedure.
B. Prescribe prophylactic antibiotic therapy only for tooth extractions.
C. She does not need prophylactic antibiotic therapy.
D. Ask her to call the clinic if she develops a fever after the dental procedure.

CHAPTER 105 | Pharmacologic Therapy for Adult Congenital Heart Disease

ANSWERS

105.1 The correct answer is D.
Rationale: This patient likely has Wolff-Parkinson-White syndrome. AV nodal blocking agents should be avoided in these patients to avoid triggering tachyarrhythmia across accessory pathways. Procainamide or other antiarrhythmics can be safely used in such patients.

105.2 The correct answer is C.
Rationale: Ideally, for simple complexity congenital lesions, such as ASD, VSD, Ebstein anomaly, and Class IC antiarrhythmic agents, such as flecainide and propafenone, can be used. Complex lesions with arrhythmias are treated with Class III antiarrhythmic agents such as amiodarone and sotalol.

105.3 The correct answer is A.
Rationale: Patients with complex congenital heart disease with arrhythmias should be treated with Class III antiarrhythmic agents such as amiodarone and sotalol.

105.4 The correct answer is B.
Rationale: Intra-atrial reentrant tachycardia or "incisional tachycardia" is the most common tachyarrhythmia observed in adult patients with congenital heart disease. It can be similar to typical atrial flutter. It can be managed with antiarrhythmics; however, often rate controlling agents are needed. Anticoagulation should be initiated in these patients depending on their prothrombotic risk factors. Radiofrequency ablation is also an option to help manage this tachyarrhythmia.

105.5 The correct answer is C.
Rationale: Adult patients with a known history of Fontan palliation that have a history of a prior pulmonary embolism or deep venous thrombosis should be on long-term systemic anticoagulation with warfarin (Class I recommendation).

105.6 The correct answer is B.
Rationale: This patient likely has a large VSD that may have led to the development of Eisenmenger syndrome given chronic hypoxia features on physical examination such as digital clubbing. Adult patients with congenital heart disease with pulmonary hypertension are at a particularly increased risk for pulmonary arterial hemorrhage and rupture and thus, anticoagulation and antiplatelet use should be used with caution.

105.7 The correct answer is D.
Rationale: Patients with right-to-left shunting should not have their BP controlled with agents that can reduce afterload as this may worsen the right-to-left shunting and thus exacerbate cyanosis. This patient should immediately be referred for cardiac catheterization for assessment of PVR and possible consideration of ASD repair if PVR is less than 6 to 8 wood units.

105.8 The correct answer is A.
Rationale: Patients with any congenital heart disease that is unrepaired should be prescribed prophylactic antibiotic therapy before any dental procedure as these patients are at a higher risk for infections and endocarditis post procedure.

SHUNT LESIONS

Samuel Kim and Joshua Schulman-Marcus

CHAPTER 106

QUESTIONS

106.1 Which of the following statements regarding a shunt is **NOT TRUE**?
  A. Left-to-right shunts may go unnoticed for many years.
  B. Right-to-left shunts involve the mixture of deoxygenated blood with oxygenated blood after passing through a communication.
  C. Left-to-right shunts result in cyanosis.
  D. Right-to-left shunts are rarely found as a single isolated anatomic lesion.

106.2 A 45-year-old male presents to your cardiology clinic to establish care. He states that he was told he had an atrial septal defect (ASD) that was incidentally discovered. He has no additional medical history **EXCEPT** for dyslipidemia. Which of the following statements is **TRUE** regarding ASDs?
  A. The most common form is primum ASD.
  B. The most common presenting symptom is palpitations.
  C. Electrocardiogram (ECG) will likely have left bundle branch morphology.
  D. Early-onset atrial fibrillation may be present.

106.3 A 19-year-old female presented to the hospital with dyspnea on exertion. She has no medical history. Her workup thus far has been unrevealing **EXCEPT** a transthoracic echocardiogram reveals a dilated right atrium and ventricle. You suspect a potential ASD. What additional workup should be considered at this time?
  A. Transesophageal echocardiogram
  B. Right heart catheterization
  C. Cardiovascular magnetic resonance (CMR)
  D. All of the above

106.4 Which of the following statements regarding ventricular septal defects (VSDs) is **INCORRECT**?
  A. Hemodynamically significant VSD results in left-sided cardiac chamber dilation.
  B. Progressive aortic valve insufficiency may occur as a consequence of a VSD.
  C. VSDs produce a murmur throughout all parts of the cardiac cycle.
  D. Inlet VSDs are associated with atrial and atrioventricular (AV) valve abnormalities.

*Questions and Answers are based on Chapter 106: Shunt Lesions by Zachary L. Steinberg, Mathias Possner, and Yonatan Buber in Cardiovascular Medicine and Surgery, First Edition.

106.5 An 8-year-old male with Down syndrome is accompanied by his mother and brought to your cardiology clinic to establish care. The mother states that her son was born with an endocardial cushion tissue defect that includes an inlet VSD as well as valve abnormalities she is unable to recall. Which of the following is **MOST LIKELY** present in this patient?

A. Bicuspid aortic valve
B. AV canal defect
C. Ebstein anomaly
D. Tricuspid atresia

106.6 A 23-year-old male with a past medical history of perimembranous VSD and asthma presents to your cardiology clinic to reestablish care. He was last seen when he was 17 years old and has been lost to follow-up since then after leaving for college. He expresses a desire for closure as the internet suggests that the VSD may negatively impact his heart. You suggest obtaining an echocardiogram. Which of the following is **INCORRECT** regarding an indication for VSD repair?

A. VSD repair is indicated in the presence of attributable symptoms.
B. VSD repair is indicated when pulmonary vascular resistance (PVR) is 2/3 of systemic vascular resistance (SVR).
C. VSD repair is indicated in the setting of left ventricular dilation.
D. VSD repair is indicated in the setting of left ventricular systolic dysfunction.

106.7 You are reviewing an echocardiogram that was obtained on a 22-year-old with a muscular VSD who was referred for closure. You review the images and note that the inferior vena cava's maximal diameter is 1.8 cm with a minimum of 0.7 cm. The peak flow velocity across the VSD into the right ventricle is 5 m/s. The patient's blood pressure at the time of the examination is 120/70 mm Hg. What is the estimated right ventricular systolic pressure (RVSP)?

A. 20 mm Hg
B. 115 mm Hg
C. 5 mm Hg
D. 100 mm Hg

106.8 Which of the following regarding patent ductus arteriosus (PDA) is **INCORRECT**?

A. It is associated with a continuous systolic and diastolic murmur that is described as "machine-like."
B. May result in left-sided chamber enlargement
C. ECG is often unremarkable but the most common abnormality is evidence of left atrial enlargement.
D. Shunt quantification with invasive oximetry is reliable.

106.9 Which of the following regarding a surgical shunt is **INCORRECT**?

A. Surgical shunts are most commonly used in patients with complex congenital heart disease accompanied by undercirculation of the pulmonary system.
B. Waterson and Potts shunt create a communication between the pulmonary artery and aorta.
C. Blalock-Taussig shunt connects the subclavian artery and pulmonary artery.
D. Most surgical shunt procedures are performed when no further interventions and repairs are planned.

106.10 Which of the following ASD can be closed with transcatheter techniques?
A. Primum ASD
B. Secundum ASD
C. Sinus venosus defect
D. Unroofed coronary sinus

ANSWERS

106.1 The correct answer is C.
Rationale: A left-to-right shunt does not present with hypoxemia and thus may go unnoticed for many years. It can result in an increase in pressure and volume through the pulmonary vasculature and cardiac chambers through which the shunted blood travels and results in irreversible physiologic perturbations.

Right-to-left shunts may result in cyanosis due to significant hypoxemia and are often diagnosed early in life. They are rarely found as an isolated anatomic lesion and more often occur because of a constellation of intracardiac abnormalities.

106.2 The correct answer is D.
Rationale: Atrial septal defects can be further subdivided with secundum ASD being the most common. Primum ASD results from the incomplete septation at the point of where the AV valves, atria, and ventricular septa meet and are a part of a constellation of abnormalities known as endocardial cushion defects. Sinus venosus ASDs are located at the junction of the vena cava and the roof of the right atria because of a deficiency in the development of the wall that separated the pulmonary vein from the vena cava. Unroofed coronary sinus is the least common and due to septal tissue deficiency surrounding the coronary sinus ostia resulting in communication between the atria.

Most patients with ASDs are asymptomatic; mild to moderate exertional dyspnea is the most common symptom. With larger shunts, symptoms of heart failure may manifest and are also associated with early-onset atrial arrhythmia (eg, atrial fibrillation).

ECG manifestation for ASDs includes right atrial enlargement and a right bundle branch block ± right axis deviation except for septum primum defects (right bundle branch block with LEFT axis deviation). Sinus venosus defects may have an ectopic atrial rhythm.

106.3 The correct answer is D.
Rationale: A significantly dilated right ventricle without an obvious intracardiac pathology detected by transthoracic echocardiogram should raise concerns and prompt further investigation.

Transthoracic echocardiography generally can establish the diagnosis of ASDs with the demonstration of color flow with color Doppler through the atria. However, certain subtypes of ASD are difficult to visualize with this modality, such as sinus venosus defect and associated anomalous pulmonary venous return, and thus further imaging with either transesophageal echocardiogram, cardiac computed tomography angiography (CTA), and/or cardiac magnetic resonance imaging (MRI) should be pursued.

Cardiac catheterization can assist with the detection of a shunt and provide additional information that may assist in determining treatment decisions once the diagnosis has been established. For example, the presence of significant pulmonary hypertension with PVR greater than 2/3 of SVR would deter closure for most patients and should be comanaged with a pulmonary hypertension specialist.

106.4 The correct answer is C.

Rationale: In patients with a VSD, a harsh holosystolic murmur may be appreciated throughout the precordium but may be loudest along the left sternal border. In those with larger shunts, S2 may also be split as well.

In the absence of other associated congenital heart disease, VSDs will result in the dilation of the left atrium and ventricle. As a result of the Venturi effect, the aortic valve cusps may also prolapse and result in progressive aortic valve insufficiency (**Table 106.1**).

TABLE 106.1 Echocardiographic Assessment of Patients With a Ventricular Septal Defect

Location and size of VSD	• Perimembranous VSD: Located in the membranous septum. Best visualized in the parasternal long-axis view. In a parasternal short-axis view below the aortic valve, the defect is typically located at 11 o'clock. • Muscular VSD: Located in the muscular septum, oftentimes occurs as multiple lesions. Color Doppler has a higher sensitivity than two-dimensional echocardiography in the detection of small muscular VSDs. • Conoventricular VSD: Located in the right ventricular outflow tract portion of the ventricular septum. Shunts are typically visualized in the parasternal short-axis just below the aortic valve with shunt flow directed into the right ventricular outflow tract at 1 o'clock. • Inlet VSD: Part of atrioventricular septal defects. The defect is best visualized in the apical four-chamber view, adjacent to the mitral and tricuspid valve.
Flow direction and pressure gradient	• In small, restrictive VSDs, peak velocity can be used to estimate right ventricular pressures: RVSP = systolic blood pressure − 4 × (peak flow velocity across VSD)^2. • The flow pattern is important for the evaluation of left-to-right, bidirectional, or right-to-left shunt.
Left atrial and ventricular size	• Hemodynamically significant shunts result in dilation of the left atrium and ventricle.
Left ventricular function	• Left ventricular systolic function typically is preserved. • Left ventricular dysfunction can occur because of aortic regurgitation or after VSD closure in patients with prolonged left ventricular volume overload.

TABLE 106.1	Echocardiographic Assessment of Patients With a Ventricular Septal Defect
Aortic valve	• Because of the Venturi effect, aortic valve cusps may prolapse into the VSD resulting in progressive aortic valve regurgitation.
Tricuspid valve	• Tricuspid valve leaflet tissue may prolapse into the VSD, providing either a partial or complete seal of the defect.
Right ventricle	• Small, restrictive VSDs may promote muscle bundle hypertrophy resulting in partitioning of the right ventricular chamber (also known as a double-chambered right ventricle) and subpulmonic stenosis. • Right ventricular dysfunction may result from severe pulmonary hypertension in patients with excessive pulmonary circulation.
Pulmonary pressures	• Estimation of pulmonary artery systolic pressures via tricuspid regurgitation or VSD peak velocities is important for the detection of pulmonary hypertension.

RVSP, right ventricular systolic pressure; VSD, ventricular septal defect.

106.5 The correct answer is B.

Rationale: Endocardial cushion defects are a group of lesions that affect the AV junction and thereby affect the interatrial septum, the interventricular septum, and AV valves. Two pathologies that belong to this group include inlet ventricular septal and AV canal defects. A higher prevalence of AV canal defects has been observed in patients with trisomy 21.

106.6 The correct answer is B.

Rationale: VSDs shunt blood generally from the left to the right ventricle and result in long-standing volume load within the pulmonary circulation and result in irreversible pulmonary arteriolar hypertension. The presence of pulmonary hypertension can be evaluated by both echocardiograms through the estimation of pulmonary artery systolic pressure with the use of tricuspid regurgitation or VSD peak velocities. In the presence of significant pulmonary hypertension (PVR 2/3 of SVR), VSD repair is contraindicated. As such, careful evaluation of the pulmonary vasculature is required in determining the candidacy of this procedure.

In the absence of severely elevated PVR, VSD repair is indicated in the presence of symptoms, left chamber enlargement, and/or left ventricular systolic dysfunction.

106.7 The correct answer is A.

Rationale: In small, restrictive VSD, the peak velocity can be used to estimate the right ventricular systolic pressure with the formula RVSP = systemic systolic blood pressure $- 4 \times$ (peak flow velocity across VSD)^2.

By inputting the values, RVSP = 120 mm Hg $- 4 \times$ (5 m/s)^2 = 120 $- 4 \times$ (25) = 120 $-$ 100 = 20 mm Hg.

106.8 The correct answer is D.
Rationale: Cardiac catheterization with serial oximetry may assist with confirming the diagnosis of PDA with the usage of serial oximetry and passage of the catheter across the PDA. The procedure also provides additional useful information, such as assessing left-sided filling pressures, evaluation of PVR, and calculation of cardiac output. However, shunt quantification with oximetry is unreliable due to the unequal shunt distribution within the pulmonary artery branches and the absence of a distal mixing chamber from which a mixed pulmonary artery oxygen saturation is sampled from.

106.9 The correct answer is D.
Rationale: Surgical shunts are generally performed as a temporary solution for hypoxemia in early childhood while pending definitive repair. They are created to increase pulmonary blood flow while simultaneously attempting to minimize exposure of the pulmonary vasculature to excessive pressure.

106.10 The correct answer is B.
Rationale: ASD closure is recommended in all patients with impaired functional capacity, evidence of right atrial and/or ventricular enlargement, right ventricular dysfunction, or concerns of paradoxical embolism. As part of the workup, careful evaluation of PVR is essential for patients as it may pose harm to those with significant elevations. For ASD closure, surgical techniques have been developed and remain the mainstay of therapy for most with one exception. Transcatheter ASD closure is the treatment of choice when anatomically feasible for secundum ASDs as it has been demonstrated to have a high rate of success with a low risk of complications when there is adequate circumferential tissue.

LEFT-SIDED OBSTRUCTIVE LESIONS*

Anojan Pathmanathan, Niranjan Ojha, and Robert L. Carhart

CHAPTER 107

QUESTIONS

107.1 A 24-year-old male with no significant medical history is referred to the cardiology clinic due to concerns of elevated blood pressure and murmur. He is currently in college and denies any chest pain, shortness of breath, headaches, visual changes, dizziness, fevers, excessive stress, or caffeine use. He further denies any illicit drug use or over-the-counter medication or herbal supplements. When asked about his exercise regimen, he states that he is active and regularly plays recreational basketball but notes he has lower extremity pain while playing. Blood pressure is 179/89 and 128/72 in his left arm and left leg, respectively. Auscultation revealed clear S1 and S2 heart sounds with a low-grade systolic ejection murmur. There are diminished lower extremity pulses bilaterally. Transthoracic echocardiogram (TTE) confirms a bicuspid aortic valve (BAV) with mild-moderate aortic stenosis. What other finding is expected for this patient?

A. A "diastolic tail" in abdominal aorta in pulse-wave Doppler studies
B. An aortic valve regurgitant fraction of 54% and effective regurgitant orifice area (EROA) of 0.5 cm^2
C. Diffuse circumferential thickening of the aortic wall
D. An inspiratory reduction in mitral peak E-wave velocities of 32% on Doppler studies

107.2 A 64-year-old male is referred to the cardiology clinic after concern of exertional dyspnea that has been worsening over the last 4 months. He has a significant medical history of morbid obesity, lower extremity arthritis, tobacco use, hypothyroidism, and hyperlipidemia. Physical examination findings include a single-second heart sound, prominent S4, and systolic ejection murmur over the precordium. Echocardiographic evaluation revealed normal left ventricular systolic function with left ventricular hypertrophy as well as thickening and doming of a BAV. Doppler studies of the aortic valve are suggestive of severe stenosis. Which of the following pathologies is most often associated with the BAV?

A. Ventricular septal defect
B. Patent ductus arteriosus
C. Coarctation of the aorta (CoA)
D. Dilated ascending aorta

---

*Questions and Answers are based on Chapter 107: Left-Sided Obstructive Lesions by Lauren Andrade and Yuli Y. Kim in Cardiovascular Medicine and Surgery, First Edition.

107.3 A 70-year-old female with a medical history of hyperlipidemia and hypertension presents to the cardiology clinic after an abnormal electrocardiogram (ECG) result. She initially presented to the emergency department last month with fever and diarrhea secondary to gastroenteritis. A routine ECG on that visit was significant for left ventricular hypertrophy. She denies any chest pain, diaphoresis, palpitations, or swelling. She does report mild fatigue and shortness of breath with slight limitations in her daily activities. Physical examination reveals a systolic murmur loudest over the midsternal border with radiation to the suprasternal notch. She does **NOT** have an elevated jugular venous pulse or peripheral edema. Chest x-ray showed no significant pathology. Echocardiogram showed normal systolic function and concentric left ventricular hypertrophy. Multiple pulse-wave Doppler reveal flow acceleration originating from a left ventricular outflow tract obstruction. Maximum gradient across the obstruction is 35 mm Hg. What is the next step in management?

A. Clinical follow-up every 6 to 12 months with ECG and TTE every 12 months and exercise test every 2 years
B. Balloon dilation
C. Clinical follow-up every 2 years with ECG, echocardiogram and exercise stress test
D. Surgical resection

107.4 A 73-year-old female with a history of hypertension, type 2 diabetes, and recently diagnosed paroxysmal atrial fibrillation presented to the hospital for a scheduled electrocardioversion. A transesophageal echocardiogram (TEE) was performed to rule out intracardiac thrombus and incidentally revealed a supravalvular aortic stenosis. She underwent cardioversion successfully and now presents to the clinic for follow-up. She performs all activities of daily living without incident and goes on walks around her neighborhood every other day. She denies any chest pain, shortness of breath, syncope, lightheadedness, or fatigue. TTE showed normal systolic function. Doppler evaluation was significant for a mean gradient of 56 mm Hg and a peak velocity of 4.2 m/s across the supravalvular obstruction. What is the next **BEST** step in further evaluating her supravalvular stenosis?

A. Follow-up in cardiology clinic in 3 years
B. Refer for surgical intervention.
C. Refer for cardiac catheterization.
D. Exercise stress testing.

107.5 A 66-year-old male with a history of hypertension, patent foramen ovale, and coronary artery disease (CAD) presents to the cardiology clinic for follow-up. He now reports lower extremity edema and shortness of breath on exertion along with occasional palpitations. Physical examination reveals a low-pitched mid-diastolic murmur. ECG reveals atrial fibrillation. Repeat TTE demonstrates an ejection fraction of 40%, an enlarged left atrium, and a parachute-like appearance of the mitral valve. What **BEST** explains the physical echocardiogram findings?

A. Rheumatic mitral stenosis
B. Mitral stenosis from an abnormality of the left ventricular papillary muscles
C. Supravalvular mitral stenosis
D. Flail mitral leaflet

107.6 A 37-year-old African American male with a history of hypertension is referred to the cardiology clinic for refractory hypertension. Patient reports that he was first evaluated by his primary physician who initiated an angiotensin-converting inhibitor, calcium channel blocker, and diuretic therapy without significant reduction in his blood pressure. The patient denies any chest pain, shortness of breath, headaches, visual changes, nausea, or vomiting. Renal artery stenosis was ruled out with ultrasound sonography. Auscultation examination is significant for an S4 and continuous ejection murmur heard over the left upper chest. Blood pressures from a sitting position were obtained and are as follows:

Right arm	144/98
Left arm	142/95
Right leg	126/89
Left leg	129/84

Which chest x-ray finding **BEST** correlates with his **MOST LIKELY** diagnosis?
A. Straightening of the left heart border
B. Pulmonary venous congestion
C. Notching of the inferior surface of the fourth and eighth ribs
D. An enlarged aortic knob

107.7 A 30-year-old male is referred to the cardiology office for a murmur identified in a preemployment physical examination. He denies any chest pain, shortness of breath, or palpitations. He does **NOT** smoke and reports occasional alcohol and marijuana use. The patient's family history is significant for hypoplastic left heart syndrome in his father. Physical examination is significant for an early systolic ejection to click with a crescendo-decrescendo murmur that radiates to the carotids. TTE shows a fish-mouth appearance of the aortic valve in the parasternal short-axis acoustic window. Doppler studies across the aortic valve show a mean gradient of 24 mm Hg and a peak velocity of 2.1 m/s. What is the appropriate next step in the management of his diagnosis?
A. Screen all first-degree relatives with TTE.
B. Left cardiac catheterization to further evaluate the transvalvular gradient
C. Cardiac magnetic resonance imaging (MRI)
D. Repeat TTE in 1 to 2 years.

107.8 A 33-year-old male with a history of Williams syndrome and hyperlipidemia presents to the cardiology clinic for evaluation of new onset chest pain. He states that he is finding it harder to exercise on his treadmill due to mild dull chest pain but is able to get through his normal routine. The pain does **NOT** radiate and is relieved with rest. ECG shows sinus rhythm with inverted t waves across the precordial leads along with voltage criteria met for left ventricular hypertrophy. TTE is significant for an ejection fraction of 40% with hypokinesis of the anterior left ventricular wall. It also demonstrates hypertrophied tissue at the sinotubular junction with flow acceleration noted on Doppler studies in the same area. What is the next **BEST** step in the evaluation of his chest pain?

A. Cardiac catheterization
B. Transesophageal echocardiography
C. Genetic testing for first-degree family members and 6 months follow-up
D. Computed tomography (CT) scan of the coronary arteries

107.9 A 44-year-old male with a history significant for BAV and CoA presents to the cardiology clinic for follow-up. He was diagnosed with BAV and CoA 15 years ago and has remained asymptomatic until recently. He is hypertensive on examination and now reports claudication during his daily jogs associated with worsening shortness of breath. Echocardiogram demonstrated normal left ventricular function with a mean gradient of 23 mm Hg across the aortic valve and a peak-to-peak coarctation gradient of 26 mm Hg. Sagittal MRI of the aorta demonstrates that the area of coarctation is in close proximity to the left subclavian artery. What is the appropriate next step in management?

A. Catheter-based stenting of the coarctation
B. Surgical coarctation repair
C. Follow-up in 3 to 6 months with ECG and transthoracic echo every 12 months
D. Transcather aortic valve replacement

107.10 A 67-year-old male presents to the cardiology clinic for a follow-up of mild BAV stenosis. He currently denies any symptoms. The patient also has a CoA with a peak-to-peak coarctation gradient of 12 mm Hg and previously repaired atrial septal defect (ASD). Repeat echocardiography showed no significant changes from his last examination. Defects in what gene have been linked to the congenital abnormalities found in this patient?

A. Elastin gene
B. PDGFRA gene
C. NOTCH1 gene
D. MYH7 gene

ANSWERS

107.1 The correct answer is A.
Rationale: This patient has clinical symptoms and signs of CoA. On Doppler studies, aliasing across the area of aortic narrowing, a delayed systolic forward flow, and continuation of forward flow with the absence of flow reversal during diastole ("diastolic tail") are key diagnostic findings in hemodynamically significant CoA. The diastolic tail is largely due to continuous collateral flow.

An aortic valve regurgitant fraction greater than 50% and EROA greater than 0.3 cm^2 meet the criteria of severe aortic regurgitation. Diffuse circumferential thickening of the aortic wall is seen in aortitis. An inspiratory reduction in mitral peak E-wave velocities greater than 25% on Doppler studies is consistent with cardiac tamponade. The patient does not exhibit the signs or symptoms of these conditions.

KEY POINTS

✓ Common symptoms of CoA include claudication, weakness, headache, chest pain, and dyspnea. Findings include higher upper versus lower extremity blood pressures, diminished lower extremity pulses, and an associated BAV (>50% of cases). Key diagnostic findings of CoA include abdominal aorta Doppler studies showing aliasing across the area of aortic narrowing, a delayed systolic forward flow, and the continuation of forward flow with the absence of flow reversal during diastole ("diastolic tail").

107.2 The correct answer is D.

Rationale: BAV is the most common congenital cardiac abnormality affecting approximately 1% of the population with a higher prevalence in males. It is most often associated with aortic valve stenosis, as in this patient, or aortic insufficiency. Thoracic aortic aneurysms are the second most frequent complication occurring in up to 50% of patients with BAV. This close association is likely secondary to increased shear stress on the walls of the proximal aorta from hemodynamic flow disturbances and genetic factors resulting in predisposed weakness of the aortic wall. As a result, there is an 8.4-fold higher risk of aortic dissection than the general population.

Ventricular septal defects and patent ductus arteriosus are associated in approximately 20% of patients with BAV. Although patients with CoA have an associated BAV in greater than 50% of cases, the opposite is false with primary BAV having an association with CoA in less than 10% of cases.

KEY POINTS

✓ Aside from aortic valve dysfunction, the most common association of BAV is thoracic aortic aneurysms. In asymptomatic or symptomatic patients with BAV, aortic sinus or ascending aorta diameters greater than 5.5 cm require replacement.

107.3 The correct answer is C.

Rationale: This patient's echocardiogram findings are significant for subvalvular aortic stenosis which comprises approximately 10% to 20% of all aortic stenosis and is most common in males. Unlike other types of aortic stenosis, it is not seen in neonates and is thus thought to be an acquired lesion. Management and follow-up patient care are largely dependent on the severity of the subvalvular obstruction and the presence of symptoms. Along with this patient's objective findings, she presents with NYHA FC II (New York Heart Association Functional Classification II) symptoms and mild hemodynamic sequelae (mild ventricular enlargement) indicative of a Stage B physiologic state. According to AHA/ACC (American Heart Association/American College of Cardiology) guidelines, she requires follow-up every 2 years with a clinical visit along with ECG, TTE, and exercise stress test (6-minute walk test or cardiopulmonary exercise test).

Clinical follow-up every 6 to 12 months with ECG and TTE every 12 months and exercise test every 2 years is required for patients with more advanced subvalvular obstruction (Stage C). Unlike valvular aortic stenosis, subvalvular aortic stenosis does not respond to balloon dilation. Definitive therapy consists of surgical resection which is indicated for patients with a subvalvular maximum gradient of 50 mm Hg or more and symptoms attributable to the obstruction or maximum gradient less than 50 mm Hg with heart failure or ischemic symptoms and/or left ventricular systolic dysfunction attributable to subvalvular aortic stenosis.

KEY POINTS

- ✔ Definitive therapy for subvalvular aortic stenosis may involve surgical resection of a discrete subaortic membrane, removal of muscle in the left ventricular outflow tract, or removal of a subaortic ridge of tissue. Patients who do not meet the criteria for surgery or postsurgical patients require clinical follow-up with objective testing that is dependent on the severity of the stenosis and the presence of symptoms.

107.4 The correct answer is D.

Rationale: This patient has an incidental finding of severe supravalvular aortic stenosis. Patients with asymptomatic aortic stenosis can have masked symptoms due to inactivity or lack of exertion often seen with aging. In these patients, stress testing may unmask symptoms of hemodynamically significant obstruction which would warrant intervention.

Follow-up patient care would be appropriate if the patient remains asymptomatic during stress testing. Surgical intervention would be warranted if the patient is found to have symptomatic aortic stenosis on stress testing. Referral for cardiac catheterization is recommended before surgical intervention to identify any concurrent CAD that may need revascularization. Furthermore, in patients with supravalvular aortic stenosis, cardiac catheterization can carry the excess risk of ischemia due to catheter manipulation in the possible setting of coronary ostial stenosis and periprocedural effects of anesthesia. CT coronary imaging may be a more appropriate modality to assess for CAD.

KEY POINTS

- ✔ Exercise testing can be helpful in risk-stratifying patients with left-sided obstructive lesions who have severe stenosis but are asymptomatic.

107.5 The correct answer is B.

Rationale: Congenital mitral valve stenosis can arise from dysplasia of the valve itself or a region above the valve. A parachute-like appearance of the mitral valve on TTE suggests that there is a single papillary muscle to which all the mitral valve chordae are attached to. This feature may or may not result in mitral stenosis. Obstruction of mitral inflow can cause elevated left atrial and pulmonary artery pressures depending on the severity of the narrowing.

Characteristic echocardiogram findings of rheumatic mitral stenosis include diastolic doming of the mitral leaflets or a hockey-stick shape appearance. Supravalvular mitral valve stenosis could be secondary to a membrane or supramitral ring just above the mitral annulus. Mitral regurgitation results from a flail mitral leaflet due to chordae rupture.

KEY POINTS

✔ A parachute-like appearance of the mitral valve on TTE suggests that there is a single papillary muscle to which all the mitral valve chordae are attached to. Parachute mitral valves are prone to stenosis. In cases of severe mitral stenosis (<1.5 cm^2), surgical management involves the division of the single papillary muscle.

107.6 The correct answer is C.

Rationale: This patient has a long-standing unrepaired CoA based on the objective findings. Chest x-ray in CoA may demonstrate dilation of the aorta before and after the obstruction. This can create a "3" appearance as well as notching of the inferior surface of the ribs created by intercostal collateral vessel development. The fourth and eighth ribs are usually involved.

Straightening of the left hard border on chest x-ray and pulmonary venous congestion are hallmarks of mitral stenosis due to underfilling of the left ventricle and aorta. Pulmonary venous congestion is seen in cases of elevated left atrial and pulmonary pressures. An enlarged aortic knob is suggestive of aortic stenosis along with a dilated aorta, widening of the mediastinal silhouette, and displacement of the trachea.

KEY POINTS

✔ Young patients with refractory hypertension should be evaluated with a thorough physical examination and imaging modalities to evaluate for CoA. Chest x-ray may reveal a "3" appearance of the aorta due to pre- and post-coarctation dilation as well as notching of the inferior surface of the ribs created by intercostal collateral vessel development. Further evaluation of CoA includes a TTE and/or cardiac MRI or CT imaging.

107.7 The correct answer is A.

Rationale: This patient's TTE shows a BAV. BAVs are often linked with a number of congenital heart defects and left-sided obstructive lesions that can present simultaneously with a strong genetic link (NOTCH-1 gene). Thus, the AHA/ACC guidelines state it is reasonable (Class IIa) to screen all first-degree relatives of those with BAV. Approximately 10% of first-degree family members of those with BAV have it themselves.

Cardiac catheterization may be utilized in complex valvular lesions when noninvasive modalities cannot estimate a true transvalvular gradient or if there are multiple levels of obstruction. Cardiac MRI and CT are reserved for lesions not well seen on echocardiography. MRI and CT are beneficial to follow a dilated ascending aorta associated with BAV. This patient has progressive class B aortic stenosis (mild severity, V_{max} 2.0-2.9 m/s) and thus, TTE is recommended every 3 to 5 years.

KEY POINTS

✔ Studies have shown that BAV has a male predominance and is prevalent in 10% of first-degree family members. The AHA/ACC guidelines state it is reasonable (Class IIa) to screen all first-degree relatives of those with BAV.

107.8 The correct answer is D.

Rationale: This patient's echocardiogram findings are indicative of supravalvular aortic stenosis. Furthermore, his symptoms of angina and the regional wall motion abnormalities are concerning for myocardial ischemia. About half of all patients with supravalvular aortic stenosis have Williams syndrome. Patients with Williams syndrome have an autosomal dominant defect in the elastin gene (7q11.23) that leads to abnormally thick and hypertrophied tissue just above the aortic valve. Due to this abnormality and the close proximity to the coronary artery ostia, patients with supravalvular aortic stenosis are at high risk for limited diastolic flow through the coronary arteries leading to ischia and possible sudden death. Therefore, it was very important to manage risk factors of CAD in these patients, identify significant coronary lesions, and pursue percutaneous or surgical revascularization if warranted. In patients with supravalvular aortic stenosis, cardiac catheterization can carry the excess risk of ischemia and periprocedural cardiac arrest from catheter manipulation in an already stenosed coronary origin as well the added effects of anesthesia on diastolic blood pressure. In these cases, cardiac CT imaging may be a better option to visualize the coronary arteries.

Transesophageal echocardiography would provide no additional benefit in this patient as the left-sided obstruction was identified clearly on TTE. Although there is a genetic link between Williams and supravalvular aortic stenosis through the elastin gene, delaying further ischemic workup is not recommended in a patient with confirmed supravalvular stenosis and signs of ischemia.

KEY POINTS

- Approximately half of all patients with supravalvular aortic stenosis have Williams syndrome. Special concern in patients with angina and syncope due to the increased risk of coronary ischemia and sudden death. Coronary CT imaging may be a preferred modality to evaluate for significant CAD as cardiac catheterization has an increased risk of ischemia due to catheter manipulation in obstructed coronary ostia (from a thickened sinotubular junction) or decrease in diastolic blood pressure from anesthesia.

107.9 The correct answer is B.

Rationale: According to current guidelines, catheter-based or surgical intervention is recommended in cases of hypertension and evidence of significant aortic coarctation with a coarctation gradient greater than 20 mm Hg. This gradient can be obtained via cuff blood pressure, catheterization, or Doppler gradient. Concurrent left ventricular dysfunction with a lower coarctation gradient cutoff can also be accepted for intervention. When deciding between surgical versus catheter-based intervention, it is important to consider the location of the coarctation and the proximity to any neck vessels. This can be best identified by CT or MRI. Stenting of a coarctation in close proximity to a neck vessel has the potential to cover and jail its origins. In these cases, surgical correction including end-to-end anastomosis after coarctation resection, bypass grafting, or subclavian flap repair is more favorable. Anatomy not amenable to stenting or surgical intervention can be considered for balloon angioplasty.

For a patient with hypertension and coarctation gradient greater than 20 mm Hg, further intervention should be considered rather than clinical follow-up. This patient has mild aortic stenosis which does not require intervention.

KEY POINTS

- Catheter-based or surgical intervention is recommended in patients with aortic coarctation with a coarctation gradient greater than 20 mm Hg. Determining which patients are candidates for catheter-based versus surgical intervention depends upon the proximity of the coarctation to any neck vessels or the need to enlarge a more significant segment of a hypoplastic aortic arch.

107.10 The correct answer is C.

Rationale: Mutations in the NOTCH1 gene have been linked to nonsyndromic congenital heart disease primarily affecting the cardiac outflow tract and semilunar valve. This can lead to abnormalities such as BAV, aortic valve stenosis, hypoplastic left heart syndrome, tetralogy of Fallot, pulmonic valve stenosis, and atrial or ventricular septal defects.

In the context of left-sided cardiac obstructions, the elastin gene is a link between Williams syndrome and supraventricular aortic valve stenosis. The PDGFRA gene is associated with total anomalous pulmonary venous return. The MYH7 gene is strongly linked with Ebstein anomaly, left ventricular noncompaction cardiomyopathy, hypertrophic cardiomyopathy, and dilated cardiomyopathy.

KEY POINTS

- The NOTCH1 gene has been linked to BAV, aortic stenosis, hypoplastic left heart syndrome, and other congenital cardiac abnormalities.

RIGHT-SIDED LESIONS

Atika Azhar, Meet Patel, and Robert L. Carhart

CHAPTER 108

QUESTIONS

108.1 A 34-year-old man presents to the emergency department with complaints of chest pain and difficulty breathing. He has a history of congenital heart disease involving the right ventricle (RV), with previous surgical repair of a double-chambered right ventricle (DCRV). Physical examination reveals elevated jugular venous pressure and a prominent right ventricular impulse. Electrocardiogram (ECG) shows evidence of right ventricular hypertrophy. Doppler echocardiography shows a peak velocity of greater than 3 m/s signifying moderate obstruction of blood flow within the subinfundibular ventricle. What is the most appropriate next step in his management?

A. Repeat echocardiogram in 1 month.
B. Initiation of anticoagulation therapy
C. Cardiac catheterization with balloon valvuloplasty
D. Coronary angiography
E. Administration of metoprolol for rate control

108.2 A 22-year-old asymptomatic woman presents to the cardiology clinic for routine follow-up. She has a history of repaired tetralogy of Fallot with residual mild-to-moderate pulmonary regurgitation. Physical examination reveals a systolic murmur along the left sternal border and a prominent pulmonary component of the second heart sound. ECG shows evidence of right ventricular hypertrophy. Echocardiography demonstrates mild-to-moderate pulmonary regurgitation with dilatation of the RV. What is the most appropriate next step in her management?

A. Initiation of beta-blocker therapy
B. Surgical repair of tetralogy of Fallot
C. Echocardiographic surveillance every 3 years
D. Administration of diuretics for symptom relief

108.3 A 24-year-old man presents with a history of dyspnea, syncope, and chest pain on exertion. On examination, there is a prominent "A" wave in the jugular venous pulse, an RV heave on palpation, and an ejection click that decreases in intensity with inspiration. A Doppler echocardiogram shows a peak velocity of 4 m/s with a peak gradient of greater than 60 mm Hg through the pulmonic valve. Which of the following is the most appropriate next step in management?

*Questions and Answers are based on Chapter 108: Right-Sided Lesions by Margaret M. Fuchs, C. Charles Jain, and Heidi M. Connolly in Cardiovascular Medicine and Surgery, First Edition.

A. Medical management with diuretics and beta-blockers
B. Immediate referral for percutaneous balloon valvuloplasty
C. Initiation of anticoagulation therapy with warfarin
D. Cardiac catheterization for further evaluation of the coronary arteries
E. Monitoring with serial echocardiograms every 6 months

108.4 A 36-year-old woman presents with a new diagnosis of valvular pulmonary stenosis. She has no symptoms at rest or with exertion. Physical examination is normal. A Doppler echocardiogram confirms the diagnosis of valvular pulmonary stenosis peak gradient of less than 36 mm Hg. Which of the following is the most appropriate initial management strategy for this patient?

A. Observation and regular follow-up with echocardiograms every 3 to 5 years
B. Medical management with diuretics and calcium channel blockers
C. Cardiac catheterization for evaluation of the coronary arteries
D. Referral for pulmonary valve replacement surgery
E. Initiation of anticoagulation therapy with warfarin

108.5 A 32-year-old patient with a history of Alagille syndrome presents with exertional dyspnea, peripheral edema, and a continuous murmur on examination. ECG shows right ventricular hypertrophy, and chest x-ray shows a relatively small vascular pedicle and increased lung lucency. Transthoracic echocardiography is challenging due to poor two-dimensional visualization of the pulmonary arteries. What is the most appropriate diagnostic modality for confirming the diagnosis of peripheral pulmonary artery (PA) stenosis in this patient?

A. ECG
B. Chest x-ray
C. Transthoracic echocardiography
D. Computed tomography (CT) scan
E. Cardiac catheterization with pulmonary angiography

108.6 A 25-year-old man with a past medical history of pulmonary atresia and surgical palliation presents with dyspnea on exertion and palpitations. Physical examination reveals a systolic ejection murmur along the left upper sternal border and normal breath sounds. ECG shows an irregular rhythm without p waves. Chest x-ray shows decreased pulmonary vascular markings. Echocardiogram reveals a small hypoplastic RV with an absent pulmonary valve and intact ventricular septum. Which of the following is the most appropriate management strategy for this patient?

A. Surgical placement of a systemic-to-pulmonary shunt
B. Initiation of a direct oral anticoagulants (DOAC)
C. Coronary angiography
D. Transesophageal echocardiogram

108.7 A 32-year-old woman presents with chest pain and palpitations. She has a history of repaired pulmonary atresia with right ventricular outflow tract reconstruction at the age of 4 years old. She has been asymptomatic since then but now has developed new symptoms. Echocardiogram shows a dilated RV with moderate pulmonary regurgitation. ECG shows normal sinus rhythm with the right bundle branch block. Which of the following is the most appropriate management strategy for this patient?

A. Initiation of anticoagulation therapy
B. Cardiac catheterization
C. Transthoracic echocardiogram
D. Surgical reintervention on RV-PA conduit
E. Amiodarone 200 mg daily

108.8 A 25-year-old woman presents with palpitations, dyspnea on exertion, and lower extremity edema for the past 3 months. On physical examination, the patient has a split first heart sound and systolic ejection click. Chest x-ray shows marked cardiomegaly with a narrow vascular pedicle. ECG shows right bundle branch block, PR segment prolongation, and low voltage QRS in the right-sided chest leads. Transthoracic echocardiography is performed, and the diagnosis of Ebstein anomaly is confirmed, with apical displacement of the tricuspid septal leaflet measuring 10 mm/m^2 on the displacement index. Multiple jets of tricuspid regurgitation are also visualized. What is the next **BEST** step in the management of this patient?

A. Cardiac magnetic resonance imaging (MRI)
B. Cardiac CT scan
C. Surgical intervention
D. Medical management with diuretics
E. Serial echocardiographic follow-up

108.9 A 34-year-old male with a known history of Ebstein anomaly presents to the adult congenital heart disease clinic for routine follow-up. He has been asymptomatic and has been on annual surveillance with echocardiogram, ECG, and exercise testing. His latest echocardiogram shows worsening tricuspid regurgitation and right heart enlargement compared to the previous year. He denies any symptoms of heart failure or arrhythmias. What is the most appropriate next step in his management?

A. Repeat echocardiogram in 12 months.
B. Initiate diuretic therapy.
C. Referral to an electrophysiologist for arrhythmia evaluation
D. Cardiac MRI every 1 to 2 years

ANSWERS

108.1 The correct answer is C.
Rationale: This patient presents with symptoms and findings consistent with obstruction of blood flow within the subinfundibular ventricle, which is characteristic of a DCRV. The most appropriate next step in management would be to perform cardiac catheterization with balloon valvuloplasty to relieve the obstruction and improve blood flow. Repeat echocardiogram in 1 month (option A) would not be appropriate as the patient is symptomatic and requires immediate intervention. Anticoagulation therapy (option B) would not be indicated in this case as there is no evidence of thrombus formation. Coronary angiography (option D) would not be necessary as

there is no suspicion of coronary artery disease in this patient. Metoprolol for rate control (option E) would not be effective in relieving the obstruction and improving blood flow in the RV.

108.2 The correct answer is C.
Rationale: This patient presents with residual pulmonary regurgitation and dilatation of the RV, which are known complications of repaired tetralogy of Fallot. The most appropriate next step in management would be echocardiographic surveillance every 3 years to monitor the progression of the disease and assess the need for intervention. Initiation of beta-blocker therapy and surgical repair may be considered for symptomatic patients. Similarly, diuretics may be considered in patients with heart failure with signs of volume overload.

108.3 The correct answer is B.
Rationale: The clinical presentation and echocardiogram findings are consistent with severe valvular pulmonary stenosis, and the most appropriate next step in management would be immediate referral for percutaneous balloon valvuloplasty.

The patient's history of dyspnea, syncope, and chest pain on exertion, along with the physical examination findings of a prominent "A" wave in the jugular venous pulse, an RV heave on palpation, and an ejection click that decreases in intensity with inspiration, all suggest significant obstruction of the right ventricular outflow tract due to valvular pulmonary stenosis. These symptoms and findings indicate that the patient is likely experiencing severe obstruction of blood flow from the RV to the PA, leading to right ventricular hypertrophy and impaired cardiac function. Echocardiography confirms the diagnosis of valvular pulmonary stenosis with severe obstruction of the right ventricular outflow tract. Medical management with diuretics and beta-blockers may be useful in managing symptoms and stabilizing the patient's condition temporarily, but it is not a definitive treatment for severe valvular pulmonary stenosis. Anticoagulation therapy with warfarin is not indicated in this case as there is no evidence of associated thromboembolic risk. Cardiac catheterization for evaluation of coronary arteries is not necessary as the patient's symptoms and echocardiogram findings are consistent with valvular pulmonary stenosis and not coronary artery disease. Serial echocardiograms every 6 months would not be appropriate as the severity of the condition requires immediate intervention.

The most appropriate next step in management for this patient is immediate referral for percutaneous balloon valvuloplasty, which can effectively relieve the obstruction and restore normal blood flow from the RV to the PA, thus improving symptoms and preventing further complications associated with severe valvular pulmonary stenosis.

108.4 The correct answer is A.
Rationale: The most appropriate initial management strategy for this patient with mild valvular pulmonary stenosis and no symptoms would be observation and regular follow-up with echocardiograms every 3 to 5 years.

This patient is asymptomatic and there are no signs of severe right ventricular hypertrophy or impaired cardiac function on physical examination or echocardiography.

Based on the clinical presentation and echocardiogram findings, the patient's condition is stable and does not require immediate intervention such as pulmonary valve replacement surgery. Medical management with diuretics and calcium channel blockers is not indicated in this case as the patient is asymptomatic. Cardiac catheterization for evaluation of coronary arteries is not necessary as there is no evidence of associated coronary artery disease. Anticoagulation therapy with warfarin is not indicated as there is no evidence of thromboembolic risk.

108.5 The correct answer is E.
Rationale: Clinical explanation: In patients with suspected peripheral PA stenosis, direct measurement of pressure gradients in the cath lab can be very helpful to simultaneously assess the severity of stenosis and identify its precise location with pulmonary angiography. Transthoracic echocardiography may raise suspicion for increased pressures in the main PA, but cross-sectional imaging with CT or MRI and cardiac catheterization with pulmonary angiography are generally required to confirm the diagnosis.

108.6 The correct answer is B.
Rationale: This patient with a history of pulmonary atresia presents with findings consistent with atrial fibrillation. Atrial arrhythmias are common in patients with palliated pulmonary atresia with intact ventricular septum. Therefore, therapeutic anticoagulation should be considered unless contraindicated. Options A, C, and D are not appropriate management strategies for this condition as the patient already had surgical palliation.

108.7 The correct answer is D.
Rationale: This patient has a history of repaired pulmonary atresia and intact ventricular septum and is now presenting with chest pain and palpitations. The most appropriate management strategy for this patient would be the surgical repair of the right ventricular outflow tract, as evidenced by the dilated RV with moderate pulmonary regurgitation. Cardiac catheterization and transthoracic echocardiogram may be helpful in further evaluating the anatomy and function of the right ventricular outflow tract, but surgical repair would be the most appropriate intervention in this case. Anticoagulation therapy and amiodarone are not indicated based on the information provided.

108.8 The correct answer is C.
Rationale: The management of Ebstein anomaly depends on the severity of the disease and the presence of associated anomalies. In symptomatic patients with severe Ebstein anomaly, surgical intervention may be required. This can involve repair of the tricuspid valve or replacement with a prosthetic valve. In some cases, additional procedures such as closure of atrial septal defects or arrhythmia ablation may also be needed. Cardiac MRI and CT scans may provide additional information about the anatomy and function of the heart, but they are not typically used as the first-line diagnostic tests for Ebstein anomaly. Medical management with diuretics may be used to manage symptoms of heart failure, but it is not a definitive treatment for

Ebstein anomaly. Serial echocardiographic follow-up is important to monitor disease progression and response to treatment, but it is not the next best step in the management of this patient with severe symptomatic Ebstein anomaly.

108.9 The correct answer is C.

Rationale: Patients with Ebstein anomaly should be monitored closely for the progression of symptoms and worsening of cardiac function. In this case, the patient's echocardiogram shows worsening tricuspid regurgitation and right heart enlargement, indicating potential progression of the disease. Referral to an electrophysiologist with experience in congenital heart disease is appropriate to evaluate for the presence of arrhythmias, especially given the patient's history of ventricular tachycardia risk factors. Cardiac MRI every 1 to 2 years may be helpful in patients with functional impairment, but in this case, the patient is asymptomatic and does not require frequent imaging. Diuretic therapy may be considered if the patient develops heart failure symptoms, but it is not the next best step in this case. Repeat echocardiogram in 12 months may be appropriate in some cases, but given the patient's worsening tricuspid regurgitation and right heart enlargement, further evaluation for arrhythmias is warranted.

COMPLEX LESIONS

Ronald Russo, Philip Chebaya, and Robert L. Carhart

CHAPTER 109

QUESTIONS

109.1 A 55-year-old male with a history of D-transposition of vessels requiring surgical repair presents to your office with a 1-month history of progressive fatigue, presyncope, and shortness of breath, particularly on exertion. Prior to this visit, the patient had been doing well and able to perform all her everyday tasks on her own with no concern. Patient's last echocardiogram was performed 3 years ago and was considered unremarkable at the time. Due to the patient presentation, you decide to order an ECHO which demonstrated severe new aortic regurgitation with moderate right ventricular (RV) dilation and neoaortic dilation.

Which of the following is the next **BEST** step in her management for this patient?
A. Surgical valve replacement
B. Metoprolol
C. Supervised exercise program
D. Start direct oral anticoagulant (DOAC).
E. Advise patients to avoid activity and remain sedentary until symptoms improve.

109.2 A 23-year-old male presents with complaints of progressive swelling of the upper extremities including his head with associated headache, shortness of breath, and blurred vision. His medical history is most significant for D-transposition of the great arteries (D-TGA) status post an atrial switch repair at 6 months of age. Other medical history includes Mobitz type II atrioventricular (AV) block status post dual chamber pacemaker 2 years ago. On examination, blood pressure (BP) was found to be 95/60 mm Hg, heart rate (HR) 60 beats per minute (bpm), respiratory rate (RR) 25 breaths/min, and saturation of 94% on 2 L O_2. His physical examination is most significant for facial plethora, nonpulsatile but distended neck veins, 2+ pitting edema in the bilateral upper extremities, and rales in the bilateral lung bases. In the above clinical setting, what would be the next most appropriate diagnostic step?
A. Transesophageal echocardiogram (TEE)
B. Transthoracic echocardiogram (TTE)
C. Computed tomography (CT) scan
D. Cardiac magnetic resonance imaging (CMRI)

*Questions and Answers are based on Chapter 109: Complex Lesions by Jeannette Lin, Prashanth Venkatesh, and Weiyi Tan in Cardiovascular Medicine and Surgery, First Edition.

109.3 A 22-year-old male presents to the emergency department (ED) with severe shortness of breath that had been progressing over several weeks, however, acutely worsened this morning. His medical history is most significant for D-TGA with an intact ventricular septum status post repair at 6 months of age with an arterial switch operation. TTE and CMRI are obtained and reveal evidence of supravalvular pulmonary artery (PA) stenosis without regurgitation. The mean gradient across the valve was found to be 52 mm Hg. The RV was also found to be dilated with reduced global systolic function. Electrocardiogram (ECG) demonstrates sinus tachycardia at a rate of 113 bpm with complete right bundle branch block (RBBB) and nonspecific ST-T wave abnormalities. What would be the next most appropriate step?

A. Surgical valve replacement
B. Coronary angiogram with left heart catheterization
C. Right heart catheterization with vasoreactivity testing
D. Intravenous (IV) loop diuretics
E. Transcatheter balloon angioplasty and stenting of the PA

109.4 A 35-year-old female presents to the office for routine follow-up. She was born with a hypoplastic RV and subsequently underwent lateral tunnel Fontan palliation. She has done well and continued to follow up regularly; however, over the past 3 weeks, she has noticed episodes of palpitations lasting minutes to hours at a time. She denies any syncope but does notice during these episodes that she becomes short of breath and experiences episodic lightheadedness. ECG in the office today reveals atrial fibrillation with a HR of 98 bpm. What is the next **BEST** step in managing her new-onset atrial fibrillation?

A. Start a vitamin K antagonist and proceed with TEE-guided electrical cardioversion.
B. Start a vitamin K antagonist alone.
C. Start a vitamin K antagonist with metoprolol bid.
D. Start an alternative oral anticoagulant (OAC) with metoprolol bid.
E. Start an alternative OAC alone.
F. Start metoprolol bid alone.

109.5 A 48-year-old male presents to the ED with complaints of abdominal bloating and confusion. His medical history is most significant for tricuspid atresia status post a right atrium (RA)-PA Fontan palliation. The patient has **NOT** followed up regularly with physicians in over 10 years. Vitals signs while in the ED are significant for an RR of 22 breaths/min, HR of 102 bpm, and BP of 102/55 mm Hg. On examination, the patient can state his name but is **NOT** oriented to time or place. Here is a prominent jugular venous distension (JVD) with hepatojugular reflex. Heart sounds are distant but with an irregularly irregular rhythm. Lung sounds are diminished at the bases with bilateral rales present. The abdomen is protuberant with a significant fluid wave, and the skin overlying the abdomen has significant blanchable telangiectasias. There is 3+ bilateral lower extremities (LE) edema. What treatment could have slowed the progression of his underlying disease process?

A. Vitamin K antagonist
B. Compression stockings
C. Oral budesonide and albumin infusions
D. Oral metoprolol

109.6 An 18-year-old patient is referred from his pediatric cardiologist to your adult office as a new patient. The patient was born with hypoplastic left ventricle (LV) syndrome and underwent a typical staged palliation. What would be the expected staged surgical procedures for this patient in chronologic order?

A. Glenn shunt at birth, Norwood procedure at 2 to 6 months, and Fontan completion with a lateral tunnel at 18 months (about 1 and a half years)
B. Norwood procedure at birth, Glenn shunt at 2 to 6 months, and Fontan completion with a lateral tunnel at 18 months (about 1 and a half years)
C. Fontan completion with a lateral tunnel at birth, Glenn shunt at 2 to 6 months, and Norwood procedure at 18 months (about1 and a half years)
D. Norwood procedure at birth, Fontan completion with a lateral tunnel at 2 to 6 months, and Glenn shunt at 18 months (about 1 and a half years)

109.7 Primary surgical repair of truncus arteriosus includes all of the following **EXCEPT**:

A. The pulmonary arteries are mobilized from the truncus and, subsequently, typically reattached to a RV to PA conduit.
B. Opening and repair of the truncus with either a patch of pulmonary homograft material or pericardium
C. Pulmonary arterial banding, which restricts pulmonary overcirculation
D. Closure of the ventricular septal defect with a prosthetic patch

ANSWERS

109.1 The correct answer is A.
Rationale: A patient who develops severe symptomatic neoaortic regurgitations status post atrial switch procedure due to congenital transposition of vessels should be offered immediate valvular replacement as it is the only curative therapy. TEE is a great initial evaluation of a patient with a history of transposition of vessels as it allows for the best visualization. However, once the diagnosis of severe neoaortic valve regurgitation is made, surgery is the option.

KEY POINTS

- The addition of a beta-blocker is not recommended in those with decompensated heart failure, especially those with aortic valve pathology.
- Supervised exercise programs and DOACs have not been shown to be beneficial in severe neoaortic valve regurgitation.
- Patient symptoms will not improve until intervention is performed.

109.2 The correct answer is D.
Rationale: The atrial switch repair involves the creation of intracardiac baffles to divert deoxygenated blood from the inferior vena cava (IVC) and superior vena cava (SVC)

across the mitral valve into the subpulmonary LV, and oxygenated blood from the pulmonary veins across the tricuspid valve into the subaortic RV. This patient is suffering from obstruction of an intracardiac baffle with a possible leak affecting the SVC limb of the baffle mimicking SVC syndrome. Stenosis of the baffles is a known complication and depending on the location of the obstruction can mimic SVC syndrome. If the obstruction occurs at the IVC limb level, it may result in examination findings such as hepatic congestion, abdominal bloating, early satiety, and LE edema.

CMRI is an excellent modality for the evaluation of RV size and function, baffle stenoses, and baffle leaks, specifically when combined with four-dimensional (4D) flow. CT scans are reasonable, particularly in patients with implantable devices that are not compatible with CMRI. This patient's device is only 2 years old, thus it is reasonable to believe that he has a CMRI-compatible device. TEE is superior to TTE for visualization of the baffles.

KEY POINTS

✓ CMRI with cine and 4D flow is the preferred imaging modality in patients with a history of D-TGA with atrial switch repair in whom there is a concern for RV failure, baffle stenoses, and baffle leaks. Although echocardiogram remains the imaging modality for patients with complex congenital heart disease (CHD), advanced imaging with CMRI is essential for evaluation of anatomy that is not well visualized by echocardiography including complex baffles.

109.3 The correct answer is E.

Rationale: This patient has evidence of severe supravalvular PA stenosis due to his previous arterial switch operation. A mean gradient greater than 50 mm Hg is considered severe whereas the moderate range is between 25 and 50 mm Hg, and mild less than 25 mm Hg. Transcatheter balloon angioplasty and stenting are preferred over surgery for treating PA stenosis. When there is evidence of severe neoaortic valvular regurgitation with root dilation, surgical valve replacement with concomitant aortic grafting would be preferred. During the arterial switch procedure, the coronary arteries are translocated and reimplanted along with islands of pericoronary sinus tissue, whereas the PA is moved anterior to the aorta. Ostial stenosis of the reimplanted coronary buttons may occur, but this would be accompanied by angina, heart failure, or ventricular arrhythmia.

KEY POINTS

✓ Severe PA stenosis following an arterial switch procedure without evidence of concomitant regurgitation is best treated with transcatheter balloon angioplasty and stenting over surgery.

109.4 The correct answer is A.

Rationale: As mentioned in the question stem, the patient is experiencing new-onset atrial fibrillation with associated symptoms. Her history of a hypoplastic RV and lateral tunnel Fontan palliation makes her new-onset atrial arrhythmia concerning. Severe dilation of the RA over time in these patients leaves them prone to atrial arrhythmias, and the low-flow state increases the risk of thrombus formation. The risk of thrombus formation is lower in patients with the lateral tunnel or extracardiac Fontan than those with an RA-PA Fontan, however, persists due to the persistent low-flow state. Atrial arrhythmias even at low HRs are poorly tolerated due to the preload-dependent nature and an inability to easily increase cardiac output. Restoring sinus rhythm should be undertaken given her symptoms despite her being stable. The anticoagulant of choice should be a vitamin K antagonist as alternative oral anticoagulants have not been adequately studied in this patient population. If electrical cardioversion fails, the patient should be referred for an electrophysiology study and ablation.

KEY POINTS

- ✔ Patients with Fontan palliation (including RA-PA, lateral tunnel Fontan, and extracardiac Fontan) are at increased risk for atrial arrhythmias and thromboembolic events due to the low-flow state. Atrial arrhythmias are usually poorly tolerated and should be managed aggressively to restore sinus rhythm.

109.5 The correct answer is C.

Rationale: The patient described is most likely experiencing Fontan-associated liver disease (FALD). After the first decade of life with a Fontan circulation, most patients develop at least mild hepatic fibrosis, and some may develop cirrhosis after several decades of chronic hepatic congestion. Hepatocellular carcinoma is reported in this patient population and screening protocols incorporate efforts to ensure early diagnosis. He is also experiencing protein-losing enteropathy, another known complication of longstanding Fontan circulation, and can be diagnosed with a 24-hour stool alpha-1 antitrypsin test. The etiology is not well understood, but the contributing factors include poor cardiac output, venous congestion, and lymphatic dysfunction. Treatment for this consists of oral budesonide and albumin infusions to help offset protein loss and maintain intravascular oncotic pressure. Liver imaging including ultrasound, CT, and MRI are studies of the recommended surveillance of stable adult Fontan patients. This patient's lack of follow-up resulted in a 10-year gap in care during which early identification of his liver pathology could have occurred.

KEY POINTS

- ✔ Patients with Fontan palliation typically will develop liver fibrosis and are at increased risk of developing cirrhosis. Ongoing surveillance of the adult patient is strongly recommended. Concomitant protein-losing enteropathy is common with liver disease. Treatment for this consists of oral budesonide and albumin infusions to help offset protein loss and maintain intravascular oncotic pressure.

109.6 The correct answer is B.

Rationale: Hypoplastic left heart syndrome is a rare congenital heart defect with modern surgical advancements allowing patients to live into adulthood. The traditional staged palliation consists of three stages:

1. Stage 1, birth: Norwood procedure which typically involves disconnecting the right/left PA from the native PA, atrial septectomy, anastomosis of the main PA, and the hypoplastic native aortic arch to create a neoaorta, aortic arch augmentation, and a modified Blalock-Taussig or Sao shunt (RV to pulmonary circulation)
2. Stage 2, 2 to 6 months: Glenn shunt
3. Stage 3, 18 to 48 months: Fontan completion with a lateral tunnel or extracardiac conduit

An alternative or hybrid approach exists to reduce mortality in frail neonates.

1. Stage 1, birth: hybrid procedure, involving PA banding, maintaining patency, of the ductus arteriosus with stenting or prostaglandin infusion, and balloon atrial septostomy or surgical atrial septectomy
2. Stage 2, 3 to 8 months: Norwood procedure with reconstruction of the aortic arch and Glenn shunt
3. Stage 3, 18 to 48 months (about 4 years): Fontan completion with a lateral tunnel or extracardiac conduit

109.7 The correct answer is C.

Rationale: Primary surgical repair is performed while patients are in deep hypothermia and placed on low-flow continuous cardiopulmonary bypass or intermittent periods of circulatory arrest.

The procedure encompasses the following steps:

- The pulmonary arteries are mobilized from the truncus and, subsequently, typically reattached to a RV to PA conduit.
- Repair of the truncus with either a patch of pulmonary homograft material or pericardium
- Closure of the ventricular septal defect with a prosthetic patch

An alternate surgical option is initial palliative pulmonary arterial banding, which restricts pulmonary overcirculation, allowing the infant to grow larger. Complete repair is then deferred until later. This procedure requires two operations and does not provide any benefit in regard to long-term mortality and morbidity. In general, primary repair is the preferred approach.

PULMONARY ARTERIAL HYPERTENSION ASSOCIATED WITH CONGENITAL HEART DISEASE*

CHAPTER 110

Nathan Centybear and Naveed M. Akhtar

QUESTIONS

110.1 Which of the following is **TRUE** regarding pulmonary arterial hypertension associated with congenital heart disease (PAH-CHD)?

A. They have the highest survival compared to other forms of PAH.
B. Pulmonary vasodilators have not been shown to have benefit.
C. Individuals with isolated pre-tricuspid defects have the highest risk for development of PAH.
D. Individuals with isolated pre-tricuspid defects who developed PAH have a higher survival rate.

110.2 A 49-year-old male patient comes to your office after a recent diagnosis of pulmonary arterial hypertension (PAH) by a pulmonologist. A transthoracic echocardiogram (TTE) shows a ventricular septal defect (VSD) of 0.7 cm. He otherwise has normal ventricular anatomy, his left ventricular (LV) function is normal, and there is no valve disease. Which statement is **TRUE** regarding the management of this patient?

A. The defect should be closed to prevent development of Eisenmenger syndrome.
B. He should be treated according to current PAH guidelines.
C. He is unlikely to benefit from a pulmonary vasodilator.
D. He should not undergo an acute vasoreactivity test.

110.3 A 30-year-old female patient with Eisenmenger syndrome comes to your office for a routine visit. She has been stable on bosentan for the past year. Her laboratory results show a hematocrit of 60%. She is asymptomatic. Which of the following is the **BEST** next step in the management of this patient?

A. Perform phlebotomy to prevent complications of hyperviscosity.
B. Start an antiplatelet agent to prevent complications of hyperviscosity.
C. Start apixaban to prevent complications of hyperviscosity.
D. Advise the patient to avoid dehydration to avoid complications of hyperviscosity.

110.4 The patient in **Question 110.3** inquires about having children. Of the following, what is the **BEST** advice to give to this patient?

A. She can become pregnant with acceptable risk if she is monitored closely.
B. An estrogen oral contraceptive would be advisable to avoid pregnancy.
C. A hormonal intrauterine device (IUD) would be advisable to avoid pregnancy.
D. Egg retrieval with surrogacy is a safe alternative to pregnancy.

*Questions and Answers are based on Chapter 110: Pulmonary Arterial Hypertension Associated With Congenital Heart Disease by Nils Patrick Nickel, Richard A. Lange, Christine Bui, and Anitra W. Romfh in Cardiovascular Medicine and Surgery, First Edition.

110.5 The same patient in **Questions 110.3 and 110.4** comes to the office 6 months later for preoperative counseling. She is scheduled to have elective cholecystectomy for recurrent gallstones. Her hematocrit is now 66%. Her symptoms have remained stable since her last visit. Which statement regarding surgery is **CORRECT**?

   A. In preparation, she should undergo prophylactic phlebotomy.
   B. Laparoscopic surgery may worsen left-to-right shunting.
   C. Prophylactic anticoagulation should be used due to the high risk of thrombus formation.
   D. A slightly negative serum pH is preferable as it dilates the pulmonary vasculature.

110.6 Riociguat is a/an:

   A. Endothelin receptor antagonist
   B. Phosphodiesterase-5 inhibitor (PDE-5)
   C. Guanylate cyclase stimulator
   D. Guanylate cyclase inhibitor

110.7 A patient presents to your office for evaluation of dyspnea. Which of the following examination findings is **NOT** consistent with Eisenmenger syndrome?

   A. Cyanosis of the lower extremities but not the upper extremities
   B. A harsh, pansystolic murmur heard at the left lower sternal border that does not change in intensity with inspiration
   C. A prominent, split S2
   D. Digital clubbing

110.8 A patient with Eisenmenger syndrome presents to your clinic for initial evaluation. His physical examination is notable for right ventricular (RV) heave, fixed split S2, and digital clubbing. He has had a recent echocardiogram, which was notable for a 1.2-cm VSD. His basic metabolic panel (BMP) is unremarkable, and his complete blood count (CBC) is notable for a hematocrit of 63%. He is **NOT** on any medications, but he has received phlebotomy several times for polycythemia. Which of the following is appropriate in the management of this patient?

   A. Iron studies
   B. Start on PAH combination therapy.
   C. Order phlebotomy.
   D. Start treatment with intravenous epoprostenol.

110.9 You are seeing a patient in the clinic who was recently diagnosed with Eisenmenger syndrome. The decision is made to start medication. Which of the following medications should be initiated as part of treatment?

   A. Bosentan
   B. Sildenafil
   C. Tadalafil
   D. Beraprost

110.10 Which of the following should be performed before initiation of vasodilator therapy in the patient from **Question 110.9**?

   A. And exercise stress test
   B. Pulmonary function test
   C. 6-minute walk test
   D. A ventilation/perfusion (V̇/Q̇) scan

ANSWERS

110.1 The correct answer is A.
Rationale: Individuals with PAH-CHD have a higher survival rate than patients with idiopathic or connective tissue disease-associated PAH, possibly due to an adaptive response in early life. Vasodilators are the mainstay of medical therapy in these patients and studies have shown clinical benefit. Pre-tricuspid defects have a lower risk of development of PAH than post-tricuspid defects, and individuals with pre-tricuspid defects who do develop PAH have worse survival rate, possibly because they have an underlying pulmonary vascular disease process independent from CHD.

110.2 The correct answer is B.
Rationale: This patient has a small (VSD <1 cm, atrial septal defect [ASD] <2 cm) cardiac defect. PAH with small, coincidental defects have a clinical picture similar to idiopathic PAH and should be treated according to current PAH guidelines, which includes pulmonary vasodilators. Defect closure is contraindicated as it may increase RV preload and cause RV failure. As the cause of this patient's PAH has not been identified, an acute vasoreactivity test should be considered (**Table 110.1** and **Figure 110.1**).

TABLE 110.1 Clinical Classification of Pulmonary Arterial Hypertension Associated With Congenital Heart Disease

Classification	Definition	Features
Eisenmenger syndrome	Includes all large intra- and extracardiac defects that begin as left-to-right shunts and progress to severe elevation of PVR and reversal (right-to-left) or bidirectional shunting	Cyanosis, secondary erythrocytosis, gout, and multiple organ involvement
PAH associated with prevalent left-to-right shunts • Correctable[a] • Noncorrectable	Includes moderate to large defects, PVR is mildly to moderately increased, and left-to-right shunting is still prevalent.	Cyanosis at rest is not a feature.
PAH with small/coincidental defects	Marked elevation in PVR in the presence of small cardiac defects (ie, VSD <1 cm or ASD <2 cm[b]), which themselves do not account for the development of elevated PVR	Clinical picture is very similar to idiopathic PAH. Closing the defects is contraindicated.
PAH after defect correction	Congenital heart disease is repaired, but PAH persists immediately after correction or recurs/develops months or years after correction.	No significant postoperative hemodynamic lesions

ASD, atrial septal defect; PAH, pulmonary arterial hypertension; PVR, pulmonary vascular resistance; VSD, ventricular septal defect.
[a]With surgery or percutaneous procedure.
[b]Size applies to adult patients.

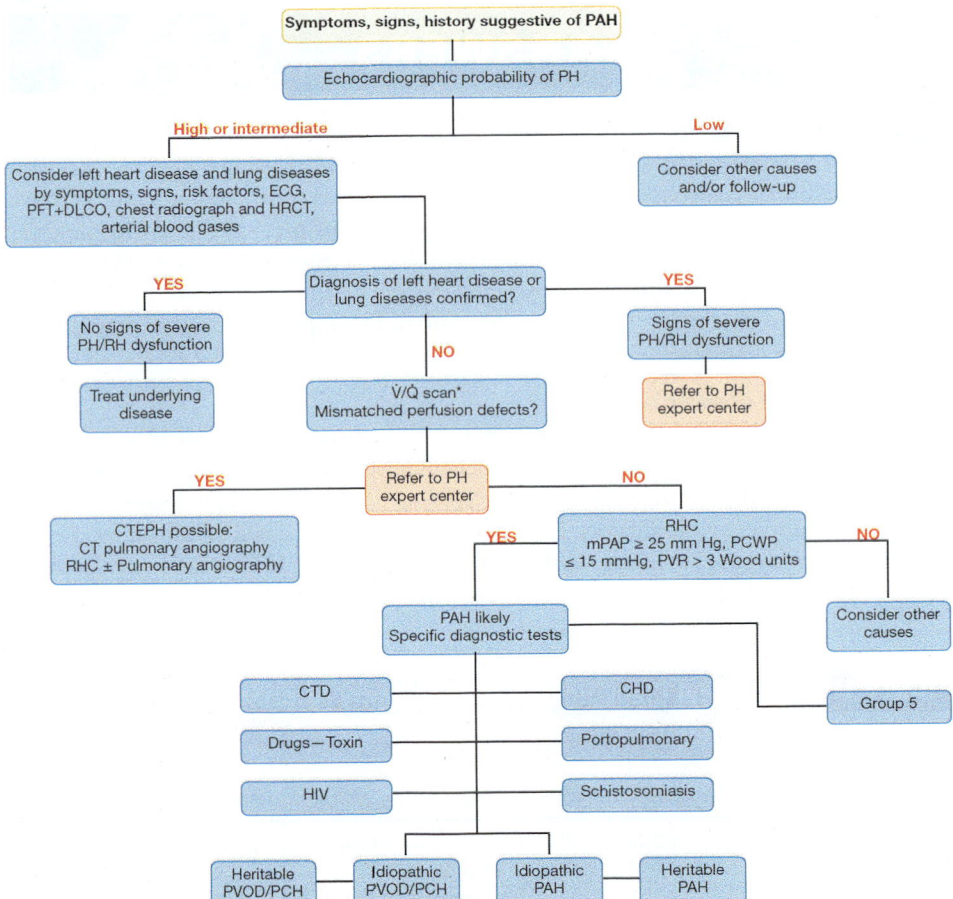

Figure 110.1 Diagnostic algorithm of PAH. CHD, congenital heart diseases; CT, computed tomography; CTD, connective tissue disease; CTEPH, chronic thromboembolic pulmonary hypertension; DLCO, carbon monoxide diffusing capacity; ECG, electrocardiogram; HIV, human immunodeficiency virus; HRCT, high-resolution CT; mPAP, mean pulmonary arterial pressure; PAH, pulmonary arterial hypertension; PCWP, pulmonary capillary wedge pressure; PFT, pulmonary function tests; PH, pulmonary hypertension; PVOD/PCH, pulmonary veno-occlusive disease or pulmonary capillary hemangiomatosis; PVR, pulmonary vascular resistance; RHC, right heart catheterization; RV, right ventricular; V̇/Q̇, ventilation/perfusion. *CT pulmonary angiography alone may miss diagnosis of chronic thromboembolic pulmonary hypertension. (From Galie N, Humbert M, Vachiery JL, et al; ESC Scientific Document Group. 2015 ESC/ERS Guidelines for the diagnosis and treatment of pulmonary hypertension: the Joint Task Force for the Diagnosis and Treatment of Pulmonary Hypertension of the European Society of Cardiology (ESC) and the European Respiratory Society (ERS): Endorsed by: Association for European Paediatric and Congenital Cardiology (AEPC), International Society for Heart and Lung Transplantation (ISHLT). *Eur Heart J.* 2016;37(1):67-119. Reproduced by permission of European Society of Cardiology & European Respiratory Society.)

110.3 The correct answer is D.

Rationale: Patients with Eisenmenger syndrome develop erythrocytosis due to arterial desaturation, resulting in hyperviscosity. Phlebotomy with isovolumic replacement should be performed in patients with moderate or severe symptoms. It should be avoided in patients with mild or no symptoms to prevent iron deficiency, which can worsen symptoms of hyperviscosity. Antiplatelets and anticoagulants should be avoided because they exacerbate hemorrhagic diathesis. Dehydration should be avoided, along with diuretics, because this will increase blood viscosity.

110.4 The correct answer is C.

Rationale: Pregnancy is contraindicated for women with Eisenmenger syndrome due to the high risk of maternal mortality. Non-estrogen-containing contraceptives should be used due to the increased thrombotic risk with estrogen. Progestin-only contraceptives, such as hormonal IUDs or the "minipill," are preferable. Egg retrieval has associated thrombotic risks due to the high levels of estrogen administration required for egg removal.

110.5 The correct answer is A.

Rationale: Patients with a hematocrit above 65% should undergo prophylactic phlebotomy with isovolumic replacement to reduce the risk of thrombotic complications. Laparoscopic surgery using carbon dioxide for insufflation can reduce the serum pH which constructs pulmonary vasculature and can worsen right-to-left shunting, not left-to-right. Anticoagulants exacerbate the hemorrhagic diathesis and should be avoided.

110.6 The correct answer is C.

Rationale: Riociguat is a guanylate cyclase stimulator (resulting in vasodilation) used in the treatment of PAH. It was assessed in a randomized trial that included patients with PAH/CHD (8% of the total patient population) and was found to improve right heart hemodynamics, exercise capacity, and functional capacity and reduce time to clinical worsening.

Sildenafil/tadalafil are examples of PDE-5 inhibitors.

Endothelin receptor antagonists (not agonists), such as bosentan, are also used in the treatment of pulmonary hypertension. Bosentan has been studied in a randomized, double-blind, placebo-controlled trial (BREATHE-5 [Breathing Restoration and Exhalation Alleviation Therapy & Healing Enhancement-5]) in 54 patients with Eisenmenger syndrome; patients with patent ductus arteriosus (PDA) and complex CHD were excluded. Compared with placebo, Bosentan therapy was associated with improved right heart hemodynamics and increased exercise capacity.

110.7 The correct answer is B.

Rationale: Although the pansystolic murmur of tricuspid regurgitation (TR) is consistent with Eisenmenger syndrome, a TR murmur increases in intensity with inspiration. The murmur described in the answer choice is consistent with a small VSD, which is less likely to lead to the development of Eisenmenger syndrome. A large VSD is more likely to lead to Eisenmenger syndrome development, at which point the murmur usually disappears due to pressure equalization between the RV and LV. Cyanosis of the lower extremities is consistent with a PDA, which may lead to and be present with Eisenmenger syndrome. Digital clubbing is associated with chronic hypoxia that may be present with Eisenmenger syndrome. A fixed, split S2 is a sign of pulmonary hypertension.

110.8 The correct answer is A.
Rationale: This patient has had phlebotomy for treatment of polycythemia which can result in iron deficiency. Because iron-deficient erythrocytes are less deformable, iron deficiency can worsen symptoms of hyperviscosity. Insufficient data exist on combination therapy in PAH-CHD; therefore, it is not recommended as initial therapy. Additional phlebotomy can worsen iron deficiency and should be avoided except before surgery, and only if hematocrit is greater than 65%. Intravenous epoprostenol should be avoided due to the risk of embolism with indwelling lines.

110.9 The correct answer is A.
Rationale: Bosentan, an endothelin receptor antagonist, is currently the only pulmonary vasodilator with a Class I indication for Eisenmenger syndrome. Choices B and C are both PDE-5 inhibitors. PDE-5 inhibitors are commonly prescribed for Eisenmenger syndrome, but survival benefit has not been shown in prospective randomized controlled trials. Hence, there is no convincing data or consensus that therapy improves the survival of patients with Eisenmenger syndrome. Beraprost, an oral prostacyclin analogue, was studied in a randomized trial in which 18% of the study population had PAH-CHD and did not show benefit in patients with PAH-CHD.

110.10 The correct answer is C.
Rationale: Before initiation of vasodilator therapy, patients with Eisenmenger syndrome should undergo a 6-minute walk test. The other options are not routinely performed in patients with Eisenmenger syndrome once they already have the diagnosis.

NONCARDIAC SURGERY IN THOSE WITH ADULT CONGENITAL HEART DISEASE*

CHAPTER 111

Atika Azhar and Robert L. Carhart

QUESTIONS

111.1 A 34-year-old woman with a history of congenital corrected transposition of the great arteries presents for noncardiac surgery. She has a history of palpitations and sustained ventricular tachycardia. Preoperative electrocardiogram shows right bundle branch block and ventricular preexcitation. She has an implanted epicardial pacing system. Which of the following is the most appropriate next step in her perioperative management?

- A. Ambulatory cardiac rhythm monitoring
- B. Exercise testing
- C. Electrophysiology study
- D. Reprogramming of the pacing system
- E. Withholding beta-blocker and calcium channel blockers

111.2 A 45-year-old man with a history of mechanical mitral valve replacement on chronic warfarin therapy presents for emergent appendectomy due to acute appendicitis. He has no history of bleeding or thromboembolic complications. The surgery team needs to determine the **BEST** approach for managing his anticoagulation during the perioperative period. Which of the following is the most appropriate next step in his management?

- A. Continue warfarin therapy throughout the perioperative period with close monitoring of international normalized ratio (INR) levels.
- B. Discontinue warfarin therapy 4 to 5 days before surgery and initiate bridging anticoagulation with heparin.
- C. Discontinue warfarin therapy 48 hours before surgery and monitor activated partial thromboplastin time (aPTT) intraoperatively.
- D. Discontinue warfarin therapy and initiate direct thrombin inhibitor or factor Xa inhibitor as bridging anticoagulation.
- E. Discontinue warfarin therapy and initiate vitamin K, fresh frozen plasma, and prothrombin complex concentrate intraoperatively in case of bleeding.

111.3 A 42-year-old man with a history of coarctation of the aorta repair presents for elective hernia repair surgery. He has been experiencing progressively unstable angina and has decreased ventricular function on echocardiography. His past medical history is otherwise unremarkable. What is the next **BEST** step in his preoperative assessment?

*Questions and Answers are based on Chapter 111: Noncardiac Surgery in Those with Adult Congenital Heart Disease by Dana Irrer and Joseph D. Kay in Cardiovascular Medicine and Surgery, First Edition.

A. Coronary angiography
B. Transthoracic echocardiogram
C. Computed tomographic imaging
D. Optimization on pulmonary vasodilator support
E. Proceed with hernia repair surgery without further evaluation.

111.4 A 35-year-old woman with a history of single-ventricle palliation presents for elective knee surgery. She has no symptoms of heart failure and has normal ventricular function on echocardiography. She is **NOT** on any pulmonary vasodilator support. What is the next **BEST** step in her preoperative assessment?

A. Coronary angiography
B. Transthoracic echocardiogram
C. Computed tomographic imaging
D. Optimization on pulmonary vasodilator support
E. Proceed with knee surgery without further evaluation.

111.5 A 40-year-old man with a history of a single-ventricle physiology due to Fontan procedure presents for elective knee surgery. The anesthesia team is planning his perioperative management. Which of the following considerations is important in the anesthetic management of this patient?

A. Avoiding hypercarbia and acidosis
B. Reprogramming of pacemaker/implantable cardioverter-defibrillator (ICD)
C. Administering inhaled nitric oxide for pulmonary vasodilation
D. Securing intravenous (IV) filters on all lines to reduce the risk of systemic air embolism
E. Maintaining elevated aortic root pressure to maintain coronary perfusion

111.6 A 28-year-old woman with Eisenmenger syndrome presents for elective abdominal surgery. The anesthesia team is planning her perioperative management. Which of the following considerations is important in the anesthetic management of this patient?

A. Avoiding hypothermia
B. Maintaining volume overload
C. Administering vasoactive medications to increase systemic vascular resistance
D. Maintaining elevated aortic root pressure to maintain coronary perfusion

111.7 A 35-year-old man with a history of supravalvar aortic stenosis presents for elective hernia repair. The anesthesia team is planning his perioperative management. Which of the following considerations is important in the anesthetic management of this patient?

A. Avoiding hypercarbia and acidosis
B. Reprogramming of pacemaker/ICD
C. Administering inhaled nitric oxide for pulmonary vasodilation
D. Maintaining volume overload
E. Securing IV filters on all lines to reduce the risk of systemic air embolism

111.8 A 35-year-old woman with Eisenmenger syndrome is scheduled for surgery. Which of the following is indicated to specifically prevent the worsening of right-to-left shunting and hypoxemia?

A. Avoidance of hypovolemia
B. Use of inhaled nitric oxide for pulmonary vasodilation
C. Maintenance of hypercarbia
D. Induction of hypothermia

111.9 A 28-year-old male with Fontan physiology presents to the hospital for noncardiac surgery. He has a history of recurrent sternotomies and thoracotomies over the course of staged palliation. The anesthesia team is planning for general anesthesia. Which of the following is the most appropriate intraoperative management for this patient?

A. Maintenance of mild hypercarbia and acidosis
B. Prolonged positive pressure ventilation to improve oxygenation
C. Inhaled nitric oxide to reduce systemic venous return
D. Intra-abdominal pressures less than 10 mm Hg during laparoscopic procedures

111.10 A 35-year-old female with Eisenmenger syndrome is scheduled for noncardiac surgery. She has a history of chronic cyanosis, fluid shifts, and bleeding risk. Which of the following is the most appropriate perioperative management for this patient?

A. Platelet transfusion before surgery
B. Administration of vitamin K to correct clotting abnormalities
C. Routine postoperative chest physiotherapy to prevent atelectasis
D. Continuous monitoring of oxygen saturation during surgery
E. Aggressive fluid resuscitation during surgery

ANSWERS

111.1 The correct answer is D.
Rationale: This patient with congenital corrected transposition of the great arteries and a history of palpitations, sustained ventricular tachycardia, and an implanted epicardial pacing system requires careful perioperative management. Electrocautery during surgery may interfere with the pacing system function, leading to unnecessary shocks or inappropriate pacemaker inhibition. Therefore, reprogramming of the pacing system to prevent such issues is crucial before proceeding with noncardiac surgery. Ambulatory cardiac rhythm monitoring and exercise testing may be appropriate in some cases, but in this patient with a history of sustained ventricular tachycardia and an implanted pacing system, reprogramming of the pacing system is the most appropriate next step. Electrophysiology studies may be considered in select cases, but reprogramming of the pacing system should be prioritized first. Withholding beta-blockers and calcium channel blockers should be avoided without careful consideration of the patient's overall cardiovascular condition and the risks and benefits of discontinuing these medications.

111.2 The correct answer is B.
Rationale: Patients with mechanical heart valves on chronic warfarin therapy may require bridging anticoagulation during the perioperative period to reduce the risk of bleeding at the time of surgery. This is particularly important in patients with additional

risk factors for thromboembolism, such as atrial fibrillation, prior stroke, systemic ventricular dysfunction, hypercoagulable state, or older-generation prosthetic valves with a less favorable thrombosis profile. Discontinuing warfarin therapy 4 to 5 days before surgery and initiating bridging anticoagulation with heparin is a common approach for mechanical mitral valve while bridging may not be necessary with mechanical aortic valve unless additional risk factors for thromboembolism are present. Direct thrombin inhibitors or factor Xa inhibitors may also be used as bridging anticoagulation, but they should be discontinued 48 hours before surgery when possible. Intraoperative monitoring of aPTT for heparin or prothrombin time for direct thrombin inhibitors or factor Xa inhibitors is recommended. Vitamin K, fresh frozen plasma, and prothrombin complex concentrate may be used intraoperatively in case of bleeding. Continuing warfarin therapy throughout the perioperative period with close monitoring of INR levels is not recommended, as the risk of bleeding may be increased.

111.3 The correct answer is A.

Rationale: This patient has a history of coarctation of the aorta repair, which puts him at increased risk for coronary artery disease. He is also experiencing progressively unstable angina and has decreased ventricular function on echocardiography, indicating a higher risk for perioperative complications. According to ACC/AHA (American College of Cardiology/American Heart Association) guidelines, coronary angiography is reasonable in patients with unstable angina or other objective evidence of ischemia, and decreased ventricular function before noncardiac surgery. Transthoracic echocardiogram could provide additional information about his ventricular function, but coronary angiography would provide a more accurate assessment of his coronary artery disease status. Computed tomographic imaging would not be the first choice in someone with unstable angina. Optimization on pulmonary vasodilator support may be considered for patients with pulmonary hypertension, but it is not the most appropriate next step in this patient's management. Proceeding with hernia repair surgery without further evaluation would not be ideal considering his increased risk for coronary artery disease and presentation with unstable angina.

111.4 The correct answer is E.

Rationale: This patient has a history of single-ventricle palliation but is asymptomatic and has normal ventricular function on echocardiography. According to the provided content, patients with complex adult congenital heart disease (ACHD) lesions, such as those with single-ventricle palliation, have an overall lower burden of coronary artery disease compared to the general population. Therefore, further evaluation such as coronary angiography or transthoracic echocardiogram may not be necessary in this patient. Computed tomographic imaging and optimization on pulmonary vasodilator support are not indicated based on the given history. Proceeding with knee surgery without further evaluation is appropriate in this case.

111.5 The correct answer is A.

Rationale: In Fontan physiology, care must be taken to avoid hypercarbia and acidosis, which can elevate pulmonary pressures and severely limit passive blood flow to the lungs and cardiac output. Reprogramming of pacemaker/ICD may not be necessary in this case. Inhaled nitric oxide may be needed for pulmonary vasodilation in the setting of suprasystemic pulmonary pressures but this is not mentioned in the stem. Securing IV filters on all lines to reduce the risk of systemic air embolism is important in patients with right-to-left intracardiac shunts. Maintaining elevated aortic root pressure to maintain coronary perfusion may be necessary in patients with supravalvar aortic stenosis.

111.6 The correct answer is A.
Rationale: Hypothermia is poorly tolerated in patients with Eisenmenger syndrome because of worsening right-to-left shunting. Volume overload is not well tolerated in patients with a single ventricle, so maintaining volume overload may not be appropriate. Administering vasoactive medications to increase systemic vascular resistance may not be appropriate in patients with Eisenmenger syndrome. Maintaining elevated aortic root pressure to maintain coronary perfusion may be necessary in patients with supravalvar aortic stenosis.

111.7 The correct answer is A.
Rationale: Avoiding hypercarbia and acidosis. Patients with supravalvar aortic stenosis can be at risk of myocardial ischemia during induction of anesthesia due to their elevated aortic root pressure requirement for coronary perfusion. Avoiding hypercarbia (high levels of carbon dioxide in the blood) and acidosis (low pH in the blood) can help minimize the risk of further compromising coronary perfusion and myocardial oxygen supply-demand balance during anesthesia. Avoiding hypercarbia and acidosis is also important in Fontan physiology. Reprogramming of pacemaker/ICD is not relevant to the management of supravalvar aortic stenosis. Administering inhaled nitric oxide for pulmonary vasodilation is not typically used in the management of supravalvar aortic stenosis. Securing IV filters on all lines to reduce the risk of systemic air embolism is not specifically mentioned as a consideration in the management of this patient.

111.8 The correct answer is B.
Rationale: In patients with Eisenmenger syndrome, inhaled nitric oxide should be readily available for pulmonary vasodilation during anesthesia to prevent the worsening of right-to-left shunting and hypoxemia. Avoidance of hypovolemia, maintenance of normocarbia, and avoidance of hypothermia are also important perioperative considerations for these patients; however, inhaled nitric oxide prevents worsening of right-to-left shunting by pulmonary vasodilation.

111.9 The correct answer is D.
Rationale: Fontan patients are intolerant of high intrathoracic and intra-abdominal pressures and maintaining intra-abdominal pressures less than 10 mm Hg during laparoscopic procedures is recommended to minimize the negative effects on systemic venous return. Maintaining mild hypercarbia and acidosis, prolonged positive pressure ventilation, and inhaled nitric oxide may not be appropriate for Fontan patients as it can further reduce systemic venous return and pulmonary blood flow.

111.10 The correct answer is D.
Rationale: Patients with Eisenmenger syndrome have increased bleeding risk due to collateralization of blood vessels, platelet dysfunction, and alterations in the clotting cascade. Continuous monitoring of oxygen saturation during surgery is important to detect any changes in oxygenation and manage accordingly. Platelet transfusion, administration of vitamin K, routine postoperative chest physiotherapy, and aggressive fluid resuscitation may not be appropriate or necessary for perioperative management in a patient with Eisenmenger syndrome.

INDEX

Note: Page numbers followed by *t* indicate table and those followed by *f* indicate figure.

A

AAA. *See* Abdominal aortic aneurysm (AAA)
AAI. *See* Atrial pacing, atrial sensing, inhibition (AAI)
AAIR⇔DDDR (programmable mode), 396, 398
AAR. *See* Area at risk (AAR)
ABCDE model, 153
Abdominal aortic aneurysm (AAA), 500, 504
　Duplex ultrasound, 514, 516, 519
　flowchart for evaluation of, 520–521*f*
　MDCT angiography, 515, 522
　mortality of, 515, 519
Abdominal hernia repair, 143
Abdominal pain, differential diagnosis of, 544
ABI. *See* Ankle-brachial index (ABI)
ACC. *See* American College of Cardiology (ACC)
Accelerated idioventricular rhythm (AIVR), 39, 44, 500, 504
ACE. *See* Angiotensin-converting enzyme (ACE)
Acetazolamide, 482, 486
ACHD. *See* Adult congenital heart disease (ACHD)
ACLS recommendations. *See* Advanced cardiac life support (ACLS) recommendations
ACM. *See* Arrhythmogenic cardiomyopathy (ACM)
Aconite poisoning, 167, 169
Acromegaly, 124, 125*t*
ACS. *See* Acute coronary syndrome (ACS)
Action potential duration (APD), 316–319
Acute aortic dissection, 7
　CT chest/abdomen/pelvis with contrast, 577, 579
Acute cerebrovascular accident (CVA), 513, 515
Acute coronary syndrome (ACS), 26–27, 159, 382, 385
　clinical management of, 33
Acute decompensated heart failure (ADHF), 481, 484
　clinical examination findings, 481, 484, 485*t*
　clinical trials for, 488–490*t*
　rehospitalization for, 483, 491
　Stevenson clinical profiles, 481–482, 484, 486*f*
Acute limb ischemia
　endovascular aneurysm repair (EVAR), 523–524, 526
　Rutherford classification for, 526*t*
　"six Ps" of, 523, 526
Acute lymphocytic myocarditis, 468, 470–471
Acute mesenteric ischemia
　characteristics of, 541, 543
　treatment for, 542, 545–546*t*
Acute mitral regurgitation (MR), 13*t*, 12, 16
Acute myocardial infarction (AMI), 137, 156, 237
　complications of, 41–43
Acute pancreatitis, 541, 544
Acute pericarditis, 83, 85
　in adults, initial treatment, 85*f*, 86
Acute rheumatic fever, 52
Acute tricuspid regurgitation, 13*t*, 12, 16
Adaptive servoventilation (ASV), 163
Adenosine, 221, 276, 279
ADHF. *See* Acute decompensated heart failure (ADHF)
Adult-acquired tricuspid and pulmonary valve disease, 68–70
Adult congenital disease, 100–102
Adult congenital heart disease (ACHD), 714
Advanced cardiac life support (ACLS) recommendations, 360
AF. *See* Atrial fibrillation (AF)
AFD. *See* Anderson-Fabry disease (AFD)
AHA. *See* American Heart Association (AHA)

AHA/ACC (American Heart Association/American College of Cardiology) guidelines, 600, 688, 690
　for ARAS, 539*t*
　for the Diagnosis and Management of Aortic Disease, 580
AHI. *See* Apnea-hypopnea index (AHI)
AI. *See* Aortic insufficiency (AI)
AIVR. *See* Accelerated idioventricular rhythm (AIVR)
AL. *See* Amyloidosis (AL)
Alagille syndrome, 694
Alcohol, 129, 130*t*
Alcohol septal ablation (ASA), 144
　complication of, 298, 302
　contraindications for, 297, 300, 300*t*
　for coronary artery disease, 299, 302
　favoring factors, 297–298, 300–301, 301*t*
　indications for, 300*t*
　mechanism of, 299, 303
　mortality for, 297, 300
　outcomes of, 298–299, 302
　procedure, 298, 301–302
Alcoholic cardiomyopathy, 473, 477
Alfieri stitch, 284, 286
Alpha-actin gene, 417, 419
Alteplase (tPA), 39
ALVC. *See* Arrhythmogenic left ventricular cardiomyopathy (ALVC)
Alveolar edema, 192
American College of Cardiology/American Heart Association (ACC/AHA) Guidelines, 63, 116, 299, 18
AMI. *See* Acute myocardial infarction (AMI)
Aminophylline, 278
　physiologic effect, 338, 339
Amiodarone, 179, 349–350, 352–353, 357, 358, 361–364, 366–368, 389
　contraindications, 364, 367
　side effects, 366, 369
Amlodipine, 231, 383
Amlodipine-benazepril, 225
Amprenavir, 157, 159, 160*t*
Amyloid cardiomyopathy, 172–181
　atrial fibrillation in, 179
　evaluation, algorithm for, 177, 177*f*
　transthyretin amyloidosis therapy, 179, 180*t*
Amyloidosis (AL), 125–126, 172, 177, 251
　transthyretin and light-chain, 442, 445, 447
Andersen-Tawil syndrome, 322, 324
Anderson-Fabry disease (AFD), 235
Anesthesia, 712
　avoiding hypercarbia and acidosis, 715
Angiography, 270, 273
Angiotensin-converting enzyme inhibitors (ACEIs), 27, 117, 509, 652
Angiotensin II receptor blockers (ARBs), 153
Angiotensin receptor blocker (ARB), 652
　therapy, 27, 117
　inhibitor, 509
Angiotensin receptor neprilysin inhibitors (ARNI), mechanism of, 492, 495
Ankle-brachial index (ABI), 524, 526, 583, 587
　exercise, 524–525, 527
Annual visit, 660
ANP. *See* Atrial natriuretic peptide (ANP)

717

Anthracycline-associated cardiomyopathy, 153
Anthracycline-based chemotherapy, 113
Anthracycline cardiotoxicity, 153
Anthracycline-induced cardiomyopathy, 214
Anthracycline-induced chemotherapy, 475, 478–479
Anthracycline therapy, 154
Anti-glutamic acid decarboxylase (anti-GAD) antibodies, 639
Antiarrhythmics, 179
Antiphospholipid syndrome (APS), 122
Antiretroviral drugs, and cardiovascular risk, 159, 160t
Antithrombotic effect, 31
Antithrombotic medical regimens, 528t
Aortic aneurysm, 126
Aortic aneurysm rupture, 149
Aortic dissection, 126, 578, 581
    acute type B
        management of, 513, 515–516
    antihypertensive agents for, 517–518t
    complications of, 513, 515
Aortic insufficiency (AI), 283, 285
Aortic regurgitation, 12, 14t, 15–16
Aortic stenosis, 13t, 12, 16, 64, 291, 292
Aortic valve area (AVA), 62
Aortic valve calcifications, 193
Aortic valve disease, 62–67
Aortic valve regurgitation, 126
Aortic valve replacement (AVR), 289, 291
    in aortic regurgitation, 65f, 66
    in aortic stenosis, 63f, 65
    approach and timing for, 568, 570
    indications for, 569, 570t
Aortic valve stenosis
    class I recommendations for, 567, 569
    cross-clamp, 568, 571
    interventions, 568, 571
    longer cardiopulmonary bypass, 568, 571
    physical examination, 567, 569
    Society of Thoracic Surgeons (STS) risk score, 567, 569
    stages of, 567, 569
    surgical aortic valve replacement (SAVR), 567, 569
    transcatheter aortic valve replacement (TAVR), 567, 569
APD. *See* Action potential duration (APD)
Apixaban, 59, 350, 353, 550, 552
Apnea-hypopnea index (AHI), 166
APS. *See* Antiphospholipid syndrome (APS)
ARAS. *See* Atherosclerotic renal artery stenosis (ARAS)
ARB. *See* Angiotensin receptor blocker (ARB)
Area at risk (AAR), for infarction, 243
Argatroban, 33
ARNI. *See* Angiotensin receptor neprilysin inhibitors (ARNI), mechanism of
Arrhythmias, 113, 113f, 238, 239t
Arrhythmogenic cardiomyopathy (ACM), 417, 419
Arrhythmogenic left ventricular cardiomyopathy (ALVC), 417, 419
Arrhythmogenic right ventricular cardiomyopathy (ARVC), 201, 236, 419
Arsenic poisoning, 170
Arterial switch procedure, 702
ARVC. *See* Arrhythmogenic right ventricular cardiomyopathy (ARVC)
ASA. *See* Alcohol septal ablation (ASA)
ASCVD. *See* Atherosclerotic cardiovascular disease (ASCVD)
ASD. *See* Atrial septal defect (ASD)
ASH (American Society of Hematology) guidelines, 557
Aspirin, 2, 17, 22, 47, 85, 117, 145, 148, 353
Asthma, 660
ASV. *See* Adaptive servoventilation (ASV)
Asymptomatic sinus bradycardia, 315, 317
Asynchronous mode (DOO), 396, 398

AT. *See* Atrial tachycardias (AT)
Atazanavir, 159, 160t
Atenolol, 105
Atherosclerosis, 623
Atherosclerotic cardiovascular disease (ASCVD), 626, 627, 629, 638, 650
    risk score, 17, 225, 628
Atherosclerotic renal artery stenosis (ARAS), 535
    AHA/ACC recommendations, 539t
    history of, 535, 538
    management of, 535–536, 538
    pathogenesis of, 536, 540
    predictors of, 536, 539
Atorvastatin, 2, 22, 157, 159, 363, 367
Atrial fibrillation (AF), 117, 129, 316, 318, 322, 324, 406, 408, 449, 451
    alcohol consumption and, 349, 351–352
    catheter ablation, 348–349, 351
    class Ic drugs, 352–353
    direct oral anticoagulant (DOAC), 353
    flecainide, 350, 352–353
    management of, 348–349, 351
    permanent, 394–397, 426, 434
    postoperative, 353
    potential triggers for, 346
    propafenone, 350, 352–353
    rhythm control therapy, 349–350, 352, 352f
    risk factors for, 351
    source of triggers for, 372, 374
    thromboembolism and, 353
    warfarin, 353
Atrial flutter, risk factors for, 351
Atrial myxoma, 7, 139–140
Atrial natriuretic peptide (ANP), 436, 439
Atrial pacing, atrial sensing, inhibition (AAI), 395, 396, 398
Atrial septal aneurysm (ASA), 294, 296
Atrial septal defect (ASD), 12, 14t, 16, 100, 284, 287, 676, 678, 680, 687
    contraindications for, 294, 295–296
    indications for, 293, 295
    magnetic resonance imaging (MRI) for, 294, 296
Atrial septal occluder device, postoperative management, 294, 295
Atrial tachycardias (AT), 345
Atrial tumors, 12, 14t, 16
Atrioventricular (AV) block
    clinical scenarios, 337, 339
    first-degree, 337, 339
    second-degree, 337, 339
    third-degree, 337, 339
Atrioventricular (AV) nodal disease
    etiology, 336, 338–339
    isoproterenol, 336, 339
Atrioventricular nodal reentrant tachycardia (AVNRT), 332, 334, 342, 345, 346
Atropine, 170
    physiologic effect, 338, 339
Autonomic dysfunction, 7, 166, 173
AVA. *See* Aortic valve area (AVA)
AVNRT. *See* Atrioventricular nodal reentrant tachycardia (AVNRT)
AVR. *See* Aortic valve replacement (AVR)
Azathioprine, 212, 470

B

B-type natriuretic peptide (BNP), 173
Balloon valvuloplasty, 55, 288, 291
BAV. *See* Bicuspid aortic valve (BAV)
Benign early repolarization, 310, 312
Benign fasciculation syndrome, 500, 504

Bentall procedure, 102
Beta-blockers, 47, 86, 166, 430, 452
　for CPVT, 321, 324
　effects of, 316–317, 318
Beta-receptor signaling, 411, 414
Bicuspid aortic valve (BAV), 684, 687, 690
Bioprosthetic aortic valve stenosis, 74
Biphasic shock, 387, 389
Birth defect, 665
Bivalirudin, 33
Biventricular pacemaker, 395, 397
Blood testing, 95, 95t
BMI. *See* Body mass index (BMI)
BMP. Basic metabolic panel
BNP. *See* B-type natriuretic peptide (BNP)
Body mass index (BMI), 2, 143
Bone marrow max, 618
Boston criteria, 406, 408
Bradyarrhythmias, 7, 278
Bradycardia, symptomatic, 394, 395, 396, 397
Brain natriuretic peptide (BNP), 436, 439, 440
Brain-type natriuretic peptide (BMP), 204
BrS. *See* Brugada syndrome (BrS)
Brugada syndrome (BrS), 310, 312, 322, 324, 368, 391, 416, 418
Bumetanide, 482, 486, 492, 495

C

C-reactive protein (CRP), 53
CABG. *See* Coronary artery bypass graft (CABG)
CAC. *See* Coronary artery calcium (CAC) scores
CAD. *See* Coronary artery disease (CAD)
Calcifications, 74, 193
Calcium, in cardiac function and heart failure, 411, 415
Calcium channel blockers (CCBs), 91, 452, 653
cAMP. *See* Cyclic adenosine monophosphate (cAMP)
Camphor, 170
Canadian Cardiovascular Society (CCS), 4–5t
Cangrelor, 39
Carcinoid, 124, 125t
Carcinoid heart disease, 462
Cardenolides, 169
Cardiac amyloidosis, 125, 240, 240f, 460
　ATTR, 463–464, 466
　ATTRh, 463–464, 466
　ATTRwt, 463–464, 466
　diagnosis of, 458–459, 465
Cardiac Arrhythmia Suppression Trial (CAST), 357, 361, 367
Cardiac auscultation, 16
Cardiac catheterization, 384, 385
　and hemodynamic assessment, 257–262
　　right atrial pressure waveform and, 259, 260t
Cardiac catheterization lab drug, 31
Cardiac computed tomography, 225–233
Cardiac concussion, 135
Cardiac magnetic resonance (CMR) imaging, 95, 95t, 234–244, 251, 251f, 254
　acquired diseases of the vessels, 238, 239t
　cardiac masses characterization, 238, 239t
　clinical indications for, 238, 239t
　with dobutamine or perfusion stress, 23, 23t
Cardiac metastasis, 141
Cardiac MIBG scintigraphy, 165
Cardiac murmurs, 12, 13–14t, 16
　diastolic murmurs, 12, 14t, 16
　differentiating them, 12, 13–14t, 16
　early systolic, 13t, 12, 16
　late systolic, 12, 14t, 16
　mid-systolic, 13t, 12, 16
　pansystolic, 12, 14t, 16
　systolic murmurs, 12, 13–14t
Cardiac myxomas, 139–140
Cardiac resynchronization therapy (CRT), 120, 443, 446, 503
　complications of, 499, 503
　indications for, 502t
Cardiac resynchronization therapy, 506, 509
Cardiac resynchronization therapy with defibrillator (CRT-D), 498–500, 502
Cardiac sarcoidosis, 126, 251, 455, 460, 461
Cardiac sympathetic denervation, 166
Cardiac syncope, 2
Cardiac syndrome X, 40
Cardiac tamponade, 7
Cardiac transplantation, 468, 471
Cardiac trauma, 132–135
　management of, 134, 135f
Cardiac tumors, 136–142
　cardiac fibroma, 139, 139f
　cardiac leiomyoma, 139, 139f
　cardiac lipoma, 139, 139f
　cardiac lymphoma, 139, 139f
　cardiac myxoma, 139, 139f
　cardiac papillary fibroelastoma, 139, 139f
　cardiac sarcoma, 139, 139f
Cardio-oncology, 151–155
Cardiomyocytes, automaticity of, 316, 318
Cardiomyopathies, 238, 239t
Cardiomyopathy
　etiology of, 474, 478
　genes associated with, 420–423t
　genetics of, 416–423
Cardiopulmonary exercise testing, 95, 96t
Cardiopulmonary resuscitation (CPR), 36, 132, 387
Cardiorenal syndrome, 484
Cardiovascular (CV) death, hospitalizations and, 427, 434
Cardiovascular (CV) function, 196
Cardiovascular disease (CVD), 168
　environmental exposures and, 167–171
　heart failure with preserved ejection fraction (HFpEF), 114
　nontraditional risk factors, 113, 113f
　risk, 156
　traditional risk factors, 113, 113f
　in women, 113, 113t
Cardiovascular imaging, 182–187
Cardiovascular system
　action of cocaine on, 473, 477
Carfilzomib, 155
Carney complex, 139–140
Carotid artery stenting (CAS), 591, 597–599
Carotid Doppler ultrasound, 592, 593
Carotid intima-media thickness (CIMT) scores, 629
Carotid sinus baroreceptors, 162, 164
Carotid sinus massage (CSM), 162, 383, 386
Carotid sinus syndrome, syncope with, 383, 386
CARPREG (CARdiac disease in PREGnancy) risk score, 104, 107–108, 108t
CARPREG II risk score, 104, 108, 108t, 668
Carvedilol, 22, 207
CAS. *See* Carotid artery stenting (CAS)
CAST. *See* Cardiac Arrhythmia Suppression Trial (CAST)
Catecholaminergic polymorphic ventricular tachycardia (CPVT), 201, 317, 318–319, 321, 322, 324
Catheter ablation therapy
　benefits of, 372–375
　risks of, 372–375
　transthoracic echocardiography, 371, 373
Catheter-based/surgical intervention, 692
Cavo-tricuspid isthmus, 343–344, 347
CBC. *See* Complete blood count (CBC)
CCBs. *See* Calcium channel blockers (CCBs)

Index

CCTA. *See* Coronary computed tomographic angiography (CCTA)
Cerebral hypoperfusion, 7
CFV. *See* Common femoral vein (CFV)
CHA2DS2-VASc score, 327, 329, 353
Chagas disease, 462
CHD. *See* Coronary heart disease (CHD)
Chemotherapy, 474–475, 478
    anthracycline-induced, 475, 478–479
    echocardiographic surveillance on, 475–476, 479
    -induced cardiomyopathy, 207
    -induced cardiotoxicity, 154, 155
Chest pain, 693
    characteristics, 309, 312
    differential diagnosis of, 6–7*t*
    electrocardiogram (ECG), 309*f*
Chest radiography, 189–195
Chest x-ray
    3-sign, 666–667
CHF. *See* Congestive heart failure (CHF)
Chloroquine, 478
Chlorthalidone, 2
Cholesterol, 643
Chord-sparing MV replacement, 573, 576
Chromium, 170
Chronic hemodialysis, 79
Chronic kidney disease (CKD), 2, 183
Chronic kidney disease (CKD) stage 2, 615
Chronic limb-threatening ischemia (CLTI), 525, 528
Chronic mesenteric ischemia
    diagnosis of, 541, 543
    first-line intervention for, 542, 544
    treatment for, 542, 545–546*t*
    weight loss, 541, 544
Chronic MR, 12, 14*t*, 16
Chronic stable angina, 5
Chronic thromboembolic pulmonary hypertension (CTEPH), 20, 95, 207
Chronic total occlusion (CTO), 47*f*, 49
Chronic tricuspid regurgitation, 12, 14*t*, 16
Chronic viral cardiomyopathy
    causes of, 468, 471
Cilostazol, 525, 527, 584, 588
CIMT. *See* Carotid intima-media thickness (CIMT) scores
Cine-cardiac computed tomography (cine-CCT), 227, 232
CKD. *See* Chronic kidney disease (CKD)
Clinical Outcomes Utilizing Revascularization and Aggressive Drug Evaluation (COURAGE) trial, 26, 119
Clinical pharmacology, 17–20
Clopidogrel, 148
Clopidogrel, 19, 22, 31–32, 40, 117, 145, 148, 562, 565
CLTI. *See* Chronic limb-threatening ischemia (CLTI)
CMP. *See* Comprehensive metabolic panel (CMP)
CMR. *See* Cardiac magnetic resonance (CMR) imaging
COACT. *See* Coronary Angiography After Cardiac Arrest (COACT)
Coarctation, covered stent for, 290, 292
Cobalt ingestion, 170
Cocaine, 129, 130*t*
    on cardiovascular system, 473, 477
Colchicine therapy, 85
Colorectal cancer, 541, 544
Combined postcapillary and precapillary PH (Cpc-PH), 99
Common cardiovascular (CV) manifestations, 126
Common femoral vein (CFV), 594
Common medications, 596–597
Commotio cordis, 134
COMPLETE. *See* Complete versus Culprit-Only Revascularization to Treat Multivessel Disease After Early PCI for STEMI (COMPLETE) trial
Complete blood count (CBC), 23, 366, 368
Complete versus Culprit-Only Revascularization to Treat Multivessel Disease After Early PCI for STEMI (COMPLETE) trial, 282
Comprehensive metabolic panel (CMP), 23
Computed tomography (CT), 95, 95*t*, 136, 245, 251, 251*f*, 506, 509, 531, 534
Computed tomography angiography (CTA), 145, 157, 253, 529, 532
Computed tomography perfusion (CTP), 229–230
Congenital bicuspid aortic stenosis, 15
Congenital heart disease, 105, 238, 239*t*
Congestive heart failure (CHF), 170
Constrictive-effusive pericarditis, 462
Constrictive pericarditis (CP), 84
Continuous positive airway pressure (CPAP), 166
Contrast echocardiography, 140
Contrast-induced nephropathy, 264–265, 268
Cor triatriatum, 661
Coronary angiography, 714
    diagnostic, indication for, 263, 265–266
    femoral artery access, location for, 263, 265, 266*f*
    four corners/around the world approach, 266, 267*f*
    left radial approach, criteria for, 263, 265–266
Coronary Angiography After Cardiac Arrest (COACT), 40
Coronary artery anomalies, 265, 268
Coronary artery bypass grafting (CABG), 27, 226, 266, 277, 281
    beta-blocker for, 562–563, 566
    candidacy for, 562, 564
    cardiovascular risk factors, 565
    clinical scenario, 561, 563
    clopidogrel, 562, 565
    conduits for, 561, 564
    emergency, 564
    intensive lipid management, 566
    intervention, 562, 565
    management of, 562, 565
    procedure, 615, 616
    revascularization, method for, 563, 566
Coronary artery calcium (CAC) score, 186, 225, 622–623, 629
Coronary artery disease (CAD), 3, 21, 116, 152, 182, 218, 392, 714
    alcohol septal ablation for, 299, 302
    reporting and data system, 229, 229*t*
Coronary Artery Disease-Reporting and Data System (CAD-RADS) classification, 225
Coronary artery stenosis, invasive physiologic indices to assess, 280–281*t*
Coronary computed tomographic angiography (CCTA), 119, 184, 225, 246, 250, 250*f*
Coronary dominance, 264, 267
Coronary fractional flow reserve measurements, hyperemic agents used in, 279*t*
Coronary heart disease (CHD), 5
Coronary revascularization, 27
Cost-minimization analysis, 19
Cost-utility analysis, 19
COURAGE trial. *See* Clinical Outcomes Utilizing Revascularization and Aggressive Drug Evaluation (COURAGE) trial
COVID-19 pandemic, 470, 655
CP. *See* Constrictive pericarditis (CP)
CPAP. *See* Continuous positive airway pressure (CPAP)
CPK. *See* Creatine phosphokinase (CPK)
CPR. *See* Cardiopulmonary resuscitation (CPR)
CPVT. *See* Catecholaminergic polymorphic ventricular tachycardia (CPVT)
Creatine phosphokinase (CPK), 299, 303
CRP. *See* C-reactive protein (CRP)

CRT. *See* Cardiac resynchronization therapy (CRT)
Cryoablation *vs.* radiofrequency (RF) ablation, 371, 374
CSM. *See* Carotid sinus massage (CSM)
CT. *See* Computed tomography (CT)
CTA. *See* Computed tomography angiography (CTA)
CTEPH. *See* Chronic thromboembolic pulmonary hypertension (CTEPH)
CTO. *See* Chronic total occlusion (CTO)
CTP. *See* Computed tomography perfusion (CTP)
CVD. *See* Cardiovascular disease (CVD)
CyBorD. *See* Dexamethasone, cyclophosphamide, and bortezomib (CyBorD)
Cyclic adenosine monophosphate (cAMP), 334
CYP2C19 gene, 19
Cytochrome P-450 system, 19, 31, 159

D

D-dimer, 129, 207, 214
D-transposition of the great arteries (D-TGA), 699, 700
Dabigatran, 59, 549, 552
Dacron graft, 578, 582
DADs. *See* Delayed afterdepolarizations (DADs)
DANISH (Danish Study to Assess the Efficacy of ICDs in Patients With Nonischemic Systolic Heart Failure on Mortality) trial, 377, 379
Dapagliflozin, 427, 434
DAPT. *See* Dual antiplatelet therapy (DAPT)
Darunavir, 159, 160*t*
DASH (Dietary Approaches to Stop Hypertension) diet, 11, 383, 386
Daunorubicin therapy, 152
DCM. *See* Dilated cardiomyopathy (DCM)
DCRV. *See* Double-chambered right ventricle (DCRV)
Decompression sickness, 294, 296
Deep sternal wound infection (DSWI), 619
Deep vein thrombosis (DVT), 3
 catheter-directed thrombolysis (CDT), 548, 552
 dabigatran, 549, 552
 edoxaban, 549, 552
 enoxaparin, 549
 management of, 549–553, 550*f*
 risk factor for, 548, 551
 thrombectomy, 548, 551
 Wells Scoring System for, 552, 551–552*t*
Defibrillation, 387, 389
Defibrillators in Non-Ischemic Cardiomyopathy Treatment Evaluation (DEFINITE) trial, 377, 379
Delayed afterdepolarizations (DADs), 315, 317–318
Deoxyglucose, 222
DES. *See* Drug-eluting stent (DES)
Dettol poisoning, 170
Device thrombosis, 68
Dexamethasone, cyclophosphamide, and bortezomib (CyBorD), 179
Dexrazoxane, 153, 207, 214, 442, 445
DI. *See* Dimensionless index (DI)
Diabetes mellitus (DM), 622, 637
 risk score, 628
 type 2 (DMT2), 9, 17–18, 23, 622
Diagnostic coronary angiography
 indication for, 263, 265
Diastolic murmurs, 12, 14*t*, 16
 early diastolic, 12, 14*t*, 16
 mid-diastolic, 12, 14*t*, 16
Diet-controlled type 2 diabetes, 47
Diets, 632–633
Diflunisal, 179, 180*t*, 443, 447
DiGeorge syndrome, 665
Digoxin, 179, 367, 443, 446, 468, 470, 494, 497
Dihydropyridine calcium channel blockers, 59

Dilated cardiomyopathy (DCM), 126, 441, 444
 chemotherapy-related, 445
 defined, 444
 diagnosis of, 441, 444
 incidence of, 441, 444
 medications not used, 468, 470
 myocarditis and, 467, 469
Diltiazem, 50, 105, 452
Dimensionless index (DI), 205
Dinitrate, 50, 444, 446
Dipyridamole, 221, 562, 565
Direct oral anticoagulant (DOAC), 353
Direct oral anticoagulants (DOACs), 149
Disopyramide, 452
Diuretic resistance, contributing factor, 482, 486
Diuretics, 452, 506, 509
 avoidance of, 383, 386
Diverticulitis, 541, 544
DM. *See* Diabetes mellitus (DM)
DOAC. *See* Direct oral anticoagulant (DOAC)
Dobutamine, 26, 64, 221, 276, 279, 483, 487, 579, 582
 echocardiography, 22*t*, 23, 26
Doppler echocardiography, 608, 693
Doppler parameters for PHV regurgitation, 75, 75–76*t*
Double-chambered right ventricle (DCRV), 693
Down Syndrome, 12, 665, 666, 679
Doxazosin, 119
Doxorubicin, 153, 207, 475, 478–479
Doxycycline, 179, 180*t*, 443, 447
Dronedarone
 contraindications, 364, 367
Drug-eluting stent (DES), 144
Drug-resistant HTN, 653
DSP (desmoplakin), 418, 419
DSWI. *See* Deep sternal wound infection (DSWI)
Dual antiplatelet therapy (DAPT), 144
Dual-chamber pacemaker, 326, 329
Dual-chamber pacing, 165
Duchenne muscular dystrophy, 419
Duke Clinical Score, 1, 7
Duke Treadmill score, 213, 216
DVT. *See* Deep vein thrombosis (DVT)
Dysautonomia, 162–166
Dyslipidemia, 21, 104, 236, 643
Dyspnea, 1–2, 85, 693
Dystrophic calcifications, 193

E

EAM. *See* Electroanatomic mapping (EAM)
EAST. *See* Eastern Association for the Surgery of Trauma (EAST)
Eastern Association for the Surgery of Trauma (EAST), 134
Ebstein anomaly, 667, 695, 697–698
ECG. *See* Electrocardiogram (ECG)
Echocardiogram, 7, 153, 289, 291, 331, 333–334, 382, 385, 386
 bedside, 387, 390
 hypertrophic cardiomyopathy, 449, 451
 12-Lead, 391
 2D, 474–475, 478
Echocardiographic surveillance, 475–476, 479
Echocardiography, 94*t*, 95, 140, 204–216
 heart failure, 712
 stress test, 441, 444
 unstable angina, 711
ECMO. *See* Extracorporeal membrane oxygenation (ECMO)
ECP. *See* Effusive-constrictive pericarditis (ECP)
ECST. *See* European Carotid Surgery Trial (ECST)
Edema, 192
Edoxaban, 549, 552

EDPVR. *See* End-diastolic pressure-volume relationship (EDPVR)
Edwards syndrome, 12
EES slope. *See* End-systolic elastance (EES) slope
Efavirenz, 159, 160*t*
Effective orifice area (EOA), 71
Effective refractory period (ERP), 332, 334
Effective regurgitant orifice area (EROA), 63, 73
Efferocytosis, 623
Effusive-constrictive pericarditis (ECP), 84
18-Fluorodeoxyglucose (FDG), 251, 251*f*
Eisenmenger syndrome, 102, 388, 390, 612, 661, 677, 705, 706, 710, 712–713
Electrical cardioversion, for VT, 355–356, 360
Electrical storm, 387
  defined, 390
Electroanatomic mapping (EAM), 332–333, 335
Electrocardiogram (ECG), 163
  abnormalities, cause of, 310, 312
  hypertrophic cardiomyopathy, 449, 451–452
  limb lead reversal, 310, 310*f*, 312
  normal axis of heart in young individuals, 311, 312
  Q waves, 311, 313
  QT interval measurement, 311, 312
  right axis deviation, causes of, 311, 313
  ST elevations and PR depressions, 309, 309*f*, 312
  stress, for diagnosing ischemia, 311, 313
  ventricular tachycardia, diagnostic algorithms for, 354, 359*f*
Electrocardiographic exercise testing, 196–202
  exercise stress tests, 200
  nondiagnostic exercise stress test, 200
Electrolyte abnormalities, 390
Electrophysiologic study (EPS), 382, 386
Electrophysiology (EP)
  clinical scenario, 333, 335
  echocardiogram, 331, 333–334
  effective refractory period (ERP), 332, 334
  His to ventricular (HV) interval, 331, 333
  isoproterenol, 332, 334
  shortest preexcited RR interval (SPERRI), 332, 334
Electrophysiology study (EPS), 498, 501–502
Eliquis, 19
EMB. *See* Endomyocardial biopsy (EMB)
Emergency Medical Services (EMS), 601, 609
Emergency room (ER), 167
EMS. *See* Emergency Medical Services (EMS)
Enalapril, 207
End-diastolic pressure-volume relationship (EDPVR), 412, 413*f*, 415
End-stage cardiomyopathy, 460
End-stage renal disease (ESRD), 71
End-systolic elastance (EES) slope, 412, 415
Endocardial cushion defects, 682
Endocarditis, 400
Endocrine disorders, 124, 125*t*
  cardiac manifestations of, 124, 125*t*
Endomyocardial biopsy (EMB), 467–468, 470, 478
Endomyocardial fibrosis, 456, 462
Endothelial disruption, 79
Endovascular aneurysm repair (EVAR), 523–524, 526
Energy metabolism, 411, 415
Enoxaparin, 33, 549, 552
Environmental exposures and CVD, 167–171
  herbal plant consumption, heart toxicity related to, 170, 171*t*
EOA. *See* Effective orifice area (EOA)
EP. *See* Electrophysiology (EP)
Epilepsy
  syncope and, 381–382, 384
Epinephrine, 389

Eplerenone and Mild Patient's Hospitalization and Survival Study and Heart Failure (EMPHASIS-HF), 120
Eplerenone Post-acute myocardial infarction Heart failure Efficacy and Survival Study (EPHESUS), 120
EPS. *See* Electrophysiologic study (EPS)
Equilibrium radionuclide angiography (ERNA), 219
ER. *See* Emergency room (ER)
ERNA. *See* Equilibrium radionuclide angiography (ERNA)
EROA. *See* Effective regurgitant orifice area (EROA)
ERP. *See* Effective refractory period (ERP)
Erythrocyte sedimentation rate (ESR), 53
ESCAPE (Evaluation Study of Congestive Heart Failure and Pulmonary Artery Catheterization Effectiveness) trial, 483, 487, 488*t*
Esmolol, 579, 582
ESR. *See* Erythrocyte sedimentation rate (ESR)
ESRD. *See* End-stage renal disease (ESRD)
Estrogen, 709
European Carotid Surgery Trial (ECST), 597
European Society of Cardiology (ESC) criteria, 299, 406, 408
EVAR. *See* Endovascular aneurysm repair (EVAR)
Event monitor, 326, 328
EVEREST (Efficacy of Vasopressin Antagonism in Heart Failure Outcome Study with Tolvaptan) trial, 483, 487, 488*t*
Exercise, 633
Exercise echocardiography, 22*t*, 23
Exercise electrocardiography (ECG), 21, 22*t*, 23
Exercise myocardial perfusion imaging, 21, 23, 23*t*
Exercise stress echocardiography, 21, 23, 213
Exercise stress test, 200, 384, 385
Extracorporeal membrane oxygenation (ECMO), 259
Ezetimibe, 646

F

F-fluorodeoxyglucose positron emission tomography (^{18}F-FDG PET), 213, 219, 222
Fabry disease, 463
FALD. *See* Fontan-associated liver disease (FALD)
False-positive PYP scan, 178
Fatigue, 1
FDG. *See* 18-Fluorodeoxyglucose (FDG)
Femoral arterial plaque burden scores, 629
FFA. *See* Free fatty acid (FFA)
FFR. *See* Fractional flow reserve (FFR)
Fibrinolytic therapy, 117, 119
Fibroelastomas, 139
Fibromas, 139
Fibromuscular dysplasia, 114, 535, 538
Fibrous adhesions, 401, 403
Finerenone, 494, 497
5 METs (metabolic equivalent of task), 201
Flecainide, 357, 358, 361–364, 367, 368
  contraindications, 364, 367
Fluid restriction, 430
Fondaparinux, 33
Fontan-associated liver disease (FALD), 703
Fontan palliation, 676, 703
Fontan physiology, 714–715
  noncardiac surgery, 713
Fontan procedure, 609, 612
Fosamprenavir, 159, 160*t*
Four corners/around the world approach, 266, 267*f*
Foxglove, 170, 171*t*
Fractional flow reserve (FFR), 246, 276, 278–279
  vs. angiography for multivessel evaluation (FAME) trial, 185
  hyperemic agents used in measurements, 279*t*
  vs. instantaneous wave-free ratio, 276, 280
Framingham criteria, 406, 408
Free fatty acid (FFA), oxidation, 411, 415
Furosemide, 482, 486

G

Ganglion plexus ablation, 166
GAS. *See* Group A beta-hemolytic streptococci (GAS)
GAS antigen test, 52–53
Gastroesophageal reflux disease (GERD), 2, 9, 227
Gastrointestinal bleeding, 506, 511
GCM. *See* Giant cell myocarditis (GCM)
GDMT. *See* Guideline-directed medical therapy (GDMT)
Gene mutation, 417, 419, 448, 450
General cardiovascular examination, 9–16
Genetic testing, 417, 419
 hypertrophic cardiomyopathy, 449, 452
GERD. *See* Gastroesophageal reflux disease (GERD)
Ghosts, 401, 403
Giant cell myocarditis (GCM), 467, 468, 470, 471–472
Global longitudinal strain (GLS), 152
GLS. *See* Global longitudinal strain (GLS)
Glucagon, physiologic effect, 338, 339
Glucose homeostasis, 411, 415
Glycosylation, 411, 415
Goal-directed medical therapy, 476
Gold therapy for rheumatoid arthritis, 170
Gothenburg criteria, 406, 408
Gout, 9
Grayanotoxin, 169
Great vessel disorder, 7
Group A beta-hemolytic streptococci (GAS), 51
Guideline-directed medical therapy (GDMT), 179, 500, 504

H

H$_2$FPEF score, 425, 429
Hakki equation, 258, 261
Hazard ratio (HR), 158
HCM. *See* Hypertrophic cardiomyopathy (HCM)
HDL. *See* High-density lipoprotein (HDL)
Heart catheterization, 478
Heart failure (HF), 113, 113*f*, 117, 638
 acute and chronic, 413*f*
 beta-blockers (BB), use of, 493, 496
 beta-receptor signaling in, 411, 414
 calcium in, 411, 415
 exacerbation, cause of, 474, 477
 Framingham criteria, 406, 408
 functional classification of, 405, 407
 with improved ejection fraction, 410, 413
 incidence of, 426, 430
 initial hemodynamic adaptive response in, 410, 414
 management of, 494, 497
 mortality, 406, 408
 NYHA class II, 498, 501–502
 NYHA class III, 502
 NYHA class IV, 502
  palliative care consultation for, 503
 pathophysiology of, 410–415
 prevalence of diagnosis, 405, 407
 routine evaluation, 494, 497
 symptomatic, guideline-directed management of, 446*f*
 in women, 481, 484
Heart failure association diagnostic algorithm of heart failure with preserved ejection fraction (HFA-PEFF) score, 425–426, 429–430
Heart failure with preserved ejection fraction (HFpEF), 114, 406, 407, 481, 484
 causes of rise in end-diastolic pressure in, 424, 428
 diagnostic test of, 425–426, 429–430
 endothelial inflammation contributing to, 424–425, 428
 etiologies of, 427–428*t*

H$_2$FPEF score, 425, 429
HTN leading to, 426, 430
medications or interventions improving morbidity and mortality in, 426, 430
risk factor for, 424, 427
treatment of, 431–434*t*
Heart failure with reduced ejection fraction (HFrEF), 406, 407, 408, 412, 415
 cycle of neurohormonal activation in, 414*f*
 improving mortality, 437, 440
 pathophysiology of, 410, 413
 risk of, 435, 438
Heart-healthy diet, 634, 635
Heart-to-mediastinum ratio (HMR), 223
Hematocrit, 706
Hemodialysis, 169
Hemodynamic collapse, assessment of, 264, 267–268
Hemoglobin A1c (HbA1c), 619
Hemolytic anemia, 74
Hemostasis, 149
Henbane, 170, 171*t*
Hepatocellular carcinoma, 154, 703
Herbal plant consumption, heart toxicity related to, 170, 171*t*
Hereditary hemochromatosis, 455–456, 461–462
HF. *See* Heart failure (HF)
HFpEF. *See* Heart failure with preserved ejection fraction (HFpEF)
HFrEF. *See* Heart failure with reduced ejection fraction (HFrEF)
High-density lipoprotein (HDL), 22, 523, 525
High-density lipoprotein cholesterol (HDL-C), 112
High-sensitivity C-reactive protein (hs-CRP), 159
His-Purkinje system, 45, 339
His to ventricular (HV) interval, 331, 333
His troponin-I levels, 246
HLD. *See* Hyperlipidemia (HLD)
HMR. *See* Heart-to-mediastinum ratio (HMR)
"Hockey stick" movement, 53
HOCM. *See* Hypertrophic obstructive cardiomyopathy (HOCM)
Hodgkin lymphoma, 152
Holt-Oram syndrome, 12, 666
Holter monitor, 325, 328, 345, 382, 384, 385
Home-based cardiac rehab, 656
HR. *See* Hazard ratio (HR)
HTN. *See* Hypertension (HTN)
Human immunodeficiency virus infection, cardiac disease in, 156–160
 antiretroviral drugs and, 159, 160*t*
Hybrid and multimodality imaging correlation, 245–252
 computed tomography (CT), 245, 251, 251*f*
 hybrid x-ray fluoroscopy, 252
 magnetic resonance (MR) image fusion, 251, 251*f*
 positron emission tomography (PET), 245, 251, 251*f*
 3D echocardiography, 252
Hybrid imaging technology, 247–248
Hybrid PET/CT, 250
Hybrid x-ray fluoroscopy, 252
Hydralazine, 442–443, 444, 445, 446, 494, 496
Hydrochlorothiazide, 17, 105, 383
Hydroxychloroquine, 178
Hyperaldosteronism, 535, 538
Hypercalcemia, 73
Hyperemia, inducing agents, 276, 279
Hyperglycemia, 411, 415, 711
Hyperinsulinemia, 411, 415
Hyperkalemia, 120, 310, 312
Hyperlipidemia (HLD), 1, 10, 19, 73, 101, 146, 151, 246
Hyperlipidemia, 617

Hyperlipidemia, 736
Hyperlipoproteinemia, 9
Hypertension (HTN), 1, 3, 9, 17, 23, 101, 104, 146, 151–152, 182, 617, 622, 645, 650–655, 663, 685
    medical therapy for, 531, 534
    patient with a past medical history (PMH) of, 592
    treatment for, 537, 540
Hypertension in the Very Elderly Trial (HYVET), 118
Hyperthyroidism, 124, 125t
Hypertrophic cardiomyopathy (HCM), 104, 234, 327, 329, 418, 419, 456–457, 462–463
    arrhythmias in, 449, 451
    echocardiogram, 449, 451
    electrocardiogram, 449, 451–452
    genetic testing in, 449, 452
    histopathologic features of, 448, 450
    with left ventricular outflow tract obstruction, 448, 450
    mutations to cause, 448, 450
    sarcomeres containing mutant proteins in, 448, 450–451
    symptomatic patients, 449, 452
Hypertrophic obstructive cardiomyopathy (HOCM), 11–12, 13t, 16, 245, 253
    alcohol septal ablation and septal myomectomy in, 297–298, 300–301, 301t
Hypervolemia, 144
Hypoplastic left heart (LV) syndrome, 703
Hypotension, 166
    orthostatic, 383, 386
Hypothermia, 715
Hypothyroidism, 124, 125t, 151, 437, 440
Hypovolemia, 7
HYVET. *See* Hypertension in the Very Elderly Trial (HYVET)

I

I-metaiodobenzylguanidine (^{123}I-mIBG), 219, 222–223
Iatrogenic pneumothorax, 191
Ibuprofen, 85
ICD. *See* Implantable cardioverter-defibrillator (ICD)
ICE. *See* Intracardiac echocardiography (ICE)
IE. *See* Infective endocarditis (IE)
iFR. *See* Instantaneous wave-free ratio (iFR)
ILR. *See* Implantable loop recorder (ILR)
Immunosuppressive therapy, 468, 471
Implantable cardiac pacing, 383, 386
Implantable cardioverter-defibrillator (ICD), 189, 325, 328, 356–357, 361, 376, 378–380, 388, 390, 391, 400, 443, 446, 453, 455, 460–461
    class I indications for, 501t
    class IIa indications for, 501t
    complications of, 499, 503
    dual chamber, 499, 503
    implantation, clinical scenario, 377, 379
    for LQTS, 378, 380
    MADIT II trial, 377, 379
    Multicenter Automatic Defibrillator Implantation Trial (MADIT), 377, 379
    Multicenter Unsustained Tachycardia Trial (MUSTT), 377, 379
    primary prevention, 376, 379, 499–500, 503
    programming, 378, 380
    subcutaneous, clinical scenario, 377, 379
Implantable loop recorder (ILR), 326–327, 329, 330, 382, 385, 386
Inappropriate sinus tachycardia, 166
Indinavir, 157, 159, 160t
Infection
    lead extraction and, 401, 403
Infective endocarditis (IE), 77–82, 212
    modified Duke criteria for, 79t, 80
Inferior vena cava (IVC), 701–702

Inflammatory cardiomyopathy, 471f
Influenza A and B viruses, 469–470
Innocent murmur, 12, 14t, 16
Inotersen (Tegsedi), 179, 180t
INR. *See* International normalized ratio (INR)
Instantaneous wave-free ratio (iFR)
    vs. fractional flow reserve, 276, 280
Insulin, 641
Insulin resistance, 411, 415
Interagency Registry for Mechanically Assisted Circulatory Support (INTERMACS), 603, 604
Interlobular septa (Kerley B lines), 192
INTERMACS (Interagency Registry for Mechanically Assisted Circulatory Support) profiles, 505, 507, 507t
International normalized ratio (INR), 349, 351
Interstitial edema, 192
Intestinal arterial thromboembolism, 541, 543–544
Intestinal arterial thrombosis, 541, 543–544
Intracardiac abscesses, 82
Intracardiac echocardiography (ICE), 253
    maximal tissues penetration of, 271, 274, 274f
    mechanical/rotational, 271, 275
    phased-array, 271, 275
    types of, 271, 275
    vs. transesophageal echocardiography, 271, 275
Intramural hematoma, 578, 581
Intravascular ultrasound (IVUS), 270, 273
    criteria, 278, 282
    minimum luminal area, 270, 273–274
    vs. angiography, 270, 272
    vs. optical coherence tomography, 270–272, 272–273f, 274
Intravenous (IV) heparin, 117
Intravenous drug use (IVDU), 79, 219
Intravenous tissue plasminogen activator therapy
    indications for, 532t
Iron deficiency, 710
Ischemic cardiomyopathy, 1, 477
Ischemic heart disease, 19, 113, 113f, 238, 239t
Isolated postcapillary PH (Ipc-PH), 99
Isolated posterior myocardial infarction, 35t, 37
Isoproterenol, 332, 334, 336, 339
    physiologic effect, 338, 339
Isordil, 494, 496
Isosorbide dinitrate, 48, 442–443, 445
Isosorbide mononitrate, 48, 50, 231
Ivabradine, 48, 50, 494, 496, 497, 503
IVC. *See* Inferior vena cava (IVC)
IVDU. *See* Intravenous drug use (IVDU)
IVUS. *See* Intravascular ultrasound (IVUS)

J

Jugular venous distension (JVD), 9, 42, 127, 700
Jugular venous pressure (JVP), 15
JVD. *See* Jugular venous distension (JVD)
JVP. *See* Jugular venous pressure (JVP)

K

Kaposi sarcoma (KS), 157
KS. *See* Kaposi sarcoma (KS)
Kussmaul sign, 85, 88

L

LAA. *See* Left atrial appendage (LAA)
Labetalol, 105
LAD. *See* Left anterior descending (LAD) artery
Late gadolinium enhancement (LGE), 234
Lateral chest radiograph, 395, 397–398

LBBB. *See* Left bundle branch block (LBBB)
LBD. *See* Lewy bodies (LBD)
LDLs. *See* Low-density lipoproteins (LDLs)
Lead extraction
  fibrinous material in right atrium and superior vena cava after, 401, 403
  indication for, 401, 403
  infection and, 401, 403
  mortality with, 401, 403
  periprocedural complications of, 404*t*
  probability of major complications of, 402*t*
  surgical removal, 400, 402
  SVC balloon during, 402, 403
  transvenous, 400, 401, 402, 403
Lead micro-dislodgement, 395, 398
Lead perforation, 499, 500, 503, 504
Left anterior descending (LAD)
  artery, 41
  stenosis, 22
Left atrial appendage (LAA)
  anatomic patterns of, 304–305, 307
  with atrial fibrillation, 304, 306
  candidates for Watchman procedure, 306, 307
  complications of, 305, 307
  puncture location, 305, 307
  thrombi occur in, 304, 307
  Watchman device removal, 306, 307, 308*f*
Left bundle area pacing, 395, 397
Left bundle branch block (LBBB), 35*t*, 37, 117, 298, 302
Left circumflex coronary artery, 22
Left heart disease (LHD), 92
Left internal mammary artery (LIMA) graft, 226
Left lower sternal border (LLSB), 9
Left radial approach, criteria for, 263, 265–266
Left-to-right shunt, 680
Left ventricular (LV)
  angiography, 264, 268
  apical aneurysm, 310, 312
  function, 23, 64
  recovery
    clinical factors with, 438, 440
    definition of, 437, 440
    outcomes for, 437, 440
Left ventricular assist devices (LVADs), 411–412, 415, 601
  absolute and relative contraindications, 508, 508*t*
  complications, assessment and treatment of, 509–510*t*
  for destination therapy, 507, 511
  and gastrointestinal (GI) bleeding, 506, 511
  infections, risk factor for, 506, 511
  risk factor for, 506, 508–509
  severe aortic stenosis, 505, 508
  thrombosis, 507, 511
Left ventricular ejection fraction (LVEF), 41, 57, 62, 69, 91, 117, 151, 173, 325, 328, 332–333, 335
Left ventricular end-diastolic diameter (LVESD), 57
Left ventricular end-diastolic pressure (LVEDP), 265, 268
Left ventricular end-systolic dimension (LVESD), 64, 568, 569
Left ventricular hypertrophy (LVH), 143
Left ventricular noncompaction cardiomyopathy (LVNC), 236, 417, 418, 419
Left ventricular outflow tract (LVOT)
  beta-blockers, 297, 299–300
  obstruction, 284–285, 287
  surgical myectomy, 297, 300
Left ventricular outflow tract obstruction (LVOTO), 448, 450
Left ventricular thrombus (LVT), 140
Leiomyoma, 215

Leiomyosarcoma, 157
Leukocytosis, 205
Lev-Lenegre disease, 322, 324
Lewy bodies (LBD), 165
LGE. *See* Late gadolinium enhancement (LGE)
LHD. *See* Left heart disease (LHD)
Libman-Sacks endocarditis, 124
Lidocaine, 357, 361, 389
Life's Simple 7, 633
Lily of the valley, 170, 171*t*
LIMA. *See* Left internal mammary artery (LIMA) graft
Limb lead reversal, 310, 310*f*, 312
Limonene, 170
Lipid-mediated inflammation, 74
Lipid medications, 648–649
Lipid metabolism, 646
Lipoprotein a (Lp (a)), 623
Liposarcoma, 215
Lisinopril, 22, 145, 494, 496
LLSB. *See* Left lower sternal border (LLSB)
Long QT syndrome (LQTS), 320, 322–323
  diagnosis and treatment, 320, 323
  type 1 (LQTS1), 320, 323, 364, 367
  type 2 (LQTS2), 320, 323
  type 3 (LQTS3), 320, 323
Loop diuretics, 430, 492, 495
Lopinavir, 157, 159, 160*t*
Low-density lipoprotein cholesterol (LDL-C), 112, 159
Low-density lipoproteins (LDL), 17, 22, 523, 525
Lower extremity Doppler, 290, 292
LQTS. *See* Long QT syndrome (LQTS)
LVAD. *See* Left ventricular assist devices (LVADs)
LVEDP. *See* Left ventricular end-diastolic pressure (LVEDP)
LVEF. *See* Left ventricular ejection fraction (LVEF)
LVESD. *See* Left ventricular end-diastolic diameter (LVESD)
LVH. *See* Left ventricular hypertrophy (LVH)
LVNC. *See* Left ventricular noncompaction (LVNC)
LVOT. *See* Left ventricular outflow tract (LVOT)
LVOTO. *See* Left ventricular outflow tract obstruction (LVOTO)
LVT. *See* Left ventricular thrombus (LVT)
Lymphomas, 140

M

MAC. *See* Mitral annular calcifications (MAC)
MACE. *See* Major adverse cardiovascular events (MACE)
"Mad honey," 169
MADIT. *See* Multicenter Automatic Defibrillator Implantation Trial (MADIT)
MADIT II. *See* Multicenter Automatic Defibrillator Implantation Trial II (MADIT II)
Magnetic resonance (MR) image fusion, 245, 251, 251*f*
Magnetic resonance imaging (MRI)
  cardiac, 442, 444–445, 468, 471–472
  for ASD, 294, 296
Major adverse cardiovascular events (MACE), 159
Marfan syndrome, 102, 126, 516, 577, 580
  angiotensin receptor blockers (ARBs), 581
Marijuana, 129, 130*t*, 477
Maternal CHD, 665
MCA. *See* Middle cerebral artery (MCA)
Mean pulmonary artery pressure (mPAP), 90
Mechanical cutting tools, 400, 403
Mechanical thrombectomy, 530, 534
Mechanical/rotational ICE system, 271, 275
Medical management, 596
MERRF. *See* Myoclonus epilepsy with ragged-red fibers (MERRF) syndrome
MESA. *See* Multiethnic Study of Atherosclerosis Risk Score (MESA)

Mesenteric ischemia
  acute
    characteristics of, 541, 543
    treatment for, 542, 545–546t
  chronic
    diagnosis of, 541, 543
    treatment for, 542, 545–546t
    weight loss, 541, 544
  computed tomography angiography (CTA), 542, 544
  immediate exploratory laparotomy, 542, 544
  intervention for, 542, 548
    follow-up after, 543, 548
  intestinal arterial thromboembolism, 541, 543–544
  intestinal arterial thrombosis, 541, 543–544
  mesenteric venous thrombosis, 541, 543–544
  nonocclusive mesenteric ischemia, 541, 543–544
  revascularization, surveillance imaging, 543
Mesenteric venous thrombosis, 541, 543–544
Mesotheliomas, 140
Metabolic syndrome, 617
Metastatic breast cancer, 442, 445
Metformin, 2
Methamphetamine, 129, 130t
  induced cardiomyopathy, 128–129
  induced pulmonary arterial hypertension, 130
Methamphetamine use, 474, 477
Methicillin-sensitive *Staphylococcus aureus* (MSSA), 68, 78
Methyldopa, 105
Metolazone, 482, 486
Metoprolol, 198, 363, 367
Metoprolol succinate, 2, 145, 482, 486
Metoprolol tartrate, 579, 582
Mexiletine, 357, 358, 361, 362, 364, 367
  side effects of, 358, 362
MI. *See* Myocardial infarction (MI)
MI with nonobstructive coronary artery (MINOCA), 36
Microvascular obstruction, 244
Mid-diastolic murmur, 15
Mid-systolic high-pitched murmur, 15
Mid-systolic murmurs, 16
Middle cerebral artery (MCA), 529, 531
  emergent treatment, 530, 532, 533f
Midodrine, 177
Mild-moderate aortic stenosis, 684
Milrinone, 483, 487
MINOCA. *See* MI with nonobstructive coronary artery (MINOCA)
Mitochondrial DNA, 417, 419
MitraClip, 284, 286, 286f
  placement of, 284, 287
Mitral annular calcifications (MAC), 77
Mitral flow obstruction, 15
Mitral regurgitation (MR), 15–16, 69
Mitral stenosis, 12, 12t, 16, 59, 214
Mitral valve (MV) endocarditis, 219
Mitral valve (MV) surgery
  anatomy of, 573, 576
  Carpentier classification, 573, 576
  chord-sparing, replacement, 573, 576
  class I recommendation, 572, 574
  determinants of successful, 573, 576, 576f
  intervention for, 572, 574–575
  management guidelines, 572, 574–575, 574–575f
  predictors of potential failure of, 573, 576
  risk factor for, 573, 576
Mitral valve balloon valvuloplasty, 52
Mitral valve disease, 56–61
Mitral valve lesions, 53
Mitral valve prolapse (MVP), 12, 12t, 15–16, 126
Mitral valve stenosis, 15

M-mode echocardiography, 210
M-moiety, 53
Mobitz I heart block, 45
Mobitz II heart block, 45
Moderate aortic regurgitation, 505, 508
Modified Duke criteria, 80
  for infective endocarditis, 79t, 80
  interpretation, 79t, 80
  major criteria, 79t, 80
  minor criteria, 79t, 80
Modified World Health Organization (mWHO) classification, 107–108, 109–110t
Morphine, 584, 588
mPAP. *See* Mean pulmonary artery pressure (mPAP)
MPI. *See* Myocardial perfusion imaging (MPI)
MR. *See* Magnetic resonance (MR) image fusion
MRI. *See* Magnetic resonance imaging (MRI)
MSA. *See* Multiple system atrophy (MSA)
MSI. *See* Myocardial salvage index (MSI)
MSSA. *See* Methicillin-sensitive Staphylococcus aureus (MSSA)
Multicenter Automatic Defibrillator Implantation Trial II (MADIT II), 120, 377, 379
Multicenter Automatic Defibrillator Implantation Trial (MADIT), 377, 379
Multicenter Unsustained Tachycardia Trial (MUSTT), 377, 379, 501–502
Multiethnic Study of Atherosclerosis Risk Score (MESA), 628
Multimodality imaging probes, 247
Multiple system atrophy (MSA), 163
MUSTT. *See* Multicenter Unsustained Tachycardia Trial (MUSTT)
MVP. *See* Mitral valve prolapse (MVP)
Myalgias, 647
MYBPC3 (myosin-binding protein C), 418, 419
MYBPC3 gene, 448, 450
MYH7 (myosin heavy chain 7), 418, 419
MYH7 gene, 448, 450
Myocardial bridging, 265, 268
Myocardial calcification, 193
Myocardial infarction (MI), 1, 27, 41, 119, 123, 123f, 144, 261, 638
  thrombolysis in, 264, 267
Myocardial infarction with nonobstructive coronary arteries (MINOCA), 237
Myocardial injury, 481, 484
Myocardial perfusion imaging (MPI), 218
Myocardial salvage index (MSI), 236
Myocardial viability study, 206
Myocarditis, 238, 239t
  acute, medications not used, 468, 470
  bimodal age distribution in, 467, 469
  causes of, 467, 469–470
  diagnosis of, 468, 472
  dilated cardiomyopathy and, 467, 469
  etiology of, 467, 470
  management of, 471f
Myoclonus epilepsy with ragged-red fibers (MERRF) syndrome, 419
Myocyte hypertrophy, 448, 450
Myopathies, 251
Myxomas, 140, 215

N

Nadolol, 364, 367
NASCET. *See* North American Symptomatic Carotid Endarterectomy Trial (NASCET)
National Institutes of Health Stroke Scale. *See* NIHSS (National Institutes of Health Stroke Scale)
Nelfinavir, 159, 160t
Nephrogenic systemic fibrosis (NSF), 186

Neprilysin, 440, 492, 495
Neurally mediated syncope. See Reflex syncope
Neurofibromatosis, 124, 125t
Neurohormonal axes, stimulation of, 436, 438–439
Nevirapine, 159, 160t
New-onset atrial fibrillation, 263, 265
New York Heart Association (NYHA), 1, 4, 4–5t, 60
    class II heart failure, 498, 501–502
    class III heart failure, 502
    class IV heart failure, 502
        palliative care consultation for, 503
Niacin, 646
Nicardipine, 579, 582
Nicotine replacement therapies (NRTs), 636
Nifedipine, 50, 105
NIHSS (National Institutes of Health Stroke Scale), 530, 532, 533f
Nitroglycerin, 22, 26, 32
Nitroprusside, 276, 279
NNRTI. See Nonnucleoside reverse transcriptase inhibitor (NNRTI)
NOACs. See Novel oral anticoagulants (NOACs)
Non-nicotine oral medications, 636
Noncardiac surgery, cardiac evaluation for, 143–149
Nondiagnostic exercise stress test, 200
Noninvasive functional stress testing modalities and guideline recommendations, 23, 24–25t
Nonnucleoside reverse transcriptase inhibitor (NNRTI), 159, 160t
Nonobstructive coronary artery disease, 47
Nonocclusive mesenteric ischemia, 541, 543–544
Nonpharmacotherapy approaches, 176
Non–ST-elevation myocardial infarction (NSTEMI), 28–33, 157, 224
Non–ST-segment-elevation myocardial infarction (NSTEMI), 621, 624
Nonsteroidal anti-inflammatory drugs (NSAIDs), 46, 85f, 86, 121
Nonstroke etiologies, 529, 532
Nonsustained ventricular tachycardia (NSVT), 332–333, 335, 449, 451, 453
Noonan syndrome, 12, 665
Norepinephrine, 36, 483, 487
North American Symptomatic Carotid Endarterectomy Trial (NASCET), 597
NOTCH1 gene, 692
Novel oral anticoagulants (NOACs), 557
NRTIs. See Nucleoside reverse transcriptase inhibitors (NRTIs)
NRTs. See Nicotine replacement therapies (NRTs)
NSAIDs. See Nonsteroidal anti-inflammatory drugs (NSAIDs)
NSF. See Nephrogenic systemic fibrosis (NSF)
NSTEMI. See Non–ST-elevation myocardial infarction (NSTEMI)
NSVT. See Nonsustained ventricular tachycardia (NSVT)
N-terminal pro–B-type natriuretic peptide (NT-proBNP), 176, 439
N-3 long-chain fatty acid, 647
Nuclear cardiology and molecular imaging, 218–224
Nuclear scintigraphy/SPECT with Technetium-99m pyrophosphate, 457–458, 463–464
Nuclear stress test, 478
Nuclear technetium-99m pyrophosphate (PYP) scan, 173
Nucleoside reverse transcriptase inhibitors (NRTIs), 159, 160t
NYHA. See New York Heart Association (NYHA)
NYHA FC II (New York Heart Association Functional Classification II), 688, 690
NYHA/AHA functional classifications of heart failure, 405, 407

O

Obesity, 146, 617, 644
Obesity hypoventilation syndrome, 7
Obstructive coronary artery disease, 1
Obstructive sleep apnea, 7

OCT. See Optical coherence tomography (OCT)
Offspring inheritance, 673
Older adults and heart disease, 116–120
OMT. See Optimal medical therapy (OMT)
Onpattro. See Patisiran (Onpattro)
Opioids, 129, 130t
Optical coherence tomography (OCT), 270, 273
    vs. intravascular ultrasound, 270–272, 272–273f, 274
Optimal medical therapy (OMT), 119
Oreo cookie sign, 192
Organophosphates, 170
Orthostatic hypotension, 7, 383, 386
Pacemaker implantation, 383, 386
Orthotopic heart transplant, 605
Ostium secundum atrial septal defect, 311, 313

P

PAC. See Premature atrial contraction (PAC)
Pace mapping, 371, 374
Pacemaker implantation, 383, 386
Pacemaker-mediated tachycardia (PMT), 394, 397
Pacing system, 711, 713
PAF. See Pure autonomic failure (PAF)
PAH. See Pulmonary arterial hypertension (PAH)
Palliative radiotherapy, 141–142
Palpitations, 8
PAP. See Pulmonary artery pressure (PAP)
Papillary fibroelastoma, 139
Papillary muscle rupture, 44–45
PARADIGM-HF trial, 492–493, 495
Parasympathetic nervous system, 162, 164
Paravalvular regurgitation, 66
Parkinson disease [PD], 164
PARTNER. See Placement of Aortic Transcatheter Valves (PARTNER) trial
PASS (Pull, Aim, Squeeze, and Sweep) criteria, 306, 307
Patent ductus arteriosus (PDA), 661, 679
    contraindication, 290, 292
Patent foramen ovale (PFO)
    in adult population, 293, 295
    contraindications for, 294, 295–296
    diagnosis of, 293, 295
    in fetal development, 294, 296
    pathologic disease processes associated with, 294, 296
    treatment, 293, 295
Patient-prosthesis mismatch (PPM), 71
Patisiran (Onpattro), 179, 180t
Patisiran, 443, 447
PAWP. See Pulmonary artery wedge pressure (PAWP)
PCE. See Pooled Cohort Equation (PCE)
PCI. See Percutaneous coronary intervention (PCI)
PCP. See Primary care physician (PCP)
PCs. See Pericardial cysts (PCs)
PCSK9 inhibitors, 645
PCTs. See Primary cardiac tumors (PCTs)
PCWP. See Pulmonary capillary wedge pressure (PCWP)
PDA. See Patent ductus arteriosus (PDA)
PE. See Pulmonary embolism (PE)
Penetrating aortic ulcer, 515, 522
Penetrating arteriosclerotic ulcer, 578, 581
Pentoxifylline, 584, 588
Percutaneous coronary intervention (PCI), 277
    role of, 278, 282
    treatment strategy for, 277–278, 282
Percutaneous coronary interventions (PCIs), 18, 22, 119, 145, 159, 227, 234
Percutaneous mitral balloon commissurotomy (PMBC), 58
Percutaneous mitral valve commissurotomy (PTMC), 57, 210
Percutaneous pulmonic valve implantation, 289–290, 292
Pericardial calcifications, 194
Pericardial cysts (PCs), 138

Pericardial disease, 83–89, 238, 239*t*
Pericardial effusion, etiologies
    inflammatory, 85
    noninflammatory, 85
Pericardiectomy, 87*t*, 88–89
Pericardiocentesis, 85
Peripartum cardiomyopathy, 187
    defined, 447
    risk factors for, 103
Peripheral arterial disease (PAD), 3, 523, 525, 535, 538, 583, 585
    diagnosis of, 583, 585, 586*t*
    long-term surveillance, 584–585, 589
    management, 584, 588
    medications used for, 589*t*
    physical examination of, 583, 585, 587
    positive test for, 524, 527
    revascularization, 585, 589–590
        modalities for, 584, 588
    symptoms of, 8
    treatment for, 584, 587–588
Peripheral vascular disease, 655
    segmental volume plethysmography in, 527*f*
Periprocedural imaging, 253–255
Permanent atrial fibrillation, 394, 395, 396, 397
Permanent pacemaker
    failure of, 398
    implantation of, 394–395, 396
    leadless, 395, 397
    oversensing, 398
    sensing, 396, 398
    single- or dual-chamber, 394, 397
    undersensing, 398
    VVIR and, 394
Permanent pacing, 337, 339
PET. *See* Positron emission tomography (PET)
PFO. *See* Patent foramen ovale (PFO)
PH. *See* Pulmonary hypertension (PH)
Pharmacovigilance, 20
Phase 3 repolarization, prolongation of, 315, 317
Phased-array ICE system, 271, 275
Phenylephrine, 483, 487
Pheochromocytoma, 124, 125*t*
Phosphodiesterase 5 (PDE5) inhibitors, 32
Phrenic nerve stimulation, 500, 504
PHV. *See* Prosthetic Heart Valve (PHV) regurgitation
Physical activity/fitness, 633
    children and adolescents, 633
    intensities of, 636
Physiologic splitting, 666
PIONEER-HF trial, 483, 487
PISA. *See* Proximal isovelocity surface area (PISA)
Pitavastatin, 159
Placement of Aortic Transcatheter Valves (PARTNER) trial, 284, 287
Plakophilin-2, 416, 419
Platelet adenosine diphosphate (ADP) P2Y12 receptor, 32, 39
Platypnea-orthodeoxia, 294, 296
Plavix, 17
PLE. *See* Protein-losing enteropathy (PLE)
Pleural effusions, 192
PMBC. *See* Percutaneous mitral balloon commissurotomy (PMBC)
PMT. *See* Pacemaker-mediated tachycardia (PMT)
POINT trial, 534
Polysplenia, 659
Pooled Cohort Equation (PCE), 628
Porcelain aorta, risk factor for, 568, 571
Positron emission tomography (PET), 245, 251, 251*f*
Positron emission tomography with fluorodeoxyglucose (PET-FDG), 237
Posterior descending artery (PDA), 264, 267

Posteroanterior (PA) chest radiograph, 395, 397–398
Postural orthostatic tachycardia syndrome (POTS), 165–166
POTS. *See* Postural orthostatic tachycardia syndrome (POTS)
PPD. *See* Purified protein derivative (PPD) result
PPM. *See* Patient-prosthesis mismatch (PPM)
Prasugrel, 28–29, 31–32, 39–40
Pravastatin, 157, 159
Pravastatin or Atorvastatin Evaluation and Infection Therapy–Thrombolysis In Myocardial Infarction 22 trial (PROVE IT-TIMI 22), 32
The PREDIMED (Prevention with Mediterranean Diet), 635
Prednisone, 470
Pregnancy
    adults with congenital heart disease, 670
    CARPREG II and ZAHARA studies, 671
    CT in, 670
    and heart disease, 103–110
        cardiac medications, 105–106*t*
        physiologic changes during, 103
Pregnancy history/delivery course, 607
Premature atherosclerosis, 124
Premature atrial contraction (PAC), 146
Premature ventricular contractions (PVCs), 184
Primary cardiac tumors (PCTs), 136
Primary care physician (PCP), 11, 650
Primary surgical repair, 701
Pro B-type natriuretic peptide (proBNP), 144, 204, 207
Procainamide, 357, 361, 365, 368
Propafenone, 363, 367
Propranolol, 165
Proprotein convertase subtilisin/kexin type 9 (PCSK-9), 18
Prosthetic Heart Valve (PHV) regurgitation, 75, 75–76*t*
Prosthetic valve dysfunction, 71–76
Protein-losing enteropathy (PLE), 610, 613–614
Proximal isovelocity surface area (PISA), 73
Pseudo-severe aortic stenosis, 211
Pseudoaneurysm, 578, 581
Pseudoaortic stenosis, 64
PTMC. *See* Percutaneous mitral valve commissurotomy (PTMC)
PTPN11 gene, 665
Pulmonary arterial hypertension (PAH)
    clinical classification of, 707
    diagnostic algorithm of, 708
    pulmonologist, 705
Pulmonary arterial hypertension associated with congenital heart disease (PAH-CHD), 705
Pulmonary artery (PA) stenosis, 700
Pulmonary artery hypertension (PAH), 18, 166
Pulmonary artery pressure (PAP), 90
Pulmonary artery wedge pressure (PAWP), 257
Pulmonary atresia and surgical palliation, 694
Pulmonary capillary wedge pressure (PCWP), 90
Pulmonary congestion, treatment for, 482, 486
Pulmonary embolism (PE), 7, 86, 390
    classification of, 559*t*
    D-dimer assay for, 555, 557
    diagnosis of, 554, 557
    management of, 555, 557
    predisposing factor for, 554, 556
    revised Geneva clinical prediction rule for, 556, 558*t*
    risk factors of, 555, 557
    rivaroxaban, 556, 557
    thrombolytic therapy, 555, 557
    thrombus formation, common sites of, 554, 556
Pulmonary hypertension (PH), 7, 90–99
    blood testing, 95, 95*t*
    cardiac magnetic resonance, 95, 95*t*
    cardiopulmonary exercise testing, 95, 96*t*
    chest x-ray, 94*t*, 95
    computed tomography, 95, 95*t*

electrocardiography, 94t, 95
  hemodynamic classification of, 90
  pulmonary function testing and blood gases, 94t, 95
  right heart catheterization, 95, 96t
  six-minute walk test, 95, 95t
  testing modalities in, 95, 96–97t
  ultrasonography, 95, 95t
  WSPH clinical classifications of, 92t, 93
Pulmonary regurgitation, 614
Pulmonary stenosis, 11t, 12, 16
Pulmonary vascular resistance (PVR), 90
Pulmonary veno-occlusive disease (PVOD), 95
Pulmonic stenosis, 16
Pulse volume recording (PVR), 524, 526, 527f
Pure autonomic failure (PAF), 165
Purified protein derivative (PPD) result, 191
Purkinje fiber disease, 333
PVCs. See Premature ventricular contractions (PVCs)
PVOD. See Pulmonary veno-occlusive disease (PVOD)
PVR. See Pulmonary vascular resistance (PVR)
Pyrethroid insecticides, 168, 170

Q

QALYs. See Quality-adjusted life years (QALYs)
QSART. See Quantitative sudomotor axon reflex test (QSART)
QT prolongation, 391
Quality-adjusted life years (QALYs), 18
Quantitative sudomotor axon reflex test (QSART), 163, 165
Q-waves, 85

R

RAAS. See Renin-angiotensin-aldosterone system (RAAS)
Race/ethnicity, 622
Radiation exposure, reducing, 263, 266
Radiofrequency (RF) ablation
  vs. cryoablation, 371, 374
Radiofrequency catheter ablation (RFCA), 298, 302
RALES. See Randomized ALdactone Evaluation Study (RALES)
Randomized ALdactone Evaluation Study (RALES), 120
Randomized controlled trials, 536, 538
Ranolazine, 22, 26, 48–50, 231, 584, 588
Rapid ventricular response (RVR), 675
RAS. See Renin-angiotensin-system (RAS) antagonists, side effects of
Raynaud disease, 535, 538
RBBB. See Right bundle branch block (RBBB)
RCA. See Right coronary artery (RCA)
RCM. See Restrictive cardiomyopathy (RCM)
RCRI. See Revised Cardiac Risk Index (RCRI) scoring system
Reentrant tachycardia, 316, 318, 344, 347
  conditions for, 316, 318
  functional, 316, 318
Reflex syncope, 384
Refractory angina, 47–50
  characteristic of, 47
Regadenoson, 221
REHEARSE-AF trial, 327, 329
REMS. See Risk Evaluation and Mitigation Strategies (REMS)
Renal artery stenosis, 535, 538, 686
Renal cell carcinoma, 154
Renal Doppler ultrasound, 537–538, 540
Renal Optimization Strategies Evaluation. See ROSE (Renal Optimization Strategies Evaluation) trial
Renal sympathetic denervation, 166
Renin-angiotensin-aldosterone system (RAAS), 410, 414, 436
  antagonists, 430
Renin-angiotensin-aldosterone system, 124
Renin-angiotensin-system (RAS) antagonists, side effects of, 493, 495
Repolarization, phase 3, prolongation of, 315, 317
RESPECT trial, 294, 296

Restricted Adempas (riociguat) REMS program, 20
Restrictive cardiomyopathy (RCM), 84, 87t, 88–89, 248
  causes of, 417, 419
  diagnosis of, 454, 459–460
Reteplase (rPA), 39
Return of spontaneous circulation (ROSC), 388
Revascularization, 27, 31
Reverberation artifact, 187
Revised Cardiac Risk Index (RCRI) scoring system, 147
Revised Jones criteria, 52t, 53
RF. See Radiofrequency (RF) ablation
RFCA. See Radiofrequency catheter ablation (RFCA)
Rhabdomyoma, 139
Rhabdomyosarcoma, 157
RHC. See Right heart catheterization (RHC)
Rheumatic heart disease, 51–55, 105
Rheumatic mitral stenosis intervention, 58f, 59
Rheumatoid arthritis, 124, 168
Rheumatologic disorders, 113
Rhododendron species, 169
Rifampin, 19
Right bundle branch block, QRS duration, 337, 339
Right bundle branch block (RBBB), 262, 298, 302
Right coronary artery (RCA), 144
Right heart catheterization (RHC), 90, 95, 96t, 288, 291
Right-sided regurgitant valve lesions, 68t, 70
  etiologies, 68t, 70
  iatrogenic, 68t, 70
  pathogenesis of, 68t, 70
  primary causes (25%), 68t, 70
  secondary causes (75%), 68t, 70
Right-to-left shunts, 680
Right ventricle (RV)
  congenital heart disease, 693
  pulmonary atresia, 694–695
  tetralogy of Fallot, 693
Right ventricular infarction, 35t, 37
Right ventricular outflow tract (RVOT), 289–290
Right ventricular systolic pressure (RVSP), 679
Riociguat, 706
Risk Assessment and Comparative Effectiveness of Left Ventricular Assist Device and Medical Management (ROADMAP) study, 603
Risk Evaluation and Mitigation Strategies (REMS), 20
Ritonavir, 159, 160t
Rivaroxaban, 549, 552, 556, 557, 562, 565
ROSC. See Return of spontaneous circulation (ROSC)
ROSE (Renal Optimization Strategies Evaluation) trial, 483, 489t, 491
Rosiglitazone, 20
Ross-Konno procedure, 289–290
Rosuvastatin, 22, 157, 159, 563, 566
Rotational/orbital atherectomy, 271, 275
  risk of, 276, 278
Rule of "12s," 39
RVOT. See Right ventricular outflow tract (RVOT)
RVR. See Rapid ventricular response (RVR)
RVSP. See Right ventricular systolic pressure (RVSP)
R wave progression, causes for poor, 309, 312

S

Sacubitril, 440
Sacubitril-valsartan, 482, 486
Saphenous vein graft (SVG), 277, 281
Saquinavir, 157, 159, 160t
Sarcoidosis, 126, 237
Sarcomas, 140
Sarcomeric proteins, 416, 417, 418, 419
Sarcoplasmic-endoplasmic reticulum Ca^{2+} ATPase (SERCA), 411, 415

SAVR. *See* Surgical aortic valve replacement (SAVR)
SCA. *See* Sudden cardiac arrest (SCA)
SCAD. *See* Spontaneous coronary artery dissection (SCAD)
SCD-HeFT trial, 377, 379
Scopolamine, 170
SCTs. *See* Secondary cardiac tumors (SCTs)
Secondary cardiac tumors (SCTs), 141
Septal myectomy, favoring factors, 297–298, 300–301, 301*t*
Septal reduction therapy, 297, 299
SERCA. *See* Sarcoplasmic-endoplasmic reticulum Ca^{2+} ATPase (SERCA)
Serum and urine protein electrophoresis, 465
Serum-free light chains, 458, 464–465
Serum protein electrophoresis and immunofixation (SPEI), 173
7-day cardiac event monitoring, 341, 345
Severe aortic stenosis, 505, 508
Severe calcific/senile aortic stenosis, 666
Severe mitral stenosis, 505, 508
Severe tricuspid regurgitation, 505, 508
Sheath, rotational mechanical cutting, 400, 403
SHEP. *See* Systolic Hypertension in the Elderly Program (SHEP)
Shock, biphasic, 387, 389
Short QT syndrome (SQTS), 322, 324
    type 1 (SQTS1), 321, 323
Shortest preexcited RR interval (SPERRI), 332, 334
Sick sinus syndrome, 401, 403
Simple traction, 401, 403
Simvastatin, 157
Singh-Vaughan Williams classification, of antiarrhythmic drugs, 369–370*t*
Single-modality imaging, 248
Single-photon emission computed tomography (SPECT), 173, 184, 219, 221–223, 245
    Tc-99m sestamibi scan, 213
Sinoatrial nodal dysfunction, 329
Sinus bradycardia, 315, 317
Sinus node dysfunction, 336, 338
    permanent pacemaker implantation, indications for, 336, 338
Sinus rhythm, amiodarone for, 366, 369
Sinus tachycardia, 135
Six-minute walk test, 95, 95*t*
SLE. *See* Systemic lupus erythematosus (SLE)
SLGT2 inhibitors, 641
SMART. *See* Strategies for Management of Antiretroviral Therapy (SMART)
Smoking cessation, 632, 650
    medical therapy for, 531, 534
Society of Thoracic Surgeons. *See* STS (Society of Thoracic Surgeons)
Society of Thoracic Surgeons (STS) risk score, 567, 569
Sodium-glucose cotransporter 2 (SGLT2) inhibitor, 364, 367, 430, 434
Sodium-glucose cotransporter 2 inhibitors (SGLT2i), 411, 415, 494, 496–497
Sodium-glucose transporter 2 (SGLT2) inhibitor, 486
Sotalol, 357, 358, 361, 362, 363, 367
    contraindications, 364, 367
SPECT. *See* Single-photon emission computed tomography (SPECT)
SPEI. *See* Serum protein electrophoresis and immunofixation (SPEI)
SPERRI. *See* Shortest preexcited RR interval (SPERRI)
Spinal flexion, 8
Spinal stenosis, 8
Spironolactone, 482, 486
Spontaneous coronary artery dissection (SCAD), 34, 112
SPRINT. *See* Systolic Blood Pressure Intervention Trial (SPRINT)
SQTS. *See* Short QT syndrome (SQTS)

Squill, 170, 171*t*
ST-segment elevation myocardial infarction (STEMI), 31, 34–41, 119, 157, 234, 261, 282
    electrocardiographic criteria for, 35*t*, 37
    management strategies for, 36*f*, 38
Stable coronary artery disease (CAD), 654, 655
Stable ischemic heart disease, 21–27
Stanford Type A dissections, 579, 582
Stanford Type B dissections, 579, 582
Staphylococcus species, 619
Stent placement, adulthood, 289, 292
Stevenson clinical profiles, 481–482, 484, 486*f*
Strategies for Management of Antiretroviral Therapy (SMART), 158
Stress-induced hyperglycemia, 638
Structural heart abnormalities, 7
STS. *See* Society of Thoracic Surgeons (STS) risk score
STS (Society of Thoracic Surgeons), 618
Subclavian crush phenomenon, 499, 503
Sublingual nitroglycerin, 26, 50
Substance abuse and the heart, 127–131, 130*t*
    alcohol, 129, 130*t*
    cocaine, 129, 130*t*
    marijuana, 129, 130*t*
    methamphetamine, 129, 130*t*
    opioids, 129, 130*t*
    tobacco smoking/e-cigarettes, 129, 130*t*
Sudden cardiac arrest (SCA)
    etiology of, 387, 389
    risk of, 388, 390, 392
    triggers for, 392–393*t*
Sudden cardiac death
    incidence of, 416, 418
    causes of, 340, 344–345
Superficial vein thrombosis (SVT), management of, 550, 553
Superior vena cava (SVC), 701–702
Supraventricular tachycardia (SVT), 366, 368, 449, 451, 453, 670, 675
    follow-up care, 343, 346
Surgical aortic valve replacement (SAVR), 283, 285, 567, 569
Surgical myectomy, mortality for, 297, 300
Surgical shunt, 679
Surgical site bleeding, 148
Surgical thrombus resection, 74
SVC. *See* Superior vena cava (SVC)
SVG. *See* Saphenous vein graft (SVG)
SVT. *See* Superficial vein thrombosis (SVT)
Symptomatic aortic stenosis, 211
Symptomatic bradycardia, 394, 396, 397
Synchronized cardioversion, 356, 360
Syncope, 7, 350, 353, 693
    carotid sinus syndrome with, 383, 386
    causes of, 7
    diagnosis of, 381–382, 384–385
    epilepsy and, 381–382, 384
    increased vagal tone, 381, 384
    reflex, 384
Systemic diseases, cardiac manifestation of, 121–126
    endocrine disorders, 124, 125*t*
Systemic lupus erythematosus (SLE), 121–123
Systemic sclerosis, 124
Systolic Blood Pressure Intervention Trial (SPRINT), 112, 118
Systolic Hypertension in the Elderly Program (SHEP), 118

T

TAA. *See* Thoracic aortic aneurysm (TAA)
Tachy-brady syndrome, 329
Tachyarrhythmia, 340–341, 341*f*, 345
Tachyarrhythmias, 7
Tachycardia-induced cardiomyopathy, 346

Tafamidis (Vyndaqel), 179, 180*t*, 443, 447, 457–458, 464, 465
Targeted temperature management, 391
TAVR. *See* Transcatheter aortic valve replacement (TAVR)
TAZ (tafazzin), 418, 419
TCAR. *See* Transcarotid artery revascularization (TCAR)
Technetium pyrophosphate (^{99}mTc-PYP), 219, 222–223, 233, 249
TEE. *See* Transesophageal echocardiography (TEE)
TEER. *See* Transcatheter edge to edge repair (TEER)
Tegsedi. *See* Inotersen (Tegsedi)
Tenecteplase (TNK-PA), 39
Tension pneumothorax, 390
Tetralogy of Fallot (TOF), 669
TEVAR. *See* Thoracic endovascular aortic repair (TEVAR)
Thalassemia, 235
Thermoregulatory sweat test (TST), 163
Thienopyridine drug class, 39
3D echocardiography, 252
Thoracic aortic aneurysm (TAA)
    flowchart for evaluation of, 520–521*f*
    symptoms of, 514, 516
Thoracic aortic disease
    echocardiography, 577–578, 580–581
    medical management, 578, 581
Thoracic endovascular aortic repair (TEVAR), 578, 581
Thromboembolism, 714
    apixaban, 350, 353
    and atrial fibrillation, 353
    prevention of, 349, 351
Thrombolysis, 39
Thrombolysis in myocardial infarction (TIMI), 264, 267
    risk score for NSTE-ACS, 31*t*, 31
    risk stratification tool, 28, 30
Thrombosis formation, 74
Thrombus, 74
Thyroid-stimulating hormone (TSH), 2, 121
TIA. *See* Transient ischemic attack (TIA)
Ticagrelor, 32, 39–40
Tilt-table test, 381, 383, 384, 386
TIMI. *See* Thrombolysis in myocardial infarction (TIMI)
Timothy syndrome, 322, 324
Tissue plasminogen activator (tPA), contraindication for, 530, 534
TKIs. *See* Tyrosine kinase inhibitors (TKIs)
TMLR. *See* Transmyocardial laser revascularization (TMLR)
TMVR. *See* Transcatheter mitral valve replacement (TMVR)
TNNT2 gene mutation, 416, 418
Tobacco abuse, 3
Tobacco smoking/e-cigarettes, 129, 130*t*
Tobacco use, 17, 634
Torsades de pointes, 354–355, 360, 361
Torsemide, 492, 495
Toxin-induced cardiomyopathies. *See specific cardiomyopathies*
tPA. *See* Tissue plasminogen activator (tPA), contraindication for
TPG. *See* Transpulmonary gradient (TPG)
TR. *See* Tricuspid valve regurgitation (TR)
Transcarotid artery revascularization (TCAR), 591
Transcatheter aortic valve replacement (TAVR), 63, 253, 283, 285, 567, 569
    for aortic insufficiency (AI), 283, 285
    limitation of, 283, 285
Transcatheter edge to edge repair (TEER), 254
Transcatheter mitral valve replacement (TMVR)
    challenges/complications of, 284–285, 287
    cost of, 285, 287
Transesophageal echocardiogram (TEE), 72, 77, 136, 146, 187, 212, 215, 219, 235, 253, 382, 385, 685, 686, 690
Transesophageal echocardiography (TEE), 288*f*, 305, 307
    vs. intracardiac echocardiography, 271, 275
Transient ischemic attack (TIA), 215, 327, 330, 591

Transmitral pulse wave Doppler study, 206
Transmyocardial laser revascularization (TMLR), 50
Transpulmonary gradient (TPG), 92
Transthoracic echocardiogram (TTE), 62, 68, 71, 77, 83, 144, 162, 184, 187, 212, 215, 219, 232, 234, 253, 498, 500–501, 705
Transthoracic echocardiography (TTE), 382, 383, 385–386, 680
    for catheter ablation therapy, 371, 373
Transthyretin amyloidosis (ATTR) therapy, 125, 172, 179, 180*t*
Transthyretin tetramer, 179
Transvenous pacemaker (TVP), 298, 302
Transvenous phrenic nerve stimulation, 166
Trastuzumab, 113, 155
Trastuzumab-induced cardiomyopathy, 476, 479
Trauma, 387, 389
Traumatic valve rupture, 134
Tricuspid regurgitation
    anatomy and pathophysiology of, 286*f*
    treatment of, 283–284, 286
Tricuspid valve (TV) leaflet, 68
Tricuspid valve regurgitation (TR), 68
Triple therapy, 277, 282
Tropane alkaloids, 170
Troponin, 132, 176, 356, 360, 436, 439
TSH. *See* Thyroid-stimulating hormone (TSH)
TST. *See* Thermoregulatory sweat test (TST)
TTE. *See* Transthoracic echocardiogram (TTE)
Turner syndrome, 665, 666
TV. *See* Tricuspid valve (TV) leaflet
TVP. *See* Transvenous pacemaker (TVP)
12-lead ECG, 321, 324
2016 American College of Radiology (ACR) Appropriateness Criteria, 595
2018 Physical Activity Guidelines Advisory Committee Report, 635
2018/2019 ACC/AHA (American College of Cardiology/ American Heart Association) guidelines, 626, 630–631
2019 American Diabetes Association/European Association for the Study of Diabetes (ASDA/EASD) Standards of Medical Care, 638
2019 ESC (European Society of Cardiology) guidelines, 627, 630–631
Twiddler syndrome, 398
Type 1 diabetes mellitus (T1DM), 637–639
    weight loss, 641
Type 2 diabetes mellitus (T2DM), 615, 617, 637–639, 645, 654, 655, 685
    pathogenesis of, 640
Tyrosine kinase inhibitors (TKIs), 151

U

Ultrasonography, 95, 95*t*
Unfractionated heparin, 444, 446
Unspecified hyperlipidemia, 645
Unstable angina, 28–33
UPEI. *See* Urine protein electrophoresis and immunofixation (UPEI)
Urinalysis, 610
Urine protein electrophoresis and immunofixation (UPEI), 173
Urine toxicology screen, 129
Ursodiol, 179, 180*t*
U.S. Food and Drug Administration (FDA), 670

V

VA. *See* Veterans Administration (VA)
VAD. *See* Ventricular assist device (VAD)
Vagal maneuvers, 342, 346

Vagal-mediated atrial fibrillation, 165
Vagal nerve stimulation, 166
Valsalva maneuver, 16, 166, 383
Valsartan, 119
Valvular heart disease, 113, 113f, 154, 238, 239t
Valvular pulmonary stenosis, 694
Vandetanib, 154
Vascular endothelial growth factor (VEGF), 151
Vasodilator myocardial perfusion imaging, 23, 23t, 26
Vasodilator stress echocardiography, 216
Vasodilator stress testing, 224
Vasovagal syncope (VVS), 384
VEGF. *See* Vascular endothelial growth factor (VEGF)
Velocity time integral (VTI), 211
Venous claudication, 8
Venous thromboembolism (VTE) prophylaxis, 104, 107
Ventilation-perfusion scan, 94t, 95
Ventricular arrhythmias, 170
    inducibility testing for, 332, 334–335
Ventricular assist device (VAD), 600–602
Ventricular assist devices (LVAD)
    absolute and relative contraindications, 508, 508t
    risk factor for, 506, 508–509
Ventricular-paced rhythm, 35t, 37
Ventricular septal defect (VSD), 12, 675, 676, 679, 681–682
Ventricular tachyarrhythmias, 186
Ventricular tachycardia (VT), 325, 328, 387, 450, 453
    Brugada criteria for, 354, 359, 359f
    electrical cardioversion, 355–356, 360
    electrocardiographic (ECG) diagnostic algorithms for, 354, 359f
    evaluation for, 356, 360
    implantable cardioverter-defibrillator (ICD), 356–357, 361
    management of, 355, 358, 360, 362, 363, 367
    monomorphic, 361, 388, 391
    nonsustained, treatment of, 364, 367
    synchronized cardioversion, 356, 360
    treatment of, 357, 361
Verapamil, 50, 452
Veterans Administration (VA), 158
Viral infection, myocarditis, 469–470
Virchow triad, 59
Voltage mapping, 374

VSD. *See* Ventricular septal defect (VSD)
VT. *See* Ventricular tachycardia (VT)
VTE. *See* Venous thromboembolism (VTE) prophylaxis
VTI. *See* Velocity time integral (VTI)
Vulnerable plaques, 625
VVS. *See* Vasovagal syncope (VVS)
Vyndaqel. *See* Tafamidis (Vyndaqel)

W

Warfarin, 349, 351, 353, 363, 367, 506, 509
Watchman procedure, candidates for, 306, 307
WHO. *See* World health organization (WHO)
Wildtype transthyretin amyloidosis (wtATTR), 221
Wilkins score, 60
Willebrand receptor, 79
Williams syndrome, 686, 691
Wolf-Hirschhorn syndrome, 12
Wolff-Parkinson-White (WPW) syndrome, 340–341, 345, 368, 677
Wolff-Parkinson-White pattern, 332
Women and heart disease, 111–115
World health organization (WHO), 668
    Class IV disease, 674
    maternal cardiovascular risk, 672
Worsening exertional dyspnea, 608
WPW. *See* Wolff-Parkinson-White (WPW) syndrome
wtATTR. *See* Wildtype transthyretin amyloidosis (wtATTR)

X

Xanthomas, 12
Xenoantigens, 74

Y

Yohimbe, 170, 171t

Z

ZAHARA (Zofenopril in the Management of Hypertension Associated With Pregnancy: A Randomized Clinical Trial), 668
    score, 109t
Zypitamag, 17